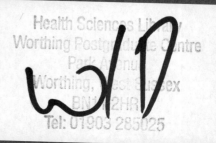

OPERATIVE SURGERY

Fundamental International Techniques

Accident Surgery

OPERATIVE SURGERY

Fundamental International Techniques

Third Edition

Under the General Editorship of

Charles Rob
M.C., M.D., M.Chir., F.R.C.S.

Professor and Chairman of the Department of Surgery,
University of Rochester School of Medicine and Dentistry,
Rochester, New York

and

Sir Rodney Smith
K.B.E., Hon.D.Sc., M.S., F.R.C.S., Hon.F.R.A.C.S.,
Hon.F.R.C.S.(Ed.), Hon.F.A.C.S., Hon.F.R.C.S. (Can.),
Hon.F.R.C.S.(I.)

Surgeon, St. George's Hospital, London

Associate Editor

Hugh Dudley
Ch.M., F.R.C.S., F.R.C.S.(Ed.), F.R.A.C.S.

Professor of Surgery,
St. Mary's Hospital, London

OPERATIVE SURGERY

Fundamental International Techniques

Accident Surgery

Edited by

P. S. London
M.B.E., F.R.C.S.

Surgeon, Birmingham Accident Hospital

BUTTERWORTHS
LONDON · BOSTON
Sydney · Wellington · Durban · Toronto

THE BUTTERWORTH GROUP

ENGLAND

Butterworth & Co (Publishers) Ltd
London: 88 Kingsway, WC2B 6AB

AUSTRALIA

Butterworths Pty Ltd
Sydney: 586 Pacific Highway, Chatswood, NSW 2067
Also at Melbourne, Brisbane, Adelaide and Perth

SOUTH AFRICA

Butterworth & Co (South Africa) (Pty) Ltd
Durban: 152–154 Gale Street

NEW ZEALAND

Butterworths of New Zealand Ltd
Wellington: T & W Young Building,
77–85 Customhouse Quay 1, CPO Box 472

CANADA

Butterworth & Co (Canada) Ltd
Toronto: 2265 Midland Avenue, Scarborough, Ontario M1P 4S1

USA

Butterworths (Publishers) Inc
Boston: 19 Cummings Park, Woburn, Mass. 01801

First Edition Published in Eight Volumes, 1956–1958
Second Edition Published in Fourteen Volumes, 1968–1971
Third Edition Published in Eighteen Volumes, 1976–1978

©
Butterworth & Co (Publishers) Ltd
1978

ISBN 0 407 00640 0

British Library Cataloguing in Publication Data

Operative Surgery: Accident surgery. – 3rd ed.
1. Surgery, Operative
I. Rob, Charles   II. Smith, *Sir* Rodney, b.1914.
III. Dudley, High Arnold Freeman   IV. London, Peter Stanford
617'.91   RD32   78-40457

ISBN 0-407-00640-0

Typeset by Butterworths Litho Preparation Department
Printed in England by The Whitefriars Press Ltd., London and Tonbridge
Bound by the Newdigate Press Ltd., Dorking, Surrey

OPERATIVE SURGERY

Volumes and Editors

ABDOMEN

Hugh Dudley, Ch.M., F.R.C.S., F.R.C.S.(Ed.), F.R.A.C.S.
Charles Rob, *M.C.,* M.D., M.Chir., F.R.C.S.
Sir Rodney Smith, K.B.E., M.S., F.R.C.S.

ACCIDENT SURGERY

P. S. London, M.B.E., F.R.C.S.

CARDIOTHORACIC
SURGERY

John W. Jackson, M.Ch., F.R.C.S.

COLON, RECTUM AND
ANUS

Ian P. Todd, M.S., M.D.(Tor.), F.R.C.S.

EAR

John Ballantyne, F.R.C.S., Hon.F.R.C.S.(I.)

EYES

Stephen J. H. Miller, M.D., F.R.C.S.

GENERAL PRINCIPLES,
BREAST AND HERNIA

Hugh Dudley, Ch.M., F.R.C.S., F.R.C.S.(Ed.), F.R.A.C.S.
Charles Rob, *M.C.,* M.D., M.Chir., F.R.C.S.
Sir Rodney Smith, K.B.E., M.S., F.R.C.S.

GYNAECOLOGY AND
OBSTETRICS

D. W. T. Roberts, M.Chir., F.R.C.S., F.R.C.O.G.

OPERATIVE SURGERY

Contributors to this Volume

R. L. BATTEN
F.R.C.S.

Consultant Orthopaedic Surgeon, General Hospital, Birmingham and Royal Orthopaedic Hospital, Birmingham

H. BOLTON
Ch.M., F.R.C.S.

Consultant Orthopaedic and Accident Surgeon to the Stockport Group of Hospitals

R. H. F. BRAIN
F.R.C.S.

Consultant Thoracic Surgeon, Guy's Hospital, London

DAVID M. CHAPLIN
M.B., F.R.C.S.

Department of Orthopaedics, University of Washington School of Medicine

J. C. CHRISTOFFERSEN
M.D., M.A.

Professor of Surgery and Director of Urology, Bispebjerg Hospital, Copenhagen

D. B. CLARKE
F.R.C.S.

Consultant Cardiothoracic Surgeon, The Queen Elizabeth Hospital, Birmingham

JOHN R. COBBETT
F.R.C.S.

Plastic Surgeon, Queen Victoria Hospital, East Grinstead

LESTER M. CRAMER
M.D., F.A.C.S.

Professor of Plastic Surgery, Temple University Health Sciences Center, Philadelphia

H. ALAN CROCKARD
F.R.C.S.

Senior Lecturer in Neurosurgery, Queen's University, Belfast; Consultant Neurosurgeon, Royal Victoria Hospital, Belfast

MALCOLM DEANE
M.B., B.S., F.R.C.S.

Consultant Plastic Surgeon, Nottingham, Derby and Mansfield Hospitals; Clinical Teacher, University of Nottingham School of Medicine

HUGH DUDLEY
Ch.M., F.R.C.S., F.R.C.S.(Ed.),
F.R.A.C.S.

Professor of Surgery, St. Mary's Hospital, London

H. H. G. EASTCOTT
M.S., F.R.C.S.

Senior Surgeon, St. Mary's Hospital, London

GEOFFREY R. FISK
M.B., B.S., F.R.C.S.,
F.R.C.S.(Ed.)

Senior Orthopaedic Surgeon, Princess Alexandra Hospital, Harlow and St. Margaret's Hospital, Epping; Hunterian Professor, Royal College of Surgeons of England

ADRIAN E. FLATT
M.D., M.Chir., F.R.C.S.

Professor of Orthopaedics, University of Iowa Hospitals, Iowa City; formerly First Assistant, Orthopaedic and Accident Department, The London Hospital

SIGVARD T. HANSEN
M.D.

Department of Orthopaedics, Harborview Medical Center, Seattle

THOMAS T. IRVIN
M.B., Ph.D., Ch.M., F.R.C.S.(Ed.)

Senior Lecturer in Surgery, The University of Sheffield; Honorary Consultant Surgeon, Sheffield Royal Infirmary

CONTRIBUTORS TO THIS VOLUME

BRYAN JENNETT
M.D., F.R.C.S.

Professor of Neurosurgery, Institute of Neurological Sciences, Glasgow and University of Glasgow

H. D. KAUFMAN
Ch.M., F.R.C.S., F.R.C.S.(Ed.)

Consultant Surgeon, Selly Oak Hospital, Birmingham

MICHAEL KNIGHT
M.S., F.R.C.S.

Consultant Surgeon, St. James' and St. George's Hospitals, London

MAGDI S. KODSI
M.D., F.A.C.S.

Assistant Professor of Plastic Surgery, Temple University Health and Sciences Center, Philadelphia

E. LETOURNEL
M.D.

Professor of Orthopaedic Surgery and Traumatology, Centre Medico-Chirurgical de la Porte de Choisy, Paris

P. S. LONDON
M.B.E., F.R.C.S.

Surgeon, Birmingham Accident Hospital

N. A. MATHESON
Ch.M., F.R.C.S.(Eng.),
F.R.C.S.(Ed.)

Consultant Surgeon, Aberdeen General Hospitals

E. TRUMAN MAYS
M.D., F.A.C.S.

Professor of Surgery, University of Kentucky School of Medicine

W. M. McQUILLAN
F.R.C.S.

Consultant Orthopaedic Surgeon, Royal Infirmary and Princess Margaret Rose Orthopaedic Hospital, Edinburgh; Senior Lecturer in Orthopaedic Surgery, University of Edinburgh

TERENCE McSWEENEY
M.Ch.(N.U.I.), M.Ch.(Orth.),
F.R.C.S.(Eng.)

Senior Consultant Surgeon and Surgeon in Charge, Spinal Injury Unit, The Robert Jones and Agnes Hunt Orthopaedic Hospital, Oswestry; Consultant Traumatic and Orthopaedic Surgeon, Leighton Hospital, Crewe and South Cheshire Hospitals

J. P. MITCHELL
T.D., M.S., F.R.C.S.,
F.R.C.S.(Ed.)

Professor of Surgery (Urology), University of Bristol; Consultant Urologist, United Bristol Hospitals and Southmead General Hospital

W. CAMERON MOFFAT
O.B.E., M.B., F.R.C.S.,
L./R.A.M.C.

Senior Consultant Surgeon, British Military Hospital, Rinteln

G. F. MURNAGHAN
M.D., Ch.M., F.R.C.S.(Ed.),
F.R.C.S., F.R.A.C.S.

Professor of Surgery, University of New South Wales; Honorary Urological Surgeon to The Prince Henry, The Prince of Wales and the Eastern Suburbs Hospitals, and Honorary Consultant Urologist to The Royal South Sydney Hospital, The Canterbury Hospital, Sydney, and The Royal Hospital for Women, Paddington, New South Wales

J. C. MUSTARDÉ
F.R.C.S.(Eng.), F.R.C.S.(Ed.)

Consultant Plastic Surgeon, West Scotland Plastic Surgery Centre, Canniesburn Hospital, Glasgow and Royal Hospital for Sick Children, Glasgow

DON H. O'DONOGHUE M.D.	*Professor of Orthopaedics, O'Donoghue Orthopaedic Clinic, Pasteur Medical Building, Oklahoma*
R. GUY PULVERTAFT C.B.E., Hon.M.D., M.Chir., F.R.C.S.	*Emeritus Orthopaedic Surgeon, Derbyshire Royal Infirmary; Honorary Civil Consultant, Royal Air Force*
POUL S. RASMUSSEN M.D.	*Orthopaedic Surgeon, County Hospital, Hellerup, Denmark*
D. A. CAMPBELL REID M.B., B.S.(Lond.), F.R.C.S.	*Consultant Plastic Surgeon, Sheffield Royal Hospital, Sheffield Royal Infirmary, Sheffield Children's Hospital, Hallamshire Hospital, Chesterfield Royal Hospital; Honorary Clinical Lecturer, University of Sheffield*
SIR RODNEY SMITH K.B.E., M.S., F.R.C.S.	*Surgeon, St. George's Hospital, London*
H. GRAHAM STACK F.R.C.S.	*Consultant Orthopaedic Surgeon, Harold Wood Hospital, Essex; Consultant in Hand Surgery, Regional Centre for Plastic Surgery, St. Andrew's Hospital, Billericay, Essex*
ARCHIE STEIN F.C.S.(S.A.)	*Baragwanath Hospital and University of Johannesburg, South Africa*
BERTIL STENER M.D.	*Professor of Orthopaedic Surgery, Sahlgren Hospital, Göteborg*
MICHAEL N. TEMPEST M.D., Ch.M., F.R.C.S.(Ed.)	*Consultant Plastic Surgeon, Welsh Regional Plastic Surgery, Burns and Maxillo-Facial Centre, St. Lawrence Hospital, Chepstow*
A. E. THOMPSON M.S., F.R.C.S.	*Consultant Surgeon, St. Thomas's Hospital, London*
JAMES P. S. THOMSON M.S., F.R.C.S.	*Consultant Surgeon, St. Mark's Hospital, London*
P. J. WHITFIELD F.R.C.S.	*Consultant Plastic Surgeon, Plastic Surgery and Burns Centre, Queen Mary's Hospital, Roehampton*
DAVID WRIGHT F.R.C.S.	*Consultant Ear, Nose and Throat Surgeon, Royal Surrey County Hospital, Guildford*

OPERATIVE SURGERY

Contents of this Volume

Introduction

It may be asked, what is accident surgery and what need is there to add a volume with this title to those that already cover all the systems and organs of the body?

Accident surgery is most informatively defined as the surgical and associated care of injured persons and whether or not the reader is prepared to accord accident surgery the status of a specialty it is liable to confront the young surgeon in training or the surgeon working in sufficient isolation to require him to deal with all-comers, as a clearly recognizable range of operative requirements at short notice. In general, the operations described are those that are likely to be required within 24 hr or so of an accident but I have not felt bound by this limit.

The purpose of this book is to provide practical advice on such parts of general and specialized surgery as are relevant to the needs of the recently injured person and to this end some chapters contributed to other volumes in the series have been reproduced in this one. However, accident surgery has its own requirements that are recognizably different from those of other surgical specialties and these are reflected in chapters written specially for this volume. Gunshot wounds of the head, for example, are no more the province of the neurosurgeon than of a surgeon of general competence working without such specialized skill at hand. Ruptures of the liver, on the other hand, can be such formidable injuries that they deserve special presentation for the surgeon who feels obliged to operate to save life but may have no special claim to abdominal expertise. Apart from these considerations, accident surgery at its best requires the skill and judgement that may owe much to specialized training but owes most to the experience gained in continually providing surgical care for injured persons.

The policy has been to try to make chapters reflect the detail or complexity of a subject, even though this may seem to unbalance the volume when taken chapter by chapter. The hope is, however, that the surgeon that turns to this volume for guidance will find that it provides the information that he seeks. To this end, standard and well tried methods are given preference, with no attempt to do more than indicate some of the other methods that are available.

Hard may be the lot of the editor of a volume with many contributors but even the hardest task-master must admire and respect the forebearance of contributors who submit to efforts to maintain a uniformity of approach and style as well as to stay the alarming debasement of the language for which medical men have much to answer. Particular thanks are due to the artists, whose interpretation of rough sketches and not always very clear photographs showed commendable perspicuity as well as skill; to my tolerant family and my secretary Miss L. E. Langley whose cheerful smile lasted a long and taxing course well and to the editorial staff of Butterworths who so effectively combined advice, sympathy and firmness.

P. S. LONDON

General Care of Wounds and Technique of Suturing

Malcolm Deane, M.B., B.S., F.R.C.S.
Consultant Plastic Surgeon, Nottingham, Derby and Mansfield Hospitals;
Clinical Teacher, University of Nottingham School of Medicine

PRINCIPLES FOR WOUND MANAGEMENT

The basic ideals in the care of wounds are (1) prevention of infection and (2) promotion of primary intention healing.

Successful wound repair, without complication, following injuries which breach the skin is essential for the restoration of function of the damaged part.

The most important complication is *infection*. If it becomes established it results in: (1) further destruction of tissue; (2) delayed healing; (3) an increase in fibrosis and scar tissue; (4) loss of function and (5) increased disfigurement.

The management of wounds is, therefore, directed towards the prevention or elimination of infection, followed by repair of injured tissues and closure of the skin.

TIMING

Ideally, the definitive treatment should take place as soon as possible after the injury is sustained; delay adds to the risk of infection. The risk varies also with the site of the wound and the means by which it was sustained.

A superficial incision caused by a clean sharp implement, sutured within 6 hr of being inflicted, stands every chance of healing without complications.

At the other end of the scale, a crushing type of injury associated with fractures, resulting in necrosis or avulsion of skin and other tissues, heavily contaminated with dirt, provides conditions in which most careful attention to the principles of wound care is essential. The difficulties are increased when there is a prolonged delay before adequate treatment can be carried out, as bacterial contamination will probably progress to established infection.

Delay may be justified, however, when a wound is associated with a potentially more serious injury, for example of the head or abdomen, which requires observation for some time before a decision regarding treatment of the various injuries can be made.

In general, most wounds less than 6 − 8 hr old can be *closed primarily* unless there is gross contamination.

This principle, therefore, applies to the majority of civilian injuries in peace time.

Under battle conditions and when delay is inevitable for other reasons, primary repair may be contraindicated even though the wound itself may appear suitable for immediate closure.

An exception to this occurs in lacerations of the face, head and neck. Because of the particularly rich blood supply to these areas they may without ill-effect be left for 24 − 48 hr before being sutured.

Initial examination and protection of the wound

Apart from the removal of loose pieces of clothing or other foreign material which can be *easily* lifted away minimal exploration or cleansing of the wound itself should be carried out on the first examination of the patient.

This inspection, related to the history of the injury is merely to ascertain whether the wound is localized and trivial or part of much more extensive and possibly life-threatening damage.

In the former instance simple clinical examination may be all that is necessary to exclude, for example, division of a nerve or tendon in the case of a cut finger.

In the latter instance it may be far more important to pay attention to the general condition of the patient, to control external haemorrhage and maintain an efficient airway, to suspect and observe for internal haemorrhage or failing consciousness.

After the preliminary examination the wound should be covered with a sterile dry dressing and gentle but firm pressure applied by means of a layer of wool or Gamgee held in place with a crêpe bandage.

1

1a & b

An injured upper limb is comfortable in a triangular bandage sling, or cradled by the other arm.

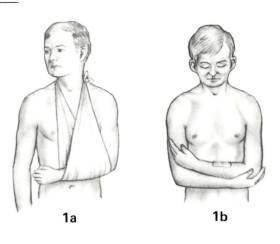

1a 1b

2

A lower limb should be kept gently elevated on a pillow, Braun's frame or Thomas' splint. This combination of pressure and elevation stops the bleeding from most wounds.

A scalp wound bleeds less if the patient is kept propped up, unless exsanguination is such that shock has supervened. In this case temporary sutures inserted to close the wound under some tension may slow the haemorrhage whilst the blood volume is being restored. It may be possible to identify a larger severed artery and apply forceps and ligate it before the definitive exploration and repair.

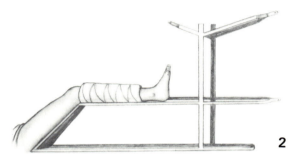

2

3

In the case of a penetrating injury of the chest-wall, the opening can be sealed effectively with a large pad consisting of several thicknesses of tulle gras under the dressings and covered with adhesive strapping whilst attention is paid to stabilizing any paradoxical movements of the rib cage. The immediate care of a person with this type of wound should also include intubation and assisted ventilation of the lungs, and the insertion of intercostal drains to the pleural cavities (*see* Chapter on 'Drainage of Pleural Space by Tube', pages 189–191).

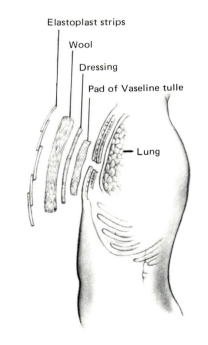

Elastoplast strips

Wool

Dressing

Pad of Vaseline tulle

Lung

3

4

Radiological investigations

It is not usually necessary to x-ray the majority of wounds except when associated fractures are suspected, or when the history suggests that there may be one or more radio-opaque foreign bodies embedded in the surrounding tissues.

It is useful, however, to x-ray a hand or foot when the wound is merely of the puncture variety if there is a suspicion that a fragment of the wounding implement or a missile is present. The position of the wound of the skin should be marked by fixing a paper-clip or similar metallic marker over it with adhesive strapping or Sellotape.

This assists in determining the approximate track of the puncture and may reduce the amount of dissection of uninjured tissues necessary to explore for and retrieve the fragment.

Although most modern glass is relatively radio-translucent fragments can usually be seen in radiographs.

A useful sign in soft-tissue x-ray films is the presence of air, which, if it is at some distance from the site of the wound, indicates that there is extensive tearing or stripping of tissues. This may not have been apparent at the initial clinical examination.

A gas bubble beneath the diaphragm in a plain radiograph of the abdomen may have got there through the wound, or may indicate a puncture of a hollow viscus.

The surgeon should not be lulled into a false sense of security if no gas is visible on x-ray films and he must always explore fully to the depths of the wound (*see* Chapter on 'General Care of Gunshot Wounds', pages 19—25).

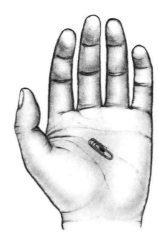

4

Contrast radiography

Occasionally an angiogram is necessary to establish the extent of arterial injury when there is no circulation distal to a wound; this is especially the case if there has not been sufficient bleeding to indicate a severed major vessel. Merely intimal damage may be present which will, however, require treatment (*see* Chapter on 'Arterial Suture and Anastomosis', pages 91—97). Rarely, a barium swallow may be useful to confirm oesophageal damage in penetrating injuries of the neck. A small split in the pharynx or oesophagus is easily missed at exploration, but may result in mediastinitis if not diagnosed, repaired and drained.

DEFINITIVE CLEANSING AND REPAIR

Essential equipment

Every surgeon must be able to carry out the repair of wounds according to the fundamental principles of the handling of tissues; muscle, fat, fascia and skin are delicate living structures and are even more delicate if injured. They must be handled with gentleness and, in order to obtain healing with the minimum of scar formation, the repair must be careful and accurate.

Few instruments are necessary, but most must be regarded as precision tools and given the appropriate care.

5a-i

Cleansing and exploration

Scrubbing brush (*a*)
Two sponge-holding forceps (*b*)
Aqueous chlorhexidine solution
Hydrogen peroxide solution 10 vol. per cent
One malleable probe (*c*)
One Volkmann's spoon curette (*d*)
Skin hooks — One pair Gillies' single hooks (*e*)
One pair catspaw retractors (*f*)
Howarth's dissector — a most useful double-ended instrument (*g*)
Haemostats (*h*)
Soft rubber tubing for finger tourniquet (*i*).

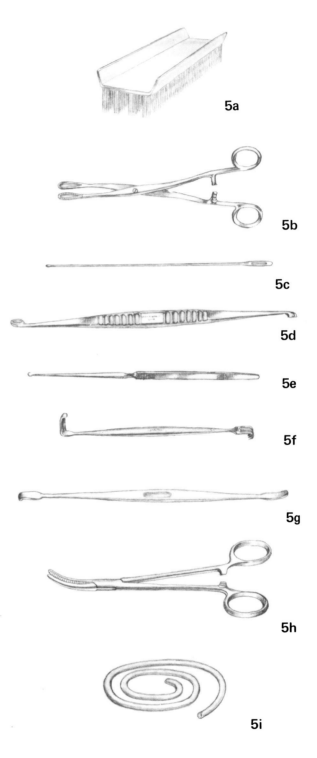

5a

5b

5c

5d

5e

5f

5g

5h

5i

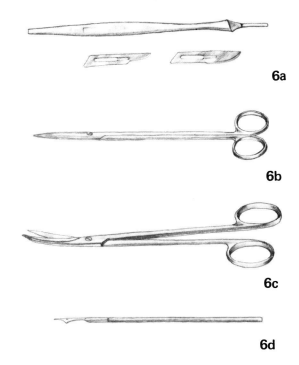

6a-d

Incision and excision

Bard-Parker's knife handle with Nos. 10 and 15 blades (*a*)
McIndoe's or Metzenbaum's scissors — excellent for trimming all tissues, including skin (*b*)
Fine curved sharp-pointed scissors (*c*)
Mapping pen (a sharpened orange-stick makes an excellent pen) (*d*)
Marking ink (made from gentian violet and brilliant green).

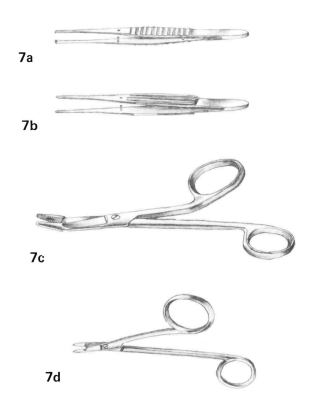

7a-d

Repair

Gillies' toothed dissecting forceps (*a*)
McIndoe's non-toothed dissecting forceps (*b*)
Gillies' needle holder (large) (*c*) or
Foster's needle holder (small) (*d*)
Suture material (*see* page 9)

With the above basic set, virtually any wound can be satisfactorily dealt with. Additional equipment such as suction apparatus, coagulation diathermy and pneumatic tourniquet is desirable when dealing with major wounds, but it is not essential.

Preparation for operation

Many minor wounds can be closed under local analgesia. However, if there is gross contamination, extensive or multiple wounds, or the possibility that important organs may have to be repaired, general or regional anaesthesia should be employed. Removal of dressings and cleansing of the skin around the wound should be delayed until after general anaesthesia has been induced.

The skin is wiped or scrubbed with an antiseptic/detergent solution; hair is cropped short. It is better to avoid contact of the antiseptics with the raw surfaces of the wound, and to cleanse this area with copious quantities of water or saline. Loose foreign bodies may be removed by this washing and the surgeon may learn much during this preliminary inspection about the nature and extent of the wound, and of the many problems that may confront him in the later excision and repair. He should not delegate this early important task to a junior or a nurse. A pneumatic tourniquet may be necessary to arrest copious haemorrhage started by the cleaning procedure after removal of pressure dressings.

Sterile drapes are then applied round the part.

Treatment of specific injuries

8

Abrasions

If the skin is abraded but not through its full depth, healing will occur rapidly, and any dirt remaining on the surface may be incorporated beneath the new epithelium and result in tattooed scarring or tattooing without scar. This is unsightly and difficult to eradicate secondarily; it can be prevented by the correct treatment of the fresh injury.

Deep abrasions, of the face in particular, from being scraped along the road or from explosions in coal mines often have dirt and dust embedded in the raw dermis. This can only be removed by vigorous scrubbing with a brush, usually under general anaesthesia. A soft wire brush as commonly used for cleaning suede shoes is the ideal instrument.

Irrigation with hydrogen peroxide 10 vol. per cent assists in floating debris away and also acts as a haemostatic agent for the raw area, which may then be covered with antibiotic powder to form a protective crust.

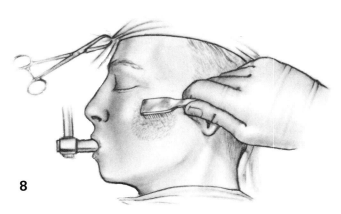

8

Incised wounds and lacerations without skin loss

9a & b

If the edges of the wound are more or less perpendicular to the skin surface, minimal or no excision of tissue will be necessary and the incised layers may each be sutured in turn.

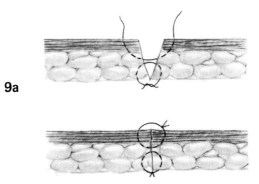

9a

9b

10a & b

If the edges are steeply shelving, and if there is sufficient laxity of surrounding skin, a better cosmetic result can be obtained by excising the skin edges at right angles.

A scalpel is usually employed, though for minor trimming, especially at the corners of the wound, curved sharp-pointed scissors are satisfactory, and easier to use.

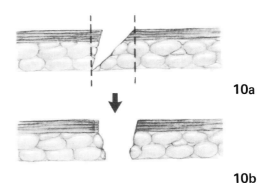

10a

10b

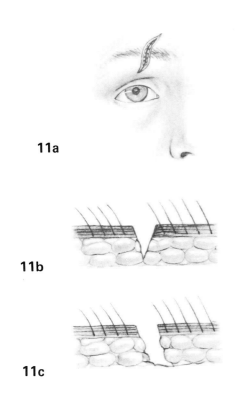

11a

11b

11c

11a, b & c

An exception to this general principle is the wound involving the eyebrow. Here the hair follicles lie obliquely in the skin. Trimming of the skin edges of a wound where it passes through the eyebrow should be parallel to the hair follicles on each side; failure to do this, or mistakenly to excise perpendicularly results in destruction of follicles and an unsightly hairless area on either side of the scar.

12a & b

Ragged and complex wounds can be simplified by excising some of the irregular skin tags, but it is often better to err on the side of conservation, unless the wound is small or the flaps obviously dead.

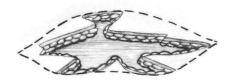

12a

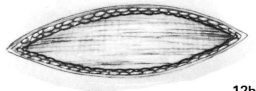

12b

13

A common and difficult wound is the small, usually superficial slicing injury occurring on the face and forehead in windscreen accidents. A C-shaped or U-shaped flap of skin has been raised on a narrow pedicle like a trap door and may be less than full skin thickness for most of its length.

If it is sutured without trimming, a heaped up area of skin results from contracture of the deep and surrounding scar tissue. However, excision may become unacceptably radical for a small wound if an attempt is made to convert it to a straight-edged incision, and may be impracticable if, as is often the case, there are numerous similar wounds within a relatively small area of skin.

A less than perfect result from the immediate closure may have to be accepted, and the contour irregularities dealt with later.

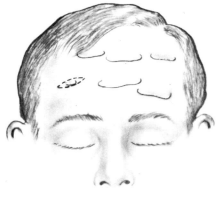

13

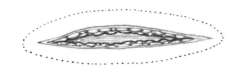

14a

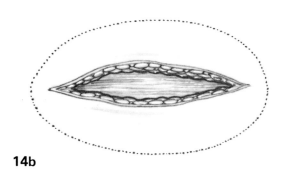

14b

14a & b

Undermining

As a general principle, undermining the skin edges should be restricted to the minimum necessary to obtain easy closure.

Dissection for 1 or 2 mm — more a mobilization of the actual skin edges than a true undermining — assists in the correct placement of the sutures to ensure proper eversion, and should be carried out in most cases unless the subcutaneous tissue is particularly soft and lax.

Where tension exists the undermining must proceed further under the skin from the wound margin; the greater the tension, the more widely mobilization becomes necessary.

A common error is insufficient undermining, thus failing to equalize (and reduce) tension along the wound's length. It must be remembered that the greater the tension the greater the risk to the blood supply of the skin edges. However, undermining increases the danger to the viability of the skin whilst reducing the tension, and the dissection should take place at the same level throughout in the upper subcutaneous tissues, but sparing the main blood vessels to the skin, which lie in the subdermal plexus.

There is an arbitrary point at which skin viability is in sufficient jeopardy that simple suture will result in marginal necrosis and closure by other means, either local re-arrangement or free graft, is necessary to achieve healing without complication.

Haemostasis

Haematoma is probably the commonest cause of wound infection, disruption and skin necrosis.

Haemostasis should be as complete as possible before closure of the wound, using fine-tipped forceps, which grasp only the blood vessel itself with as little as possible of the surrounding tissue.

Larger vessels should be ligated using unabsorbable (linen) or absorbable (polyglycolic acid) ligatures.

Small vessels may be electrocoagulated either by touching haemostats already applied or by carefully picking up the bleeding vessel in fine-tipped insulated diathermy dissecting forceps. This method is rapid and efficient.

Blood clots and any debris from trimming of skin edges or fat can be washed from the wound with 10 vol. per cent hydrogen peroxide.

This also helps to control capillary oozing.

Suture materials

The finest gauge possible should be used, commensurate with the part of the body to be sutured.

Polypropylene monofilament suture is ideal as it is stronger, relative to its size, than other materials, is soft, not irritant, knots easily and is simple to remove.

Polyglycolic acid suture is absorbable but less irritant than catgut or collagen. It is much stronger, relative to its gauge, than catgut.

	Eyelids and Face	*Hands*	*Limbs and Trunk*
Subcutaneous tissue suture	5/0 Polyglycolic acid	5/0 PGA	3/0 or 4/0 PGA
Intradermal suture ('Subcuticular')	5/0 or 4/0 Polypropylene	—	3/0 or 2/0 Polypropylene
Skin suture	6/0 or 5/0 Polypropylene	5/0 Polypropylene	4/0 or 5/0 Polypropylene
	on 11 or 15 mm curved cutting needles	15 mm curved cutting needle	15 or 25 mm curved cutting or 50 mm straight for subcuticular

Its only disadvantage lies in the fact that it is braided and not smooth and, therefore, tends to cut soft and thin tissues like a band saw when pulled through under any tension.

For the same reason care must be taken to ensure that knots have slid up to their correct tightness.

It can be used as a skin suture but in most cases should be removed as it may persist for up to 6 weeks and so leave stitch marks.

It should not be used on the face for this purpose, but is useful in the postauricular sulcus.

TECHNIQUE OF SUTURING

The accurate approximation of skin edges with minimal tension assures primary healing with little scarring.

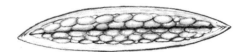

15a & b

When necessary, fascial layers and subcutaneous tissues should be brought together with interrupted absorbable sutures to reconstitute the layers, obliterate dead space and support the skin repair.

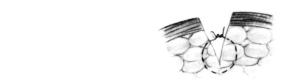

15a

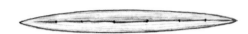

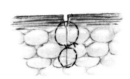

15b

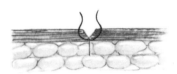

16a

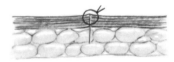

16b

16a & b

The everting interrupted suture is most frequently employed. The needle is inserted through the skin close to the wound edge, diverging away from it as it passes more deeply in order to encircle a greater amount of tissue deeply than near the surface. This ensures eversion of the edges.

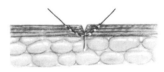

17a

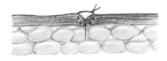

17b

17a & b

The converse results in inversion.

18

Stitches should be placed close together to reduce tension and allow even apposition.

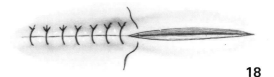

18

19a & b

Intradermal sutures are used when there is tension, and always on the face. They allow tension-free skin closure.

The knots are placed downwards to lie beneath the dermis.

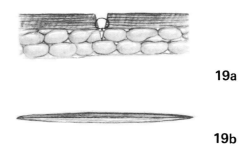

19a

19b

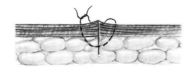

20a

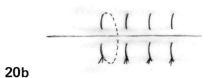

20b

20a & b

Occasionally interrupted mattress sutures may be used to assist in maintaining skin eversion. They may be placed deeply to help in obliterating dead space when subcutaneous sutures cannot be effectively used, for example when the adipose layer is thick, friable or oedematous.

21

A simple continuous running suture is effective and rapid. If good tension-free apposition of the skin edges has been achieved with intradermal stitches, and the surgeon is confident that deep closure and haemostasis are adequate, this suture gives excellent approximation, especially on the face. Theoretically, at least, it should cause less skin ischaemia at the site of each spiral turn than the partial ligature effect of an interrupted stitch.

A continuous stitch must not be used if the wound has been heavily contaminated and is potentially infected, as it may be necessary to remove one or two interrupted stitches to release haematoma or pus, should sepsis become established.

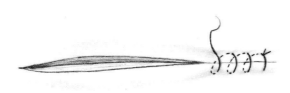

21

The subcuticular suture

This is not commonly used in the repair of fresh injuries, although it is occasionally useful when there is considerable tension, especially in children. This suture can remain in place for a longer period, to allow the scar tissue to strengthen without the risk of causing stitch marks.

22

It consists of a continuous intradermal suture using monofilament material on a curved or straight needle.

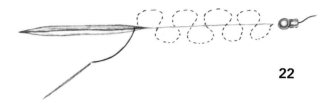

22

23

If the wound is long, or sharply curved or angled, it is wise to bring the stitch to the surface at intervals so that it can be cut and easily removed. It is fixed at each end by knotting or by compressing a soft alloy sleeve above a bead onto the thread.

Care must be taken over the adjustment of the tension of the suture to avoid puckering the skin.

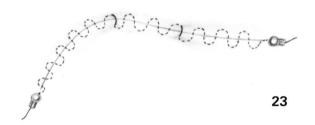

23

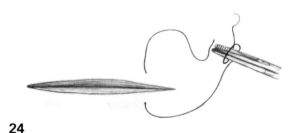

24

Technique of tying knots

24

One turn round the needle holder followed by another turn in the opposite direction, ties a reef knot.

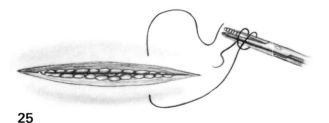

25

25

The surgeon's knot is created by two turns at the beginning.

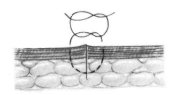

26a

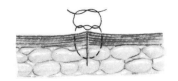

26b

26a & b

Care should be taken to pull the ends in the correct direction so that each layer lies flat.

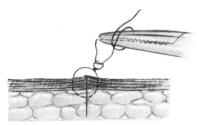

27a

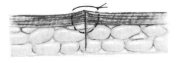

27b

27a & b

A third turn should be made to ensure against slipping. The knot should rest over the entry or exit hole.

Dressings

A smear of Polyfax antibiotic ointment along a suture line of monofilament polypropylene has greatly reduced the incidence of inflammation at the stitch holes.

Twice daily applications are all that are required for most facial wounds, which often cannot be adequately covered with occlusive dressings.

Twenty-four to forty-eight hours of cover with eyepad, wool and crêpe bandage helps to prevent further bruising and swelling after repair of eyelid lacerations.

Firm dressings of dry gauze, wool and crêpe bandage should be applied to all other wounds. They support the soft tissues and prevent haematoma formation: any bleeding occurring in the few hours after repair will be discharged through the suture line into the dressings which can remain undisturbed for 4 — 7 days.

Earlier inspection of the wound and change of dressings is indicated if there is increasing pain, soaking through with blood or serum or whenever there is any doubt about the viability of the skin.

Haematoma should be evacuated as soon as it is discovered.

Removal of a few sutures may be necessary to accomplish this, after which firm pressure is re-applied.

Suture removal

If stitches are removed within 4 days, no marks should remain. In some instances sutures can be taken out within 48 hr. In certain cases removal must be delayed for 7 — 10 days.

It is often better to remove the sutures a few at a time over the course of 4 or 5 days, rather than take out all of them at once.

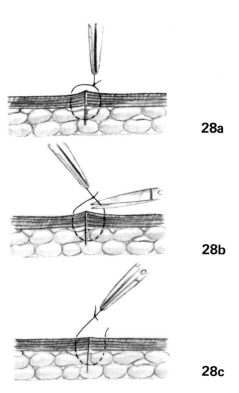

28a

28b

28c

28a, b & c

The knot is lifted up and the thread cut with sharp pointed scissors below it, close to the skin. The buried part is then pulled through towards the incision scar. Strong traction is never necessary with monofilament synthetic materials.

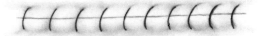

29a

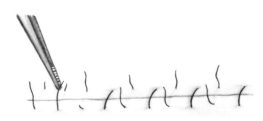

29b

29a & b

Alternate loops of a continuous suture are cut, each piece being removed by lifting the intervening loop.

It may be difficult to withdraw a subcuticular suture until 2 or 3 weeks after insertion. This is not important as no stitch-marks are left.

30a & b

It is often wise to support the repair with transverse and oblique adhesive strapping, especially if stitches are removed early.

Steristrip skin closures are ideal.

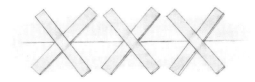

30a

Later management

The usual red, indurated scar occurring after wound repair may progress to hypertrophic or frankly keloidal tissue.

Regular grease massage using olive oil, lanolin or cold cream assists in the resolution of the reactive scar and may partly prevent progress to keloid. If the latter occurs, however, the natural process of settling can be accelerated by massage with a steroid cream such as Betnovate or Synalar Forte.

Secondary corrective surgery for the scars should be withheld until induration has mostly subsided — often 6–9 months or more.

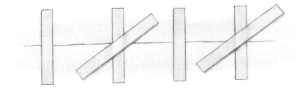

30b

ADDITIONAL TECHNIQUES TO OBTAIN CLOSURE

Correction of dog-ear

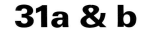

31a

31a & b

The result of slight inequalities in the length of the two sides of the wound becomes apparent as skin closure nears completion.

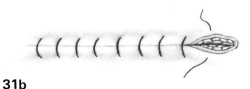

31b

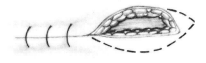

32a

32a & b

Simple excision of the peak in an ellipse solves the problem.

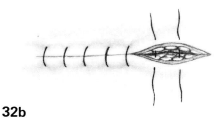

32b

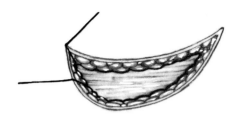

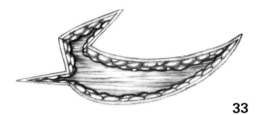

33

33 & 34

Unequal sides

If the wound is crescent-shaped, ordinary closure would result in a very large dog-ear. Plan two incisions, more or less at right angles to each other.

(*a*) One lengthens the short side by creating a defect.

(*b*) The other creates a triangular flap to transpose into the defect without lengthening the long side further.

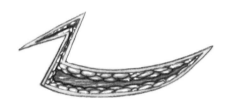

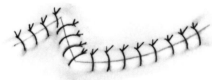

34

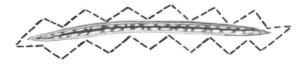

35a

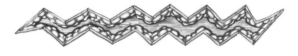

35b

Breaking a straight line and redistributing tension

35a & b

The W-plasty

A zig-zag excision of the wound margins creates a series of small triangular flaps which interdigitate with those on the other side.

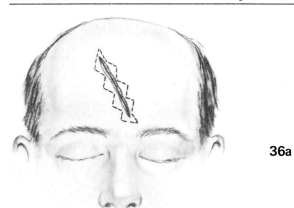

36a

36a & b

It is useful when a wound is clearly crossing the skin-crease lines (the lines of minimal tension).

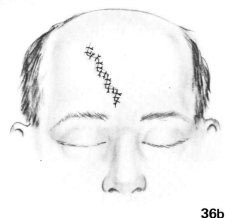

36b

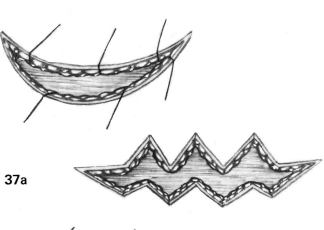

37a

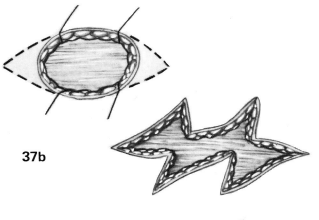

37b

37a, b & c

Modifications of the W-plasty are sometimes employed in the closure of curved unequal-sided wounds, or narrow oval or circular defects.

The secrets of success in these repairs are careful planning, measuring and marking, and undermining well beyond the bases of the triangular flaps.

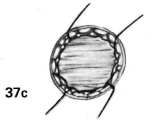

37c

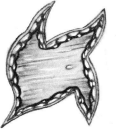

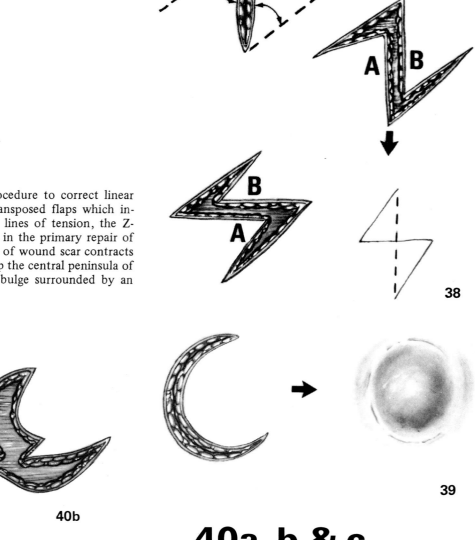

The Z-plasty

38 & 39

More often a secondary procedure to correct linear scar contracture by two transposed flaps which increase length and alter the lines of tension, the Z-plasty is occasionally useful in the primary repair of C-shaped wounds. This type of wound scar contracts around its curve and raises up the central peninsula of skin to form an unsightly bulge surrounded by an apparently depressed scar.

40a

40b

38

39

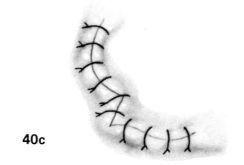

40c

40a, b & c

This unsatisfactory result may be prevented at the original repair by incorporating one or more small Z-plasties along the circumference of the wound.

An incision is cut at 60° to each skin edge to create an equilateral triangle shaped flap on either side of the wound.

Each flap is widely undermined and transposed across the wound to lie in the defect left by the other.

This manoeuvre breaks the line of the resultant scar.

[The illustrations for this Chapter on General Care of Wounds and Technique of Suturing were drawn by Mr. G. Lyth.]

General Care of Gunshot Wounds

Colonel W. Cameron Moffat, O.B.E., M.B., F.R.C.S., L./R.A.M.C.
Senior Consultant Surgeon, British Military Hospital, Rinteln

GENERAL CONSIDERATIONS IN WOUND CARE

The object of wound care is to achieve sound healing in the shortest time compatible with safety. The enemy of sound wound healing is infection. All wounds should be regarded as contaminated and potentially infected. Established infection is more likely to occur if the wound is first dealt with more than 6 hr after its infliction, and is virtually certain if primary treatment fails to remove dead and damaged tissue, foreign bodies and blood clot.

All wounds require careful inspection and exploration to determine their depth, extent and nature. Only when the full extent of the wound has been visually explored will the detailed diagnosis be made and the opportunity for correct treatment be presented.

In the case of penetrating or perforating wounds particular attention should be directed to the detection of associated fracture, major vessel or nerve injury or injury of internal organs. Such injuries may not be obvious on pre-operative clinical assessment, and it should not be forgotten that penetrating injuries rarely occur when the patient is in the 'anatomical' position and wound tracks are unpredictable and often bizarre. Wounds caused by missiles, and particularly those from high velocity bullets or fragments, are especially dangerous.

They are usually much more extensive than is immediately apparent; all are grossly contaminated and frequently contain large amounts of dead and damaged muscle with other tissue debris and foreign material.

The penalties for incorrect treatment are high because not only is serious local sepsis inevitable but also the patient's life may be lost from systemic infection.

PRE - OPERATIVE

Pre-operative assessment

A wound must not be regarded as an isolated phenomenon but the whole patient must be examined and treated. The airway must be secure and ventilation and circulation receive attention as necessary. Vital signs should be recorded and a rapid general neurological examination carried out and noted. A search should be made for other injury, especially in the abdomen and chest and posterior aspect of trunk and limbs. Dressings should be disturbed as little as possible, compatible with thoroughness, because brisk bleeding may recur. A record should be made of relevant peripheral pulse and nerve function. X-rays may be helpful in demonstrating associated fractures or foreign bodies and can be invaluable in the assessment of chest and abdominal wounds. The use of contrast media, for example excretion pyelography or arteriography, can be most helpful in appropriate cases, but such examinations should not be allowed to delay treatment unduly.

Anaesthesia

Many wounds can be adequately cared for using local or regional anaesthesia but when there is any doubt as to the depth or extent of a wound general anaesthesia should be employed. The presence of a large wound or multiple wounds makes general anaesthesia particularly desirable. Wound treatment is likely to be more thorough when general anaesthesia is used, especially in the very young or unduly apprehensive patient.

Position of patient

This will depend on the site of the wound and the probability of the need for extending incisions. Head-up or head-down tilt can be helpful in limiting haemorrhage. The surgeon should always be able to work comfortably and with good lighting. Where intricate repair work is required he should if possible be seated.

Cleansing the wound area

A detergent antiseptic should be used to clean a wide area round the wound. The damaged tissues should be shielded with gauze swabs during initial cleansing. If there is gross wound contamination it may be helpful to wash out the wound with a copious flow of normal saline prior to towelling. The towels should be placed to allow of generous wound extension if necessary.

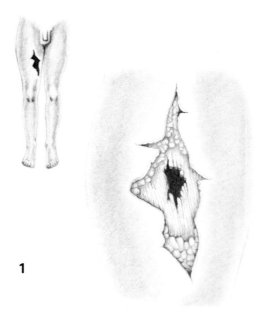

1

THE TWO - STAGE OPERATION

1

Primary wound excision and delayed primary closure

This is the procedure of choice for all heavily contaminated wounds, for all wounds seen late and for all penetrating wounds caused by missiles, especially those caused by fragments or high velocity bullets.

PRIMARY WOUND EXCISION

2&3

Wound extension

Since it is necessary to inspect all of the wound under vision extending incisions will often be required.

These should be made in the long axis of the limb except where joint creases are crossed, when S-shaped incisions are used. Where there is probability of neurovascular damage the incisions should be planned to give appropriate access.

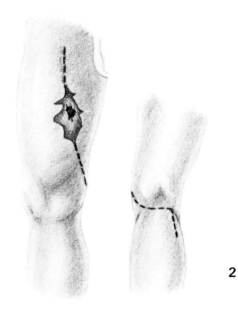

2

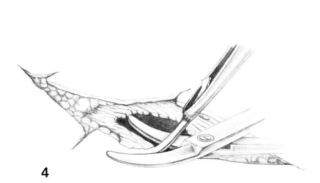

3

4

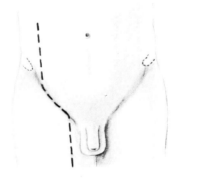

4&5

Excision of damaged skin

Skin is elastic and remarkably resistant to damage. All viable skin must be preserved. Damaged skin should be trimmed away to leave a clean healthy edge. This may be done with the knife or with sharp curved scissors, depending on the surgeon's preference and experience.

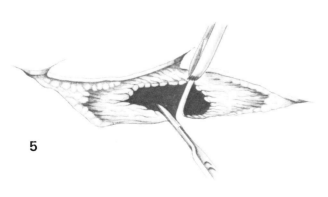

5

6

Superficial and deep fascia

Superficial fat should be widely removed because its blood supply is poor and it harbours foreign material easily. Deep fascia should be widely incised to expose the deeper parts of the wound and release tension on the underlying muscles. This is the true act of 'debridement' or unbridling of the wound. Damaged deep fascia should be excised.

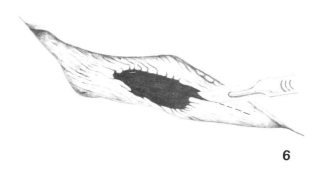

6

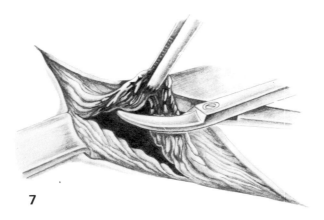

7

7

Excision of muscle

Good retraction and good lighting are essential. All dead and damaged muscle must be removed. This includes muscle which does not bleed when cut, which does not contract when pinched with forceps or which is of mushy consistency and unhealthy colour. Bruised muscle may be viable but must be excised if there is doubt. Excision must continue until only healthy muscle remains. Foreign material is removed concomitantly with the muscle excision.

8

Bone

Bone is valuable and must be preserved if possible. Small unattached cortical fragments should be removed. Larger fragments are likely to have some muscle attachment and blood supply and must be preserved undisturbed as far as possible. Dirt and debris may have to be curetted and washed from such fragments.

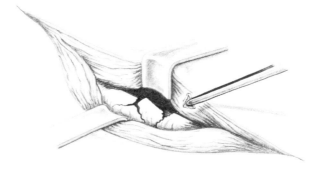

8

9

Major vessels and nerves

These structures should be carefully inspected and any damage dealt with appropriately. Immediate nerve repair in heavily contaminated wounds is inadvisable. Repair of major vessels may be essential but it is best to avoid the use of synthetic implants.

General rule

Tissues of great structural or functional importance should be preserved if there is a prospect that they will survive whereas tissues of no great functional or structural importance should be discarded if there is a chance that they will die or are already dead.

Haemostasis

At the conclusion of wound excision haemostasis must be achieved as completely as possible. Fine catgut ligatures accurately placed kill less tissue than diathermy generously used. Ligatures on major vessels should be of unabsorbable material doubly tied and cut short.

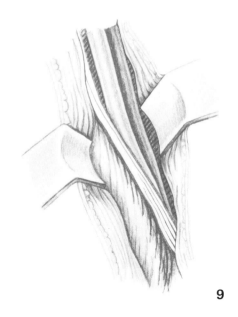

9

10

Dressing

After primary excision the wound is not closed but left widely open to promote free drainage. Joint synovium, pleura, peritoneum and dura mater must be closed but the muscle and fascial layers left unsutured.

Additional drains should be unnecessary. Fine mesh gauze is laid onto the wound surface. Packing should not be employed and in particular paraffin gauze should not be used. Fluffed up fine absorbent gauze should be arranged lightly over the entire wound area and the whole dressing covered with a generous amount of absorbent, sterile wool.

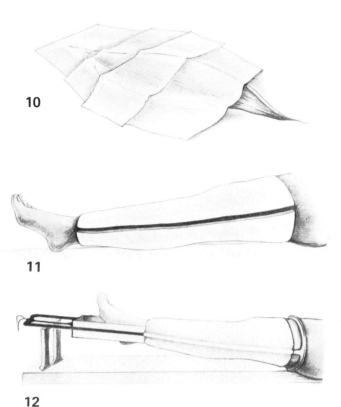

10

11

12

11 & 12

Splinting

Even in the absence of fracture the wounded part should be adequately supported. Circumferential elastic bandages bring the danger of restriction of circulation and should be used with caution. Plaster casts should be split immediately. For wounds in the lower limbs the application of plaster over a well-padded Thomas's splint in the form of a 'Tobruk' splint is particularly useful if the patient is to be transported.

DELAYED PRIMARY CLOSURE

After excision and dressing as described above, the wound should preferably be left undisturbed for a period of 4 or 5 days. At the end of this time the patient is returned to theatre and the wound inspected. If it is clean and early healthy granulations are present it is sutured exactly as it would have been had primary wound closure been employed. Any deep dead space should be obliterated with absorbable sutures. The skin edge should come together without tension. A small amount of undermining of the skin edge is permissible but if skin closure cannot be accomplished without tension an appropriate area of the wound should be covered with a split skin graft.

The skin stitches should remain in place for 14 days. If the wound is unhealthy when inspected it must not be closed. Necrotic tissue must be excised and sepsis drained. When conditions have improved and the wound is suitable it will be closed by secondary suture or grafting.

13

THE ONE - STAGE OPERATION

13

Wound toilet and primary closure

This is the method usually employed for all minor wounds and for those wounds which are seen early and which are not grossly contaminated, for example, those caused by knives or broken glass or by low-velocity missiles. It is the desirable procedure for wounds of the head and face. Although the threat of sepsis still exists the main danger is that the full extent of the damage is not discovered.

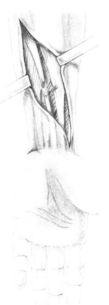

14

14

It is necessary to explore even small wounds thoroughly under direct vision, and for this purpose wound extension may be required.

The condition of muscles, tendons, major vessels and nerves should be verified, and dealt with accordingly. If wound exploration confirms the absence of unhealthy tissue primary closure may be carried out. The wounded part should be dressed and supported as necessary.

STAB WOUNDS

15

It is usually very difficult and always very dangerous to attempt to assess the extent of the wound clinically. When stab wounds of the abdomen are explored it is better to make a formal laparotomy incision away from the original wound. The line of the wound track can then be more easily followed.

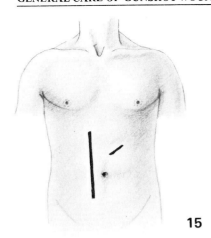

15

SPECIAL POSTOPERATIVE CARE AND COMPLICATIONS

The principles of good general nursing care, good nutrition and rest for the injured part apply. If the wound has been grossly contaminated antibiotics should be given. The choice of antibiotic will be influenced by local conditions and practice but it is important to give one which acts effectively against gram positive anaerobes and of these crystalline penicillin or cloxacillin is usually best.

If there has been much blood loss then whole blood or red cells should be given to correct the haemoglobin at least above 11g/100 ml.

The special complications are those of inadequate primary treatment.

Reactionary haemorrhage

Fresh bleeding from the wound within 24 hr of operation is usually due to slippage of a ligature on a major vessel. It is obviated by careful double ligation.

Secondary haemorrhage

Brisk bleeding from the wound at any time after 24 hr is usually due to erosion of a major vessel by sepsis. It is obviated by thorough primary wound care.

In either case the wound must be re-opened and the vessel ligated accurately if possible. Packing the wound firmly will control bleeding but carries additional risks of further sepsis.

Sepsis

The most serious form of sepsis is that due to the clostridial anaerobes of gas gangrene and tetanus. The former is a specific infection of skeletal muscle which commences in dead tissue and proceeds to kill and invade living muscle. In established cases the mortality is high in spite of further wide excision, amputation, antibiotics or hyperbaric oxygen. It must be distinguished from anaerobic cellulitis, which is rarely lethal and which requires less aggressive treatment. A wide range of other organisms is capable of causing serious local or general sepsis with consequent morbidity and mortality. Thorough primary wound excision should prevent serious wound sepsis but, should it occur, it is important to make the diagnosis early. Patients at risk should be carefully observed for any deterioration in general condition, rise in pulse rate, or sustained fever or onset of pain or heaviness in the wound. If suspicion exists the wound should be inspected in the operating theatre with the patient prepared for general anaesthesia, and appropriate measures taken.

[*The illustrations for this Chapter on General Care of Wounds were drawn by Miss A. Barrett.*]

Free Grafts

Malcolm Deane, M.B., B.S., F.R.C.S.
Consultant Plastic Surgeon, Nottingham, Derby and Mansfield Hospitals;
Clinical Teacher, University of Nottingham School of Medicine

INTRODUCTION

Free grafts may be (*a*) 'partial-thickness' or 'split-thickness' skin grafts; (*b*) full-thickness skin grafts or; (*c*) composite grafts.

As their name implies, free grafts have been severed from their blood supply and have to rely on nourishment by the raw area first for their survival and then for healing.

A graft is said to have *taken* when it appears vascularized and healthy and is adherent to the bed of the defect; it is said to have *failed* if it remains loose and appears pale and sodden, or is obviously dead.

Both appearances can be present in the same skin graft, depending on the success with which various parts of the graft have revascularized.

Tissues which will accept a free graft

(*1*) Healthy young (not more than 48–72 hr old) granulation tissue.
   (2) Muscle.
   (3) Fasciae, nerves, blood vessels, paratenon; that is, any vascular tissue or organ normally covered by a layer of areolar tissue.

   (*4*) Periosteum.
   (*5*) Cancellous bone.
   (*6*) Membrane bone of orbit, maxillary sinus, etc.
   (*7*) Pleura, peritoneum, meninges, dermis.

Tissues which will less readily accept a free graft (those with a rather poor blood supply)

(*1*) Fat.
   (*2*) Joint capsule and ligaments.

Tissues which will not accept a free graft

(*1*) Bare tendon (except in very young children).
   (*2*) Bare cortical bone.
   (*3*) Hyaline cartilage.
   (*4*) An open synovial joint.
Defects with these structures exposed usually require a flap for cover.

Factors affecting healing of free grafts

Movement

It is important to immobilize the defect as far as possible and in particular to prevent shearing movements between the graft and its bed. Any sliding action completely disrupts the attempts of capillaries to bridge the gap.

Haematoma

Blood collecting beneath a graft prevents the healing process and the overlying area of graft usually dies. A small collection of tissue juices ('seroma'), however, is less destructive and the skin graft forming its roof may survive for a few days, and still take when the liquid is released.

Infection

Haemolytic streptococcal contamination results in total failure of the graft. Certain staphylococci have a similar effect. Most other pathogens, although reducing the chances of success, are not usually so harmful. The pseudomonas species can cause up to 50 per cent failure, but this may be related to the presence of dead tissue in the wound and thus an avascular bed rather than the bacteria's effect on the graft and healing process.

Choice of graft

A split-thickness graft is the one most commonly used to close skin defects resulting from injury or burns.

Its advantage lies in the ease of take in most situations, and the fact that the donor area heals with little or no scarring. The latter factor is important in large burns because available donor sites may be limited. If very thin grafts are removed, healing is such that a further crop of grafts can be taken from the same area within 2 weeks or so.

The disadvantage of very thin grafts is that the quality of their texture remains poor and they are subject to marked contracture of the underlying healing scar, especially across concavities and flexion sites.

When the defect is smaller or localized, medium split-thickness grafts are used — the most common type of graft.

The thickest partial-thickness grafts should be confined to the palms of the hands and the face because it is important from the functional and cosmetic points of view that the least possible shrinkage of the healed graft occurs.

The indications for a full-thickness free graft and a composite graft will be considered in the next sections.

Pinch grafts are mentioned only to be condemned. *They have no place in modern skin grafting techniques.*

1

Thickness of the free graft

A thin split-skin graft has a low metabolic requirement and a high concentration of capillaries within it (and hence more open ends in the cut dermis for anastomosis with those in the granulation tissue bed). These desirable factors are progressively reduced if the graft is cut thicker. A full-thickness skin graft, with an intact dermis, has relatively few open capillaries on its deep surface; it also contains complete hair follicles and sweat glands, which increase its metabolic demand.

The chance of partial failure of a thick graft is consequently greater than that of a thin one.

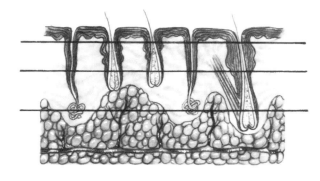

1

SPLIT-THICKNESS SKIN GRAFTS

Immediate primary free skin grafting

If the toilet and repair of an injury leaves a raw surface that will take a free graft this should be applied at once, but if complete haemostasis is not achieved, grafting should be delayed for a few days.

Delayed primary skin grafting

When capillary oozing is persistent or the raw area consists of the less hospitable tissues, it is better to dress the wound, with firm pressure, for 24—48 hr, by which time bleeding will have stopped and granulation tissue will be forming over the whole defect.

Split-skin grafts taken at the original operation and stored can then be applied to the wound with a much greater chance of success.

Secondary skin grafting

A previously sutured wound may break down because of haematoma, infection, ischaemia or unsuspected skin damage, resulting in a raw defect after removal of dead and infected tissues. When this is granulating satisfactorily it is often preferable to apply free skin grafts rather than wait for epithelialization from the edges or attempt a secondary suture.

DONOR SITES

Usually convex surfaces of the body are chosen, in particular the thighs, from which large sheets of split-skin can be removed.

2a & b

If it is important that the graft should not grow hair, less hirsute areas such as the inner aspects of the arms, or the buttocks are selected as donor sites.

Whenever possible in female patients, the buttocks should be used so that any scarring occurring in the healed donor site will be less noticeable than on the thighs or upper limbs.

Grafts may be cut from the front and back of the trunk when other donor sites are insufficient or unavailable, but special instruments are necessary because of the yielding and irregular contours of these areas.

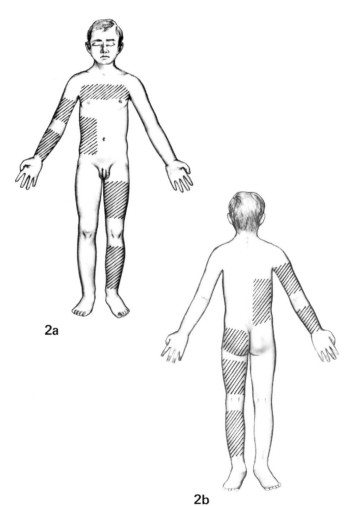

2a

2b

3

The dorsum of the proximal segment of the injured finger yields sufficient skin to graft onto a small finger-tip loss.

The skin tends to be thinner on the inner aspects of the thighs and upper arms; it is generally thickest on the buttocks, back and extensor surfaces of the limbs.

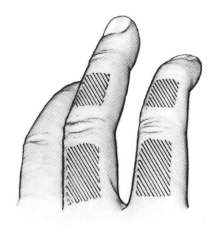

3

INSTRUMENTS

In addition to that required for wound cleansing, excision and repair, the following equipment is required for split-skin grafting.

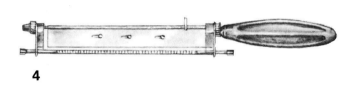

4

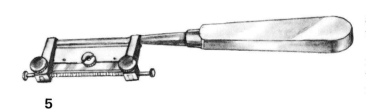

5

4 & 5

Graft-cutting knife

This has an adjustable roller or bar above a disposable blade so that the thickness of the graft being cut can be controlled and varied.

Several modifications of this basic design are available, most of them quite satisfactory for routine use.

A miniature form — Silva's knife, utilizing ordinary razor-blades is a useful addition, and adequate for taking small grafts from the forearm or dorsum of the finger.

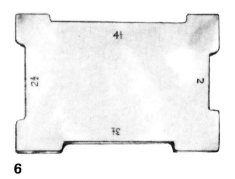

6

6

Gabarro's board

Used to stretch the skin and present the appropriate width of donor surface to the approaching knife.

7

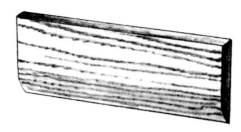

7

Hardwood boards

Used in conjunction with, or instead of Gabarro's board.

Sterile liquid paraffin

Used to lubricate the knife blade and roller, and the skin surface, thus easing the graft-cutting action.

Large hardwood board or other firm flat surface upon which to spread the grafts.

Vaseline gauze

Long strips, 8 inches (20 cm) wide are best for dressing the donor sites and on which to spread the grafts.

Bowl of sterile normal saline solution

Sterile cotton wool

Sterile sheets of polyethylene sponge (0·5 inches (12 mm) thick and up to 12 inches (300 mm) square).

Sterile screw-top jars. Used for storage of skin grafts.

Two other graft-cutting devices — dermatomes — may be found in certain operating theatres.

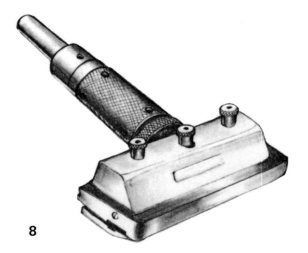

8

8

The electric dermatome

This is used particularly in large burns when difficult or small donor sites, such as small areas of trunk are the only ones available.

9

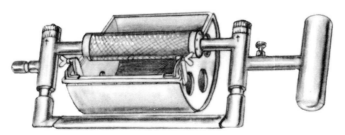

9

The Padgett dermatome

This is also known as a drum and very even grafts can be cut. The drum is fixed to the skin with special adhesive in order to lift the skin to be cut.

These machines are not strictly necessary in the early management of most wounds, so will not be described in further detail.

TAKING A SPLIT-THICKNESS SKIN GRAFT

10

The donor site (usually a limb) is shaved and the skin cleansed in the usual way. Drapes are applied so that the limb is freely mobile.

Unless only a small graft is necessary, the whole circumference of the limb should be made available.

Usually general anaesthesia is employed, but if the wound requiring the graft is being dealt with under local or regional block, it is possible to take smaller grafts with local infiltration only.

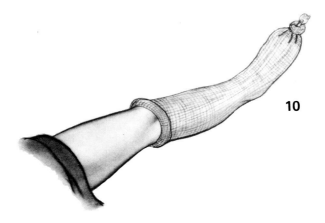

10

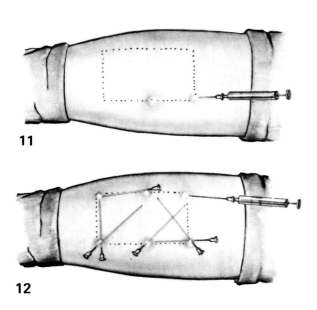

11

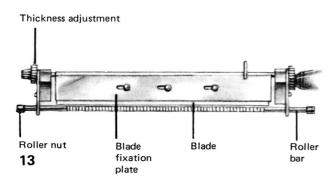

12

11 & 12

An area of skin slightly larger than the proposed graft is marked on the thigh. Blebs of skin are raised at appropriate sites with local analgesic solution then the whole area infiltrated with lignocaine 0·5 per cent solution in a criss-cross manner just below the dermis, using a long needle.

13

Setting the knife

Roller knives have minor variations but the principles of usage are the same. Care must be taken to ensure that the whole framework of the knife is rigid, and that the blade has been inserted and fixed correctly. The nuts or screws of the roller assembly should be tested for tightness: an embarrassingly deep incision can occur if the roller comes adrift whilst cutting the graft.

The calibrations on the thickness adjustment are merely for guidance in setting each end of the roller. They do not indicate actual widths of opening, and vary from knife to knife.

Thickness adjustment

Roller nut   Blade   Blade   Roller
13   fixation   bar
              plate

14

Gauging the position of the setting is a matter of experience and judgement, of familiarity with the knife, and variations in the donor site.

It is helpful to hold the knife up to a light so that the gap between the edge of the blade and the roller can be estimated more clearly. One should err on the side of thinness to start with: if the graft is obviously too thin it is easy to stop and start again after adjusting to a thicker slice.

The medial and flexor surfaces of the limbs tend to be covered by thinner skin than the extensor surfaces and an allowance must be made for this.

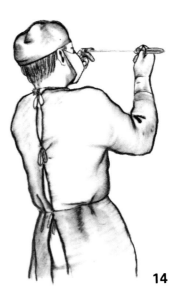

14

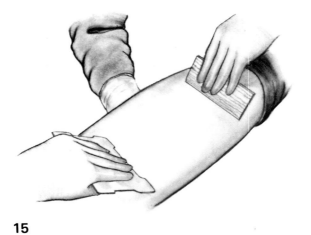

15

15

Cutting the graft

The donor site and the back of the knife blade, and also the edge of the Gabarro board are lubricated with sterile liquid paraffin. An assistant puts the skin on the stretch and creates a flat surface by placing a wooden board, or the edge of his hand on the skin, and applying traction away from the proposed donor site.

It may also be necessary for the assistant to place a hand beneath the limb to press the tissues upwards, thus creating a broader surface from which the graft can be cut.

The surgeon then places the knife parallel and with its back close up to the board, and applies counter-traction with the Gabarro board held in his left hand, just in front of the cutting edge. This presents a flat, firm, steady and stretched surface of skin to the knife.

16

The blade is held at an acute angle to the skin. This angle varies with the thickness of the graft and the type of knife, but should never be more than about 25–30°.

16

17

The graft is then cut with a gentle sawing action, maintaining a steady forward progression and moderate downward pressure.

The Gabarro board should progress at the same rate, remaining about 1 cm ahead of the cutting edge and parallel to it.

Sometimes, if a long strip of graft is being cut, or if the limb is obese, it is necessary for the cutting action to cease momentarily in order to allow the assistant to move his counter-traction board forwards over the donor site to a new position close behind the knife, thus maintaining stability of the surface.

The graft usually collects in folds on the top of the knife blade, but occasionally it is necessary for another assistant to hold it gently stretched with forceps in order to prevent it wrapping itself around the roller.

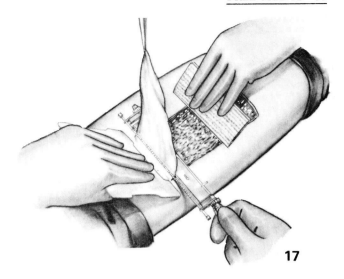

17

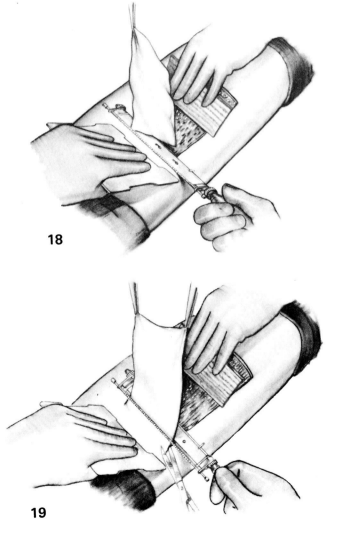

18

19

18 & 19

When sufficient graft has been removed it is completely severed from the donor site by turning the knife so that the blade approaches the surface. Alternatively, the knife can be withdrawn slightly and the graft cut with scissors.

If further strips of split-skin are to be taken, the donor limb is rotated and held by the assistants in such a way that the surgeon can cut the next graft as near as possible to the edge of the preceding one.

Dressing the donor site

Donor sites bleed briskly from incised capillaries, and if large areas of graft have been cut, blood loss may be significant, especially in children.

Gauze swabs soaked in 10 vol. per cent hydrogen peroxide can be applied immediately, to be quickly replaced by firm pressure dressings consisting of at least two layers of vaseline gauze, then dry gauze, cotton wool and crêpe bandage. This can be further fixed with adhesive strapping so that the whole dressing can remain intact for 10–12 days, by which time re-epithelialization should be complete and the dressing removed with relatively little discomfort.

Donor sites are extremely painful, especially when dressings stick to them and various so-called 'non-adherent' dressings and membranes have been devised. For the average donor site, few offer significant advantages over the above traditional method.

Preparation of the grafts

As the pieces of skin are removed they are placed in sterile normal saline until they can be prepared for application to the defect.

20 & 21

Single sheets of Vaseline gauze are placed on the large wooden board. The grafts are then spread, cut surface upwards, on the gauze, which thus supports the thin slice of skin. Non-toothed forceps, and if necessary, fingertips are used, taking care to avoid contamination of the cut surface with vaseline.

(The Vaseline acts as a loose adhesive only and if the graft has been cut too thick, it will tend to curl up at its edges rather than lie flat. In these circumstances it is better to discard the gauze and suture the graft directly to the defect).

The Vaseline gauze is then trimmed with scissors round the pieces of skin, which are covered with saline-dampened swabs until all the grafts have been prepared for application or storage.

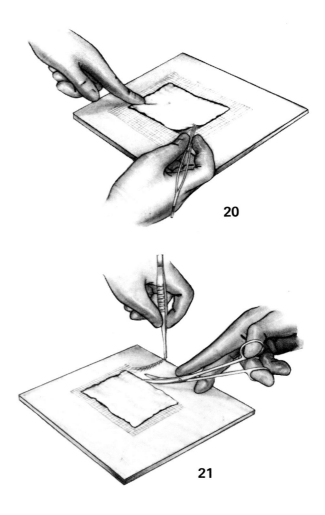

20

21

Storage of split-skin graft

The skin, mounted on Vaseline gauze can be stored in an ordinary domestic refrigerator at 4°C for up to 3 weeks, after which time any grafts unused should be discarded as they no longer take.

The pieces of skin are folded so that cut surfaces come together in order to protect them from Vaseline contamination, and placed in sterile storage jars containing one or two drops of normal saline.

Several pieces can be stored in a single jar, but they should not be packed tightly. The jars are then labelled with the patient's name and the date.

Application and fixation of split-skin graft

They may be applied immediately to the defect at the initial operation, or at the first dressing of the wound 24 or 48 hr later.

Immediate grafting

22

If the defect is small, for example on the back of a hand, and haemostasis is satisfactory, the graft may be sutured edge-to-edge with continuous 5/0 polypropylene after trimming to the appropriate shape.

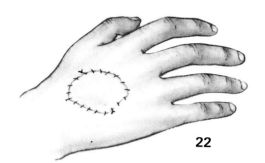

22

23

Larger defects may require more than one piece of skin. Separate strips are then fitted edge to edge over the defect, with a little overlap of the wound sides. Care is taken to ensure that sufficient graft is used to avoid tenting over irregular concave areas of the wound.

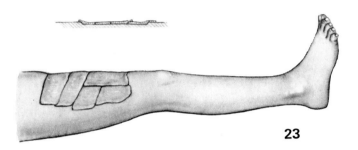

23

24

Another layer of Vaseline gauze is then placed over the grafts.

Small pieces of cotton wool wrung out in saline are gently pressed into the concavities to ensure complete apposition of the grafts to the raw area, and the contour built up with successive layers of wet wool. Even pressure is maintained by a thick layer of dry cotton wool held in place by a crêpe bandage.

Further immobilization can be obtained, and is certainly desirable in small children, by means of a few turns of a plaster of Paris bandage.

Dry gauze   Wet wool   Crêpe bandage

Dry cotton wool

24

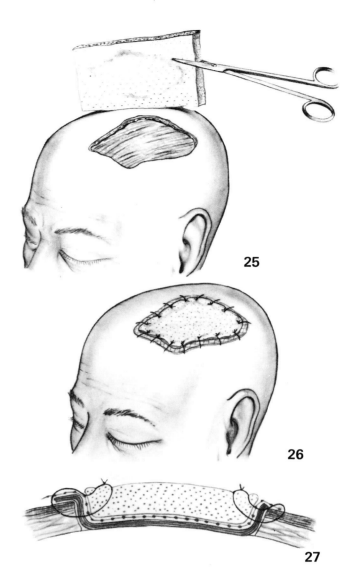

25

26

27

25, 26 & 27

Skin grafts can be easily held in place on certain smooth convex defects such as in the scalp or over the fasciae of the limbs by means of 1 cm thick polyethylene foam sponge.

A piece of sponge is pressed onto the defect in order to take an exact pattern, which is then cut out.

The sponge is applied to the skin grafts and stitched in place with mattress sutures passing through the sponge, the graft, the skin edge then back through the graft and the sponge. Wool and crêpe bandage are then applied.

Delayed grafting

This may be done 24 or 48 hr after excision of the wound, when the possibility of further tissue necrosis, the presence of undue oozing of blood, or a poorly vascularized bed, such as fat, contra-indicate immediate grafting.

Wound dressings are removed and if a satisfactory granulating wound is present grafts may be applied in the ways described above.

The exposure method

Pressure is not necessary for a graft to take.

The pieces of skin are applied to the raw area without fixation other than, perhaps, a further single layer of Vaseline gauze. The grafted part is immobilized by being supported on a Thomas's splint, blocks of polyethylene sponge or in a plaster cast, as appropriate to the injury.

The advantages of this method are:

(*1*) without dressings the graft is cooler, and therefore has a lower metabolic demand;

(*2*) regular inspection is possible and any collection of haematoma beneath the graft can be expressed.

Exposed grafts are found to be adherent to the bed within 4–6 hr of application (though not of course yet taken).

28

Postage stamp grafting

Thought at one time to be essential for satisfactory take, the use of small rectangles of split-skin graft, rather than larger sheets is only an advantage when the base of the wound is extremely irregular, when there is residual serous oozing or when established infection with purulent discharge is present. The grafts are applied with small gaps in between to allow escape of exudate. They are small enough to conform to most irregularities, and too small to tent over and retain exudate which might otherwise result in loss of portion of the graft.

The cosmetic result of small grafts, with many intervening marginal scars between them, is poor in comparison with larger sheets of skin.

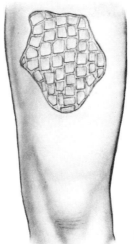

28

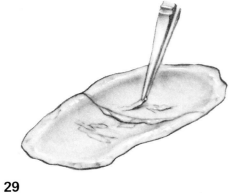

29

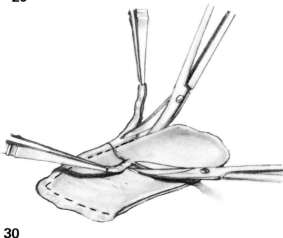

30

Subsequent management

29 & 30

Pressure dressings, sponge, Vaseline gauze and sutures are removed 4 days after grafting.

Skin that has taken will be pink and firmly adherent to the underlying raw area, and if forcibly lifted, bleeding will result.

There is usually a thin layer of separating epidermis, which should be gently peeled away where it is loose.

Surplus graft overlapping either healed graft or the wound's edge should be cut away with fine, sharp-pointed scissors.

31

In some areas the graft may have been lifted by an underlying haematoma or seroma. If this is released by the fourth day so that the skin can come into contact with the bed, healing may still take place.

The bleb should be opened with a knife blade or scissors, and the liquid expressed through the incision by gentle pressure with a cotton bud or similar small swab. Aspiration by syringe and needle is insufficient.

Liquid beneath a graft exposed from the onset is similarly released, but it may be possible, on the first or second day to express it by rolling it towards the edge of the graft, without actually making an incision.

Depending on the circumstances, the healing graft may be completely redressed with Vaseline gauze, wool and bandages or merely covered with a single layer of Vaseline gauze.

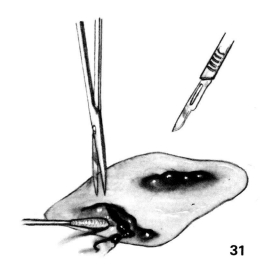

31

32a

32b

32a & b

The areas are then inspected every day or on alternate days, with removal of epidermis, crusts and fluid collections until all parts are healed, or there is a clear indication that portions of the graft have failed to take.

Any graft which appears dead and is loose, or floating on pus, should have been removed by the seventh day.

The resulting areas of granulation should be cleaned with saline solution, and if more than 1 cm in diameter should be regrafted with pieces of stored skin. Often these small patches may be applied and left exposed.

Smaller areas of granulation can be expected to heal from the edges of healed graft, though this process is slow if the granulations are heaped up, as they tend to remain exuberant.

They can be flattened by regular applications of hypertonic saline, or 1 per cent hydrocortisone cream or ointment, after which final healing is rapid.

After-care

Two weeks after the successful application of grafts, consolidation has usually progressed far enough for the grafts to be exposed, though in practice a light dry dressing is often used for protection for a few days or weeks, depending on the site and the patient's occupation.

Grafts on the lower limb tend to become purple and congested on adoption of the upright posture; gradual lowering of the limb to a dependent position for a few minutes each hour is advisable during the first week after healing, progressing to full activity if the graft appears satisfactory. Lower limb grafts should have firm elastic bandage or stocking support for a few weeks until their venous drainage has matured to the extent that congestion no longer occurs.

Regular daily gentle massage with lanolin cream helps to soften the graft and its marginal scars.

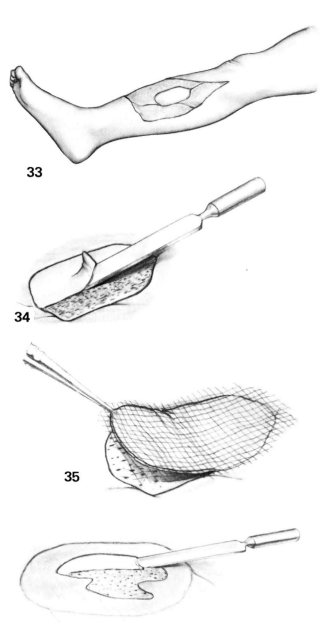

33

34

35

36

33-36

Split-skin grafting onto cortical bone

Although bare cortical bone will not support a large skin graft, small areas of exposed bone, for example on the subcutaneous surface of the tibia, can be covered by graft if the exposed bone is freshened with a gouge or chisel. The surface of the bone is clearly avascular, but if a sliver of bone is removed to a depth of 1—2 mm bleeding points in the underlying bone may be observed. Split-skin graft applied to this bone will take, at least in part. One week later, any remaining bone exposed through graft failure should be treated in the same way, and at similar intervals until healing is complete.

This is a particularly useful procedure to cover over a fracture site when multiple injuries or other factors temporarily prevent more complicated surgery to obtain a definitive skin repair.

FULL-THICKNESS FREE GRAFTS (WOLFE GRAFTS)

These are usually employed to cover limited defects in special sites, when normal thickness of the skin, minimal shrinkage and good colour-match are desirable.

Such sites are the lower eyelids, the lips, nose and other areas of the face where mobility without distortion is important.

Some surgeons also prefer full-thickness grafts for the repair of slicing injuries of the distal finger pulps, though thick split-skin grafts are equally satisfactory and re-innervation is sometimes superior.

Donor sites

A full-thickness skin defect is created and sites are, therefore, chosen where direct closure of the area can be achieved.

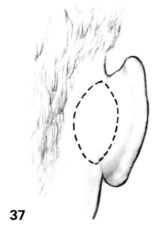

37

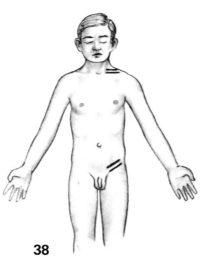

38

37 & 38

(*1*) *Postauricular skin* is hairless and of excellent texture and colour-match for eyelid and small nasal defects.

(*2*) *Supraclavicular skin* is suitable for larger defects on the face. There is good colour-match, though not as good as with postauricular skin in white skinned people. This is the donor area of choice in coloured races, because colour match is better than with postauricular grafts, which may become more deeply pigmented than the surrounding normal skin.

(*3*) *The groin* provides soft, thin skin but offers no advantage, except possibly convenience, when taking graft for an area such as a hand, where colour-match is less important.

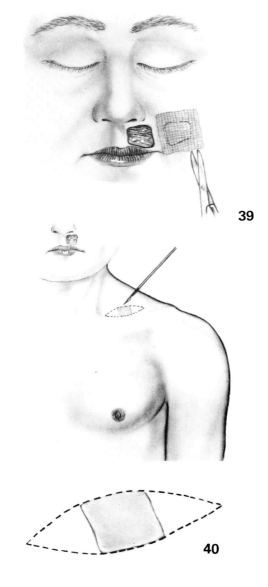

39

40

CUTTING A WOLFE GRAFT

39 & 40

An exact pattern of the defect is drawn on jaconet or paper, cut out and arranged appropriately on the donor site. The pattern is then drawn on the donor site, adding orientation marks to the outlined graft, if necessary. It is convenient to mark and cut the final ellipse at the same time if it is clear that simple straight line suture of the donor defect will be possible. The graft outline is then incised only as deep as the thickness of the skin.

There are two ways of taking the graft. The first is elegant but difficult.

41

One corner of the graft is picked up with a skin hook and by sharp dissection at exactly the level of the deepest part of the dermis the graft is separated from the underlying subcutaneous fatty tissue.

Shape and tension are maintained by the finger tips of the hand holding the hook.

It is easy to button-hole the graft accidentally.

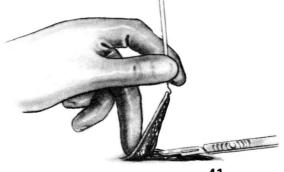

41

42

The second method consists of a simple excision of the outlined skin with no attempt at avoiding taking subcutaneous tissue, which thus remains in variable amounts on the deep surface of the graft.

The fat has then to be excised, so far as possible, using curved scissors. The graft is supported on a convex surface such as a finger in order to facilitate this removal.

Care must be taken to ensure that skin hooks do not tear the graft. Forceps should be used as little as possible.

The donor site is then sutured in layers. Wide undermining to mobilize the skin edges and allow closure with minimum tension is often necessary.

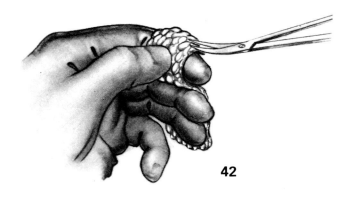

42

Application of the graft

Absolute haemostasis on the recipient defect is essential.

The graft's natural elasticity causes it to curl up and apparently shrink. However, if the dimensions are correct, the graft will be under correct tension when sutured into place.

43 & 44

Interrupted stitches of 5/0 polypropylene should be used and as few as possible to achieve exact edge-to-edge apposition.

One end of each suture is left 5—10 cm long, for tying over the dressing.

One layer of Vaseline gauze is applied and then firm pressure and splintage of the graft maintained by tying the long ends of the sutures over a pad to hold it in place. The pad may be either saline-soaked cotton wool, a dental roll, or a piece of shaped polyethylene sponge, depending on the size of the graft and the contour of the bed of the defect. As with split-skin grafts, it is essential that the graft is in contact with the defect over its whole area.

Further firm padding and fixation with bandage or strapping is applied as appropriate and is left undisturbed for 7 days.

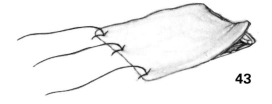

43

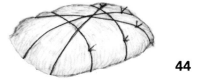

44

Subsequent management

The tie-over dressing and alternate sutures are removed after a week, the remainder being removed 3 or 4 days later.

A successful graft will appear rather plum-coloured at this stage.

Darker bluish-black areas in the graft indicate haematoma beneath it, and some loss may be inevitable.

If one of these areas is close to the edge of the graft, very gentle pressure may expel the haematoma. Any other interference probably does more harm than good, and the graft should be disturbed as little as possible at the first dressing.

Polyfax antibiotic ointment and a dry dressing should be applied.

Further dressings are carried out as necessary, and the graft can usually be exposed after 14—18 days on the face, though longer protection is normally necessary for grafts on the hands. Physiotherapy may then be required to restore full mobility.

THE PRINCIPLES OF THE WOLFE GRAFT APPLIED TO CERTAIN SKIN INJURIES

Flap wounds

If an injury raises a flap which is short in length and proximally based, the chances are that the flap is viable and can be sutured back after only sparingly trimming of torn subcutaneous tissues.

If, however, the flap is long, and always if its base is distal, the skin should be considered as unlikely to survive in its entirety, although, on occasions, and unpredictably, it may do so. If the skin is clearly badly damaged it should be excised, and the appropriate free graft applied.

If, however, it is relatively free of contusions and contamination then it can be salvaged with a reasonable prospect of successful healing.

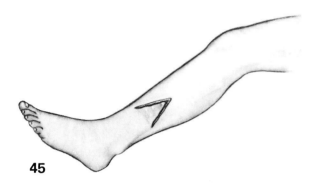

45

A common example is the triangular, distally-based flap on the lower part of the leg, simple suture of which invariably results in at least partial necrosis, possibly with subsequent infection, and requiring secondary excision and skin grafting. At the initial operation the flap should be lifted and all the fat on its deep surface and also all the fat overlying the fascia beneath the flap should be carefully trimmed away.

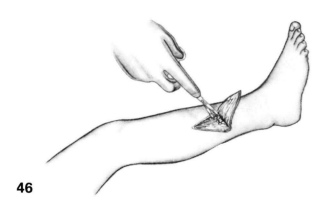

46

This creates a full-thickness skin graft, but still attached by its base.

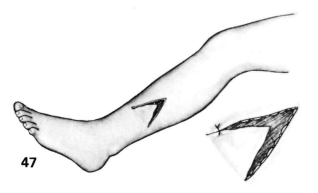

47

Haemostasis is secured, and the flap-graft laid in place without tension, being held there with a few sutures. Often a small V-shaped defect remains.

Split-skin grafts should be taken and stored for application to this defect later.

The wound is then dressed with Vaseline gauze and wet wool packing.

After 48 hr the wound is inspected and the split-skin grafts applied to the residual defect. The defatted flap will be found to have taken, mainly as a full-thickness graft.

Major undermining skin injuries (partial avulsion or flaying)

These often result from run-over accidents by which much of the skin of a limb may be torn from its subcutaneous attachments.

48

Even without a wound, the skin of almost the whole circumference of the limb may be separated from the underlying fascia by a large haematoma (closed flaying).

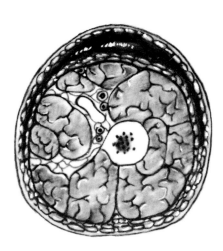

48

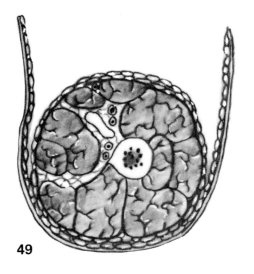

49

49

The presence of a wound will reveal the extent of the avulsion.

Much of this undermined skin will inevitably die because of crushing and damage to its arterial supply and venous drainage — particularly the latter, though the doomed areas are not necessarily apparent for a few days.

If the patient's condition and other injuries allow a prolonged procedure, much healing time can be saved and later morbidity prevented at the initial operation.

Grossly damaged skin is excised. The undermined flaps are turned back and fat excised from the deep surface and from the fascia.

50

If the flaps are held on only by narrow pedicles, it is easier to excise the skin flaps completely and spread them out on a board to facilitate the defatting procedure. A skin-grafting knife with the gap set as wide as possible is a useful instrument for carrying out the excision of fat down to the deep surface of the dermis.

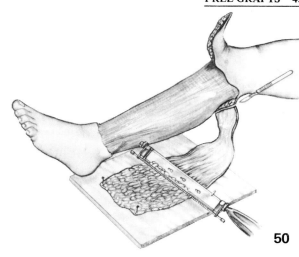

50

A special machine with a longer blade than a graft knife has been devised by Gibson to carry out this procedure on large pieces of skin.

The defatted flaps, or free full-thickness grafts, are replaced on the limb and held in place, without tension, using 3/0 polyglycolic acid sutures.

Split-skin grafts are taken and stored for application to remaining raw areas.

51

If small amounts of full-thickness skin remain after excision, these should be applied to parts of the limb, such as around the knee joint or ankle, which would most benefit from full-thickness cover, assuming replaced skin survives.

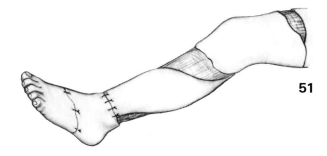

51

The usual dressings of Vaseline gauze, dry dressings and wool are applied and the limb elevated.

Subsequent management

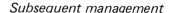

The dressings are removed on the fourth or fifth day. Further excision of dead tissue is carried out if necessary, including any of the replaced skin flaps which have not become attached.

In a large wound such as this, excision must be radical if gross infection is to be prevented. It is better to remove too much skin than too little.

If infection is not severe and residual raw areas are granulating, the stored split-skin can be applied.

Patching of areas of loss is carried out at subsequent dressings, using split-skin, as described on page 34.

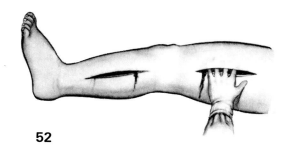

52

52

In a case of closed flaying, appropriate incisions are made in order to evacuate the haematoma, explore the extent of the undermining, and turn back the skin flaps so that adequate excision of fat can be performed.

COMPOSITE GRAFTS

As the name implies, these are free grafts of more than one tissue.

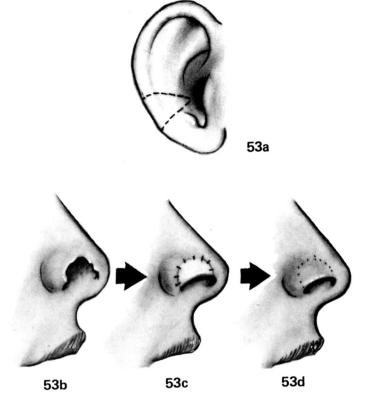

53a

53a-e

The common one is a portion of an ear margin, consisting of a sandwich of cartilage between two layers of skin and subcutaneous tissue, used to reconstruct a defect of the ala of the nose. Only small grafts from vascular donor sites can be used, and must be inserted into defects in similarly vascular areas, otherwise death of the relatively bulky graft is likely.

Another example is a graft of nasal septal cartilage and overlying mucosa, to restore conjunctiva and tarsal plate in eyelid losses.

Because of the complexities of preparation of the defect and the grafted tissue, composite grafts are not used in the initial management of injuries, but are part of the armamentarium in correcting secondary defects and deformities which result from simpler and more appropriate primary repairs.

53b　　**53c**　　**53d**

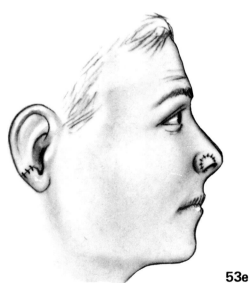

53e

[*The illustrations for this Chapter on Free Grafts were drawn by Mr. G. Lyth.*]

Skin Flaps

Malcolm Deane, M.B., B.S., F.R.C.S.
Consultant Plastic Surgeon, Nottingham, Derby and Mansfield Hospitals;
Clinical Teacher, University of Nottingham School of Medicine

INTRODUCTION

The previous chapter lists a variety of tissues which, if exposed on a raw surface would, by virtue of their avascularity, be unable to support a free graft.

It is necessary for healing and function that important structures such as tendon, joints and important tactile areas such as finger tips should have adequate supple skin cover. Furthermore, the lack of sub-cutaneous fat in free grafts results in dense adhesion of the skin to the underlying tissue, with reduction of mobility and loss of protective padding.

For these reasons, when confronted with such a wound, the necessity for repair with a flap must be considered.

Characteristics of a flap

A flap consists of (*1*) skin and (*2*) subcutaneous tissue. It may also contain (*3*) deep fascia and (*4*) muscle. It must have (*5*) an adequate blood supply and drainage.

A flap is basically a rectangular segment of skin, free on three of its sides, and remaining attached by its fourth, *the pedicle*, through which it receives its blood supply and venous and lymphatic drainage.

1

So that the bulk of tissue is not too great for the available blood vessels a guiding rule for a flap raised on any part of the body is that it should not be longer than it is wide.

In general, this is a safe proportion when the blood supply is from a random network of cutaneous vessels.

On the head and neck this ratio is unnecessarily cautious, and longer, narrower flaps may be raised— 2:1 and sometimes longer.

On the upper limb, flaps with their pedicles based proximally may also break the rule, but only perhaps 3:2.

These conditions are reversed, however, on the leg. Here the flaps should be twice as wide as long, owing to the generally lower vitality of the skin.

TYPES OF FLAPS

A flap is created to transfer skin cover from a place where it is available to an area where it is needed.

It may be (*1*) local or (*2*) distant.

LOCAL FLAPS

The ideal condition exists when skin adjacent to a defect can be made into a flap to cover the raw area.

The advantages of a local flap are; (*a*) cover is restored in a one-stage procedure and (*b*) quality, texture, thickness and colour are the same as the skin which was lost.

A local flap can be moved into the defect in one of three ways.

2a & b

Advancement

The flap is designed in such a way that its distal end merely moves forwards into the defect. Undermining the skin edges round a wound before suturing it is in effect forming two advancement flaps.

3

Transposition

Here the flap pivots on one corner of its pedicle when it is swung into the defect. Note that the flap must be longer than the defect in order to reach the further corner of the defect without tension. Note also the inevitable 'dog-ear' resulting from the excess when a long side is sutured to a shorter one.

Finally, note also that a *secondary defect* has been created and that it usually requires split-skin cover.

4a, b & c

Rotation

Here the flap is more or less semicircular in shape, so that as it moves into the defect the secondary defect is distributed evenly along the curve.

However, the secret of rotation with minimal tension lies in the back-cut, which must be made with care because it is reducing the pedicle. When the horizontal back-cut is sutured vertically the flap is pushed further round into the defect.

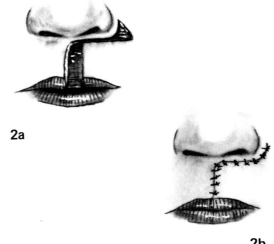

2a

2b

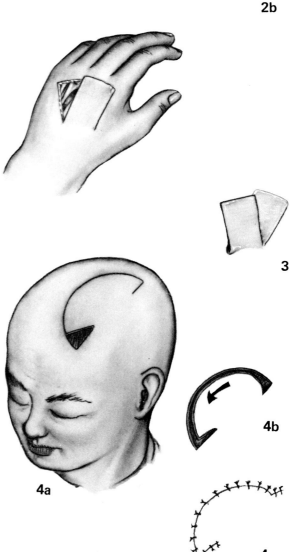

3

4b

4a

4c

DISTANT FLAPS

The transference of skin from one part of the body to another requires at least two operations, and occasionally six or seven and may take several weeks to complete.

DIRECT TRANSFER

A flap is raised, being designed in such a way that it can be accurately placed on the defect when the two parts are brought close together. Immobilization must then be sufficient to allow healing without traction, torsion, tension, pressure or kinking at any part of the flap, particularly across the pedicle.

Whilst healing is taking place the tissues of the flap rely on the blood supply through the pedicle, but gradually this dependence diminishes as vascular anastomoses develop between the recipient defect and the flap. The pedicle can then be divided, freeing the two parts: the flap survives on its newly developed blood supply.

Depending on the site and size of the flap, and the relative vascularity of the defect, this process takes between 2 and 4 weeks.

This type of repair is the most commonly used flap in traumatic lesions and includes thenar, palmar and cross-finger flaps for distal pulp injuries, inframammary, groin and cross-arm flaps for finger and hand injuries, abdominal and flank flaps for upper limb defects and cross-leg flaps for skin lost from the lower leg and foot.

FLAPS FOR DISTAL FINGER PULP LOSSES

5

The best replacement skin comes from the thenar eminence and palm. Dorsal finger skin is also satisfactory, although tactile sensory return is not quite so good. However, these areas should not be used in the presence of arthritic conditions. The finger tips must reach the donor site easily. They must not be forced into position and held there as permanent stiffness of the interphalangeal joints may result.

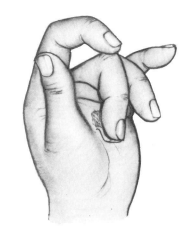

5

6

Thumb

A palmar flap based on the lateral side of the hand, distal to the head of the second metatarsal, is convenient.

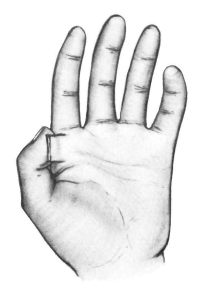

6

7

Index, middle and ring fingers

A thenar flap may be used. The donor site scar can sometimes be tender.

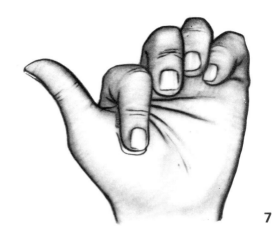

7

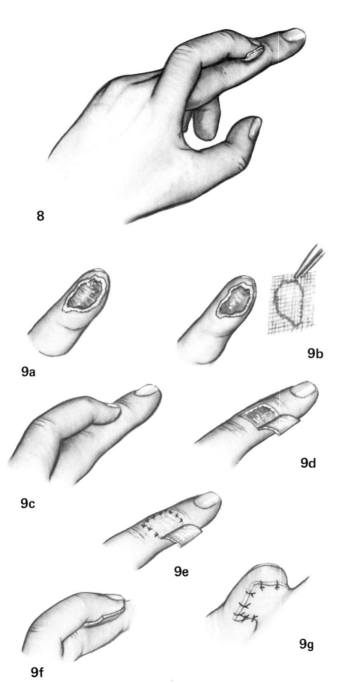

8

9a

9b

9c

9d

9e

9f

9g

8

Middle, ring and little fingers

Cross-finger flaps are useful for volar and lateral pulp injuries. These laterally-based flaps should not encroach anteriorly beyond the mid-lateral line of the donor finger.

9a-g

Technique

The principles for all these flaps are the same. Local analgesia may be employed.

The wound edges are cleaned and trimmed. A pattern of the defect is made, the digit and the pattern are put into position, and the pattern is then transferred to the donor site (planning in reverse).

The flap is marked, and raised with a thick layer of subcutaneous tissue.

The donor defect is repaired with a Wolfe graft taken from the forearm or groin.

A bulky tie-over dressing should not be used; 0·25 inches (6 mm) polyethylene sponge cut to shape and held with adhesive strapping is an excellent support for the graft.

The graft should also be adequate to cover raw areas of the flap not in contact with the wound.

The flap is then sutured to the pulp defect and the digit held in position with elastoplast strapping.

Small flaps such as the above examples can usually be divided at 14 or 18 days.

The pattern is once again applied to the flap, the pedicle is divided and the wound closed.

Other finger and hand injuries

When the defect is too large for the above flaps, or when the injured digit cannot flex comfortably to the donor site, remote flaps must be used, which means that the quality of sensibility in the repaired area is inferior to that obtained with thenar or palmar flaps.

Patterns and careful position planning are vital to a satisfactory flap transfer.

Donor sites may be closed either directly, or covered with split-skin graft.

Fixation is adequate using elastoplast strapping.

10

The submammary flap

Useful because the donor site scar is concealed beneath the breast.

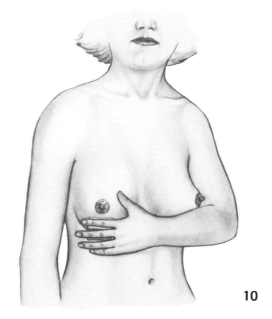

10

11

The cross-arm flap

Useful for thumb web defects, but much reduces the patient's independence.

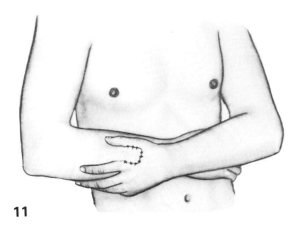

11

12

The groin flap

This will cover quite large dorsal or volar defects. Because it contains the superficial circumflex iliac artery, this flap can be made three or four times as long as its width.

All three flaps can be divided and inset at 17–18 days.

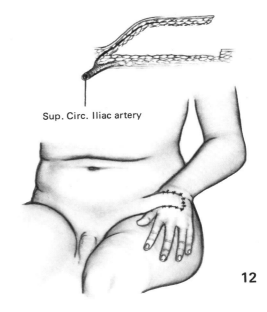

Sup. Circ. Iliac artery

12

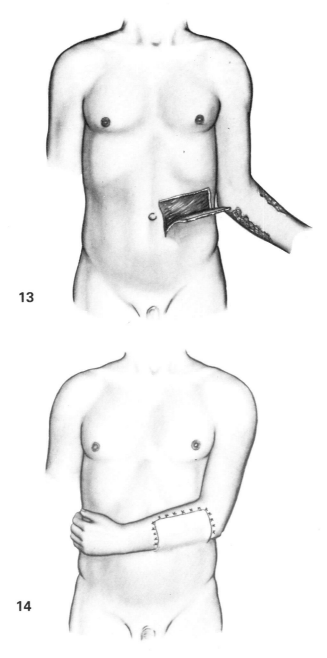

13

14

13 & 14

Upper limb defects

Large areas of skin lost from the elbow and forearm and requiring flap cover can be repaired using flank or abdominal flaps.

Again, accurate reversed planning with a paper or jaconet pattern is important to ensure that the limb lies easily against the trunk and the donor site.

THE CROSS-LEG FLAP

This is the commonest flap used to cover defects involving the subcutaneous surface of the tibia, heel, ankle joint or dorsum of the foot. Even if primary healing can be achieved using split-skin grafts, the resultant scarring and adherent grafts may be inadequate to withstand normal wear and tear and full-thickness cover is necessary.

However, it is rare for a cross-leg flap to be contemplated as a primary procedure; bleeding, swelling,

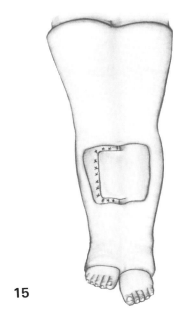

15

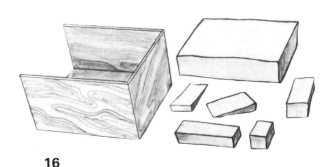

16

injuries to other parts of the body, including the donor leg, and head injury are complicating factors which could, in the early stages prevent a satisfactory flap transfer.

The operation is usually carried out as an elective procedure from a few days to several months after the injury, depending on the site and other complicating factors. All lower limb fractures should be rigidly fixed, usually by plates or medullary nails; external fixation devices obstruct the approximation of the limbs in most cases.

15

Fixation of the two joined limbs

Many methods have been devised including a complete swaddling 'mermaid' plaster of Paris, numerous turns of elastoplast bandage, and interosseous fixation.

The difficulty lies in the small amount of leeway available in movement of one leg in relation to the other. There is often little difference between the perfect position and the one in which traction or kinking is endangering the flap.

Adjustment is often quickly necessary as normal muscle tone returns to the awakening patient, but it can be awkward or impossible without completely dismantling and starting again.

The method described here avoids these disadvantages, and is reasonably comfortable.

16

An open-ended, open-topped box of plywood 18 inches wide, 18 inches high and 24 inches long (45 cm, 45 cm and 60 cm) with a floor raised 6 inches (15 cm) is constructed.

Sheets of 10 and 15 cm thick polyethylene foam sponge sufficient to fill the box are obtained. One sheet remains as the base mattress, the others are removed and cut up into various sizes of block and wedge.

In the ward, a rough pattern of defect and proposed flap is cut in paper or jaconet and the appropriate position of the two limbs arranged within the box as it lies on fracture boards on the bed. The legs are then supported and held in position by means of the sponge blocks and wedges.

The patient spends at least one night in this position before the operation in order to become accustomed to it.

The sponge blocks are then marked to identify their positions, and sterilized ready for use.

The operation

The usual exact pattern and reverse planning are carried out after the patient is anaesthetized.

17

Most defects lie on the front of the injured limb. The flap is therefore usually anteriorly based, on the medial aspect of the donor leg.

Whenever possible, the flap should be raised so that the intact long saphenous vein runs close to its base and so ensures good venous drainage.

It is dangerous to exceed the 2 : 1 width to length ratio, and careful planning is of the greatest importance. The legs usually lie closely side to side with variable amounts of knee flexion.

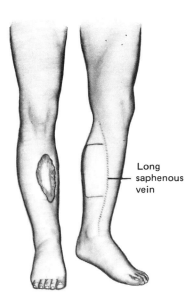

Long saphenous vein

17

18

The defect is prepared by excising scar tissue and skin graft and by freshening exposed bone. Skin edges are narrowly undermined.

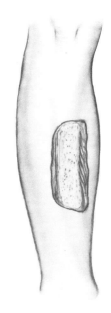

18

19

The flap is raised by dissecting it off the deep fascia and perforating vessels are ligated.

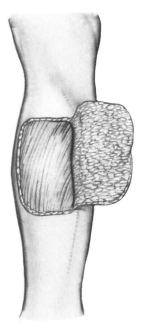

19

20

The donor defect is covered with a split-skin graft taken from the thigh of the injured limb or the buttocks. It should not be taken from the thigh of the donor leg because dressings may obstruct the venous return of the flap.

The graft is sutured under sponge and, if possible, graft is also applied to the undersurface of the pedicle.

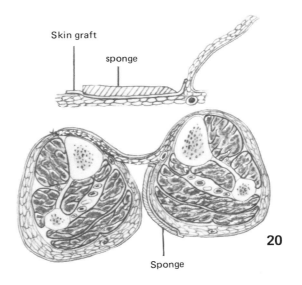

21 & 22

The flap is then sutured into the defect, using skin stitches only.

Two or three assistants are usually necessary to support the two legs in the correct alignment as the attachment progresses. The final position should be such that the flap is in complete contact with the whole area of the defect without tension or acute folding along its pedicle.

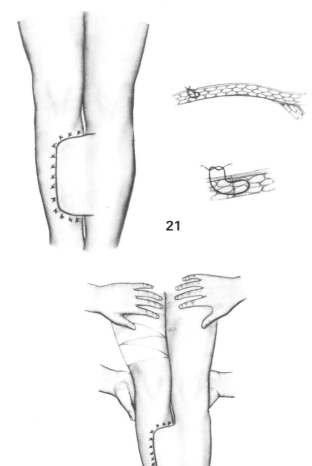

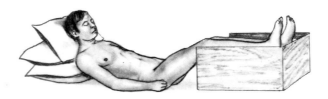

23

23 & 24

The patient is then lifted from the operating table directly into bed whilst still anaesthetized, and the joined limbs are arranged in the box on a layer of Gamgee. The sterile sponge blocks are replaced in their marked positions, further adjustments being made by adding extra wedges of sponge around and beneath the legs and feet. The alignment of the pedicle is examined frequently during this procedure.

One or two strips of elastoplast extending from one side of the box to the other and passing over the lower parts of the thighs and the knees are all the additional fixation necessary to prevent involuntary flexion and disturbance of the position.

Polyfax ointment and a light removable dressing are applied to the flap's suture line, and anaesthesia is discontinued. Careful supervision of the patient is important until full consciousness is regained.

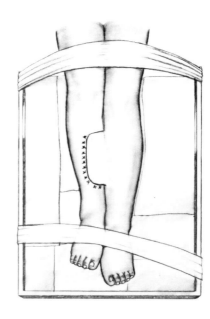

24

Postoperative care

Regular inspection of the pedicle and the flap is carried out in search of tension and haematoma.

Adjustment of the sponge fixation is easily accomplished with minimum disturbance and discomfort to the patient. Thin wedges may be necessary between knees and ankles to prevent pressure at these points.

Within a few days, when the viability of the flap is assured, the legs can be removed from the sponge blocks under the supervision of the physiotherapist, in order to exercise the knees, hips and feet, and to inspect and dress the skin graft at appropriate times.

A considerable range of movement can be achieved whilst still maintaining the correct alignment of the legs. After exercising, the limbs are replaced in the box and the sponge blocks fixation re-applied.

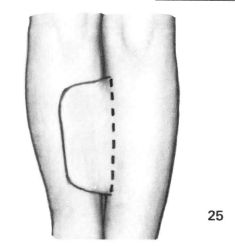

25

25 & 26

The flap is divided at 3 weeks.

Always take more flap than the pattern indicates—
at least 1 cm.

If the pedicle is not bulky, it can be inset immediately, closing the defect with skin stitches.

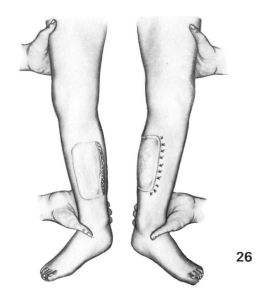

26

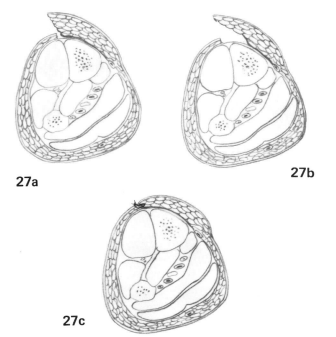

27a

27b

27c

27a, b & c

If there is a marked difference between the thickness
of the flap and that of the edge of the defect it is better
to leave the wound unsutured and merely dress it.
Three or four days later the fat can be trimmed from
beneath the flap edge and the skin closed without the
risk of ischaemia and breakdown of the margin.

Dependent mobilization of the injured limb can be
commenced when the skin has healed, but elastic
bandages should be applied for 4 weeks or so in
order to prevent congestion and swelling of the transferred flap.

INDIRECT TRANSFER

Flap repair of any type requires more specialized services, training and experience than simple free grafting procedures, so that complicated multistage planning and aftercare of the transfer of large areas of skin by means of tubed pedicles is usually carried out in plastic surgical centres. However, by applying the principles of the direct transfer of skin flaps, repair of a large defect, for example, over the subcutaneous surface of the tibia, too extensive for a cross-leg flap, may be achieved without specialized help.

THE TUBED PEDICLE FLAP

Fractures should be rigidly held by internal or external skeletal fixation.

Attempts to get the wound healed as much as possible with split-skin grafts should be continued during the stages of flap transfer, in order to reduce the level of infection.

First stage

28

The area of the defect is measured, and the dimensions marked out on one half of the anterior abdominal wall as a rectangle such that its length is not more than twice its width, or its width not less than half its length, depending on the actual measurements of the defect. The markings should not cross the mid-line.

Two incisions made along the longer side of the rectangle are carried down to the external oblique aponeurosis. The intervening skin is undermined at the level between Scarpa's fascia and the aponeurosis, thus creating a strap of skin and subcutaneous tissue commonly extending from the iliac fossa to the costal margin. This is a *bipedicled* flap.

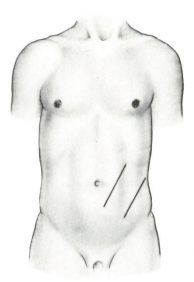

28

29, 30 & 31

After careful haemostasis of the deep surface of the flap the two free edges are sutured together, using 5/0 polypropylene, in order to form a tube of skin. No subcutaneous stitches are used. In order to avoid distortion or constriction of the two pedicles the edges should not be approximated at each end beyond the point where they can come together easily without tension. The skin edges of the donor defect are then sutured to the aponeurosis with continuous 3/0 polyglycolic acid stitches in order to immobilize the defect and avoid an ugly stepped effect. The defect is then filled with split-skin grafts sutured under polyethylene sponge, ensuring that the grafts fold over the ends of the sponge in order to cover the triangular raw areas at each end of the tubed flap, but avoiding any pressure on the deep surface of each pedicle. Gauze and wool dressings are then applied, but leaving the tube exposed so that it can be readily inspected.

Postoperative care of a tubed flap

Haematoma within the tube is the commonest cause of failure. If the tube becomes swollen, tense and discoloured, haematoma should be suspected, and released by removal of one or two sutures in the centre of the seam. The surgeon should not hesitate to take the patient to the operating theatre and completely open the tube to release haematoma if he considers that bleeding is persisting.

During the next 3 weeks the blood flow within the tube alters from an irregular random network of vessels to a linear arrangement from end to end.

Often one end is more important than the other as a source of blood supply. This is the dominant end, is usually the lower one, but not necessarily so. Plethysmography, dye injections and removal of radioactive markers have been used to establish more accurately the flow-characteristics of the tube.

In practice, however, a simple clinical test is all that is necessary prior to the next stage of the transference.

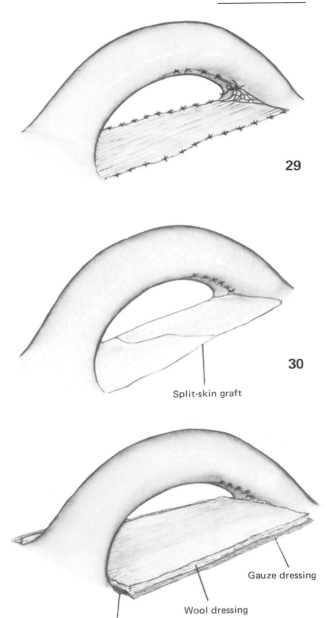

29

30

Split-skin graft

Gauze dressing

Wool dressing

Sponge

31

32

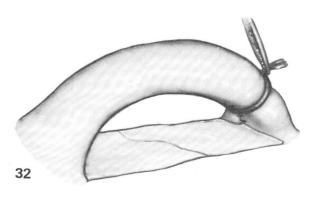

32

The 'strangle' test

A soft rubber catheter is applied fairly tightly round each end of the tube in turn, and held with a clamp to act as a tourniquet. After 10 min it is inspected. Pallor of the tube suggests that the end constricted is the one carrying the more important blood supply. The opposite end is, therefore, the one to be separated first.

Second stage

The wrist is most often used to carry a tubed pedicle flap.

Choice of side depends on the position of the defect, and it should be ascertained that the patient can adopt the final planned position with the flap attached appropriately to wrist and leg, before beginning the transference.

33, 34, 35 a & b

The subsidiary end of the tube (usually the upper) is divided from the abdomen using a curved incision. Scar tissue and skin graft are excised from the under-surface of the end so that a roughly circular raw surface results.

A semicircular incision is made on the ulnar border of the wrist, turning down a flap to create a circular raw area. The tube is then sutured to the wrist in correct alignment, using 5/0 polypropylene.

Stitch marks and excess scarring on the tube are prevented by using mattress sutures which do not pierce the skin surface on the pedicle side.

The abdominal defect is closed with skin graft or direct apposition, as appropriate.

The upper limb is fixed to the trunk in the correct position with elastoplast strapping, until the attachment has healed.

The tube must lie comfortably without tension or kinking.

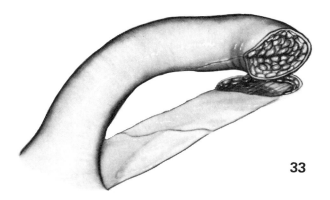

33

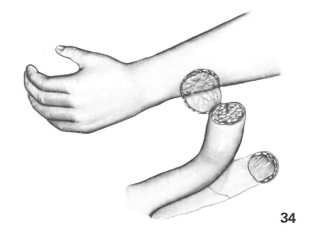

34

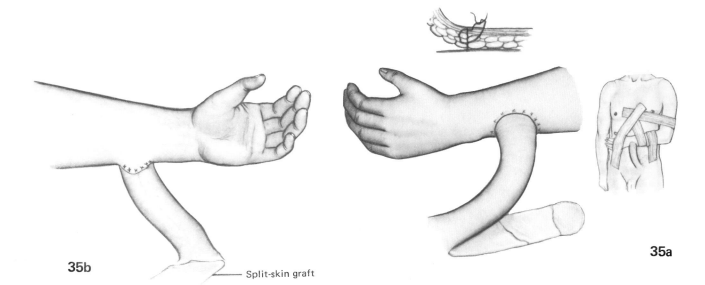

35b

——— Split-skin graft

35a

Delay incisions

After 3 weeks or so, there will be sufficient blood supply through the wrist attachment to nourish the tube. A strangle test at the abdominal end of the tube will confirm this.

It is safer, however, to separate this end in two stages, known as delays.

36

The line of incision is marked, but only half of the area of attachment is lifted, though all this area is undermined so that large blood vessels can be identified and divided. The end is thus nourished via only the dermal plexus in the intact skin bridge. The delay incision is then sutured. Four days later, the skin bridge is similarly incised, any remaining vessels entering the tube are divided, and the wound is once again closed.

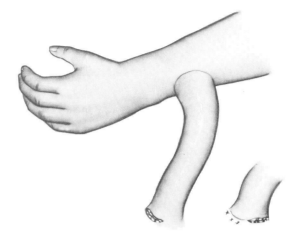

36

37 & 38

Four days later the whole tube is lifted from the abdominal wall and inset into an appropriate circular excision of scar and skin graft at the lower end of the defect on the leg.

Confirmatory strangle tests after 3 or 4 weeks show that it is safe to separate the tube from its wrist attachment, insetting its end into the upper part of the leg defect.

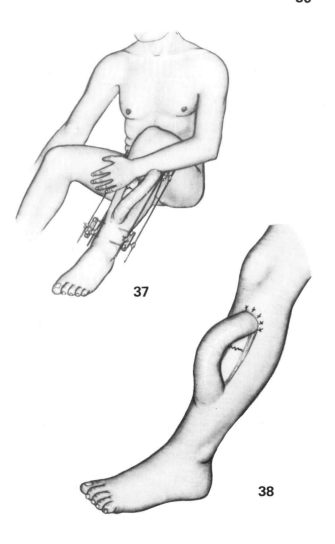

37

38

39 & 40

Approximately 6 weeks after transferring the tube, its seam can be opened to create a rectangular flap once more. This is set into the remainder of the defect after scar and skin grafts have been excised and any exposed bone freshened.

Subsequent operations whether to bone graft an ununited fracture, remove a plate or improve the contour of the flap by thinning subcutaneous tissue, are carried out by lifting the flap along one of its sides.

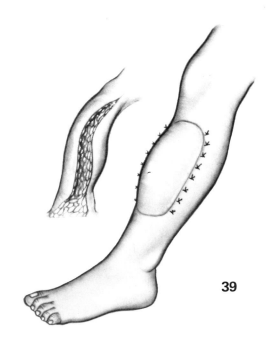

39

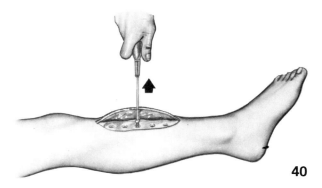

40

GENERAL CARE OF THE PATIENT

All patients subjected to the immobilization of transferred flap procedures require particular attention.

(*1*) Their position, ensuring that no danger exists to their flap by inadvertent movement. Fixation must be constantly adjusted, augmented and, if necessary, completely removed and replaced in order to maintain correct alignment.

(*2*) Pressure areas, including unsuspected sites, for example where an elbow may be pressing on a knee, or between a heel and an ankle.

(*3*) Physiotherapy, maintaining movement in as many joints as the fixation will allow. There is inevitably stiffness when fixation is removed, but its relief is assisted by attention to the problem in the early stages.

Tubed pedicle flaps often become oedematous, and gentle massage will alleviate the condition and promote their blood supply.

Short wave diathermy or ultrasound may be necessary to reduce chronic oedema in a tube if this has resulted from infection and excess scarring.

Great care must be taken in the use of these appliances, because heat is generated and can burn an ischaemic flap.

(*4*) Morale, which must be maintained by constant encouragement from all members of staff involved in patient care. Optimism in the face of set-backs and complications which are almost inevitable in a prolonged multistage procedure, is almost as important as all the above factors put together.

(*5*) Infection, which to some degree is very likely to occur because it is difficult to apply occlusive dressings to all wounds and raw areas; frequent inspection of pedicles and flaps is necessary. It is desirable to use prophylactic antibiotics during the healing stages, and local antibiotic ointment (Polyfax) to incisions to prevent minor inflammation if sutures have to remain in place longer than usual.

Pulmonary and urinary tract infection are liable to occur in the immobilized patient, and must be guarded against.

(*6*) Other dangerous complications such as thrombo-embolism and acute gastric dilatation.

Contra-indications

In general, patients over the age of 45 — 50 years are not suitable candidates for cross-leg flaps or abdominal tube pedicles to lower limb injuries because of the high risk of thrombo-embolic complications. The incidence of peripheral arterial disease also adversely affects the chances of satisfactory vascularization of flaps.

Patients with multiple injuries may not have suitable flap donor sites or carrier limbs available.

Those who cannot co-operate for neurological reasons such as coma or mental defect are also unsuitable, whilst any patient may decide, after the implications of the proposed treatment have been explained fully, against a programme of reconstruction, and may even prefer amputation.

[*The illustrations for this Chapter on Skin Flaps were drawn by M. G. Lyth.*]

Exposure of Major Blood Vessels

H. H. G. Eastcott, M.S., F.R.C.S.
Senior Surgeon, St. Mary's Hospital, London

and

A. E. Thompson, M.S., F.R.C.S.
Consultant Surgeon, St. Thomas's Hospital, London

PRE-OPERATIVE

Indications

The exposure of blood vessels is indicated under emergency circumstances for local injury and control of bleeding, or for the relief of occlusion. It is also required for very rapid blood transfusion, for the intra-arterial injection of radio-opaque contrast media, extracorporeal circulation and regional perfusion.

The major vessels are most often exposed for the elective surgical treatment of aneurysms, arterio-venous fistulae and arteriosclerotic obstruction.

Contra-indications

No major blood vessel should be exposed if the surgeon's purpose can be adequately achieved in any other way, such as by pressure in local injury for control of bleeding, or percutaneous injection for radiology. An overlying layer of infected or densely adherent tissue should not be disturbed; an alternative normal adjacent site should be chosen for the approach.

Special pre-operative treatment

Some patients will have been receiving anticoagulant drugs. It is wise to counteract these by giving the appropriate antidote: for heparin, the appropriate amount of 10 per cent protamine sulphate (2 mg protamine for 1 mg heparin); and for the pro-thrombin depressor group, such as warfarin, 20 mg of vitamin K_1.

Compatible blood transfusion should be available in adequate quantity to replace blood losses.

Anaesthesia

General anaesthesia is preferable for most patients, although local infiltration with 1 per cent Xylocaine is very suitable for limb embolectomy in patients with severe heart disease. Hypotension should be avoided in the presence of coronary or cerebrovascular disease.

Heparin

Total heparinization may be used if protracted clamping is anticipated (1·5 mg/kg body weight). Alternatively, heparin—saline solution (1:200,000) may be instilled into the arterial tree distal to the site of operation. A vasodilator (e.g. thymoxamine 30 mg) may be added to this solution to reduce vasospasm.

Exposure

'The use of wide approach for dealing thoroughly with nerves and vessels needs no defence' (Henry, 1946). When reconstructive surgery is necessary flexures may be crossed, muscles and tendons divided and the abdomen opened to its fullest extent.

THE OPERATIONS

EXPOSURE OF ASCENDING AORTA

1

The incision

This is in the mid-line extending from the suprasternal notch to just beyond the xiphisternum. The extent is dictated by the need for extracorporeal circulation. A transverse component at the upper end improves the cosmetic result.

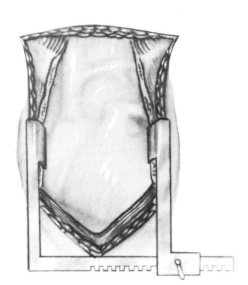

2

Entering the mediastinum

The sternum is divided with a counter-rotating power-driven saw or a Gigli saw. The line of division deviates slightly to the left in its lower half to avoid entering the right pleural cavity.

3

Deep dissection

The thymic remnant is divided and the innominate vein identified. Final access to the ascending aorta is obtained by opening the pericardium longitudinally.

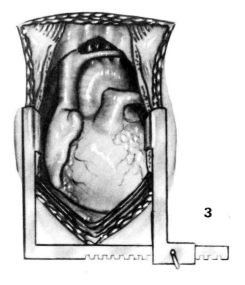

**EXPOSURE OF INNOMINATE ARTERY AND
THORACIC PART OF RIGHT SUBCLAVIAN ARTERY**

4

The incision

The shoulder girdle is displaced backwards by placing a sandbag between the patient's shoulders. The incision is centred over the right sternoclavicular joint, exposing the medial third of the clavicle, the manubrium and the first two intercostal spaces.

5

Splitting the manubrium

The manubrium is divided in the mid-line with Sauerbruch's shears or a Gigli saw. The two halves are separated with a Tuffier's retractor. Further exposure can then be obtained by transecting the sternum below the manubrium or dividing the clavicle and anterior ends of the first and second ribs.

6

Deep dissection

The thymic remnant and anterior mediastinal fat are cleared to expose the innominate vein. The anterior borders of the pleural cavities are swept away laterally.

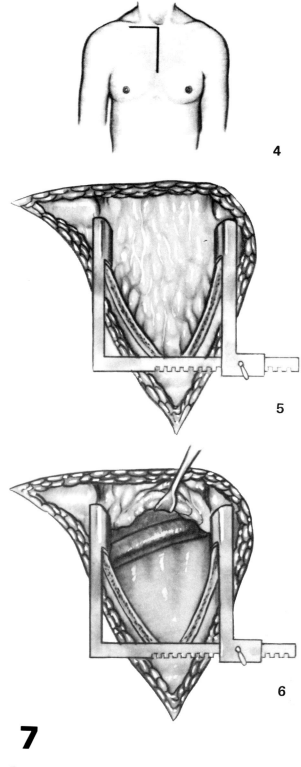

4

5

6

7

Exposure of great vessels

Mobilization of the innominate vein permits it to be retracted upwards, revealing the origins of the great vessels.

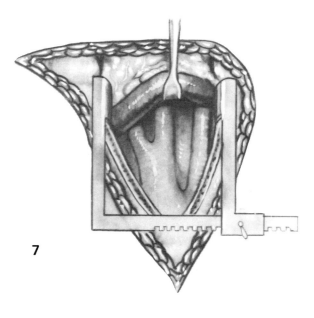

7

EXPOSURE OF THORACIC PART OF LEFT SUBCLAVIAN ARTERY

This can be exposed by modifying the approach for the innominate and right subclavian arteries (above), or by lateral approach through the fourth left intercostal space.

8

The incision

With the patient in the right lateral position a curved incision skirts the angle of the left scapula.

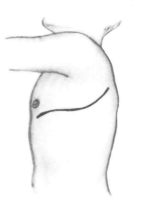

8

9

9

Deep dissection

The trapezius and serratus anterior muscles are divided and the chest is entered through an incision along the upper border of the fifth rib. Adequate exposure requires division of the fifth rib (and fourth if necessary) at the posterior end.

10

Intrathoracic exposure

The intrathoracic segment of the left subclavian artery can be exposed by incision of the overlying mediastinal pleura. The vagus nerve, the left superior intercostal vein and the thoracic duct lie close to the vessel.

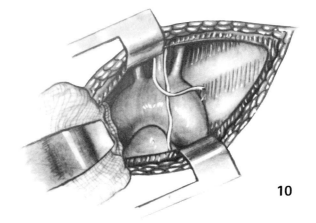

10

EXPOSURE OF CERVICAL PART OF SUBCLAVIAN ARTERY AND ORIGIN OF VERTEBRAL ARTERY

11

The incision

The patient's neck is extended and turned to the opposite side. A skin crease incision is made one finger's breadth above the middle third of the clavicle. The platysma and the clavicular head of the sternomastoid are divided.

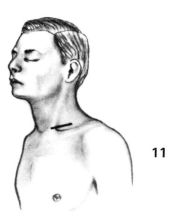

11

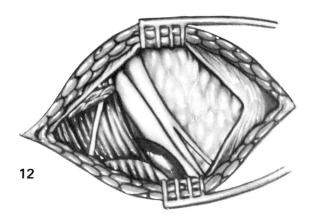

12

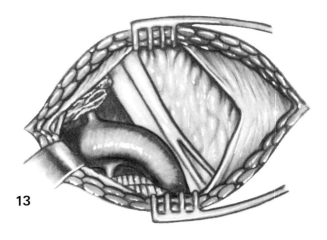

13

12 & 13

Deep dissection

The omohyoid fascia is incised and the scalenus anterior muscle exposed with the phrenic nerve on its surface. The internal jugular vein and the termination of the thoracic duct (on the left side) lie in the medial end of the field. The phrenic nerve is delicately mobilized and retracted medially, before the scalenus anterior muscle is divided piecemeal to avoid damage to the underlying vessel and its branches. The artery is finally exposed by incision of its sheath. The lower trunks of the brachial plexus lie above and lateral to the vessel.

More extensive exposure of the distal part of the vessel and the axillary artery is obtained by subperiosteal excision of the appropriate part of the clavicle.

ANOTHER EXPOSURE OF LOWER PART OF VERTEBRAL ARTERY

14

The incision

The patient's neck is extended and the head turned to the opposite side. An incision, 8 cm in length, is made over the lower third of the sternomastoid in the groove between its sternal and clavicular heads, in line with the muscle fibres. The two heads of the muscle are separated.

15

Deep dissection

The internal jugular vein is retracted medially. The triangular space between the scalenus anterior laterally and the longus colli medially is cleared to expose the artery. Division of the scalenus anterior may be required; if so, the phrenic nerve has to be preserved. Branches of the thyrocervical trunk are divided. The thoracic duct is avoided on the left side.

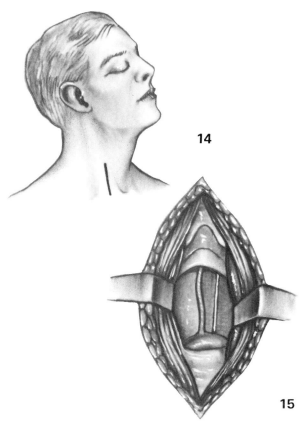

14

15

EXPOSURE OF VERTEBRAL ARTERY IN ITS CANAL

16

The incision

An incision, 8 cm in length, is made along the anterior border of the sternomastoid muscle, similar to that made for the common carotid artery.

17

Deep dissection

The sternomastoid muscle is retracted laterally and the carotid sheath medially. The scalenus anterior muscle is detached from its origin from the transverse processes of the cervical vertebra. The vessel is exposed by removal of the anterior margins of the foramina in the transverse processes. Branches of the thyrocervical trunk are ligated and the sympathetic and vagus nerves preserved.

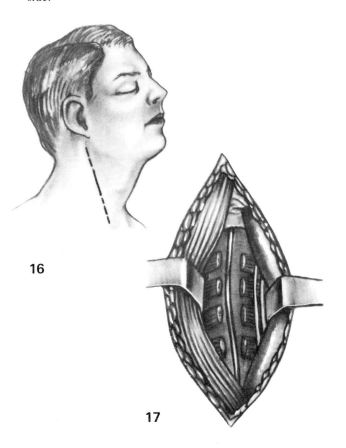

16

17

**EXPOSURE OF AXILLARY ARTERY
(FIRST PART)**

18

The incision

With the arm abducted to a right angle, the incision is made just below the clavicle and parallel to it.

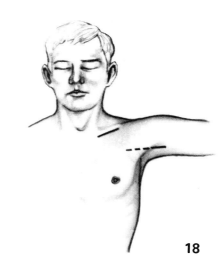

18

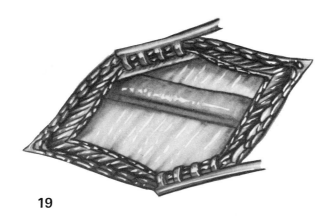

19

19

Dissection

The pectoral fascia is divided along the line of the muscle fibres of the clavicular head of the pectoralis major, which are then split to expose the vascular sheath. The pectoral branch of the acromiothoracic axis may require division.

20

Division of sheath

The pulsations of the artery are palpated and the vascular sheath is divided along the line thus indicated. Here the only other important structure is the axillary vein which lies below and medial to the artery from which it is then carefully separated. This is the site for axillofemoral bypass.

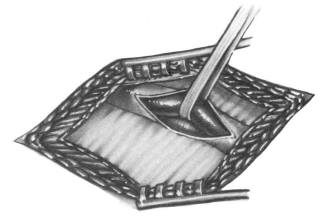

20

EXPOSURE OF AXILLARY ARTERY
(SECOND AND THIRD PARTS)

21

The incision

With the arm abducted to a right angle the incision is
made along the line of the pulsating artery up to the
lower border of the pectoralis major muscle. If the
artery is pulseless the groove between the coraco-
brachialis and triceps is the guide.

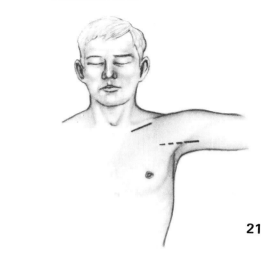

21

22

Dissection

The pectorals are retracted upwards and medially to
expose the distal two thirds of the axillary artery. If
necessary both muscles are divided and a portion of
the clavicle resected to gain exposure of the whole
subclavian–axillary axis. Sections of bone should not
be replaced (Elkin, 1946; DeBakey, 1955).

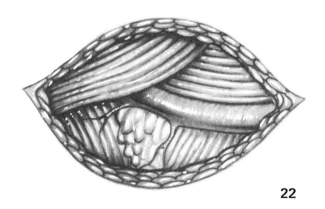

22

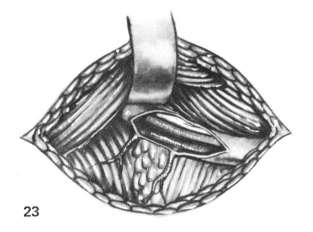

23

23

Exposure of artery

The axillary sheath is opened to reveal the vein
medially and the brachial plexus laterally. Between
these two structures the artery will be found. It can
also be identified by following the subscapular
artery to its origin.

EXPOSURE OF BRACHIAL ARTERY IN THE ARM

24

The incision

The incision is made along the line of the pulsating artery or in the line of the sulcus separating the biceps muscle from the triceps muscle. The length of the incision is governed by the procedure to be performed. A sandbag placed to support the elbow in extension facilitates exposure.

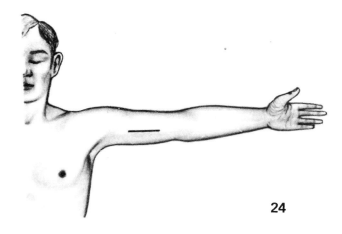

24

25

Dissection

The neurovascular sheath is opened. The veins, and the median nerve which crosses the artery from the lateral to the medial side, are separated from the artery. Care must be taken to recognize a high bifurcation of the vessel. The ulnar collateral artery and medial cutaneous nerve of the forearm lie close to the brachial artery and must not be included in clamps. The dissection is further complicated by the basilic vein which perforates the deep fascia and joins the brachial vein in this region.

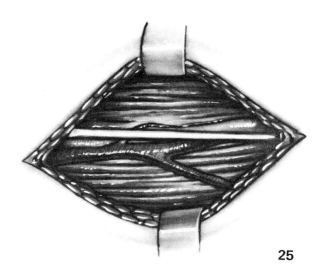

25

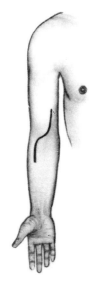

26

EXPOSURE OF BRACHIAL ARTERY AT THE ELBOW

26

The incision

A skin crease incision is made at the elbow with longitudinal extensions along the line of the brachial artery medially, and down the brachioradialis laterally. The skin should be marked to allow an accurate closure.

27

Superficial dissection

The artery is obscured by the cubital veins, the deep fascia and the bicipital aponeurosis. The two cutaneous nerves to the forearm lie deep to the veins at the medial and lateral ends of this plane of the incision and should be avoided.

28

Deep dissection

The overlying superficial veins and the bicipital aponeurosis are divided; this exposes the artery, with its accompanying deep veins, just above the bifurcation which is close to the medial side of the biceps tendon. Opening the sheath allows the vessel to be lifted away from its venae comites and the median nerve which lies on its medial side. This exposure is most commonly indicated when the brachial artery has been damaged in a supracondylar fracture. Spasm in the intact vessel can be overcome by the injection of saline into the lumen of the affected segment between arterial clamps (Mustard and Bull, 1962).

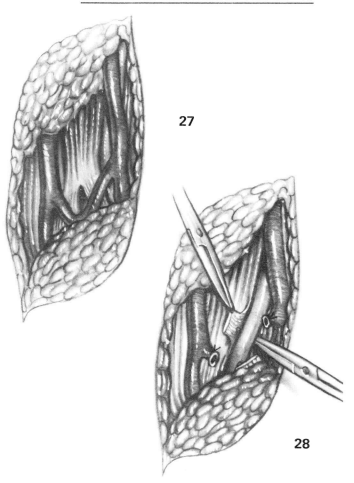

27

28

EXPOSURE OF THE RADIAL ARTERY AT THE WRIST

29

The incision

A longitudinal or transverse incision centred 3–4 cm above the radial styloid is used.

30

Dissection

The origin of the cephalic vein is found in the superficial tissues and the artery beneath the deep fascia on the ulnar side of the brachioradialis tendon. The vessels can be mobilized to allow side-to-side approximation for the construction of a fistula for dialysis.

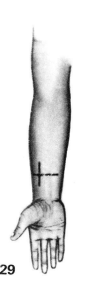

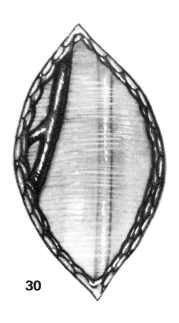

29   30

EXPOSURE OF COMMON CAROTID ARTERY

31

The incision

With the neck slightly extended, and the head turned to the opposite side, a 6 cm incision is made along the anterior edge of the sternomastoid with its centre three fingers' breadth above the clavicle.

For a wider exposure of the common carotid artery and internal jugular vein the incision is extended along the dotted lines, dividing the origin of the sternomastoid.

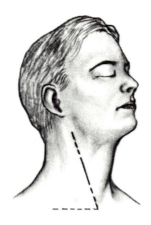

31

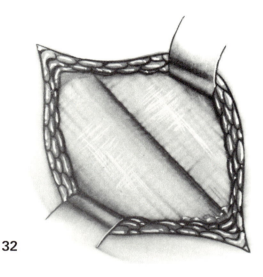

32

32

Dissection

The deep fascia is opened in the same line and the sternomastoid and infrahyoid muscles are separated from the underlying vascular sheath. This plane of dissection is bloodless except for a sternomastoid branch of the superior thyroid artery.

33

Exposure

The sheath is opened above the omohyoid. The jugular vein is dissected free and retracted laterally to isolate the artery. The vagus lies well back between the vessels, and the sympathetic trunk farther still and more medially. Lower in the neck the inferior thyroid artery crosses behind the carotid artery.

Note: Ligation produces hemiplegia in some subjects owing to defective anastomosis of the cerebral vessels through the circle of Willis. The operation should be performed under local anaesthesia and a temporary ligature applied for 5—15 min, or longer if there is any doubt.

In elderly women the common carotid artery is often dilated and tortuous, resembling an aneurysm.

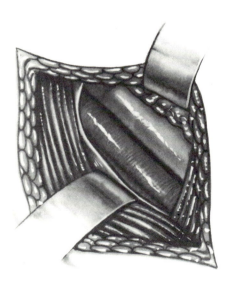

33

EXPOSURE OF INTERNAL AND EXTERNAL CAROTID ARTERIES

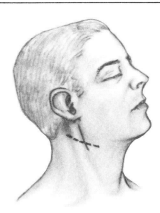

34

The incision

An incision is made along the anterior border of the sternomastoid from just above the angle of the jaw, passing downwards for 7—9 cm. For simple ligation a shorter skin crease incision may be preferred.

34

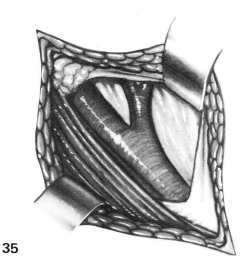

35

35

Dissection

The platysma is divided and the sternomastoid defined and retracted posteriorly. The common facial vein is divided at the upper end of the incision and the vascular sheath opened.

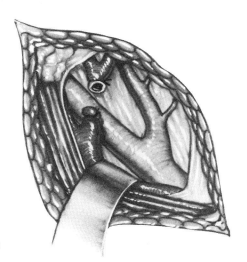

36

36

Exposure

The common carotid bifurcation usually lies much higher in the neck than is supposed. The two arteries lie close together beneath the angle of the jaw. Branches identify the external carotid, which is anterior and deeper. The hypoglossal nerve must be avoided as it crosses the vessels, and the vagus, superior laryngeal and sympathetic nerves which lie behind the bifurcation. The upper part of the internal carotid artery is difficult to expose; it runs deeply and is covered for the most part by the ascending ramus of the mandible. The sternomastoid can be detached from the mastoid process, which may itself be partly removed. The digastric muscle, the occipital artery and the styloid process are divided. This exposes the superficial aspect of the artery to some extent.
Note: The internal carotid artery may be tied for intracranial aneurysm. Hemiplegia often follows. The external carotid is ligated preliminary to radical pharyngolaryngeal or faciomaxillary operations.

EXPOSURE OF AORTIC ARCH

37

The incision

With the patient in the right lateral position the chest is opened through a long curved incision skirting the angle of the left scapula. The lateral chest wall muscles are divided in the same line.

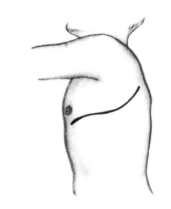

37

38

Dissection

The thorax is entered through the fourth intercostal space. Adequate exposure is obtained by division of the fifth rib (and fourth if required) posteriorly, or by division of the sternum anteriorly.

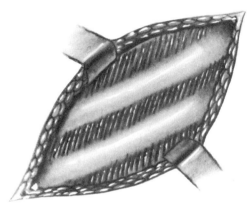

38

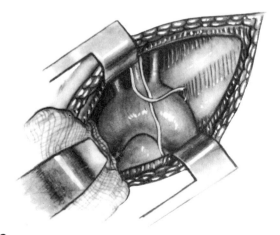

39

Exposure

The lung is retracted downwards and the arch of the aorta is seen beneath the mediastinal pleura. It is crossed on its left side by the phrenic nerve, the vagus nerve and the left superior intercostal vein. The left main bronchus and left pulmonary artery lie beneath the arch and the oesophagus and thoracic duct on the deep aspect.

39

EXPOSURE OF DESCENDING THORACIC AORTA

40

The incision

The site of the incision and the position of the patient depend upon the level of the lesion. A posterolateral incision is made over the appropriate rib space, with the patient rotated slightly backwards from the right lateral position. The chest wall muscles are incised in the same line.

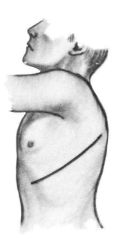

40

41

Dissection

The thorax is entered through the appropriate rib space. The incision can be extended across the costal margin into the abdomen and the diaphragm divided peripherally if necessary. The lung is emptied and retracted forwards to reveal the descending aorta beneath the mediastinal pleura. The oesophagus must be carefully avoided in mobilizing the aorta.
Note: The main blood supply to the spinal cord comes from the branches of the thoracic and upper abdominal aorta.

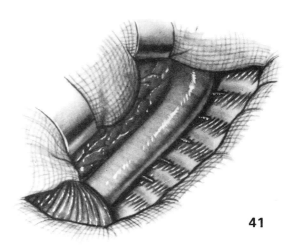

41

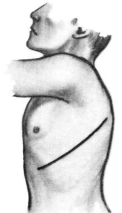

42

EXPOSURE OF AORTA ABOVE RENAL VESSELS

42

The incision

A thoraco-abdominal incision is made along the line of the eighth rib and continued into the abdomen, with the patient inclined backwards from the right lateral position. If temporary control of the upper abdominal aorta is all that is required during an operation on the distal vessel, a very long paramedian incision will suffice.

43

Deep dissection

The latissimus dorsi is divided. The chest is opened along the upper border of the eighth rib and the costal cartilage divided. The diaphragm is divided peripherally until the incision sweeps up to the aorta. The stomach, spleen and pancreas are swept forwards from the posterior abdominal wall to expose the aorta, the left kidney and the suprarenal gland. The visceral branches can be identified and controlled. Care must be taken in dividing intercostal vessels from which the spinal cord derives its blood supply. Temporary occlusion and hypothermia minimize the risk.

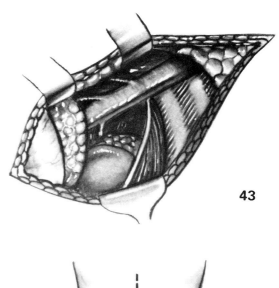

43

EXPOSURE OF RENAL ARTERIES

44

The incision

Either a mid-line upper abdominal (Morris *et al.*, 1962) or a transverse incision 1 inch (2·5 cm) above the umbilicus (Owen, 1964) gives adequate exposure.

44

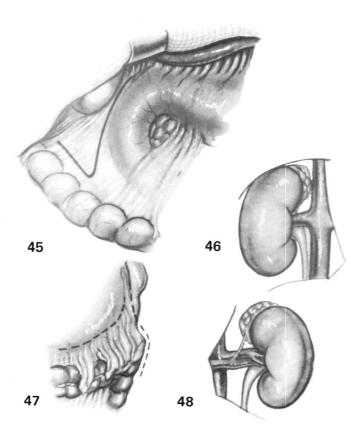

45

46

47

48

45 – 48

Deep dissection

On the right side, the peritoneum around the hepatic flexure of the colon is incised and the colon displaced downwards. The peritoneum on the right side of the duodenum is incised up to the free border of the lesser omentum. The duodenum can be displaced forwards and to the left, exposing the renal vessels, the vena cava and the aorta.

The left renal vessels are exposed by dividing the peritoneum lateral to the splenic flexure, continuing upwards behind the spleen. The spleen and colon can be displaced forwards and to the right to expose the left kidney and its vessels. The arteries lie behind the larger, more superficial, renal veins.

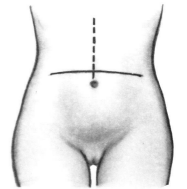

EXPOSURE OF SUPERIOR MESENTERIC ARTERY

49

The incision

A high left paramedian incision is made and the peritoneal cavity opened.

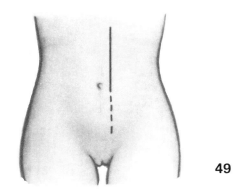

49

50

Deep dissection

The omentum and transverse colon are elevated and the posterior peritoneum incised. The superior mesenteric artery is seen where it emerges below the pancreas. The superior mesenteric vein lies on its right side. The origin of the vessel is exposed by upward dissection and retraction of the pancreas.

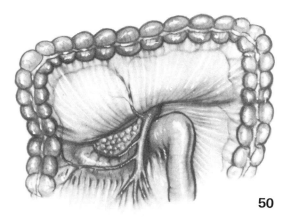

50

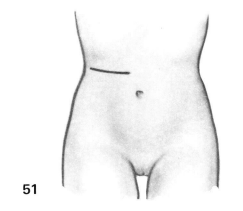

51

EXPOSURE OF THE INFRARENAL INFERIOR VENA CAVA

51

The incision

A transverse incision is made in the upper part of the right lumbar region.

52

Deep dissection

The oblique abdominal muscles and transversus are divided in line with the skin incision. The extraperitoneal space is entered and the peritoneum pushed to the left, to expose the inferior vena cava.

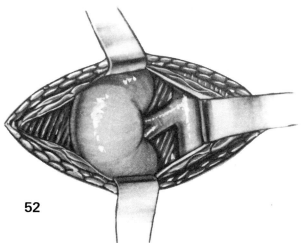

52

EXPOSURE OF ABDOMINAL AORTA BELOW RENAL VESSELS (TRANSPERITONEAL)

53

The incision

A long left paramedian or a median para-umbilical incision runs from the xiphisternum to just above the symphysis pubis. This will provide good access for most abdominal aortic grafts. Complete muscle relaxation is essential. The operator stands on the patient's left.

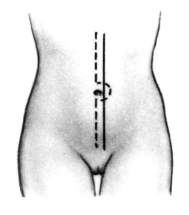

53

54

Dissection

Often it is sufficient to turn the small bowel across to the right side of the abdomen and to hold it there under a large abdominal pack with deep retraction. In very obese subjects, or where the aortic lesion is juxtarenal, it is better to mobilize the whole mid-gut loop by dividing the peritoneal reflection lateral to the right colon and round across the base of the small bowel mesentery. The intestines are then drawn up out of the abdomen and a plastic bag is placed over them.

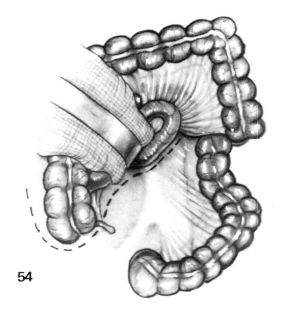

54

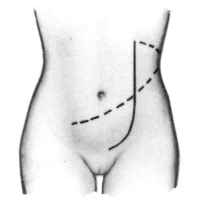

55

EXPOSURE OF ABDOMINAL AORTA BELOW RENAL VESSELS (EXTRAPERITONEAL)

55

The incision

A long J-shaped incision runs along the left linea semilunaris, and lateral to its upper half (Helsby and Moossa, 1975). The patient's left side is lifted up on a sandbag. Alternatively a more oblique incision as recommended by Rob (1963) may be preferred, running from the tip of the left twelfth rib downwards and across the lower abdomen.

56

Dissection

The oblique and transversus muscles are divided in the same line over most of the central part of the incision. They are kept intact with their nerve supply at its two ends. The peritoneal sac is then wiped off the muscles. The aortic bifurcation and iliacs are exposed. Difficulty is most likely with the lower right iliac and the upper aorta. The inferior mesenteric artery retracts with the peritoneum across the aorta to the right.

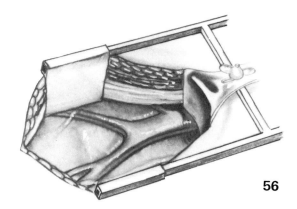

56

EXPOSURE OF THE ABDOMINAL AORTA BELOW RENAL VESSELS (BOTH ROUTES)

57

Exposure of the aorta

Whichever route has been used the deep dissection after displacing the abdominal contents consists in reflecting the duodenum over to the right. Intraperitoneally the aorta can now be isolated as far as the renal vein above. The inferior mesenteric vessels are retracted to the left, as in this diagram. With the extraperitoneal exposure the inferior mesenteric vessels are retracted up with the peritoneum across to the right as shown in *Illustration 56*. A Goligher retractor with deep blades is valuable for both routes.

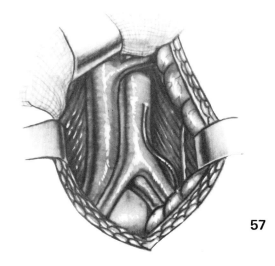

57

EXPOSURE OF THE COMMON ILIAC ARTERY (INTRAPERITONEAL)

58

The incision

A long lower left paramedian incision is required for adequate control of this vessel.

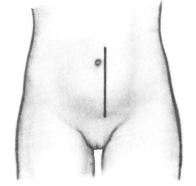

58

59

Dissection

If the need is for a good view of the lower end and bifurcation the left colon is mobilized and retracted across to the right. Similarly on the right side the caecum is lifted up and over to the left. The ureter is seen crossing the bifurcation and can be identified by its peristalsis. The internal iliac disappears on the deep surface of the bifurcation and is closely related to the pelvic veins.

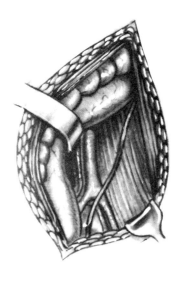

59

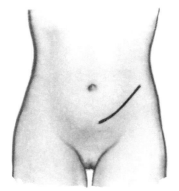

60

EXPOSURE OF THE COMMON ILIAC ARTERY (EXTRAPERITONEAL)

60

The incision

An oblique incision crosses the spino-umbilical line in its upper third.

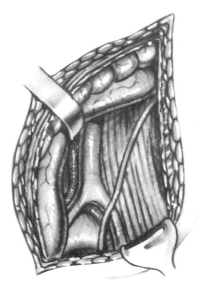

61

61

Dissection

The oblique and transversus muscles are divided in the same line. The peritoneum is carefully separated from beneath the transversus aponeurosis and the plane developed so as to displace the peritoneal sac medially. A good view is obtained of the lower part of the artery.

EXTRAPERITONEAL EXPOSURE OF EXTERNAL ILIAC ARTERY

62

The incision

The classical muscle-cutting in the iliac fossa remains the best. The deep epigastric artery at its inner end should be preserved.

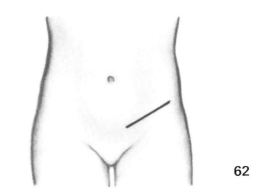

62

63

Deep dissection

The posterior parietal peritoneum is pushed up under the medial edge of the incision. The external iliac vessels are found lying on the pelvic brim on the medial side of the psoas muscle. The obturator nerve lies under the vein in its upper part and the genito-femoral nerve on the muscle lateral to the artery. The ureter is seen crossing its origin. This incision is suitable for renal transplantation.

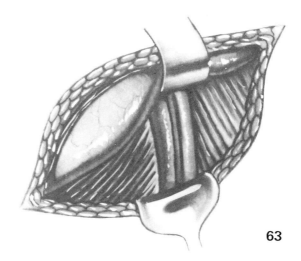

63

EXPOSURE OF COMMON FEMORAL ARTERY

64

The incision

A longitudinal incision allows adequate exposure of the common femoral artery, particularly of its deep branch, and can be extended if necessary.

64

65

Superficial dissection

The termination of the long saphenous vein is exposed and retracted medially, dividing such tributaries as required. The main vein should be preserved for grafting purposes. The superficial external pudendal artery is ligated.

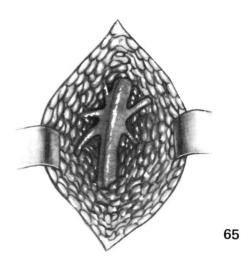

65

66

Deep dissection

The femoral sheath is opened to expose the common femoral vessels. The femoral nerve lies on the lateral side. The profunda femoris artery must be located with care. It arises from the posterior and lateral aspect of the common femoral artery. Its origin is closely related to the termination of the profunda femoris vein. A multiple origin or early branching of the vessel may cause difficulty.

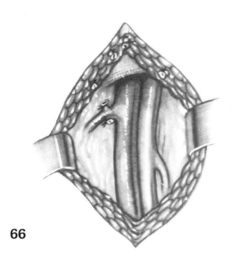

66

67

Iliofemoral junction

This can be exposed by an upward extension of the above dissection, dividing the inguinal ligament. The deep epigastric vessels are preserved. If this manoeuvre is anticipated, the S-shaped incision shown in *Illustration 64* is preferred.

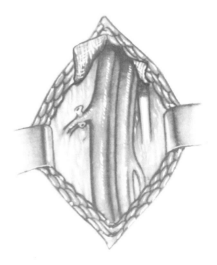

67

EXPOSURE OF SUPERFICIAL FEMORAL ARTERY IN HUNTER'S CANAL

68

The incision

This is made along the line of the anterior border of the sartorius muscle. The limb is slightly flexed and abducted, with a sandbag beneath the knee.

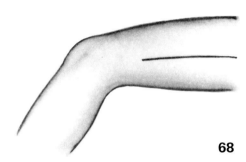

68

69

Superficial dissection

The saphenous vein is carefully preserved in the posterior flap. The fascia over the sartorius muscle is incised.

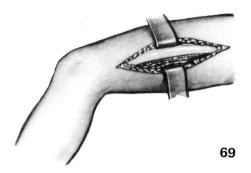

69

70

70

Deep dissection

The sartorius muscle is retracted backwards. The fascial roof of Hunter's canal is exposed and incised. The saphenous nerve is separated from the artery which is then dissected from the underlying vein. Care is taken to preserve as many collateral vessels as possible.

EXPOSURE OF THE POPLITEAL ARTERY

The medial approach is used for most bypass operations, but the posterior approach is better for direct procedures such as the repair of arterial cysts or entrapment.

Medial approach (upper)

71

The incision

The patient is placed supine with the knee flexed over a sandbag. The line of the incision should run from four fingers' breadth above the adductor opening downwards and backwards to a little behind the medial femoral condyle, avoiding the long saphenous vein.

72

Dissection

The deep fascia is incised and the anterior border of the sartorius is defined. The muscle is displaced backwards to reveal the thicker aponeurosis of the adductor canal, running into the tendon of the adductor opening. The saphenous nerve leads the dissection to the artery; the fascia is incised to free it and the artery which can then be followed downwards into the popliteal fat.

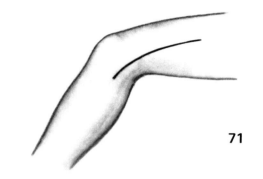

71

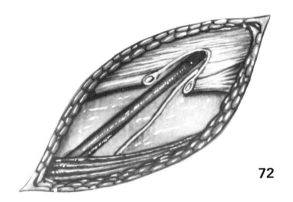

72

Medial approach (lower)

73

The incision

This is along the posterior tibial border from the lower aspect of the medial condyle, avoiding the long saphenous vein.

74

Dissection

The deep fascia, here very thick, is incised and the medial head of the gastrocnemius is displaced backwards. The loose popliteal fat is stroked free from the vascular bundle to reveal the vein, with the artery beneath it. Care should be taken not to damage the medial popliteal nerve. The bifurcation is obscured by the soleus arch and muscular veins but by division of these the posterior tibial artery can be exposed.

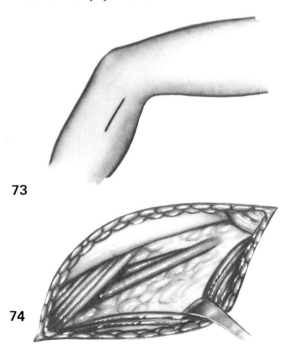

73

74

Posterior approach

75

The incision

Recurrent ulceration and contraction often complicate the vertical incision which crosses the flexure at right angles. An S-shaped incision, with its upper limit medial, avoids this. The middle portion should run in the skin crease. A vertical incision is satisfactory, however, for exposing the lower portion of the popliteal vessels. Placed between the two heads of the gastrocnemius, it commences below the flexure, and can be extended downwards to expose as much of the upper course of the posterior tibial vessels as may be necessary.

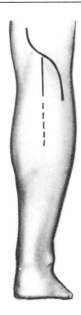

75

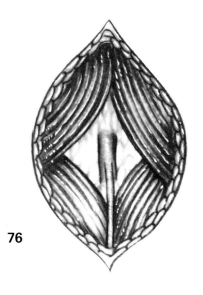

76

76

Superficial dissection

The short saphenous vein is followed through the popliteal fascia and the posterior cutaneous nerve dissected aside. The fascia, whose fibres run transversely, is split longitudinally to reveal the popliteal fat.

77

Deep dissection

The fat is cleared from the two popliteal nerves. The popliteal vein is next found, usually via one of its deep tributaries, or perhaps the short saphenous vein. The artery lies deeper still. It is crossed by a very constant leash of vessels, mainly some large veins from the medial head of the gastrocnemius; they must be divided. The short saphenous vein is preserved if possible.

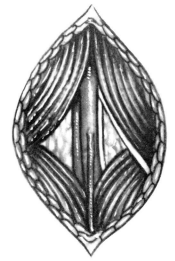

77

Extension of exposure

Upward

To reach the femoral vessels, the semimembranosus belly and tendon of semitendinosus are retracted, or divided, along the line of the artery. The tight hiatus in the adductor magnus is also cut through.

Downward

The posterior tibial artery is readily exposed by splitting the gastrocnemius and soleus fibres in its line, also the fascia which covers the vessels as they lie on the long deep flexors.

Note: These extensions of the posterior approach are limited and can be difficult. If long exposure is required the medial approach should be chosen.

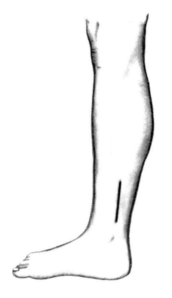

78

THE ARTERIOVENOUS SHUNT

78

The incision

To construct a shunt for access in haemodialysis the incision is centred 4–6 cm above the medial malleolous, 0·5 cm behind the posterior border of the tibia.

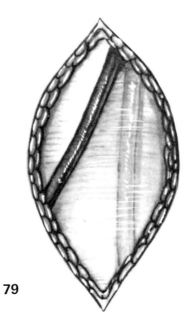

79

79

Dissection

The origin of the long saphenous vein lies in the superficial tissue in the anterior flap and the posterior tibial artery beneath the deep fascia directly under the incision. Limited mobilization of the vessels permits insertion of the silastic cannulae.

POSTOPERATIVE CARE

This depends upon the regular, detailed and careful observation of local and general signs. There must be continuity of responsibility to ensure accurate interpretation of the local and general circulation.

In the surgery of atherosclerosis it must be remembered that the disease is generalized. Hypovolaemia and hypotension must be stringently avoided. In all cases of major arterial surgery, postoperative monitoring of central venous pressure and a continuous electrocardiogram are recommended, in addition to the usual observations on pulse, blood pressure and respirations. Oxygen administration by mask or catheter maintains maximal saturation. The urine output is best collected by catheter drainage over the first 24—48 hr.

Posture

The cerebral and coronary circulations take precedence over the peripheral circulation. If postoperative shock is present or the patient has not regained consciousness, head-down tilt is required. When the central circulation is adequate, dependency of an operated extremity promotes the local arterial circulation.

Local signs

Immediately after operation, the state of the distal circulation must be established. In the extremities, the colour of the limb, the skin temperature, filling of the superficial veins and the pulses are all guides to adequate circulation.

Pulses

The distal pulses may not be felt immediately after an operation in which a limb artery is clamped. They return following improvement in the general circulation and progressive local vasodilatation. The latter can be encouraged before the closure of the arteriotomy by the injection of a vasodilator (tolazoline 25 mg, or thymoxamine 10 mg in heparinized saline) into the distal arterial tree (Hall, 1964). Intravenous infusion of low molecular weight dextran promotes capillary circulation in the operated limb.

Skin temperature

After clamping the arterial supply, the distal part of the limb becomes pale and cold. The peripheral veins are collapsed. As recovery progresses the level of transition from warm to cold skin becomes more distal, with improvement in the colour and filling of the peripheral veins.

Sensory impairment

Numbness of the skin is a serious sign, though some skin sensation will often persist in parts of a limb which are on the same level as patches of established necrosis.

Complications

Haemorrhage

The use of heparin during operation, and the presence of arterial suture lines, requires close observation of the operative site. The use of a vacuum drainage system gives early indication of undue blood loss. The effect of heparin can be reversed at the end of the operation if necessary by the injection of protamine sulphate (2 mg protamine neutralizes 1 mg heparin). If excessive haemorrhage occurs, re-exploration of the site of operation is required.

Ischaemic muscle necrosis

The musculature of a limb is more sensitive to ischaemia than most other tissues. Prolonged ischaemia of the leg may cause necrosis of muscle, particularly in the anterior tibial compartment, where the muscles are firmly enclosed by osseous and fascial boundaries. The presence of tenderness over this area and loss of dorsiflexion of the ankle demand early decompression. Delay in diagnosis or deferring active treatment will jeopardize recovery and lead to gangrene, ischaemic muscle contracture and an equinovarus deformity.

Swelling of leg

Mild oedema of the foot and leg frequently follows operations on the femoral and popliteal vessels even in the presence of normal deep veins (Husni, 1967). This disappears with increasing activity and early mobilization should be practised whenever possible.

References

Elkin, D. C. (1946). *J. Am. med. Ass.* **132,** 421
Elkin, D. C. and DeBakey, M. E. (1955). *Vascular Surgery in World War II.* Office of the Surgeon General
Hall, K. V. (1964). *Acta chir. scand.* **128,** 365
Helsby and Moossa (1975). *Br. J. Surg.* **62,** 596
Henry, A. K. (1946). *Extensile Exposure as Applied to Limb Surgery.* Edinburgh: Livingstone
Husni, E. A. (1967). *Circulation* **35,** Suppl. 1, 169
Morris, G. C., DeBakey, M. F., Cooley, D. A. and Crawford, E. S. (1962). *Surgery* **51,** 62
Mustard, W. T. and Bull, C. (1962). *Ann. Surg.* **155,** 339
Owen, K. (1964). *Br. J. Urol.* **36,** 7
Rob, C. (1963). *Surgery* **53,** 87

[*The illustrations for this Chapter on Exposure of Major Blood Vessels were drawn by Mr. G. Lyth.*]

Arterial Suture and Anastomosis

H. H. G. Eastcott, M.S., F.R.C.S.
Senior Surgeon, St. Mary's Hospital, London

and

A. E. Thompson, M.S., F.R.C.S.
Consultant Surgeon, St. Thomas's Hospital, London

PRE - OPERATIVE

Indications

Repair of a divided or injured major artery is usually preferable to tying its ends. This applies particularly in the lower limb. Trauma, surgical accident and the radical surgery of cancer, as well as the elective treatment of arterial lesions, require the surgeon to be familiar with methods of arterial suture. The methods illustrated will meet the requirements of the arterial operations shown in other sections.

Increasing surgical expertise has allowed anastomosis of very small vessels. The technique for this microsurgery is learned by experience and constant practice. Although under emergency circumstances, a surgeon may be required to attempt small vessel surgery, the techniques are believed to be outside the scope of this chapter (O'Brien, 1976).

Contra-indications

Arteries should never be sutured in the presence of infection. Severe compound or crushing injury with loss of the main artery are indications for amputation, not arterial repair. Simpler procedures are similarly necessary in treating battle casualties when tactical considerations demand early evacuation. Some viscera regularly survive arterial ligation (for example, the left colon). Arterial reconstruction under such circumstances is superfluous.

Suture materials

Fine sutures on atraumatic needles are most frequently used for arterial anastomosis. A number of mechanical devices have been developed for the same purpose. These are very useful for the anastomosis of small vessels, making them valuable in experimental surgery. They have not been widely adopted in clinical surgery. Similarly, adhesives (epoxy resins) have been tried but not found satisfactory in normal clinical practice.

Silk has been used extensively in arterial surgery. It can be obtained in varying sizes (2/0–7/0) with appropriate sized and shaped needles, depending upon the type of tissue to be sutured. It is now being replaced by man-made fibres, which are less traumatic to the arterial wall than silk. Both braided and mono-filament sutures in a wide range of sizes are available. These sutures have the advantage that the anastomosis can be tightened more easily by longitudinal tension than with silk. Monofilament fibres are crushed and weakened if grasped by instruments. Extra care is required when tying these materials to avoid loosening of knots and the ends must be cut long. Polypropylene (Prolene) is the most widely used synthetic mono-filament suture for vessels. Though less easy to handle than silk or man-made multifilamentous sutures such as Dacron it passes more easily through the tissues and engenders no reaction in them.

THE OPERATIONS

LATERAL SUTURE

1

This is a simple method of closing a longitudinal incision in the artery wall, as after embolectomy or thrombo-endarterectomy. Some narrowing of the vessel is always produced and the blood pressure tends to open the repair instead of tightening it, unlike the circumferential suture of an anastomosis. Where there is loss of substance of the arterial wall, resection and anastomosis or grafting is preferable.

A simple continuous stitch is used, rather than an everting stitch which would narrow the artery even more. A patch graft will sometimes be required.

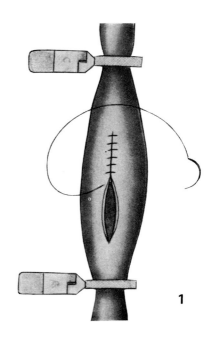

1

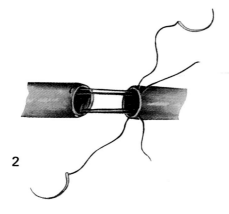

2

END-TO-END ANASTOMOSIS BY MODIFIED CARREL METHOD

2

Stay sutures

The ends of the vessels to be anastomosed are carefully cleared of excess adventitia. Inclusion of adventitia or other extraneous tissue in the suture line may promote thrombus formation. Stay sutures are placed to define the anterior and posterior aspects of the anastomosis. Everting horizontal mattress sutures are used for this purpose.

3

Continuous suture of anterior aspect

A simple continuous suture is placed along the anterior aspect at intervals of 1–2 mm, according to the size of the artery, and a similar distance from the edges which, if the wall is normal, will have already been everted by the stay sutures. These are held apart with sufficient tension to equalize the diameter of the ends of the vessels.

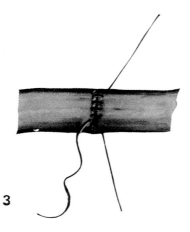

3

4

Rotation of anastomosis

The clamps and stay sutures are then used to rotate the anastomosis so that the posterior half can be seen and sutured in the same way. It is often possible to place the clamps in such a position that the anastomosis can be rotated without releasing them.

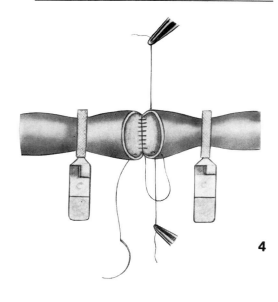

4

5

Single stitch method

If difficulty is anticipated in rotating the ends of the artery—near a large bifurcation, for example—a single continuous stitch is used. One supporting suture is placed nearest the operator and this is continued forwards from within the lumen, then back along the front of the anastomosis until the starting point is reached in an accessible position.

   This method is particularly useful in diseased arteries which will not allow the smooth pull-up of the Blalock suture.

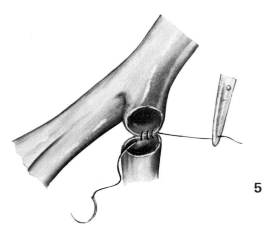

5

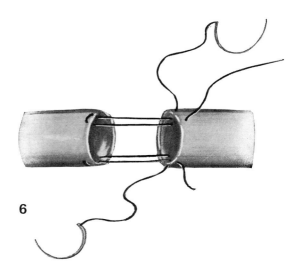

6

EVERTING MATTRESS SUTURE

This method still has some place in arterial surgery. It does evert the edges of the vessel and may therefore be chosen in circumstances where a second continuous suture is intended for haemostasis, for example in a healthy aorta. It is also useful in large arteries for ensuring haemostasis and a firm repair when suturing normal to diseased arteries.

6

Insertion of stay sutures

Two everting mattress sutures are placed as shown with the loop on the adventitia. Traction is exerted on them to equalize the diameter of the two ends.

7

Continuous everting suture

A continuous everting suture is then placed, first anteriorly, then posteriorly by rotating the anastomosis. One stay suture is passed behind the anastomosis and the ends pulled in opposite directions.

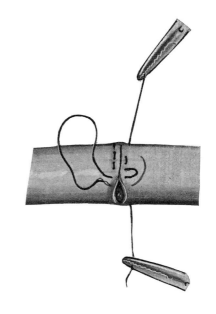

7

8

Use of interrupted sutures

Where growth of the anastomosis must be allowed for, as in coarctation of the aorta in children, interrupted everting mattress sutures may be used.

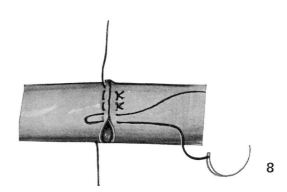

8

BLALOCK SUTURE

This is a valuable method of anastomosing normal or thin-walled arteries or veins when access to the posterior aspect of the anastomosis cannot be obtained by rotation. It is used in coarctation, Blalock's and Pott's operations, portacaval anastomoses, and in the bypass type of arterial graft.

9

Continuous everting suture

A continuous everting suture of polypropylene fibre is placed in the posterior half of the anastomosis with the loops on the adventitia. The ends are not tied.

9

10

Completion of suture

When this suture line is complete the ends are drawn together with steady traction and the edges are everted. It is then completed as a normal continuous everting stitch, maintaining the tension in the stitch throughout. The suture is finally tied to the free end.

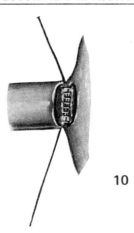

10

SUTURING THE DISEASED ARTERY

Stronger material (2/0) may be used for suturing densely sclerotic or calcified vessels. Care must be taken that the suture is not cut by a sharp plaque. A second, finer suture is recommended to ensure haemostasis.

11

Fixation of plaque

If possible the lower limit of a resected artery or an arteriotomy should be firmly sutured by several longitudinal sutures to the vessel wall, with the ligations on the outer aspect. Unsecured plaques are liable to be dissected free by the subsequent blood flow and to cause thrombosis.

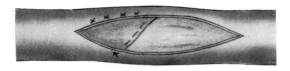
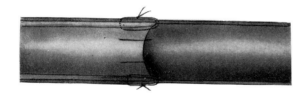

11

12

Including plaques in end-to-end suture

The anastomosis can sometimes be made to include these plaques in the suture line. The needle should be passed through the plaque from within outwards to avoid loosening the plaques.

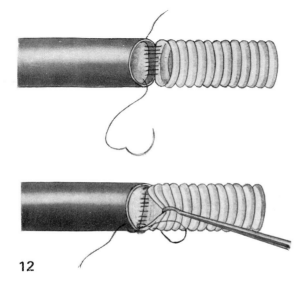

12

13

Including plaques in lateral suture

Often it is necessary to suture a synthetic graft to the side of a diseased artery, e.g. the femoral. It is here particularly important to secure the plaque at its distal end where it may easily become loose. Interrupted silk sutures hold it well.

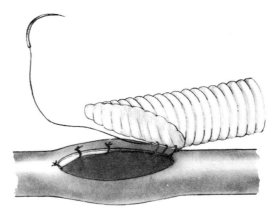

13

14

Completing lateral anastomosis to include plaques

Beginning at the proximal corner of the anastomosis a continuous suture of polypropylene is inserted from within the lumen. This effectively completes the approximation of the plaque to the arterial wall and the graft.

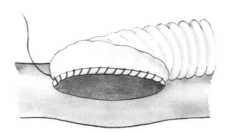

14

INVAGINATION OF GRAFT

A cloth graft or vein graft also may be sutured within the lumen of a diseased vessel using a continuous everting mattress suture. The blood flow then tends to dilate the diseased vessel, reducing the tendency to strip plaques by longitudinal pressure.

RELEASE OF CLAMPS

While the artery is clamped the peripheral vessels are constricted. Early recovery of the circulation can be promoted by instillation of a vasodilator (tolazoline 25 mg or thymoxamine 10 mg, in heparin saline) into the distal vessel before completing the anastomosis. The lower clamp is released first. This allows the air in the vessel to be expelled and the suture to take up the slack gently. It is customary to have some initial bleeding from the suture lines and the needle holes. This stops after applying steady pressure for 5—6 min over 'Surgicel' absorbable gauze. An inclination to add supplementary sutures should be resisted until an adequate period of pressure has been tried, as further stitch holes often increase rather than decrease the haemorrhage.

If haemorrhage is persistent, the possibility of the persistence of circulating heparin must be considered. The common practice is to reverse half the dose of heparin originally used with the appropriate amount of protamine sulphate (2 mg protamine sulphate neutralizes 1 mg heparin). Rarely, a second continuous suture or reinforcement of a suture line with fascia, muscle or a cloth graft may be necessary.

After prolonged arterial procedures with massive blood transfusion, an excess of fibrinolysis in the blood may cause persistent haemorrhage from the operative wounds. If this is confirmed by laboratory investigations, the effect of the increased fibrinolysis can be reversed by intravenous epsilonaminocaproic acid (0·1 g/kg body weight every 4 hr) (Nilsson, Sjoerdsma and Waldenström, 1960).

POSTOPERATIVE CARE

The measures enumerated in the previous chapter are equally applicable under these circumstances. Both the general condition of the patient and the state of the local circulation must be carefully watched.

Local circulation

Improving colour and increasing temperature of the extremity, filling of the superficial veins and peripheral pulses are indicative of satisfactory circulation.

Haemorrhage

The use of vacuum suction to drain the site of an arterial anastomosis gives early warning of excessive blood loss. There is an increased risk of haemorrhage when a grossly atherosclerotic or calcified artery is sutured. Under such circumstances it is imperative to neutralize the heparin used at operation.

Postoperative anticoagulants

It is rarely necessary to use anticoagulants post-operatively, except after embolectomy when it is wise to prevent the re-formation of propagated thrombus. Some bleeding from the suture line in a relatively healthy vessel is preferable to re-thrombosis of the peripheral arterial tree. Heparin (500 mg/24 hr) in a low molecular weight dextran by intravenous infusion is recommended. One litre of the latter is the maximum in 24 hr. Also the subcutaneous injection of 50 mg 12-hourly over the first postoperative week, or longer in poor risk subjects.

References

Carrel, A. (1905). *Ann. Med.* **10**, 284
Jahnke, E. J. and Howard, I. M. (1953). *Archs Surg.* **66**, 646
Nilsson, I. M., Sjoerdsma, A. and Waldenström, J. (1960). *Lancet* **1**, 1322
O'Brien, B. McC. (1976). *Ann. R. Coll. Surg.* **58**, 87, 171

[*The illustrations for this Chapter on Arterial Suture and Anastomosis were drawn by Mr. G. Lyth and Mr. F. Price.*]

Peripheral Nerve Injuries

W. M. McQuillan, F.R.C.S.
Consultant Orthopaedic Surgeon, Royal Infirmary and
Princess Margaret Rose Orthopaedic Hospital, Edinburgh;
Senior Lecturer in Orthopaedic Surgery, University of Edinburgh

PRE - OPERATIVE

General principles

Peripheral nerve injuries may be classified as open or closed or, according to the histological nature of the nerve injury:

(1) Lesions in continuity without distal axonal degeneration—neurapraxia—recovery is rapid.

(2) Lesions in continuity with distal axonal degeneration—axonotmesis—recovery follows the rate of nerve regeneration.

(3) Nerve division—neurotmesis; degeneration distal to the division—no recovery.

The pathology may be mixed.

Closed nerve injuries

Approximately 90 per cent of cases are lesions in continuity—neurapraxia or axonotmesis. The remaining 10 per cent are nerve divisions—neurotmesis.

Closed injuries are usually the result of fractures and dislocations and attention is directed towards the care of the skeletal injury. A conservative policy is followed in the expectation of spontaneous recovery of the nerve.

The limb has to be protected against secondary changes developing in joints and in unparalysed muscles. Anaesthesia of skin increases the risk of pressure sores. Management during the period of paralysis is therefore directed to maintaining a full range of active movement when possible and passive movement of those where paralysis is present. Splints may be applied temporarily. The patient is instructed to put his joints through a full range of passive movement.

Lesions in continuity can be expected to recover at a rate which is dependent upon the pathology. Non-degenerative lesions will recover within a few weeks while the degenerative lesions will move slowly. If recovery does not occur within a predictable period one must differentiate between the degenerative lesion in continuity and the degenerative lesion with disruption of the nerve. A period should be allowed to elapse for axonal growth at the rate of 1 mm per day to re-innervate the first motor branch distal to the site of injury. If this does not occur, an exploration is performed to find if the nerve has been divided, in which case repair will be necessary.

As a general rule, immediate or early exploration of peripheral nerve injuries associated with closed fractures or dislocation is not indicated. There are occasions, however, when early exploration is indicated, for instance when it appears probable that the nerve is being subjected to persistent compression. This may be shown by pain or severe paraesthesia in the nerve's distribution.

Open nerve injuries

In man, functional regeneration will not occur if there is a gap in excess of 1—2 mm. Following nerve division, the nerve ends invariably retract and it follows that the nerve ends must be approximated if there is to be any possibility of recovery. It is important to distinguish between two different processes, both of which are important to the functional result:

(*1*) Repair, which is a connective tissue phenomenon similar to repair of connective tissue generally.

(*2*) Nerve regeneration, a complex process which can occur only if proximal axons are in close proximity to the distal nerve sheaths.

The decision to perform primary or secondary nerve suture is based upon important prognostic factors. The prognosis of recovery after nerve division is influenced by:

(*1*) The age of the patient—the younger the patient the better the prognosis.

(*2*) The level of nerve division—the higher the level of nerve division the poorer the prognosis; the more distal, the better the prognosis.

(*3*) The nature of the nerve divided—a pure sensory nerve or a pure motor nerve has a better prognosis than a mixed nerve.

(*4*) The severity of the injury—both in regard to the extent of nerve damage and disturbance of its blood supply.

Primary nerve repair may be carried out under the following circumstances:

(*1*) Simple wounds, i.e. incised wounds rather than wounds showing considerable contusion and contamination.

(*2*) Distal nerve lesions.

Secondary nerve repair is usually indicated when the circumstances are adverse, namely:

(*1*) When delay has occurred before wound treatment begins.

(*2*) In complicated injuries, or when there is considerable soft tissue damage.

(*3*) In contaminated wounds.

(*4*) In proximal nerve injuries.

THE OPERATIONS

PRIMARY NERVE REPAIR

1

Wound excision

Under general anaesthesia and tourniquet the wound is thoroughly cleansed. A damaged skin margin is excised; deep fascia is dealt with in similar fashion.

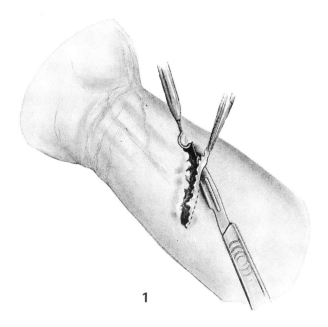

1

2

Exposure

Divided tendons and nerves may retract considerably and enlargement of the wound is necessary. S-shaped extensions are used because of the better exposure so afforded and to avoid secondary skin contractures. Extensions of the wound in T fashion should be avoided. The tourniquet is released at this stage. If multiple wounds are present care must be taken not to reduce viability of the intervening skin and to ensure that any extension of the wound does not reduce the viability of flaps. Venous drainage is as important as arterial supply. Thin bridges of skin between wounds are always of doubtful viability and careful judgement is required to know when skin bridges may be left and when excision is better. Obviously damaged muscle and tendon are excised.

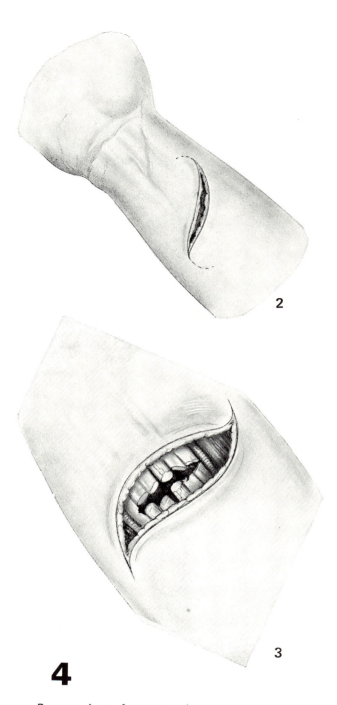

2

3

3

Identification

Divided tendons are easily identified if distal attachments are confirmed by gentle traction.

Nerve division is confirmed by identification of both ends. Considerable variation occurs in the size of peripheral nerves at different sites and also in the level of origin of branches. Care should be taken to look for undamaged branches arising from the proximal end of the nerve and also to preserve smaller branches distally. It is important to preserve any intact nerve supply. The tendons are sutured (see Chapter on 'Tendon Injuries in the Hand', pages 529–547). Having said this, it is still advisable to warn that errors of identification can and do occur.

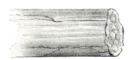
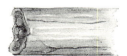
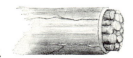
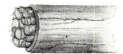

4

4

Preparation of nerve ends

The nerves are picked up gently by their connective tissue sheath (epineurium), using fine non-toothed forceps. Blood clot and damaged tissue are resected cleanly until healthy nerve is reached. Since the injured nerve is very delicate, multiple small cuts are best avoided and one clean transverse section to expose healthy bundles is all that is required. It is helpful, for the act of cutting, to compress the nerve in a loop of plastic material held by a curved artery forceps.

5

Orientation and suture

If a nerve is divided obliquely the nerve tissue at the extremes of the obliquity should be preserved because an oblique line of division can be used to ensure that the orientation of the nerve is being correctly maintained. If transverse division of the nerve has occurred the correct orientation can usually be determined by careful inspection of the nerve ends and, particularly, by comparing the pattern of vessels on the surface of the nerve. In some nerves, e.g. the median nerve, there is a vessel which can be readily discerned on the volar surface of the nerve and can be used as a reliable index of correct rotation. Sutures of 5/0 to 8/0 should be used on an atraumatic needle. The material should be inert and therefore catgut and black silk are best avoided. Stainless steel wire or nylon provides a satisfactory suture. Human hair is not suitable. The sutures should pick up the delicate epineurium and not pass through nerve bundles.

A suture is placed at each side of the nerve and tied, the ends being left long and held in bulldog clamps to serve as retractors.

The anterior surface of the nerve can then be sutured by the insertion of two or more similar sutures which will pick up only the epineural connective tissues, allowing them to be slightly infolded.

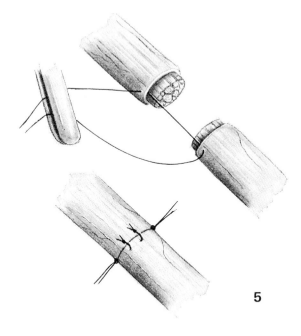

5

6

Suture

The lateral sutures can then be passed across the nerve, one in front and one behind, and the nerve rotated so that a similar number of small interrupted sutures can be inserted on the deep surface between the two stay sutures. It should be remembered that all sutures are foreign material and that an excessive number of tight sutures around a nerve should be avoided. The purpose of suture of nerve is to ensure repair of the connective tissues and closely placed sutures are unnecessary for this purpose. There should be no fascicles of nerve projecting through the suture line. Should this occur, the edges of the projecting fascicles should be trimmed back so that the nerve tissue comes to lie within the epineurium.

It is common practice, if not already done, to release the tourniquet after repairing the nerve and before closing the wound. This is a technique which is not universally recommended, but with certain nerves, e.g. the median nerve, where a large vessel is present, disruption of the suture line can occur because of arterial bleeding. It is, therefore, advisable to release the tourniquet and satisfy oneself that this is not the case before the wound is closed.

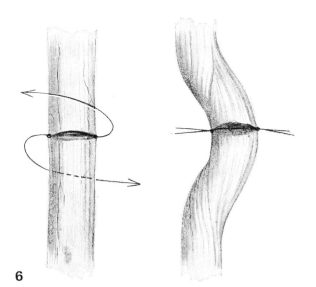

6

7

Marker sutures

Disruption of a suture line is a common cause of failure of nerve repair. The insertion of marker sutures is a useful device which will allow diagnosis of nerve disruption. On the proximal site of nerve repair two fine sutures of stainless steel wire are inserted and a further suture is inserted distal to the suture line, the distances between these three sutures being the same. X-ray examination later will show the site of these sutures. If disruption has occurred the gap between the second and third sutures is seen to be greater than the gap between the first and second.

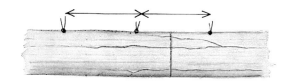

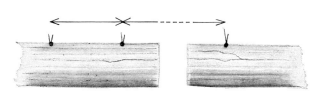

7

Splintage

The nerve suture should be protected from strain for a period of three weeks, after which there is a period of carefully controlled mobilization. In the case of the median and ulnar nerves in the forearm it is usual to ensure that no tension will occur by immobilizing the wrist in slight palmar flexion. If tendon division has occurred at the same time, immobilization of both structures can be carried out by holding the wrist in a dorsal plaster slab, including the fingers, for a period of 3 weeks. A position of excessive flexion of the joints is not necessary when primary repair is carried out.

Incomplete nerve divisions

Primary suture

At primary operation where an incomplete nerve division is found the temptation to insert sutures to pull the divided sections of the nerve together is one which should be resisted. This has only the effect of producing scarring and resultant entrapment neuropathy of the intact portion of the nerve.

One is frequently astonished at how small is the deficit in circumstances of incomplete nerve division. Where an incomplete nerve division is found at primary operation the division should be left alone or at best wrapped by Silastic sheeting to reduce the amount of neuroma formation which occurs.

No sutures should be inserted. A decision to deal with the matter secondarily should be based upon the nerve deficit which is found, by assessment at around 1 month after injury.

AIDS TO PERIPHERAL NERVE SURGERY

Magnification

Simple magnifying devices can be of considerable advantage, not only in identifying the structures of the nerve precisely but also in facilitating the insertion of fine apposing sutures. The degree of magnification which is used is a controversial subject. If magnification is used it should be on account of positive advantages which accrue from it. Magnifying devices and operating microscopes which provide magnification of greater than ×4 pose technical problems in their use, and without the addition of very delicate instruments and suture material their use is incongrous.

Nerve stimulation

A nerve stimulator is of great value in the operation of nerve repair. Its use makes it possible to distinguish motor branches and intact portions of nerve and to differentiate in anomalies of innervation. Several varieties are available.

Nerve glues

Other methods of apposition of nerve than by the use of suture have been described. In particular nerve glues, e.g. by use of thromboplastin, have achieved some popularity. This is a useful method of approximating small nerves and may also be of value in larger nerves in association with a minimum number of sutures. Glues derived from naturally occurring materials, i.e. fibrinogen and thromboplastin, are not harmful, but glues containing methylmethacrylate are cytotoxic and should not be used in peripheral nerve repair.

Nerve wrapping

Wrapping of the site of definitive nerve repair with various substances has been described for many years. Materials which have been used include vein, celluloid, rubber tubing, millipore, and more recently Silastic, which is sometimes used as a prepared nerve cuff. If such a material is to be used it must be remembered that sheathing material around the nerve may interfere with the process of nerve repair. These nerve wrapping materials, i.e. Silastic, are most useful in protecting a nerve preparatory to secondary repair. If nerve wrapping is used at the time of primary operation the risks of infection are increased.

[*The illustrations for this Chapter on Peripheral Nerve Injuries were drawn by Miss A. Brown.*]

Craniocerebral Injury

Bryan Jennett, M.D., F.R.C.S.
Professor of Neurosurgery, Institute of Neurological Sciences, Glasgow
and University of Glasgow

PRE-OPERATIVE

Only a small minority of civilian (non-missile) head injuries require operative treatment. The most common are:

(*1*) Open injuries, which must be closed to prevent infective complications.

(*2*) Intracranial haematomas, which must be evacuated to prevent irreversible pressure effects on the brain, particularly the brain stem.

Many of the patients with one or other of these two types of injury have not suffered severe initial brain damage — as evidenced by the fact that many of them have recovered to the extent of being able to talk before complications develop. Properly treated, they should therefore make a good recovery — but death or persistent disability can be the price of mismanagement.

A third of patients in hospital with head injuries have another major injury and these should be made known to the anaesthetist before embarking on cranial surgery. Chest injuries with pneumothorax, pulmonary collapse or surgical emphysema are important to him, as are fractured upper or lower jaws with the possibility of blood in the pharynx, and long bone fractures or soft tissue injuries associated with blood loss. The anaesthetist must guarantee full oxygenation and absence of straining, to avoid raising intracranial pressure and aggravating brain damage and bleeding. Controlled respiration is advised, with a mild degree of hyperventilation; the head end of the table should be elevated 15° to minimize venous congestion in the scalp and intracranially. A careful watch on blood pressure is essential because, if there has been previous blood loss, induction of anaesthesia may disturb compensatory mechanisms with resulting hypotension. Appreciable blood loss can occur during operations for haematoma, or depressed fracture involving the venous sinuses, and arrangements should always be made for blood transfusion — although this must not delay relieving acute compression from haematoma. Gunshot wounds may require very vigorous replacement of blood both in preparation for operation and during its course.

OPEN INJURIES

OPEN DEPRESSED FRACTURE OF VAULT

1

Compound depressed fracture should be suspected whenever a scalp wound goes down to bone. Inspection and probing are unreliable guides to an underlying fracture unless brain tissue or bone fragments are obvious in the wound; the contour of the outer table may suggest only slight depression, even when the inner table is considerably displaced and has lacerated the dura. The scalp is so mobile that the fracture line may not lie directly under the wound.

Because the brain damage is usually confined to the area of the fracture there may be loss of consciousness or for only a brief period, or even not at all; this contributes to the risk of overlooking this injury.

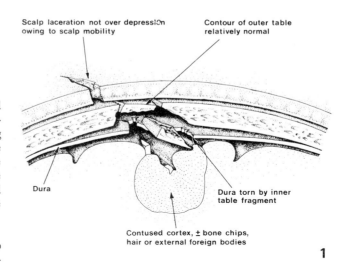

Scalp laceration not over depression owing to scalp mobility

Contour of outer table relatively normal

Dura

Dura torn by inner table fragment

Contused cortex, ± bone chips, hair or external foreign bodies

1

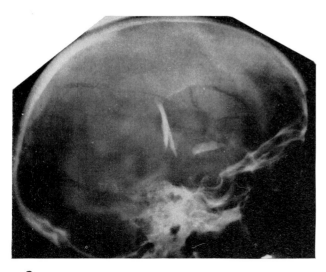

2

2

DIAGNOSIS

Diagnosis depends on good quality x-ray films, including at least two views in different planes; a fracture which looks quite innocent in one view may prove to be considerably depressed in another.

Even when angulation is not obvious depression may be deduced if a double density shadow is seen; this is produced by a fragment being displaced under the full thickness of unfractured bone.

OPERATIVE PROCEDURE

3 & 4

Scalp lacerations

All scalp wounds should be properly sutured in case there is an undisclosed fracture beneath. Ideally, suture is deferred until after x-ray, but it may have to be done first either for convenience or because bleeding cannot be controlled otherwise. Hair is shaved for 2·5 cm in all directions; either local or general anaesthetic is essential if the wound is to be adequately explored and cleaned, and accurately sutured. The scalp is so vascular that wound edges are rarely devitalized and skin excision is rarely necessary. Separate closure of the galea and skin is always preferable and, in addition, avoids the need for definitive haemostasis; if the dura is left open and the galea is neither separately sutured nor included in an 'all layers' suture there is considerable risk of a brain hernia developing.

If skin is missing, enough mobility may be gained by undercutting, and by extending the incision into an approximate 'S' shape; larger defects may require a scalp flap to be rotated or relieving incisions made to enable the bone defect and dural tear to be covered with full-thickness scalp, whilst split-skin grafts are applied to the resulting skin defects remote from the area of injury (*see* page 34).

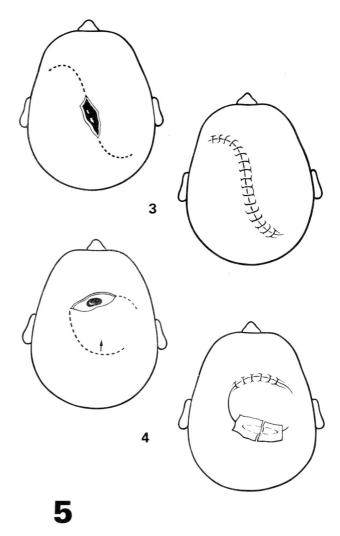

3

4

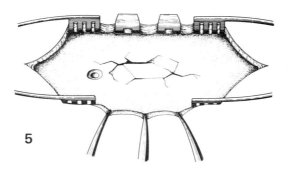

5

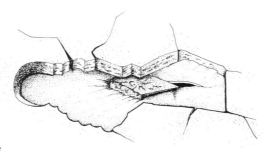

6

5

Elevation of bone fragments

Depressed fragments of bone are elevated not because pressure on the brain is harmful, but to prevent infection by disclosing dural tears and to allow removal of foreign material and devitalized brain. If the outer table is largely intact, because fragments are impacted, a burr hole is placed adjacent to the fracture and extended by nibbling until the fragments can be removed.

6

Bone removal

Bone removal must be continued to the extent of any dural tears but need not follow linear fractures extending from the depressed area.

7

Closure of dura

After damaged brain has been sucked away the torn dura is sutured if possible; if not, a double layer of surgical haemostatic gauze or a free patch of pericranium is placed over the defect. If the dura is found to be intact it should be opened only if subdural haematoma is suspected; this may be indicated by a blue appearance of the dura.

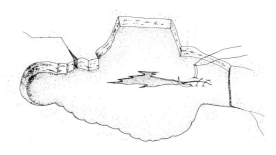

7

8

Replacement of bone fragments

Bone fragments can be replaced as a mosaic after washing them clean, even when the dura has been torn, unless the wound is grossly contaminated or exploration has been delayed more than 24 hr after injury. This saves the need for delayed cranioplasty; immediate repair with foreign material carries a high risk of infection, even in relatively clean but fresh wounds.

When a fracture clearly involves the sagittal or lateral venous sinuses elevation is avoided if possible. If elevation seems essential because of gross contamination or marked angulation, operation is postponed until there are ideal operating conditions and several pints of blood are available for transfusion.

Operation on a depressed fracture is never an absolute emergency — it is better to accept delay of 12—18 hr to ensure definitive treatment in skilled hands; the risk of infection is reduced if prophylactic antibiotics are administered as soon after injury as possible.

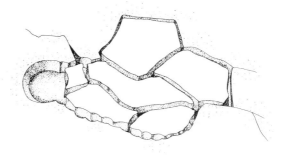

8

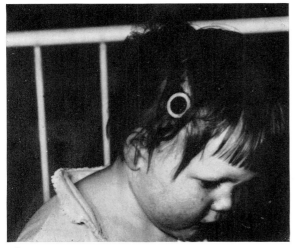

9

PUNCTURE WOUNDS

9

Patients with these injuries are frequently fully conscious, having sustained only local brain damage; the potential severity of the injury is readily underestimated, unless the injuring instrument is still in place. This child suffered a penetrating wound from a constructional toy. This type of injury requires the same treatment as a missile injury.

Particularly deceptive are puncture wounds through the eyelid. Sharp sticks, knitting needles and the like may readily penetrate through the roof of the orbit, with only a tiny external mark of entry.

BASAL FRACTURE WITH DURAL TEAR

This injury puts the nasopharyngeal cavity in continuity with the subarachnoid space, and meningitis can develop. This may be recurrent and may first occur even years after injury.

10

Anterior fossa fracture

This may be into one or more of the air sinuses. If the ethmoid is involved there is almost always anosmia, which may be unilateral.

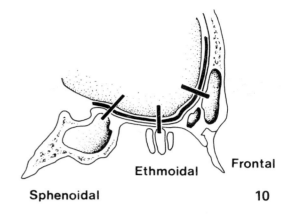

Ethmoidal   **Frontal**

Sphenoidal   **10**

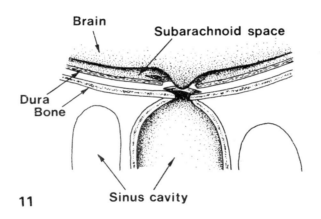

Brain

Subarachnoid space

Dura
Bone

Sinus cavity

11

11

Rhinorrhoea

Rhinorrhoea may be delayed in development or may not be recorded at all, even in patients developing meningitis. More often it occurs for a few days or a week or two and then stops. This does not necessarily mean that the tear has healed — more often a brain plug or hernia has stopped the leakage. This does not form a barrier against bacteria, and it may prevent dural healing.

12

Another clue to dural tearing is the finding of intra-cranial air on the plain skull film, usually best seen in a brow-up lateral projection. A tear should also be suspected if a broad fracture line is seen in relation to the sinuses, or an upwardly angulated spicule of bone (usually from the ethmoidal roof). However, no fracture may be seen, even though meningitis has occurred.

Aerocele with fluid level

12

13

Frontal craniotomy

Repair of the dural defect through a frontal craniotomy is the only effective prophylactic treatment.
Only one side need be explored if the fracture line or
unilateral anosmia make localization certain; a
coronal skin incision is usually made and a bifrontal
bone flap turned. This enables bilateral exploration
to be made, which is often advisable, because it is
seldom possible to be confident that tearing is confined to one side.

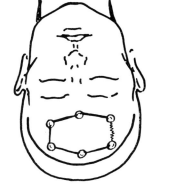

13

14

Exposure

Intradural exploration and retraction of the brain
reveals the dural defect, which is usually located by
finding a small plug of brain bulging into it.

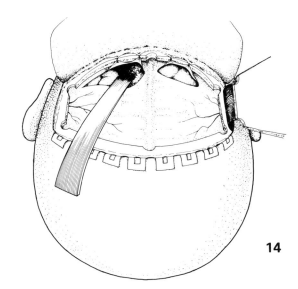

14

15

Insertion of patch

A patch of pericranium from the middle of the
bone flap will cover a small defect; larger ones call
for fascia lata from the thigh. The patch need not
be sutured in place but should extend 0·5 cm beyond
the defect in all directions.

Cerebrospinal fluid otorrhoea

Cerebrospinal fluid otorrhoea, due to a petrous
temporal fracture tearing the dura over the middle
ear cavity, usually stops spontaneously and the dura
heals naturally, because a brain hernia forms less
readily than in the anterior fossa. Occasionally delayed
meningitis develops and fascial repair is then carried
out through a lateral flap, or a craniectomy similar
to that used for trigeminal rhizotomy.

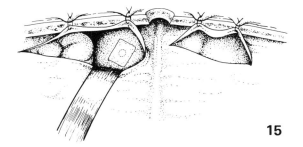

15

INTRACRANIAL HAEMATOMA

16

Many fatal head injuries are found at autopsy to have an intracranial haematoma. Although in some removal of the clot would not have saved the patient because there was serious impact injury to the brain, very often the initial injury has been mild but progressive cerebral compression then developed and could have been reversed by expeditious operation. This is especially so when extradural haematoma occurs alone; not infrequently there is intradural haemorrhage as well; it may be intracerebral or subdural, but commonly a mixture of both. The distinction between the anatomical types of acute and subacute intracranial haematoma (less than 14 days after injury) is not always as clear as text books suggest. Whenever a patient who has talked even a few mumbled words becomes less responsive, an intracranial haematoma should be suspected and immediate steps taken to verify the diagnosis. Deterioration can be very rapid and delay of an hour or so can make the difference between death and survival, or between satisfactory recovery and permanent disability.

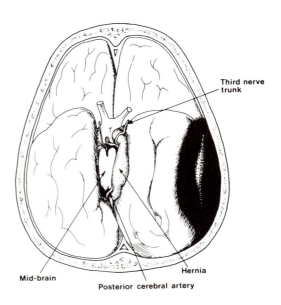

16

CLINICAL DIAGNOSIS

(*1*) Loss of consciousness or deepening coma is the one consistent feature and it is the earliest sign.

(*2*) Dilatation of the pupil on the same side as the clot, with loss of light reflex due to pressure on the third nerve, is common but not invariable.

(*3*) Contralateral hemiparesis next develops and then extensor rigidity in the same limbs; bradycardia, rising blood pressure with tachypnoea or periodic respiration are late signs which indicate critical compression of the brain stem.

Early detection of this complication depends on careful clinical monitoring, particularly of the conscious level (*see* page 114).

17

Confirmation of diagnosis

Skull fracture occurs in 80—90 per cent of patients with intracranial haematoma and the detection of a fracture is the best method of avoiding the mistake of ascribing unconsciousness to other factors such as alcohol or recent stroke. Echo-encephalography is a rapid method of detecting shift of mid-line structures. Polaroid pictures of the oscilloscopic tracing of the skull and mid-line echos, elicited in turn from right and left sides, enable the distances from each side of the skull to the mid-line of the brain to be compared. It is reliable only in the hands of those who use it frequently and are aware of artefacts.

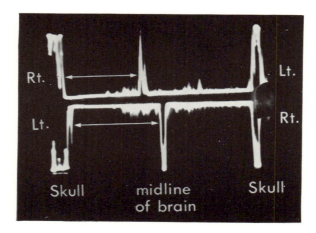

17

18

EMI (CT) scanning has revolutionized the diagnosis of intracranial haematoma, because it shows not only shift of intracranial structures but usually indicates the exact site and size of the clot. It is reliable and does not involve any invasive measures, but restless patients require anaesthesia.

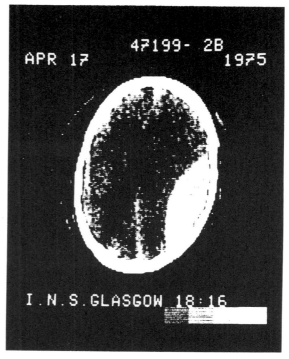

18

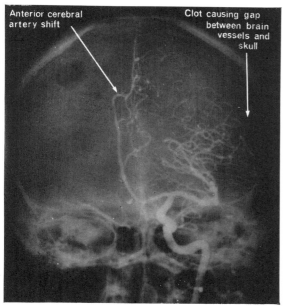

19

19 & 20

Angiography remains useful when EMI scanning is not available. The arterial phase shows mid-line shift, but the capillary phase is best for outlining the clot. Note the burr hole made on the wrong side before angiography.

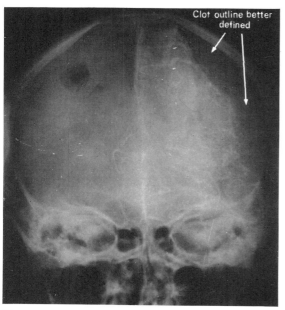

20

OPERATIVE PROCEDURE

The skull must be opened with the minimum of delay — the urgency depending on how far advanced and how rapid is the deterioration. There may not be time for neuroradiological investigations, and in that event burr holes are best made in the sites where extradural haematoma is likely to be found. In desperate circumstances only the release of such a clot is likely to result in good recovery. Both sides should be explored, but first the side of the fracture or of the fixed dilated pupil; in the absence of other evidence scalp marks, visible after shaving the head, may be of localizing value. However, burr holes frequently fail to reveal the haematoma, and radiological procedures are then needed.

Endotracheal intubation is recommended even if the patient is so deeply unconscious as not to require general anaesthesia, because inadequate ventilation leads to brain swelling and increased haemorrhage due to vasodilatation. Blood should be taken for emergency cross-matching because serious bleeding can occur, particularly in children.

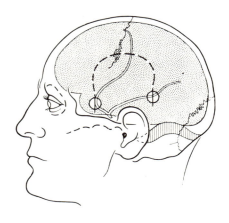

21

21

The incision

Vertical incisions should be marked over the anterior and posterior branches of the middle meningeal artery before the head is draped. A scalp flap should be scratched in lightly as this may be required if a large clot is found. Burr holes are made in the usual way.

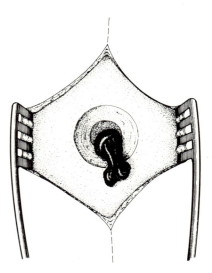

22

22

Exposure

When a burr hole is made clot may immediately begin to protrude; if none is evident a periosteal elevator is used to explore the extradural space and when clot is located the bone is nibbled in this direction. If no clot is found, but the dura is tight, further holes may be made in the frontal and parietal regions — if necessary similar openings are made on the other side. Unless the occasion is desperate, if the initial set of burr holes fails to show a clot but does indicate increased pressure, the best course is to carry out neuroradiological investigations.

23

Sufficient exposure may be obtained by continuing to nibble away bone but the resulting skull defect is permanent and may require cranioplasty; neuro-surgeons usually prefer to turn a bone flap, which gives better access and avoids a skull defect.

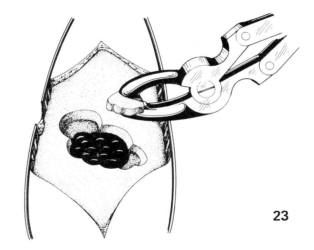

23

24

Closure

Haemostasis depends on diathermy, on packing with haemostatic gauze and on 'hitch stitches'; these run from dura to periosteum and approximate dura to bone, preferably over haemostatic gauze.

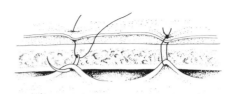

24

CHRONIC SUBDURAL HAEMATOMA

Only half the patients with this lesion can remember a head injury, which has usually been trivial and has occurred several weeks previously. Headache is the commonest complaint but a mild degree of mental confusion is frequent before drowsiness and later quiet and fluctuating stupor develops. Two-thirds of patients are over 50 years of age — inviting a differential diagnosis of diffuse cerebrovascular disease or senile dementia.

25

Although fracture is unusual x-rays may show pineal shift, as pineal calcification is the rule at this age. Echo-encephalography may show no shift because bilateral haematomas may balance each other. Angiography is the most reliable means of diagnosis — but surface clot may be obvious only in special oblique views.

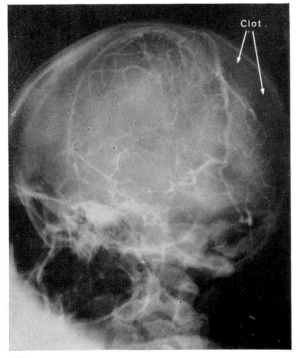

25

OPERATIVE PROCEDURE

26

Most chronic haematomas are fluid and can be evacuated through burr holes; unless angiography indicates a very local collection three holes are made on each side, one of them low in the temporal region. If a solid clot with a thick membrane is encountered a bone flap must be turned and the initial burr hole incisions should therefore be so placed that they can form part of a flap incision.

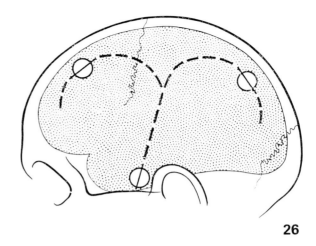

26

27

Drainage

The clot cavity is washed through with saline and the head moved around to drain the liquid away as completely as possible. Dura may remain depressed below the inner surface of bone and clot may re-accumulate; some surgeons try to prevent this by closing the scalp round a suction drain; others leave the wound open for 48 hr and nurse the patient head down; most prefer to close the wound and deal with a recollection by aspiration through a brain cannula, by re-opening one of these, or by making a fresh burr hole. Intrathecal injection of saline carries the risk of infection and is of dubious value.

Conscious level should be frequently recorded using a simple system which can be reliably interpreted by nurses and junior medical staff. The Glasgow Coma (or responsiveness) Scale was designed for this purpose — it records visually the responsiveness of the patient. It can be incorporated in a single observation chart which enables pupils, hemiparesis, temperature, pulse, blood pressure and respiration all to be recorded on the same sheet.

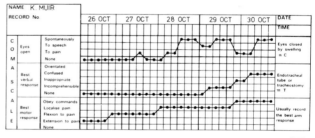

27

Intracranial pressure measurements have become routine in many neurosurgical units for severely affected patients. Usually a catheter is introduced into the ventricle through a burr hole or a twist drill hole; or else a surface sensor is put in through a burr hole. Monitoring often shows that patients with severe brain stem dysfunction do *not* have raised intracranial pressure, and that it is inappropriate to treat them as though they had. On the contrary, it may be clear that pressure is high or rising and that intervention is required.

Monitoring of conscious level and intracranial pressure

The decision to operate, or to employ non-surgical means of controlling intracranial pressure (such as osmotic diuretics, steroids or controlled ventilation) depends on detecting a deteriorating conscious level or high or rising intracranial pressure.

[The illustrations for this Chapter on Craniocerebral Injury were redrawn by Mr. J. M. P. Booth.]

Missile Injuries of the Brain

H. Alan Crockard, F.R.C.S.
Senior Lecturer in Neurosurgery, Queen's University, Belfast;
Consultant Neurosurgeon, Royal Victoria Hospital, Belfast

INTRODUCTION

The surgery of penetrating craniocerebral missile injuries is only a part of the total care of such injuries and their pre- and postoperative management is as important as the surgery itself. It is a mistake to consider these injuries as rather severe compound depressed injuries, though many of the surgical principles are applicable to both conditions. Set out below is a counsel of perfection in the treatment of such injuries; it may be impossible to follow it due to local circumstances, but is must be stated that adequate resuscitation and care of the airway are the important first steps in management; operation can be delayed and is best performed in a specialist centre.

MECHANISMS OF INJURY

Theory of missiles

When a missile strikes an object, all or part of its energy is released into the object. Missiles may be bullets, fragments from mines and antipersonnel devices, or may be stones or fragments of masonry which have become missiles either by being struck by the bullet or being close to a bomb. Missiles are classified as being of either low or high velocity, depending on whether they are faster or slower than the speed of sound (1000 feet or 300 metres/sec). Bullets from hand guns, pistols and submachine guns are low velocity missiles (600 − 900 feet or 150 − 250 metres/sec): those fired from rifles are high velocity (1000 − 2500 feet or 300 − 650 metres/sec). A bomb or mine will send numerous irregular fragments at high velocity over a short distance. As the kinetic energy possessed by the missile depends on the square of the velocity (kinetic energy = ½ mass × velocity^2), it can be appreciated that a rifle bullet or high velocity fragment from a bomb will release 10 − 16 times more energy into the brain and the injury will be correspondingly more devastating. When a missile hits the body tissue it quite literally causes an explosion within them; there is a temporary cavity maybe up to 30 times the diameter of the missile lasting a few milliseconds after impact and positive and negative pressure peaks occur in rapid succession. There will be direct damage to the skin, bone, dura and brain along the track of the injury, fragments of bone may become secondary missiles and cause further brain damage along their respective tracks. In addition to these direct local effects along the track there will be diffuse effects due to the explosive cavitation and the dissipation of the energy in a closed cavity, the skull. The outcome will depend on a series of interdependent variables, such as the energy released by the missile, the amount of brain involved and the extent and type of secondary complications.

115

Pathophysiology

On impact the energy will be dissipated throughout the dural cavity, the amount depending on the energy possessed by the missile. This will produce local and remote pathophysiological changes. There will be immediate changes due directly to the explosive force but then there will be secondary epiphenomena. Early after injury conditions are very labile. *Local effects* include areas of cell necrosis surrounded by oedema. Intracranial bleeding is not usually a major problem although external bleeding from scalp or cerebral vessels may be serious. The brain swelling may result in raised intracranial pressure (ICP), reduced cerebral perfusion pressure and, if severe enough, may completely arrest the circulation either in small parts or to the brain as a whole. The *remote effects* include the body's reaction to trauma of any kind as well as specific effects of the energy on brain stem centres. These include transient apnoea, alteration in respiratory rate and rhythm, neurogenic pulmonary oedema and aspiration of vomitus. There may be a fall in blood pressure due to marked reduction in cardiac output, transient changes in heart rate and electrocardiogram. Unlike the closed head injury, there may be no loss of consciousness initially, pin-point pupils are extremely rare, and the intracranial pressure may not be raised until some hours later, when cerebral oedema occurs. Any coughing or struggling will produce rapid deterioration in levels of consciousness and irreversible rises in intracranial pressure. It is therefore necessary to prevent any respiratory inadequacies. Signs associated with a poor prognosis are coma, any deviation of blood pressure from the normal range, and dilated pupils. Conscious or drowsy patients with normal pupils and normal pulse and blood pressure correctly treated should have a mortality of 10 per cent or less.

PREPARATION OF THE PATIENT

Reception and resuscitation

It cannot be too strongly emphasized that time and effort spent in the initial assessment and resuscitation of patients with bullet injuries of the brain is time well spent. It is only the very occasional expanding intracranial haematoma which requires emergency operation and, for the rest, operation is best delayed until conditions are stable (4 − 6 hr after injury). Unless fully conscious, the patient should be anaesthetized using intravenous drugs rather than volatile inhalation agents, a cuffed endotracheal tube passed, after the cords have been sprayed with 0·5 per cent lignocaine, and ventilation mechanically controlled following complete muscle relaxation with curare-like drugs. This is completely justified in that many of these patients, apart from the moribund, will need surgical exploration and, therefore, the loss of physical signs brought about by controlled ventilation is of theoretical interest only. Also, it is not unknown for dilated pupils to become reactive with the treatment of pulmonary problems. At least one, and perhaps two, intravenous infusions should be started because there has been much blood lost or because of the central shock due to brain stem involvement already alluded to. A central venous manometer and urinary catheter will be of great value in evaluation of fluid requirements. Initially the circulation may be replenished with 5 per cent dextrose or Hartmann's solution but not 0·9 per cent saline. Plasma expanders, plasma or unmatched group O Rh negative blood may be required if bleeding is severe. Careful records are kept of all liquids administered and if bleeding is severe all problems associated with massive transfusion guarded against, e.g. platelet and clotting factor depletion. Only after initial resuscitation and ventilation should radiographs of the skull and chest be considered. Unnecessary moving of the patient from one room to another should be avoided and so, if possible, x-ray films should be taken in the resuscitation area or even in the operating theatre. Check radiographs may be required during the operation to ensure the removal of all bone fragments. When conditions are stable and when there is adequate blood cross-matched and available, surgical treatment may be considered. If after resuscitation and controlled ventilation the pupils are still fixed and dilated, and there is either persistent hypotension in the absence of severe bleeding or hypertension, the prognosis is very poor. Through-and-through high velocity missile injuries are also invariably fatal and in such cases operation is rarely worthwhile.

Transportation

It is only after resuscitation and assessment that operation should be considered and, as already stated, this is best performed in a specialist centre. That being the case, when stable, the patient should be transferred, as quickly as possible, fully curarized and ventilated and accompanied by an anaesthetist.

Anaesthesia

In all but the fully conscious, the patient will have been previously intubated with a low-pressure cuffed endotracheal tube of suitable size. Anaesthesia should be maintained with intravenous drugs such as phenoperidine and fentanyl (0·1 mg); pancuronium bromide used to effect muscular relaxation (2—4 mg IV) repeated as required, and the patient should be ventilated in a zero to positive cycle 10—15 ml/kg body weight. Arterial blood gas analysis should be performed and ventilation adjusted to produce P_aCO_2 $30 - 35$ mmHg and P_aO_2 $150 - 200$ mmHg. The head should be elevated above the chest to reduce venous congestion. Positive end-expiratory pressure (PEEP) type ventilation should be reserved for those with severe pulmonary oedema, aspiration pneumonitis or blast lung as it raises intracranial pressure. The electrocardiogram should be recorded throughout and if possible an arterial catheter should be attached to a pressure transducer though this is useful rather than absolutely necessary. Intracranial pressure may be recorded using a subdural transducer postoperatively.

Positioning

Apart from injuries of the posterior fossa, most injuries can be adequately dealt with with the patient supine. The whole head should be shaved to allow for adequate surgical exposure and identification of small entrance wounds undetected at the time of initial examination. The area of wounds should be left to the last and only when the surgeon is ready to operate should the area round the wounds be shaved. The whole of the head should be surgically prepared using cetyl trimethyl ammonium bromide and chlorhexidine. Any facial wound can be dealt with subsequently. Skin towels are arranged so as to allow access to the whole cranium if possible. The head can be moved around therefore during the procedure without the necessity of retowelling. When there are large skin and skull defects a thigh should be prepared for skin and/or fascia lata grafting.

Basic surgical equipment

The standard instruments for a craniotomy are essential — a wide selection of bone nibbling forceps, Hudson's brace, perforator and burrs and self-retaining retractors. At least two suction sets should be available and diathermy is essential. Larger vessels can be controlled using haemostatic metal clips. Non-absorbable suture material is used. Vacuum drainage, beween dura and skin, is a desirable method of eliminating wound haematoma.

Surgery — general principles

It is best to form a large skin flap around the scalp wound to allow for a very generous craniectomy. It also facilitates the subsequent cranioplasty required by most of these patients. In general terms, exploration of the wound by enlargement of the existing injury is unsatisfactory. A wide craniectomy is effected using a perforator and burr close to the actual bony defect and this is enlarged towards the area of damage using bone nibbling forceps. The craniectomy should be large enough to expose healthy dura and brain. All bony fragments, accessible metal fragments and all necrotic brain, clot, debris, hair, etc., must be removed, for which suction is very useful. Careful haemostasis is most important. The cavity should be flushed out with hydrogen peroxide. After haemostasis, the dura must be repaired using the pericranium or fascia lata. The skin flap is sutured in layers and the original wound should have its edges excised and repaired in the conventional manner. Vacuum drainage of the wound is essential. Unless bone fragments are large and attached to the temporalis muscle, they are not preserved. It is much more satisfactory to repair the defect with titanium than with dental acrylic resin. If there is skin loss, then rotation flaps must be considered. Good skin cover is essential over the area of bony defect.

THE OPERATION

A low velocity temporoparietal injury has been chosen to illustrate the main points of the surgical procedure. Special forms of injury and treatment will be illustrated later. The entrance wound is in front of the ear.

1

The wound

After preparation of the whole head and leaving the area of the wounds to the last for shaving etc., a skin flap is planned so as to allow adequate exposure of the cranial contents. Care is taken to ensure a good blood supply to the areas between the wounds and the flap's edges. If there is active bleeding from the edges of the wounds, these may be coagulated at this stage but no attempt should be made to remove bone fragments through the wound until there is an adequate brain exposure. A skin flap is fashioned in the usual way and the temporalis muscle dissected from the bone and reflected with the skin flap, exposing healthy bone and the area of damage. Dead and damaged temporalis muscle is removed at this stage.

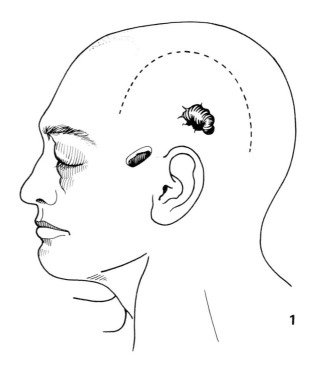

1

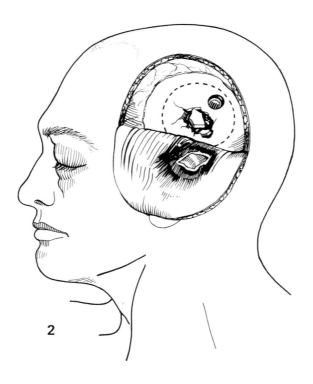

2

2

Craniectomy

If there are large bone fragments depressed into the wound these may be gently removed using the rongeurs but if the fragments are impacted it is much wiser to begin with a burr hole placed some distance away from the wound so that the bone is removed towards the area of damage. A wide craniectomy is always desirable. Great care must be taken in removing the bone fragments as within the area of damage there may still be viable intact major blood vessels, the sacrifice of which will lead to a greater deficit.

3

Exposure

A wide craniectomy has been performed exposing healthy intact dura all around the wound. The surface bone fragments have been removed. A blunt periosteal elevator is placed between the dura and the brain and the dura widely opened in a stellate fashion around the area of damage to expose normal brain all around the wound. The dural edges are sutured back over the bone edge to protect the bone and allow adequate exposure of the brain for toilet of the wound. All unhealthy portions of dura should be sacrificed.

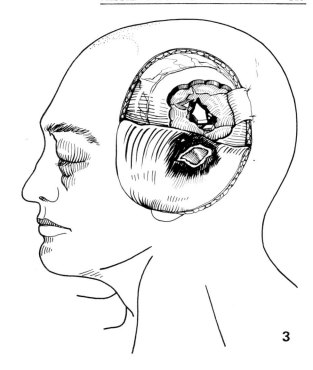

3

4

Further exposure

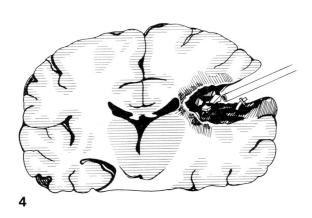

4

All damaged and dead brain should be removed. Constant checks are made with the original x-ray films to search for bone fragments which are removed with diathermy forceps or suction. Adequate haemostasis is essential. Large vessels which are actively bleeding should be stopped with haemostatic metal clips and the shaft of dead brain removed. If there is brain swelling, the surface part of the wound may close before the depths have been explored; this can be prevented by adequate removal of damaged brain at the beginning and also with gentle retraction, using malleable brain retractors. The depths of the wound must be explored completely and at the end of the procedure there should be a bloodless shaft or cavity into the depths of the brain. The cavity should be thoroughly irrigated with saline and hydrogen peroxide throughout the procedure. All hair, dirt, stones and accessible metal fragments should be removed. Metal fragments which are minute and lodged in vital structures may be left. Unless this procedure is performed adequately there is a very high incidence of brain abscess. Secondary toilet is a misnomer and indicates inadequate primary toilet.

5

Closure of the dura

The dura should be carefully closed, when necessary with a patch taken from adjacent pericranium or, for a large defect, a fascia lata graft obtained from the outer aspect of the previously prepared thigh. If the brain is swollen it is important to use a generous fascial patch to accommodate it. Non-absorbable suture material, for instance black silk (3/0), can be used as this is useful for identifying the various layers at a subsequent cranioplasty.

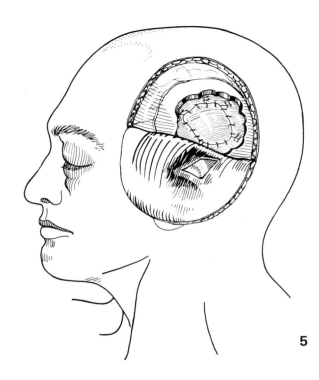

5

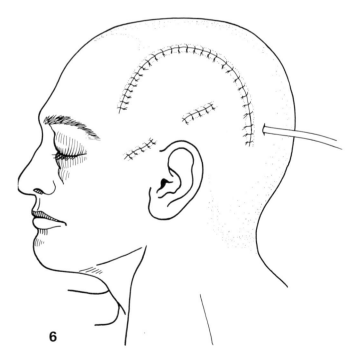

6

6

Skin closure

The wounds are carefully debrided both on the inside and the outside of the flap, and closed with interrupted silk stitches in two layers. The skin flap is closed in the usual fashion and a vacuum drain inserted into the wound. The wound should be lightly bandaged, because with large bony defects high bandage pressure will adversely affect the brain.

SPECIAL TYPES OF INJURY

7

Widely separated cranial wounds

Many injuries with widely separated cranial wounds are fatal. Through-and-through, side-to-side injuries are almost invariably fatal so that it is only occasionally that extensive operation can be justified. If the wounds are widely separated it is better to have a skin flap around each wound. The entrance wound is explored in the manner described and the pulped brain removed in the conventional way. The exit wound is explored through a similar flap and the whole missile track explored from both the entrance and the exit sites. If the ventricle has been penetrated the ventricular system must be carefully washed out to ensure that there are no clots or necrotic material within it. Gelfoam may be used as a temporary haemostatic agent but if the ventricular system has been penetrated great care must be taken to remove the Gelfoam as it may cause aqueduct obstruction and hydrocephalus.

8a&b

Extensive skin loss

If there is extensive skin loss associated with the craniocerebral injury then a transposition or rotation flap will be necessary to close the defect. A rotation flap is usually very satisfactory and the exposed pericranium can be covered with a partial-thickness skin graft obtained from the previously prepared thigh. A shotgun, if discharged from close range, will produce a devastating soft tissue injury and comparatively little intracranial damage and the problem is often one of skin cover after the necessary toilet. Radiographs may reveal 50 — 100 pellets scattered through the skin. Clearly it would be impossible to remove every pellet, so only those in the area of the brain wound need be removed. Those in important organs such as the eye will require appropriate specialized care at the same time.

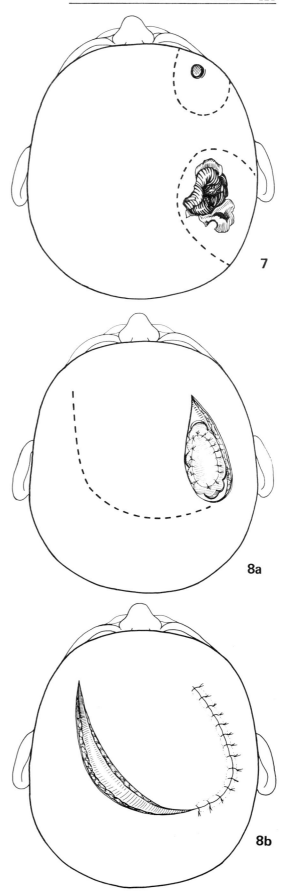

7

8a

8b

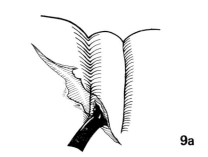

9a

9a,b&c

Bleeding from a major venous sinus

Wounds of a major venous sinus may be fatal before
the patient arrives at hospital. In the anterior third
of the sagittal sinus, little need be done other than to
ligate the venous channel. Around the torcula or
transverse sinus area or posterior third of the sagittal
sinus it is necessary to repair the vessel. The blood
loss can be controlled by temporary pressure on a
cotton pledget, adequate blood replacement must be
available, and a small patch of pericranium or dura is
sutured in position. Stay sutures (4/0 silk) are placed
and then the patch applied to the defect, held in
position with a cotton pledget and suction and then
further interrupted sutures placed around the patch
to make a watertight closure. Good team work with
the anaesthetists is absolutely vital to keep abreast
of blood loss during this procedure.

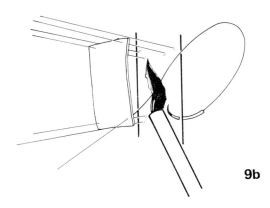

9b

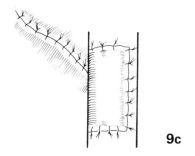

9c

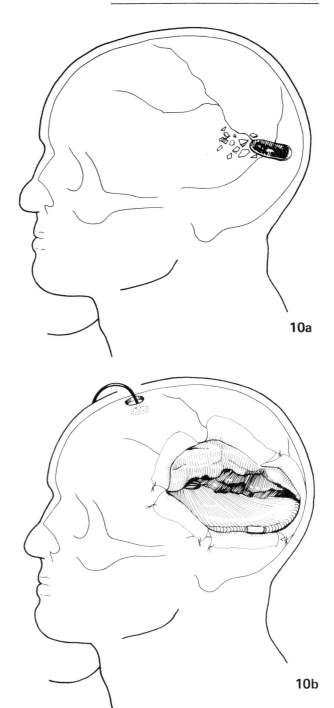

10a&b

Tangential high velocity missile injury

Due to the energy dissipated by a high velocity missile the area of damage from a tangential high velocity injury is quite enormous. Bone fragments will have become secondary missiles and penetrated deep into the brain surface. There will be extensive fractures extending over the vault and down into the base and there may be tears of the major venous sinuses. As before, adequate resuscitation and adequate toilet are the only methods of treatment of such wounds. A wide craniectomy and dural opening is necessary to expose and remove all damaged brain tissue. Following this sort of injury a large cavity is left and intracranial pressure monitoring is very useful in such cases; any significant rise in intracranial pressure in the early postoperative period is taken as evidence of haematoma accumulating in the wound and re-exploration is indicated.

Associated neck and facial wounds

If there is a bullet wound in the neck great care must be taken to evaluate adequately the major vessels and, if there is any doubt, transfemoral retrograde angiography and/or surgical exploration of the vessels should be undertaken. A delayed caroticojugular fistula may present in the postinjury period as raised intracranial pressure and with false intracranial localizing signs. Facial wounds, especially those around the eye, require early definitive attention.

POSTOPERATIVE CARE

In all but the very simple cases such patients should be ventilated for 48 hr after operation to minimize rises in intracranial pressure. Pupillary signs and intracranial pressure changes will give an indication of accumulation of an haematoma. If there is any doubt the wound should be re-explored. At the end of 48 hr ventilation the muscle relaxants are stopped and the patient assessed. Depending on the amount of postoperative brain swelling and the condition of the patient, mechanical ventilation is either discontinued or continued for another period. Antibiotics are used as is 'Decadron' and 'Aludrox'; prophylactic antiepileptic therapy may be given.

COMMON POSTOPERATIVE COMPLICATIONS

Brain swelling

The most common complication of missile injuries of the brain is also the most difficult to treat. Controlled ventilation with moderate hypocapnia is routinely used in this unit and its benefit is most easily seen in the early postinjury and postoperative stages. Every 24–48 hr the muscle relaxants are discontinued and the intracranial pressure observed during spontaneous respiration. The swelling may last for 10 – 12 days after severe high velocity injuries and a tracheostomy will be required if it is decided to continue ventilation for longer than 3 or 4 days.

Dexamethasone, 16 mg initially and 4 mg four hourly thereafter, is also used but its efficacy at this dose is debatable. Recent good reports of high dose dexamethasone therapy remain to be confirmed. Mannitol 1·5–2 mg/kg body weight has also been used but there is a danger of encouraging haematoma if used in the early postinjury period. After 48 hr, however, high dose Mannitol may be useful provided the severe potassium depletion is corrected with potassium supplements (up to 100 mEq/day).

Haematoma

This can be minimized with adequate attention to coagulation defects during massive transfusions and also adequate haemostasis at the time of surgery. Nevertheless this complication should be constantly guarded against and its treatment has already been mentioned.

Infections and brain abscesses

Adequate primary toilet will prevent this complication; so far in over 130 cases we have not had a brain abscess. An awareness of this complication and heavy antibiotic cover, including intrathecal antibiotics, will control any meningitis which develops.

Epilepsy

The risk of epilepsy following bullet injury to the brain is at least 35 per cent and in the more devastating injuries up to 60 per cent; so there is a good case for prophylactic anticonvulsants, such as phenytoin 200 mg three times daily, especially if the area around the motor strip is involved. Epilepsy early after injury may herald spreading cortical vein thrombosis, meningitis, a subdural collection of pus or intracerebral abscess and so these complications must be excluded.

Cerebrospinal fluid leaks

Otorrhoea and rhinorrhoea are common complications of tangential high velocity injuries due to the extensive fracturing of the base of the skull. Usually the fracturing in the base of the skull is so extensive that it is impractical to think of intracranial dural patching; instead the ear may be packed through the mastoid air cells with the help of the otologist, or the sphenoid air sinus may be packed through the nose. The appearance of a cerebrospinal fluid leak 10 days or so following injury may be an indication that hydrocephalus is developing due to basal adhesions. An air ventriculogram will confirm this and a thecoperitoneal shunt may relieve both the cerebrospinal fluid fistula and the hydrocephalus. If available, computerized tomography is preferable to air ventriculography.

Hydrocephalus

Unless debris has been left in the ventricular system the hydrocephalus is usually of a communicating variety, either due to adhesions around the tentorium secondary to the subarachnoid haemorrhage, or due to defective absorption with extensive damage around the arachnoid granulations. It is preferable to control this complication using a thecoperitoneal shunt in such patients, after outlining the cerebrospinal fluid pathways in an air ventriculogram or by computerized tomography.

Systemic complications

The main early postoperative complications are chest infections, inadequate respiratory function and haemorrhages from acute gastric erosions. Extensive physiotherapy and early rehabilitation are absolutely essential. Regular prophylactic antacids may minimize the chances of gastric haemorrhages, though their aetiology may be ischaemia not excess acid secretion.

Skull defect cranioplasty

When there is no further brain swelling and the wounds are well healed a cranioplasty may be considered. This ideal method for closure of these defects is a titanium cranioplasty. If small, these may be repaired using the titanium strips. However, if areas such as the eyebrow is involved or there is a large skull defect then a special plate preformed is cosmetically more useful. The original scalp flap is opened and the flap reflected. The adequate dural closure allows for a good layer dissection. The bone edges are identified and the plate screwed into place using self-tapping titanium screws of appropriate length, without disturbing the bone edge or dura.

Cortical vein thrombosis

This may often follow an apparently minor low velocity tangential injury to the vault. A recognition of the complication and conservative management is required. Usually the patient presents with small skin wounds, an intact skull and no neurological signs initially, but 12 – 24 hr later develops a progressive hemiparesis: Decadron should be prescribed.

CONCLUSION

The treatment of these devastating brain injuries is demanding in team work, resources and skills and, despite this, many will die. Nevertheless the good quality survival of many thus injured indicates that careful initial selection of patients for definitive treatment is worthwhile. Inadequate resuscitation, surgery or postoperative care minimize the patient's survival potential.

References

Byrnes, D. P., Crockard, H. A., Gordon, D. S. and Gleadhill, C. A. (1974). 'Penetrating craniocerebral missile injuries in civil disturbances in Northern Ireland.' *Br. J. Surg.* **61**, 169

Crockard, H. A. (1974). 'Bullet injuries of the brain.' *Ann. R. Coll. Surg. (Eng.)* **55**, 111

Crockard, H. A., Brown, F. D., Johns, L. M. and Mullan, S. (1977). 'An experimental cerebral missile injury model in primates.' *J. Neurosurg.* **46**, 776

Hammon, W. M. (1971). 'Analysis of 2187 consecutive penetrating wounds of the brain from Vietnam.' *J. Neurosurg.* **34**, 127

[*The illustrations for this Chapter on Missile Injuries of the Brain were drawn by Miss H. McIlhenny.*]

Fractures of the Skeleton of the Face

Michael N. Tempest, M.D., Ch.M., F.R.C.S.(Ed.)
Consultant Plastic Surgeon, Welsh Regional Plastic Surgery, Burns and Maxillo-Facial Centre,
St. Lawrence Hospital, Chepstow

SURGICAL ANATOMY

1

For practical purposes the skeletal structures of the face, in frontal view, can be divided into three regions.
(*1*) The upper third: formed by the frontal bone.
(*2*) The lower third: formed by the mandible.
(*3*) The middle third: formed by the nasal-malar-zygomatic complex (the maxillary bones, palatal shelves and pterygoid plates) all packed into the intervening space, which on lateral view has been likened to a wedge.

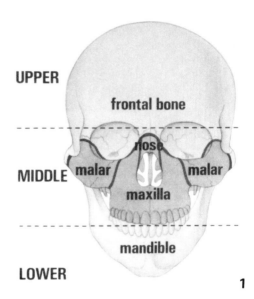

1

2

Unlike the upper and lower segments which are formed by a single strong bone, the middle third is composed of several intricate interlocking bones, some strong, some papery thin. Their structural alignment provides a set of buttresses that give excellent protection against vertical stress, but very little support against blows from the side or front. The close proximity of the eyes, nasal cavity, paranasal sinuses, cranial cavity, mouth and pharynx explain why serious complications may follow injuries to this part of the facial skeleton.

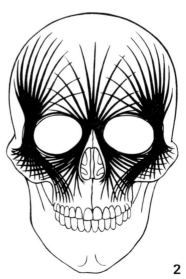

2

CLINICAL PRESENTATION

The pattern of skeletal injury may be perfectly obvious. However, local oedema and bruising may mask its extent and indeed its existence may pass unrecognized simply because it is not suspected or sought.

The bony damage may range from a simple undisplaced fracture of a single bone to gross comminution of several, sometimes so complex that it defies classification and is best described by our French colleagues as a 'disjonction cranio-faciale'. Most middle third fractures are open directly into the oral or nasal cavities or indirectly through one of the paranasal sinuses. The external tissues may be intact, contused, grossly shredded or even completely missing, as for example in gunshot wounds of the face.

PRE - OPERATIVE INVESTIGATIONS

Radiological

Good x-ray films are invaluable, particularly facial views taken with the occipitomental and 30° occipitomental projection. Poor films may be misleading and difficult to interpret accurately. Not all foreign bodies are radio-opaque and a 'clear' film does not necessarily exclude their presence. A chest film may sometimes reveal a missing tooth, a broken piece of dental plate or a bone fragment lying in the tracheobronchial tree.

Haematological

The patient's haemoglobin level and blood group should be known. Blood must be given to correct any deficit and further supplies must be available to replace any further blood lost during operation. In dark-skinned or Mediterranean peoples a screening test for sickling should be carried out.

Clinical

Patients admitted after major accidents may well have sustained other serious injuries that demand absolute priority of treatment. A severe facial injury is rarely, in itself, a threat to life *with two very important exceptions*: persistent uncontrollable bleeding and mechanical obstruction of the airway. The former may require an emergency operation to deal with the bleeding point, the latter may need endotracheal intubation and/or tracheotomy.

SURGICAL TREATMENT

As with any skeletal injury, the presence of a fracture is not necessarily an indication for any active treatment. Thus, fractures of the middle third of the face should be treated surgically only if the bones are displaced, producing disability or disfigurement. If the bony damage is complicated by extensive damage to the soft tissues, it is preferable to repair both the skeletal and soft tissue damage at the same time. The presence of an external wound does not necessarily demand immediate operation, but there are obviously times when a few well placed sutures may be required to replace some large skin flaps which are literally flapping and interfering with the management and comfort of the patient.

'Quick' operations under basal sedation or exploration under local anaesthesia in the accident department have no place in the proper management of these injuries. General anaesthesia through a cuffed endotracheal tube and with an effective nasopharyngeal pack in place, good lighting and an efficient suction apparatus in good working order are essential, minimum requirements. The operation may well prove to be complicated and lengthy. The theatre staff and the anaesthetist must be forewarned and prepared for this.

NASAL FRACTURES

The nasal anatomy must be restored to give a good airway through each nostril with the nasal bones symmetrically placed, leaning against the cartilaginous nasal septum and vomer, the septum sitting centrally in its groove on the upper surface of the hard palate.

Most nasal fractures are caused by lateral or frontal violence and show correspondingly different patterns of displacement.

3

'Lateral violence' usually produces a lateral displacement of both nasal bones and septum away from the source of injury.

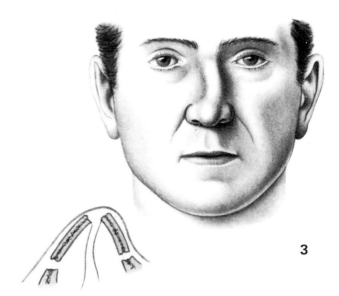

3

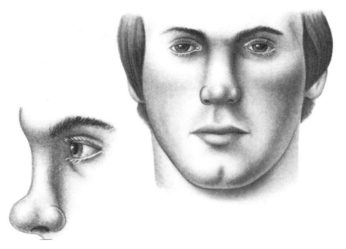

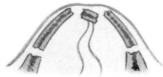

4

'Frontal violence' usually splays the nasal bones apart and the nasal septum is broken or buckled to give the typical 'saddle-nose' deformity on profile view.

4

5&6

The nasal bones may be so loose that digital manipulation and replacement is simple and may be all that is required, particularly with those injuries due to lateral violence. If simple digital pressure is ineffective, then Walsham's forceps are used to disimpact and replace the nasal bones. The unpadded rounded blade is passed upwards into the nostril, the outer, padded and flatter blade is laid externally alongside the nasolabial groove to grasp the nasal bone and the adjacent part of the frontal process of the maxilla. By a combination of rotation and leverage each nasal bone in turn is loosened and repositioned.

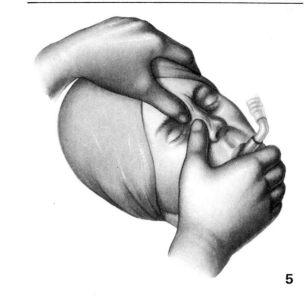

5

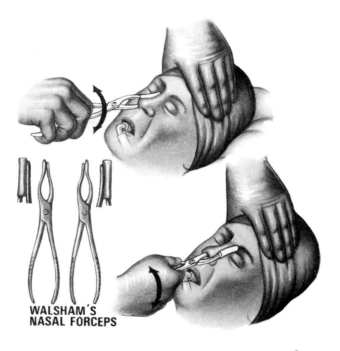

WALSHAM'S
NASAL FORCEPS

6

7&8

With most nasal fractures, and particularly with those caused by frontal violence, in which there is a saddle-nose deformity, the vomer and cartilaginous nasal septum must be lifted forwards and repositioned in the mid-line using the broad, flat-bladed, Asch's septal forceps. A nasal speculum is then passed to confirm the adequacy of the airway through each nostril and to allow blood clot and any other débris to be sucked out. Each nostril is now gently but firmly packed with ribbon gauze (0·5 inches in width) lightly impregnated with Whitehead's Varnish (Pig. Iodoform Co.). The neatest and tidiest way to pack any cavity is to place the gauze roll flat in a gallipot, soaked with the appropriate solution, and then withdraw the gauze from the *centre* of the roll. These nasal packs support the nasal structure from within, help obliterate dead space and so reduce the risk of a septal haematoma. Dry gauze should not be used for nasal packing as the stench soon becomes unbearable for patient and nurse alike. Similarly, tulle gras or paraffin gauze packs are smelly and have the added disadvantage of easily slipping out of the nostril.

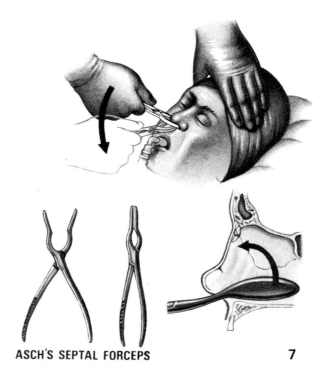

ASCH'S SEPTAL FORCEPS　　　　　7

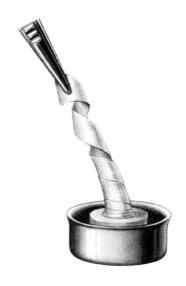

8

9 & 10

A small plaster of Paris splint is then applied externally, cut from a preformed pattern, using eight thicknesses of plaster bandage. The eyes are protected by a piece of tulle gras during the application of the wet plaster slab. After it has set, the splint is trimmed and fixed in place by several strips of adhesive strapping after cleaning and drying the skin of the forehead and cheek with a gauze swab soaked in ether. A small gauze pad is then placed under the nose to absorb any blood or exudate. The nasal packs are removed on the fifth to seventh day after softening the exposed ends with liquid paraffin: the plaster splint is removed after 10–12 days.

Occasionally the nasal bones may be extremely unstable and show a tendency to 'fall back' into the nasal cavity once the steadying finger or instrument is removed. In these circumstances the bones may be stabilized by:

(1) Direct interosseous wiring of the nasal bones to one another, the frontal bone or the adjacent maxilla.

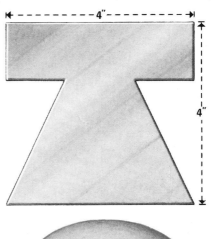

9

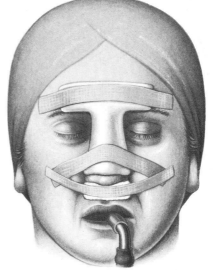

10

11

(2) The use of a pair of sutures of stainless steel wire or nylon passed through the nose on a straight needle and tied over a small pad or lead plate placed externally on the side of the nose. The lead-plate technique is not without complications for the plates may produce pressure necrosis of the skin and the sutures may leave very unpleasant stitch marks. A more satisfactory method of fixation is to introduce two straight needles across the nose through the external plaster splint whilst it is still wet and malleable, and before the nasal packs have been inserted. Two stainless steel wires can then be drawn through the nose and tied externally on the plaster of Paris splint.

If nasal fractures are seen within the first 2 or 3 weeks of the injury the simple manipulative methods mentioned above may be feasible and successful. If not, and with all nasal fractures seen late, refracture should be carried out along the lines of an elective corrective rhinoplasty.

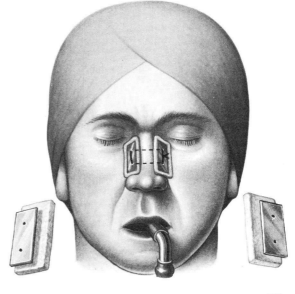

11

FRACTURES OF THE MALAR-ZYGOMATIC COMPLEX

The external Gillies-Kilner approach is the method of choice for the surgical correction of those fractures of the zygomatic arch and malar bone which are displaced and producing symptoms or disfigurement.

12a,b&c

A short oblique incision is made inside the hair-line in the temporal region taking care to avoid the superficial temporal artery. The incision is carried down to and through the temporal fascia to display the fibres of the temporalis muscle. As the temporalis fascia is attached to the upper border of the zygomatic arch, any instrument passed downwards and medially through the fascial slit will pass beneath the zygomatic arch. It can be pushed more medially still to lie underneath the malar buttress or may even enter the maxillary sinus itself with certain very comminuted fractures of the middle third of the face. Using a Bristow elevator as a lever (or even a strong flat instrument like a pair of Mayo scissors) the depressed zygomatic arch or malar complex can be lifted into place, using the fingers of the other hand to control and check the position of the fragments. Quite often these fractures can be reduced with a satisfying and audible click. The skin wound only is closed, the fascial layer is left unsutured.

Before closing the skin it is important to ensure that the corrected position of the fracture is stable; this is done by gentle but firm pressure over the cheek after releasing pressure on the proximal end of the lever. If the bone is unstable, direct interosseous wiring may be required. The most common site of instability is usually the frontomalar suture, but the infra-orbital margin or the zygomatic arch itself may also require open reduction and wiring.

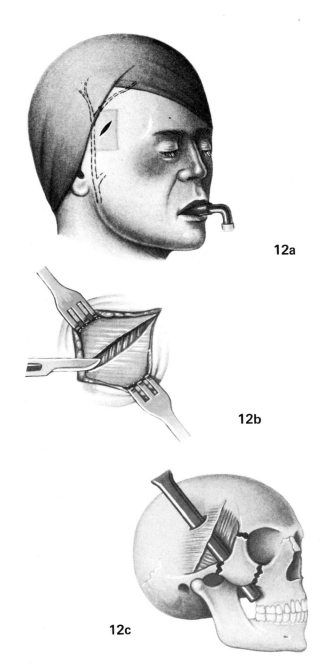

12a

12b

12c

13a,b&c

With comminuted fractures of the malar bone, the maxillary sinus and the orbital floor it may be necessary to supplement the replacement achieved by Gillies' method with a gauze pack placed in the maxillary sinus. The wall of the sinus is exposed by an incision in the upper buccal sulcus, the soft tissues and periosteum are dissected off the bone and an opening is made as low down as possible into the sinus through its thin anterior wall. Very often there is a visible crack in the bone, in which case the cavity is entered through the fracture line. Blood clot is sucked out of the sinus and the surgeon's index or little finger is then introduced into the cavity. By sweeping the digit round the cavity it is possible to detect any irregularity in its wall and to 'iron out' any protruding bony fragments, particularly in the roof (or orbital floor). The cavity is then packed with ribbon gauze soaked in Whitehead's Varnish. Its capacity is very deceptive: the adult maxillary sinus can hold as much as 12 feet of 1 inch ribbon gauze or 6 feet of 2 inch gauze. The opening in the antral wall is left open with a tiny piece of the pack protruding in the upper buccal sulcus. The pack is left in place for at least 2 weeks, and can safely be left for very much longer.

It is easy to 'overpack' the sinus and a postoperative x-ray film should be made to confirm that the fragments are properly in place and that the pack is indeed inside the sinus. If there is displacement of the level of the pupil and the patient has diplopia that was *not* present before the operation, then some of the pack should be removed.

Warning

The surgical correction of a malar-zygomatic fracture is not always a quick operation done with the proverbial 'flick of the wrist followed by an audible click'. Disimpaction of malar fractures may produce brisk nasal bleeding and it is for this reason that this operation should always be done with general anaesthesia and with a cuffed endotracheal tube in place. Bleeding may also occur rapidly into the orbital cavity. Unless this is recognized and dealt with promptly, increasing tension within the orbit may produce temporary or even permanent blindness. Similarly, when replacing some of the very comminuted fractures of the orbital floor, it is possible to dislodge a spicule of bone into the orbit and cause direct damage to the optic nerve or the associated vessels with resulting temporary or permanent blindness.

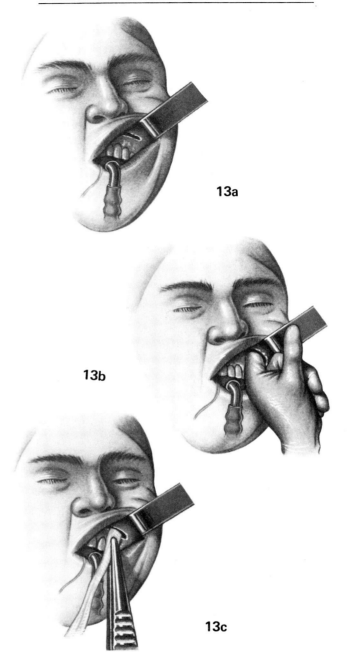

13a

13b

13c

Some oral surgeons recommend elevation of malar-zygomatic fractures by an intra-oral approach, but compared with the external Gillies' technique it is a clumsy and inefficient manoeuvre. An even more questionable procedure is the insertion of an inflatable balloon (e.g. Foley catheter) into the sinus to replace severely comminuted fractures. The technical difficulties are considerable: the risk of damage to the balloon is great, both whilst it is *in situ* and particularly during its removal, and the method has very little to commend it.

Direct wiring of facial bones

As with all operations calling for accurate osteo-synthesis, adequate exposure is essential. The bone ends are identified and approximated. Small drill holes are made in each fragment using either a dental hand piece attached to the electric motor, a pencil-like battery-driven drill or, if nothing else is available, a small hand drill. These instruments, particularly the first two mentioned, allow finger tip precision in drilling and reduce the risk of splintering the bone fragments or breaking the drill.

14, 15 & 16

Stainless steel wire (0·015 gauge) is the most suitable material for direct wiring. It is somewhat soft and springy and each short length that will be used should be stretched between two strong artery forceps for several seconds to take up this 'slack' before it is inserted into the drill holes. The wire ends should then be pulled tight after each twist to give maximum compression of the fragments at the fracture site. A simple and efficient twisting device can be made from an old pair of artery forceps by shortening and blunting the blades.

The steel wire is then cut, the protruding ends tucked against the bone and the wound closed in layers using fine suture material (4/0 chromic catgut for the sub-cutaneous tissues and 6/0 nylon for the skin).

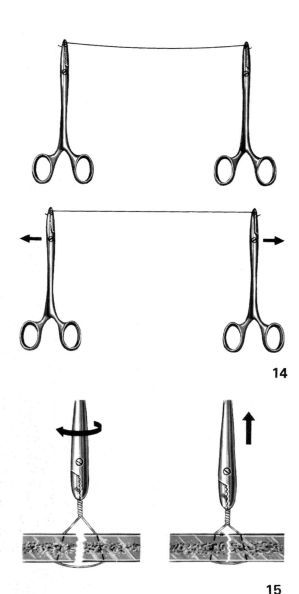

14

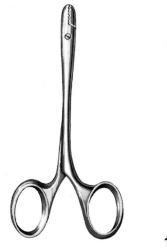

15

16

FRACTURES OF THE MIDDLE THIRD

Fractures of the middle third of the face may be relatively simple, localized injuries involving the alveolus and a few adjacent teeth; the palatal processes may be split down the mid-line and separated to produce a defect not unlike a cleft palate or alternatively the maxillary segments may show an extensive horizontal fracture line (a low-level, Le Fort type I fracture).

17a & b

In the more severe and complicated lesions, there may be associated fractures of the malar-zygomatic arch complex, the nasal bones, maxillary and frontal sinuses, orbital floor, ethmoid region and the base of the skull in the anterior cranial fossa. These are the complicated Le Fort type II and III fractures, which often show the typical backward and downward displacement of the bony fragments, which accounts for the facial flattening, the derangement of the dental occlusion, the gagging of the teeth and (at least with the high-level fractures) the escape of cerebrospinal fluid from the nose. These fractures may be solidly impacted as a 'wedge' or alternatively extremely mobile so that the whole face can be literally pushed from side to side — a true 'disjonction cranio-faciale'.

Since these fractures may involve the teeth and the patient's dental occlusion may be grossly deranged it is important to have dental help to decide on the viability of the teeth, the feasibility of dental conservation, the restoration of normal dental occlusion and the choice of the most suitable method to control the bone fragments and immobilize the jaws. It cannot be emphasized too strongly that the complicated cases should be referred to a plastic and maxillofacial unit as soon as possible. If the patient cannot be moved to the specialist unit, then the specialist team should come to the patient.

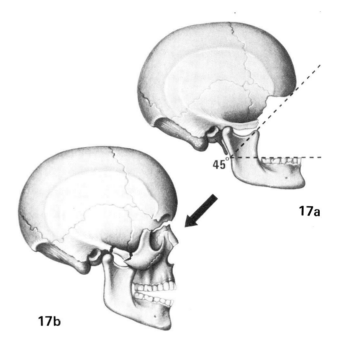

45°

17a

17b

18 & 19

In the absence of any immediate dental help the surgeon should confine his attention to:

(*1*) removing all débris and useless fragments of bone: closing the oral mucosa and approximating the gingivae with 4/0 black silk sutures;

(*2*) removing hopelessly loose and damaged teeth;

(*3*) fixing the remaining teeth which are displaced but viable with eyelet wires or simple arch bands;

(*4*) providing temporary fixation between the maxilla and mandible in those cases in which the mandible and maxilla can be brought together easily in correct occlusion without major disimpaction manoeuvres.

In the management of the complicated fractures of the middle third of the face the three essential steps are:

(*1*) To disimpact and replace the middle third of the face and then fix the maxilla in correct occlusion with the mandible, sandwiching the maxillary segments between the mandible and the skull. *In those cases in which the mandible is also broken, this bone must be stabilized first*, if need be by open operation, direct wiring, pinning or plating.

The maxilla may be fixed to the skull by zygomaticofrontal wiring; a box-frame using pins and connecting rods; cap splints cemented to the teeth fixed by connecting rods to a halo frame or to a plaster of Paris headcap; or, finally, in the edentulous patient, the fitting of Gunning's splints, which are then fastened to the halo frame or plaster of Paris headcap by connecting rods. References are given at the end of the chapter to well-illustrated accounts of the intricacies of these techniques.

(*2*) To reduce the superstructure of the face (the malar-zygomatic complex) and fix these structures by direct wiring or packing the maxillary sinus.

(*3*) To replace and fix the nasal fragments.

Leakage of cerebrospinal liquid

High-level fractures of the middle third may be associated with damage to the cribriform plate, dural tears in the anterior cranial fossa, loss of the sense of smell and leakage of cerebrospinal fluid either through the nose externally or into the nasopharynx. It is not always easy to diagnose with certainty the escape of cerebrospinal fluid during the early days following severe facial injuries, but a trickle of watery liquid, often increased in rate by flexing the head, combined with loss of the sense of smell, is strong circumstantial evidence of a dural tear. Often the flow of cerebrospinal fluid stops quite dramatically after correction and stabilization of the fracture, but unfortunately this happy event does not necessarily mean that the

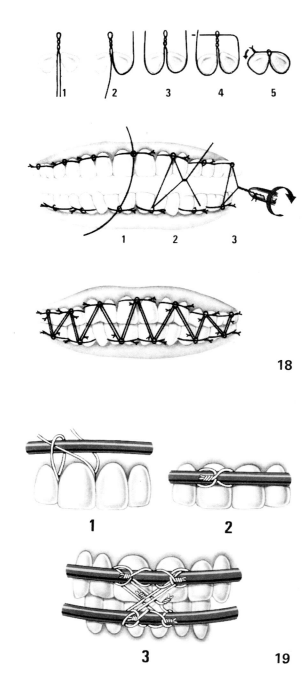

18

19

dural tear will heal completely or that the risk of subsequent intracranial aerocele or meningitis has passed. These patients should all be given prophylactic therapy with a sulphonamide preparation (sulphadiazine 2 g statim followed by 1 g 6 hourly for 5 days or longer) combined with penicillin 1 mega unit daily for the same period. A neurosurgical opinion should be sought on the need for any exploration of the frontal dural defect and the correct timing of its repair, particularly if the cerebrospinal fluid leak persists or recurs after a period of remission.

Damage to the lacrimal apparatus and the canthal ligaments

With certain high-level fractures and comminuted naso-ethmoid injuries, the inner canthal ligaments and the lacrimal apparatus may be displaced and damaged, producing gross widening of the interpupillary distance. If this condition is not treated in the early days after the accident it may be extremely difficult to repair the damage later. The key to the treatment of this condition is early exploration and fixation of the naso-ethmoid fractures by direct wiring using two transfixion wires which, as they are twisted on each side of the nose, exert compression and draw the bones and inner canthal ligaments closer to the mid-line. In certain cases it may be necessary to resuture or re-attach the inner canthal ligaments or to attempt to reconstruct the nasolacrimal duct. This can be a very complicated little exercise but is well worthwhile (Stranc, 1970).

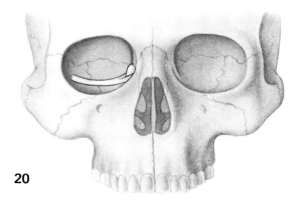

20

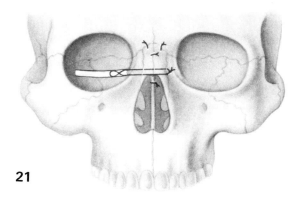

21

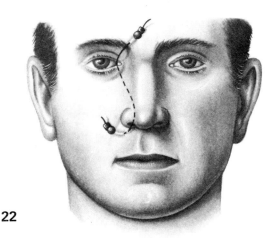

22

20,21&22

Most of the fibres of the inner canthal ligament are attached to the anterior lacrimal crest, on the medial wall of the orbit and pass in front of the lacrimal sac which lies in a bony recess from which the naso-lacrimal duct passes downwards into the nasal cavity.

If the inner canthal ligament has been severed or is detached from its bony insertion it must be sutured or re-attached. This is best done by inserting a figure-of-8 stainless steel wire suture into the divided end of the ligament: the two ends of wire are then passed across the nasal bony complex (if necessary through small drill holes) and tied against the opposite nasal bone at the correct height. If the nasal bones themselves are broken and displaced, these bone fragments must be stabilized first by interosseous wires and additional wires to fix the fragments to the frontal bone in the glabellar region.

If there is disruption of the canaliculi and the naso-lacrimal duct, continuity of the lumen must be restored by suture using fine 6/0 nylon or Dexon sutures. It is often possible to insert a length of monofilament nylon through the canaliculi, via the puncta in the eyelids, into the lacrimal sac and then pass these strands down into the nose to act as an internal splint. The upper end of the nylon 'splint' can be attached to the skin in the region of the eyebrow, the lower end to the base of the columella. This will minimize the risk of its being accidentally pulled out. The nylon strand should be left in place for at least 3 weeks.

BLOW-OUT FRACTURES OF THE ORBIT

This type of injury is caused by direct injury to the orbit, usually by a small flying object such as a tennis ball, which strikes the orbit, suddenly raises the intra-orbital tension and shatters the orbital floor, leaving the orbital margins intact. It can be easily missed in the early stages because of the intense local swelling, but once this subsides the diagnosis is easy to confirm.

23 & 24

If it is desired to explore the orbital floor, an incision is made through the skin, orbicularis muscle and periosteum at the level of the infra-orbital margin. Further dissection is carried out by lifting the periosteum off the bony fragments to display the orbital floor. The bony rim of the orbit can then be stabilized by one or two fine stainless steel interosseous wires. The orbital floor itself can usually be gently replaced and stabilized by an antral pack, but if this is impossible and there is a localized 'blow-out' fracture then a thin sheet of Silastic or nylon film can be laid on the orbital floor. The wound should be closed accurately in layers using 4/0 chromic catgut for the muscular layer and 6/0 nylon for the skin. After any intra-orbital dissection of this kind it is important to watch for any postoperative bleeding and to re-explore the wound at once at the first sign of trouble.

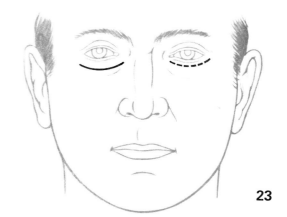

23

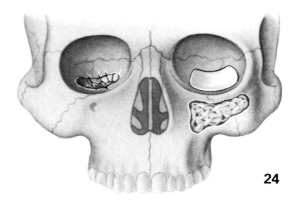

24

POSTOPERATIVE CARE

Care of the suture line

Crusts should not be allowed to form or remain for long on any facial suture line because they invite infection and will help to produce untidy and permanent stitch marks. Suture lines should be cleaned regularly and all débris removed. They can then be kept dry or alternatively a thin layer of Polyfax can be applied. Sutures should be removed as early as possible in a good light with sharp, fine instruments. The suture line should then be supported with Steristrip tape or micropore tape after cleaning and drying the adjacent skin with ether.

Danger of respiratory obstruction

In the postoperative care of any patient who is still unconscious and who has had his jaws wired together and fixed by external connecting rods, a pair of wire cutters and a box-spanner must always be provided at the bedside in case of sudden and unexpected respiratory obstruction by vomiting, bleeding or oedema. It may even be wise to fasten the wire cutters to the head of the bed by a chain to prevent their 'appropriation' by staff or visitors who may be souvenir hunters and cannot resist a good bargain. It is always safer in moments of crisis to cut the intermaxillary wires than to do a tracheotomy. It is also much quicker.

Intra-oral hygiene

The care of the mouth begins at the end of the operation, when all blood clot and adherent dried blood should be removed or washed away with plenty of water. Then mouth washes and cleaning of the teeth are required several times a day, particularly after meals. If splints have been used to achieve intermaxillary fixation they should be gently cleaned along with all the intra-oral connecting wires and arch bands. Unless this is done, the mouth can soon become a stinking cavity with unpleasant and serious consequences.

Feeding of patients with jaw injuries

The feeding of these patients, particularly if the jaws are wired together is important and requires a good deal of ingenuity. The swallowing of liquid food, prepared by a liquidiser, is usually no problem, but the diet can become monotonous unless some imagination and good sense is used by the nurse or dietician who makes up the feed. The patient can usually feed himself with straws or plastic suction tubes, but will often prefer to help himself with a spoon and cup. After every feed, the mouth must be thoroughly cleaned to avoid food débris collecting alongside the teeth and intra-oral fixation devices.

LATER SURGICAL RECONSTRUCTION

In many patients who have received skeletal injuries of the middle third of the face prompt and efficient primary treatment may be all that is ever required. However, in the complicated cases, particularly those with a good deal of soft tissue damage and destruction, further reconstructive surgical work is usually required. The timing of this work and its detailed planning and execution are the very essence of plastic surgery. Its possibilities and its limitations must be explained to the patient (and the family) in language that they can understand. The widespread belief that plastic surgeons are 'invisible menders' has been promoted so assiduously in the glossy magazines and the popular press that the management of the patient has become almost as important and as difficult as the management of the wound.

References

Gillies, H. D., Kilner, T. P. and Stone, D. (1927). 'Fractures of the malar zygomatic compound with the description of a new X-ray position'. *Br. J. Surg.* **14,** 651
Killey, H. C. (1971). *Fractures of the Middle Third of the Facial Skeleton.* Bristol: John Wright
McGregor, I. A. (1972). *Fundamental Techniques of Plastic Surgery,* 5th Edition. Edinburgh: Churchill Livingstone
Rowe, N. L. and Killey, H. C. (1976). *Fractures of the Facial Skeleton,* 3rd Edition. Edinburgh: Churchill Livingstone
Stranc, M. F. (1970). 'Primary treatment of naso-ethomoid injuries with increased intercanthal distance.' *Br. J. plast. Surg.* **23,** 8
Stranc, M. F. (1970). 'The pattern of lacrimal injuries in naso-ethmoid fractures.' *Br. J. plast. Surg.* **23,** 339

[*The illustrations for this Chapter on Fractures of the Skeleton of the Face were drawn by Mr. M. J. Courtney.*]

Injuries of the Face, Nose, Pinna and Lips

Magdi S. Kodsi, M.D., F.A.C.S.
Assistant Professor of Plastic Surgery, Temple University Health and Sciences Center, Philadelphia

and

Lester M. Cramer, M.D., F.A.C.S.
Professor of Plastic Surgery, Temple University Health and Sciences Center, Philadelphia

INTRODUCTION

The management of facial injuries has to take into account any other injuries of the head and neck as well as those of the body as a whole.

Ensuring a patent airway, replenishing the circulation and the proper assessment and management of concomitant cervical injury are vitally necessary.

The main objective in the surgical repair of soft tissue injuries of the face is to obtain primary healing of the wound. The stage has to be set for the various tissue layers to meet anatomically at the site of injury with minimal interposed foreign body and foreign tissue. This will provide the least amount of tissue reaction and so reduce deformity and scarring. The less the inflammatory reaction the less the final scarring and the more acceptable the result.

The extent of inflammatory reaction is related to:

(*1*) mechanism of injury;
(*2*) contamination;
(*3*) tissue handling;
(*4*) tension of closure;
(*5*) delayed healing resulting in extended epithelialization and granulation tissue;
(*6*) age of injury;
(*7*) age of patient;
(*8*) general condition of patient.

The wounding force causes a localized injury. The effect on the surrounding tissues of the spread of that force contributes to the extent of the immediate reaction and to the quality of healing of the wound.

Clean cuts by sharp objects do little damage apart from the division of the tissues but avulsion injuries result in a flap which has been subjected to a tearing force, with more or less damage affecting most of the flap. Although the flap usually survives it is likely to show a certain amount of oedema and contusion.

High speed accidents can cause bursting injuries in which multiple flaps result from the spread of the force through the tissues and each of the flaps usually has sustained additional damage.

Injuries by low velocity missiles do not cause the extensive surrounding destruction seen with wounds caused by high velocity missiles. Shotgun wounds at close range cause massive destruction and often loss of tissue and they may also embed in devitalized tissues the wad, which may be contaminated by clostridia. As the range increases the degree of damage diminishes to painful but perhaps harmless peppering.

Severe crushing injuries cause more extensive damage to the surrounding tissues and the greater devitalization leads to more scarring.

Dogbites cause puncture wounds, laceration or flaps. The inflammatory reaction to such injuries is increased by the inevitable bacterial contamination. Cleansing and conservative toilet aided by extensive irrigation, and the abundant blood supply of the face promote primary wound healing. Puncture wounds that trap salivary organisms are prone to more intense reaction, even if sound surgical practices are adopted. Systemic antibiotics are indicated. Rabies is a rare disease but its possibility must not be ignored, even though vaccination is very seldom indicated.

With wounds with extensive loss of skin, the need for an immediate flap or other grafting is based on:

(1) the degree of contamination of the wound;

(2) the viability of the base of the wound.

Where bone or cartilage is exposed and cannot be covered by soft tissues immediate cover by a flap is required, but the periosteum or perichondrium will accept a free skin graft.

Contamination at the time of injury is unavoidable and the sooner the wound is treated the better. Wounds closed over fewer than 10^5 organisms per gram of tissue usually do not suppurate but heal with little inflammatory reaction. The longer the interval between injury and surgical repair the more the bacteria multiply and the higher their concentration in the wound. However, if a wound cannot be treated promptly, because of associated injuries, the good blood supply of the face allows wounds to be closed primarily even after 1 or 2 days.

Associated injuries such as occur with crush and blast, produce more devitalized tissue with consequently greater likelihood of infection.

Tissues should be handled delicately at the time of toilet and repair. Copious irrigation and adequate haemostasis have to be assured, keeping the amount of surgical injury to a minimum. Closing the wound under tension may lead to strangulation and additional death of tissue. Obstruction of the upper airway with facial injuries is most frequently caused by blood, secretion, loss of support of the tongue, or aspiration of loose teeth. The airway must be cleared at once by removing debris from the pharynx, supporting the mandible, putting in an oral airway and, when feasible, turning the patient semiprone with due attention to the possibility that the cervical spine has been injured.

Clearing the airway may alleviate hypoxia, thus allaying apprehension and diminishing bleeding.

The specialized structures, bony and soft tissues of the face, require special evaluation. The distinguishing features of fractures of the mandible, maxilla, sinuses, nose and orbits, dental arches and teeth must be looked for and recorded (see Chapter on 'Fractures of the Skeleton of the Face', pages 126–139). The facial nerve, the parotid duct, the canaliculi of the eyelids, the canthal ligaments and the facial muscles can be at risk and must be examined and any injury recorded.

In examining the wound, one has to determine the depth of the injury, i.e. whether partial or the full thickness of skin or mucous membrane has been affected, or whether a through-and-through injury exists. If there is underlying skeletal injury it usually communicates with the wound. Having assessed the extent of the injury, and once the condition of the patient allows, the type of anaesthetic and its mode of administration have to be chosen carefully.

Although preservation of life is the foremost consideration, once the patient's condition allows, the wounds require the utmost care. A common error with severely injured patients is that inadequate local care is given and that disabling disfigurement occurs later.

PARTIAL THICKNESS WOUNDS

CLEAN SUPERFICIAL ABRASIONS

These are best treated by cleansing the skin with a bland antiseptic solution and the abrasion itself with sterile saline. Apply one layer of a water-miscible petrolatum gauze and add dry sterile dressings and compression.

1a & b

CLEAN DEEPER ABRASIONS

These are cleansed as the superficial ones above, following which (*a*) sterile porous paper tape is applied across the wound or; (*b*) fine sutures are inserted in the depth of the injury so as to avoid a depression when the shallow gaping wound heals.

TATTOOING INJURIES (INGRAINED FOREIGN MATTER)

2, 3 & 4

These injuries cause marks that are extremely difficult to correct later. With the fresh injury, the embedded dirt is excised and the irregular surfaces are abraded surgically, using field block anaesthesia containing epinephrine. Embedded foreign particles are removed by:
  (*a*) a brush with fine bristles;
  (*b*) a knife that can be used to excise the embedded dirt if this cannot, as is often the case, be gently scraped out;
  (*c*) a dermabrader;
  (*d*) a combination of the above.

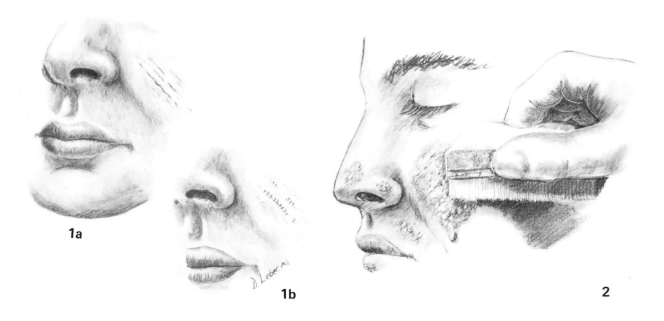

1a

1b

2

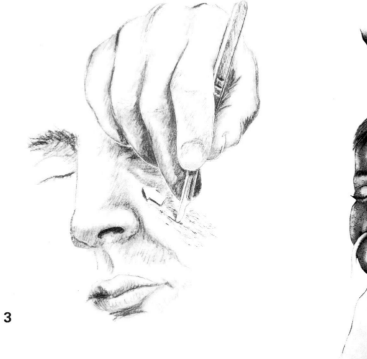

3

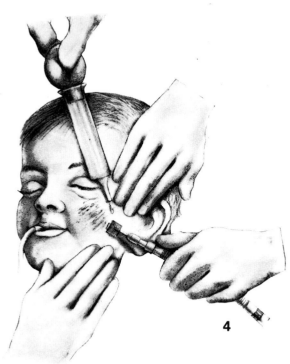

4

DEEPER INJURIES WITHOUT LOSS OF SUBSTANCE

5

Wounds running perpendicular to the lines of tension (against the grain) result in scars which hypertrophy and are objectionable. Scars running parallel to the lines of tension (with the grain) are the least noticeable.

6-9

To obtain optimum alignment of the key anatomical points when local anaesthesia is used, nerve blocks are indicated. When this is not possible a field block should be used so as not to distort the key points. Careful placing of the anaesthetic solution 0·1 ml at a time enables one to avoid distortion of the anatomical key points. *Illustrations 7, 8* and *9* show methods of nerve block of the infra-orbital distribution, the mental nerve distribution and field block for the pinna.

10, 11 & 12

The more extensive the surfaces of the wound, the more scar will form within the wound and the more contracture will occur. This is particularly true of bevelled wounds.

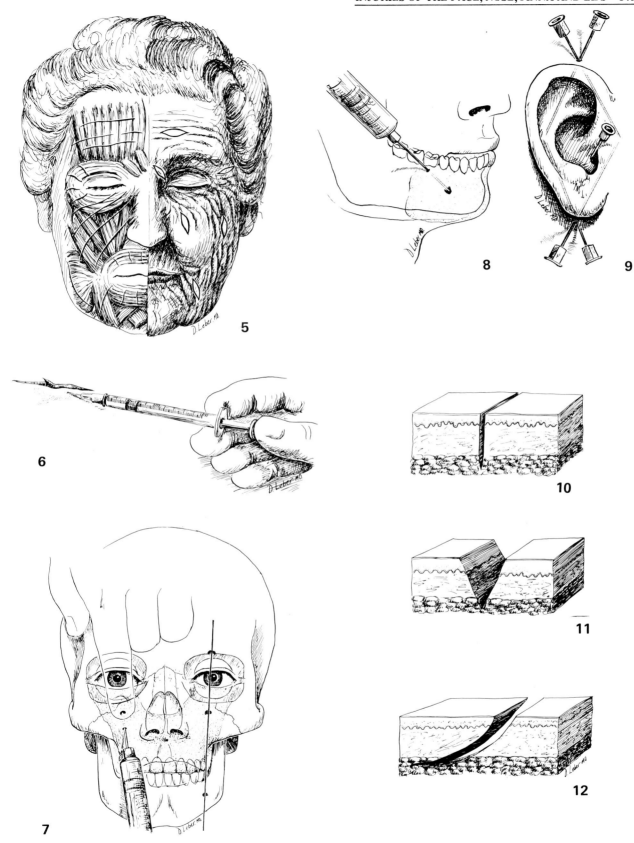

5

6

7

8

9

10

11

12

CLEAN PERPENDICULAR CUTS OF THE FACE

Cleansing the wound, adequate haemostasis, obliterating dead space and direct approximation layer by layer using the key anatomical landmarks of the region for alignment is the procedure of choice. Re-approximation of the delicate muscles of facial expression is essential in order to avoid dimples. The retraction that causes a gaping wound can give a misleading impression of loss of substance. As the interval between injury and surgical repair increases the bacterial count will increase. For wounds more than about 6 hr old systemic antibiotics are indicated and more vigorous irrigation of the wound is needed.

13-18

The repair should be done in layers with absorbable sutures on the mucosa and in the depth of the wound and close co-aptation of the subcutaneous tissue with the minimum amount of sutures and closure of the skin with fine 5/0 or 6/0 gauge non-absorbable, bland, monofilament sutures. Sutures must not be tied too tightly because of local swelling of the wound. Skin sutures should be placed 2–4 mm from the wound margin. Inversion of the edges is avoided by placing the sutures so that the distance YY is slightly longer than the distance XX. The sutures are removed at 1 week. It is undesirable to remove properly placed sutures too early. The most frequent cause of cross-hatching is a tight suture, but some cross-hatching may occur even with properly placed and tied sutures. It can be avoided only by using subcuticular pull-out sutures. These can be left much longer and are our first choice whenever possible. When sutures are removed early, sterile micropore paper tape should be applied to the wound as shown.

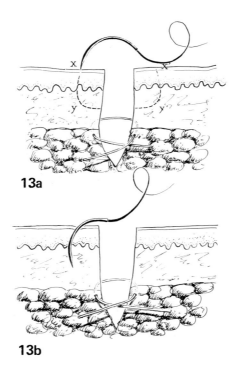

13a

13b

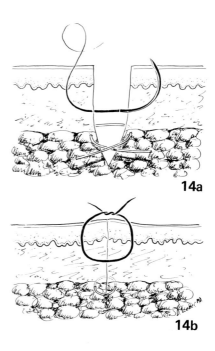

14a

14b

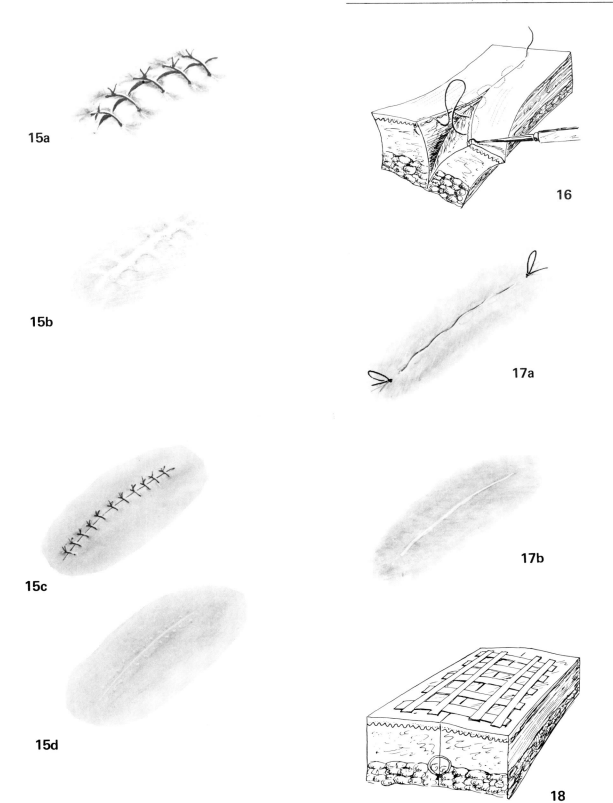

15a

15b

15c

15d

16

17a

17b

18

WOUNDS WITH IRREGULAR EDGES

19

Sharp, conservative trimming (1–2 mm) while keeping the skin taut should convert a ragged edge to a straight one. Sometimes an irregularity in the lacerated edge should be preserved because it can offer an advantage in special situations. For example, over the rim of the pinna or at the nostril's edge matching irregularities may be used to achieve a tongue-in-groove closure which could prevent notching.

BEVELLED INJURIES

20

Oblique sliced skin edges often result in step deformities; slicing, U-shaped wounds leave a semicircular scar which contracts to cause a very noticeable step and bulge. Fragments of glass from broken windshields frequently cause multiple small flaps. Special discretion is needed to decide whether to convert them to perpendicular wounds or to approximate them by accurate suturing.

21

Excision of a narrow margin can convert an oblique edge to one that is perpendicular to the surface. More skill is required for proper approximation of bevelled edges. When excision of a margin has been decided upon, one needs to be careful not to produce more tension or otherwise make the closure more difficult.

The application of a pressure bandage following repair of bevelled wounds helps to hold the undercut wound surfaces together.

The face has such a good blood supply that all tissues that might survive should be saved. Partially avulsed facial tissue should be retained if it has even a small pedicle because it may survive and be useful in any later reconstruction.

Scars must be given time to flatten and fade after a worrying stage of becoming pink and prominent.

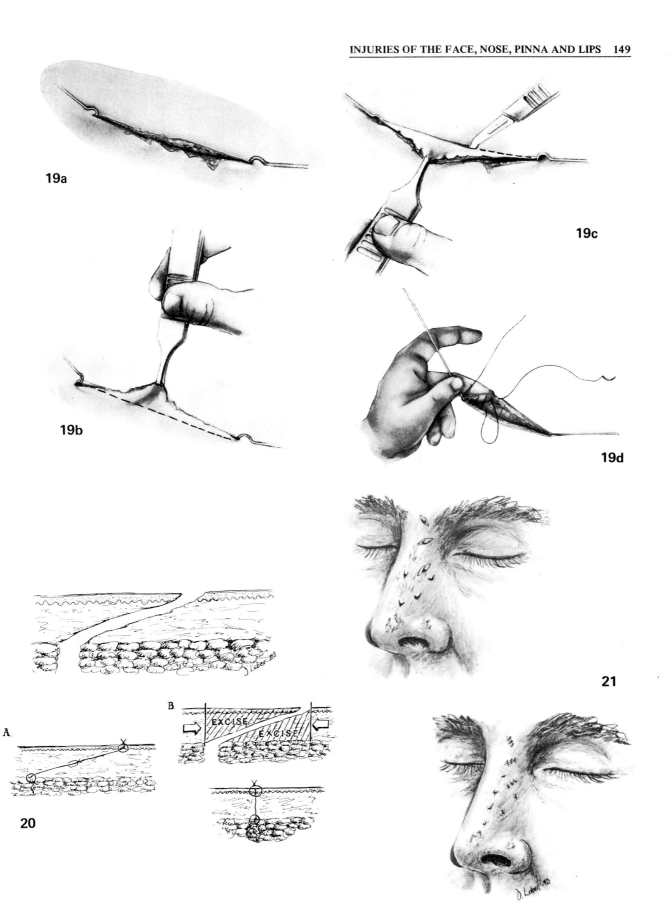

19a

19b

19c

19d

20

A.

B.

21

U - SHAPED FLAPS

22

The scar of a U-shaped flap is particularly liable to step deformity that is frequently accentuated by swelling of the flap. When small and occurring in a favourable relationship to the lines of tension, excision and primary closure should be considered. When larger, the initial approach should be proper approximation as with clean perpendicular cuts. Later revision by Z-plasty will be indicated.

When overlying the nasal skeleton, a mild nasal hump will make a step deformity much more evident so that revision will have to include lowering of the underlying skeletal framework.

INCISED WOUNDS OF THE NOSE

23-26

With cuts of the nose the nostril's rim must be accurately restored and the underlying cartilages, vestibular skin and nasal septum repaired accurately in layers.

The following stages should be adopted.

(1) Identify the extent of underlying skeletal involvement.

(2) Align cartilages and septum.

(3) Approximate mucosa in one layer, cartilages in a second layer, muscles in a third layer and skin in a fourth layer.

(4) Align the rim by guide sutures. Approximate vestibular skin. Approximate the external skin. When a nasal fracture has been reduced at the same operation, or when intranasal flaps have occurred, petrolatum gauze packing will help to splint the nose and a light plaster splint externally is used unless extensive contusion jeopardizes the vitality of the skin. If there has been loss of less than about 1 cm from the nostril's rim in an average adult, it should be treated by approximating the wound edges. If much more than 1 cm has been lost, immediate reconstruction with a flap is indicated. A composite graft is used for defects measuring $1 \cdot 0 - 1 \cdot 2$ cm. If the tip of the nose has been damaged but the perichondrium remains, a skin graft can be applied primarily. If much skin has been lost from the bridge of the nose a graft should be considered.

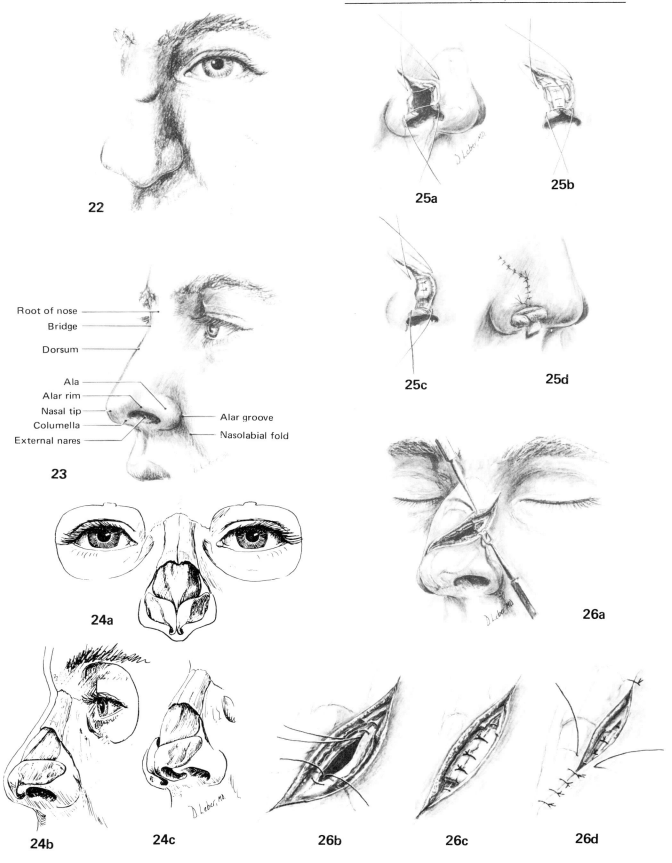

22

25a

25b

Root of nose
Bridge
Dorsum
Ala
Alar rim
Nasal tip
Columella
External nares
Alar groove
Nasolabial fold

23

25c

25d

24a

26a

24b

24c

26b

26c

26d

SLICING INJURIES OF THE PINNA

27,28&29

Align helical rim.

Align antihelix.

If a flap has been raised, it should be trimmed sparingly, replaced and approximated in layers with the cartilage as a separate layer. Apply water-miscible petrolatum gauze on both sides of the ear and dress with a contour dressing that is changed at 48 hr. Redress in the same way for at least 10 days.

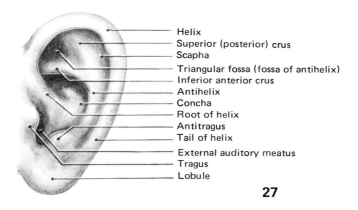

Helix
Superior (posterior) crus
Scapha
Triangular fossa (fossa of antihelix)
Inferior anterior crus
Antihelix
Concha
Root of helix
Antitragus
Tail of helix
External auditory meatus
Tragus
Lobule

27

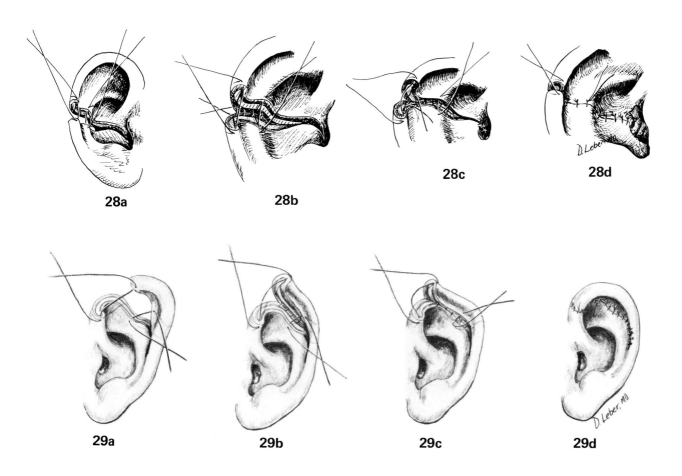

28a   **28b**   **28c**   **28d**

29a   **29b**   **29c**   **29d**

LACERATIONS WITH LOSS OF SUBSTANCE

30 & 31

When the wound leaves a defect the best treatment is to make the appropriate flap. Short of that, if the defect is equal in all components, approximation of the medial skin to the lateral skin should be the objective. This will allow earlier and easier reconstruction of the ear by the appropriate flaps in due course.

When loss of skin is more extensive on one side than on the other and the cartilage has been denuded of its perichondrium, burying the exposed cartilage in the nearby scalp will preserve the residual framework to provide the initial stage for reconstruction with a flap. If the missing segment is available it should be thoroughly rinsed in saline and kept at 4°C and moist in antibiotic solution, but not frozen. Its appearance and condition will determine whether the skin should be abraded and the whole segment buried in the postauricular region or subcutaneously in an area of the body less subject to injury. When the overlying skin of the missing fragment has been extensively damaged, the cartilaginous portion should be separated meticulously from the skin and banked in the appropriate postauricular region or subcutaneously elsewhere.

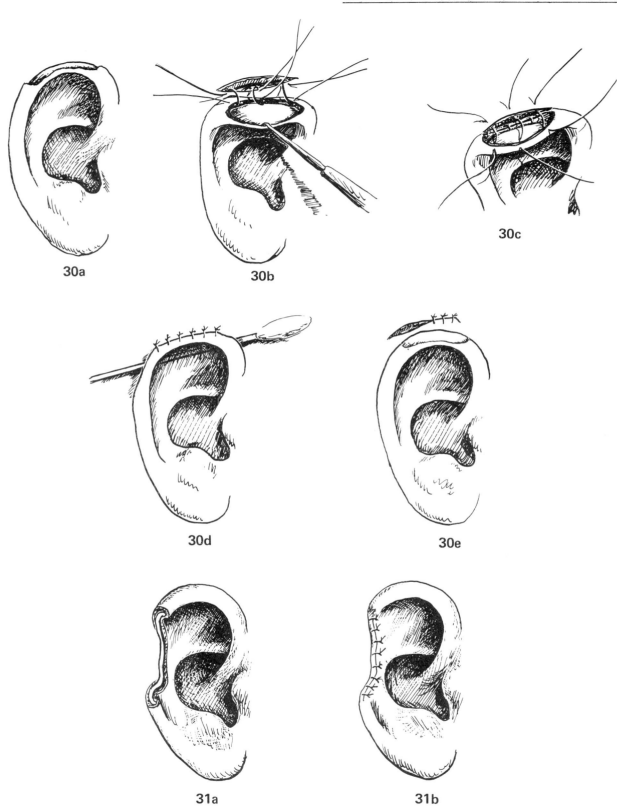

30a

30b

30c

30d

30e

31a

31b

SLICING INJURIES OF THE LIP

32

The surface markings for proper alignment of the lip are the white line at the junction of the vermilion with the skin as well as the line of junction between the vermilion and mucosa.

The Cupid's bow has to be restored. In the upper lip special attention has to be given to the philtral column. These lines should be marked before infiltration or manipulation of the wound. Guide sutures can be used for this purpose.

33a, b & c

Closure of the mucosa as a separate layer effects a water-tight seal and with particular attention to the labial sulcus it will avoid later obliteration of the sulcus. Accurate approximation of the muscle layer will control the amount of stretching of the scar and help to retain facial movements. This is followed by closure of the skin under proper tension.

With wounds that have entered the mouth systemic antibiotics are used and the mouth must be kept clean.

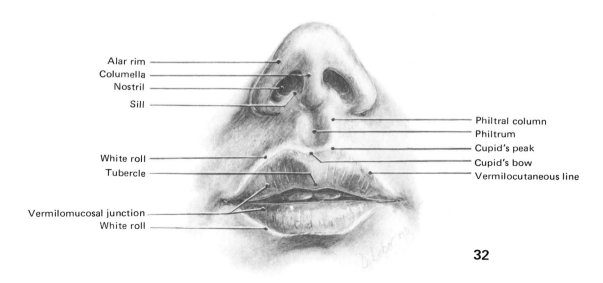

Alar rim
Columella
Nostril
Sill

White roll
Tubercle

Vermilomucosal junction
White roll

Philtral column
Philtrum
Cupid's peak
Cupid's bow
Vermilocutaneous line

32

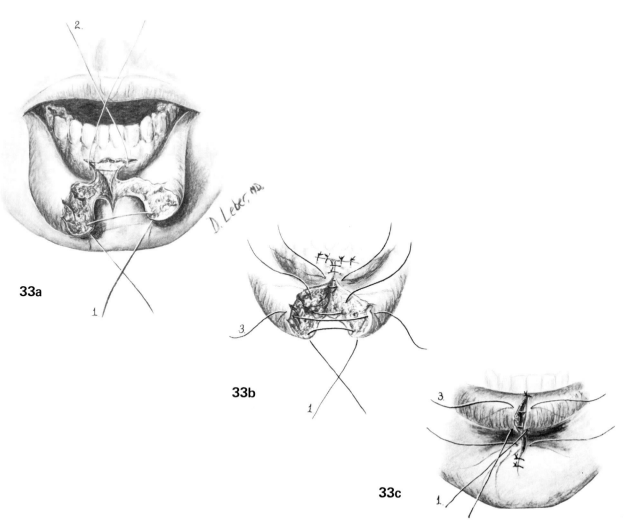

33a

33b

33c

WOUNDS WITH LOSS OF SUBSTANCE
34 & 35

While the main objective remains the achievement of prompt healing this can be obtained by direct tissue approximation by flaps or by skin grafts.

The lower lip can afford more loss of substance than the upper lip because the additional landmarks of the upper lip make any scar more noticeable and asymmetry more likely.

When the vermilion has been lost, approximation of mucosa to skin will reduce the amount of fibrosis and prepare the wound for a more definitive reconstruction.

36

With the lip, as well as with the nose and the ear, the objective should be to maintain the proper spatial relationship of the components of the organ.

In a wound with loss of different amounts of different tissues, treatment should include repair and alignment of any full thickness injury in addition to the management of the partial thickness loss as previously described.

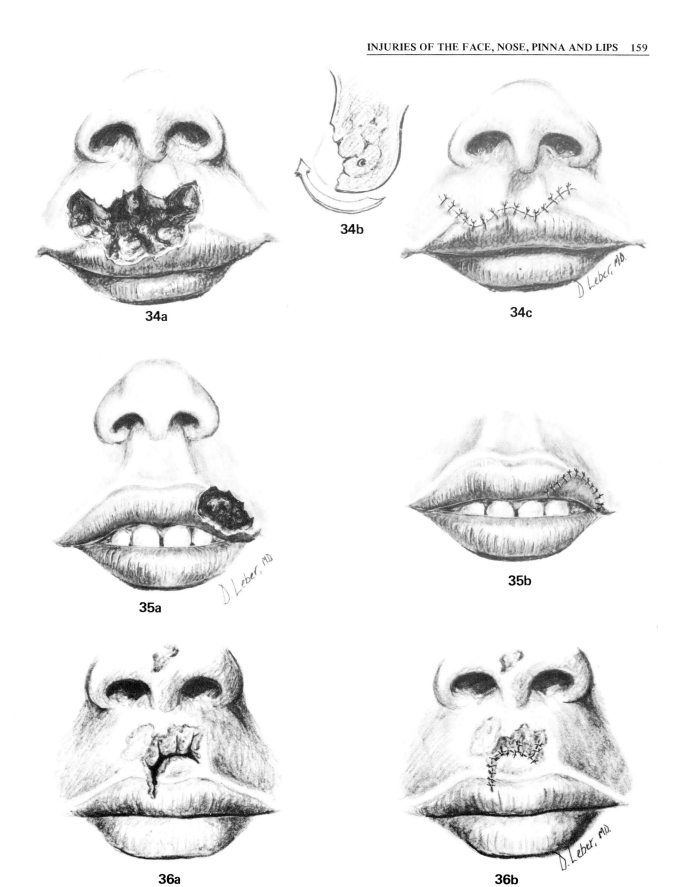

34a

34b

34c

35a

35b

36a

36b

INJURY OF THE FACIAL NERVE AND PAROTID DUCT

37

The facial nerve can be transected anywhere in its course from the stylomastoid foramen to its peripheral destination.

Primary repair of the facial nerve or its branches is indicated when it is technically possible and the wound can be expected to heal promptly. After isolation of the ends and utilizing the proper magnification, epineural sutures should be inserted using 8/0, 9/0 or 10/0 nylon.

The parotid duct lies beneath a line drawn from the tragus of the ear to the mid-portion of the upper lip. The first step in the repair is the insertion of a polyethylene tube from the duct's opening in the mouth to the wound and then into the proximal portion of the duct. This facilitates repair and serves as a support for 10 days. The edges of the duct are co-apted with interrupted sutures of 6/0 chromic catgut. The overlying wound is closed in layers and the splint is secured with a suture in the mouth.

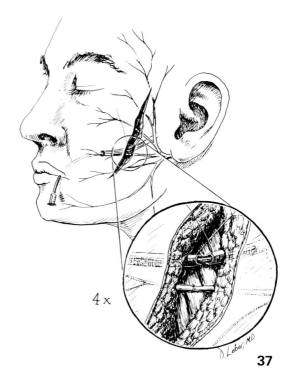

4 x

37

[*The illustrations for this Chapter on Injuries of the Face, Nose, Pinna and Lips were drawn by Dr. D. Leber, M.D.*]

Injuries of the Eyelids

J. C. Mustardé, F.R.C.S.(Eng.), F.R.C.S.(Ed.)
Consultant Plastic Surgeon, West Scotland Plastic Surgery Centre,
Canniesburn Hospital, Glasgow and Royal Hospital for Sick Children, Glasgow

INTRODUCTION

Injuries of the eyelids are particularly important because of the ever-present risk to the underlying eye, either at the time of the injury or at a later date when, due to scar contraction, the cornea may be exposed and damaged.

Because the eyelids have a 'skeletal' structure — the tarsal plate — which imparts their normal curved shape, injuries of the lids may be considered as either *partial-thickness*, i.e. involving skin and orbicularis oculi only, or *full-thickness*, i.e. involving skin, orbicularis, tarsal plate, and the closely subjacent conjunctiva.

As with all surface tissues, there are three categories of injury.

(1) Wounds without loss of tissue.

(2) Wounds with loss of tissue.

Either of these wounds may affect either only part or the whole of the thickness of the eyelid.

(3) Scars.

PARTIAL - THICKNESS INJURIES

Wounds

1a&b

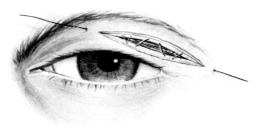

1a

Injuries caused by glass or cutting instruments may run in any direction. If the wound lies in the line of the fibres of the underlying orbicularis muscle a continuous 6/0 intradermal suture may be used, fixing both ends to the skin with squares of adhesive. Such sutures are pulled out in 5 days.

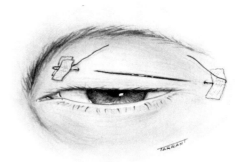

1b

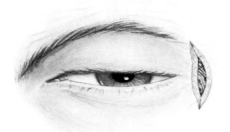

2a

2a&b

If, however, the wound lies *across* the line of the orbicularis fibres there will be retraction of the wound edges and interrupted 5/0 Prolene or silk sutures should be used to close the skin wound.

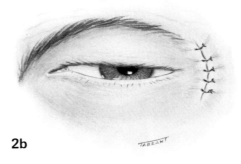

2b

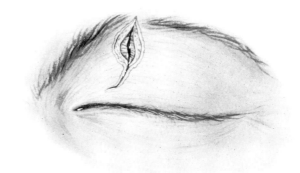

3a

3a,b&c

If the orbicularis has also been divided across its fibres it must be united with interrupted sutures of 6/0 chromic catgut. The skin sutures are removed in 5 days.

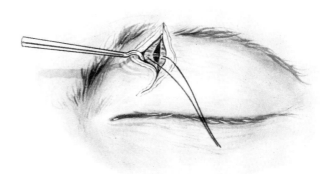

3b

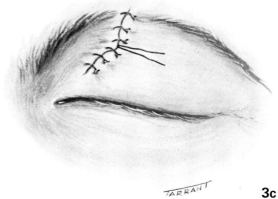

3c

Loss of tissue

Central

4 a, b & c

Partial-thickness loss of tissue of the lids may result from injury by cutting instruments, by animal or human bites, by resection of tumours or by burns. Such loss of tissue on or close to the eyelids should be dealt with by application of a skin graft. When the defect is on or close to the lower lid, in the medial canthal or the lateral canthal regions, or in the pretarsal area of the upper lid (the region immediately superficial to the tarsal plate), a full-thickness skin graft should be inserted. The most suitable skin to use, from the point of view of colour, texture, and thickness is postauricular. Upper eyelid skin is too thin to produce a satisfactory result, except in the upper lid, and, even if it is available, it is not the best material to use.

Full-thickness skin grafts should be cut to fit the defect so that edge-to-edge apposition is obtained, and there should be no overlapping of graft edges with subsequent necrosis and production of a thicker scar. In the absence of deep scarring such grafts will contract very little, but an additional amount (about 15 per cent) should be inserted to counteract the slight contraction which will take place. The whole graft is put on the stretch by leaving the sutures long and by 'overtying' these under slight tension across a pad of cotton wool. The overtied sutures are removed in 1 week, and the graft may be lightly smeared with petroleum jelly or any oily preparation for about a week.

5a, b & c

In the upper lid above the pretarsal zone, loss of tissue should be made good by using a split-skin and not a full-thickness graft. This is because split skin is more supple and will produce the normal eyelid folds more readily than the full thickness of the skin. However, as a skin graft contracts in direct proportion to its thickness the thinner split-skin graft will contract by about a third of its area; additional skin must be inserted, being kept on a slight stretch during healing by tying the sutures joining the graft and the wound edges over a suitably large cotton wool pad.

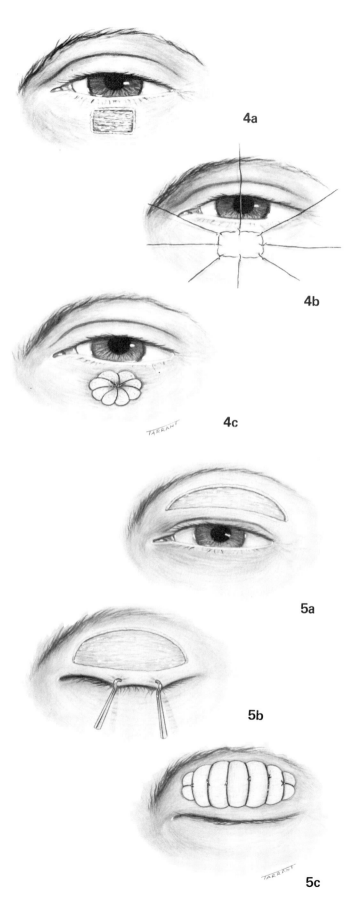

4a

4b

4c

5a

5b

5c

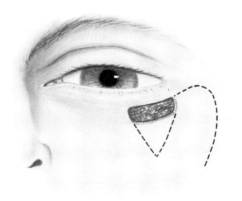

6a

Peripheral

6a&b

If the loss of tissue involves the peripheral parts of the orbit, e.g. the malar prominence, where the skin is thicker and there is a layer of subcutaneous fat, insertion of even a full-thickness skin graft into the defect will result in a sunken appearance of the graft. In resurfacing peripheral areas of the orbit, flaps of skin and subcutaneous tissue should be brought into the site. Skin of a similar texture, colour and thickness should be used, so that local flaps, such as rotation flaps should be employed wherever this can be done.

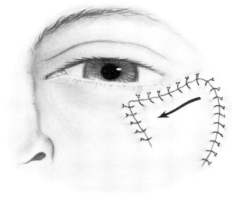

6b

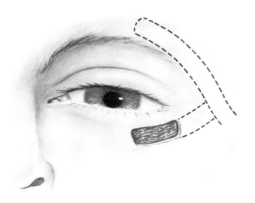

6c

6c&d

Such flaps are usually obtainable in regions below, lateral to, and above the orbit, but if local rotation flaps are not for some reason available, a flap may have to be transferred from another area.

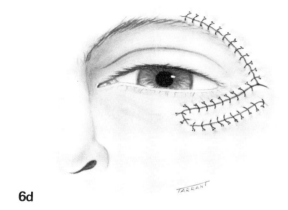

6d

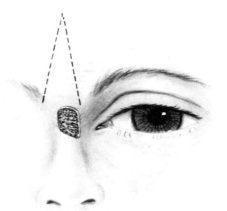

7a

7 & 8

For defects in the peripheral part of the medial canthal region it is best to bring down some skin and subcutaneous tissue from the centre of the forehead, either using the V—Y procedure, or by turning down a long flap on a pedicle, the latter being divided after a 2 week interval.

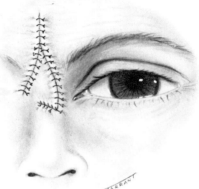

7b

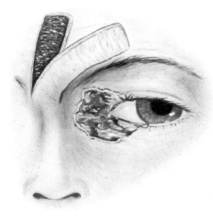

8a

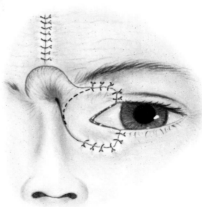

8b

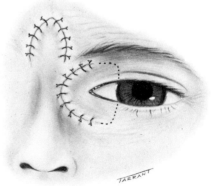

8c

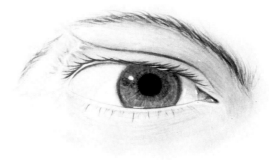

9a

9a, b & c

Scars

Contraction of partial-thickness scars running between the lid's margin and the periphery of the orbit may cause the margin to turn out, producing ectropion. Scars of the eyelid skin are seldom thick enough to require excision, and any tight line or scar causing such an ectropion should, after scar contraction has ceased some 6—9 months after injury, be broken up by the use of a Z-plasty confined to the skin. There is seldom troublesome scarring in the orbicularis layer so that it is usually unnecessary to include it in the Z.

Gross superficial scarring of a lid may require to be resected *en bloc,* producing a loss of tissue — which may have been the original clinical condition. The defect is then treated as described above.

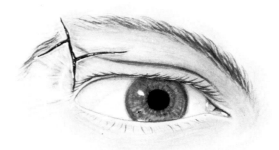

9b

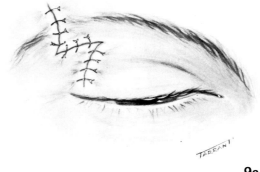

9c

FULL - THICKNESS INJURIES

Wounds

10a

Full-thickness injuries of the eyelids caused by cutting instruments may run in any direction but generally speaking they are oblique because the lids are protected from vertical slashes by the more prominent eyebrows and cheeks. With such injuries there is always a possibility that the underlying cornea has been damaged so it must be examined carefully, after inserting a drop of 1 per cent fluorescein.

The essential requirement in closing a full-thickness wound of the eyelid is to re-align the divided tarsal plate. If this alignment is carried out accurately there will be no deformity of the lid's margin, but if it is incorrectly carried out a deformity will result no matter what normally unnecessary adjuncts, such as inter-marginal sutures, are used.

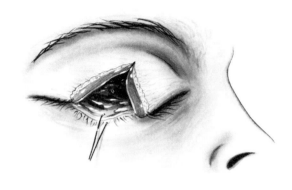

10a

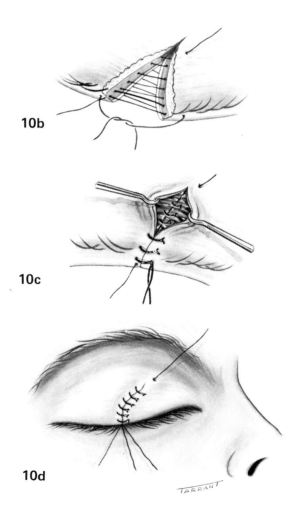

10b

10c

10d

10 b, c & d

The two edges of the tarsal plate (and its closely applied layer of conjunctiva) are carefully approximated using a 6/0 running suture of monofilament material such as Prolene, commencing by passing the suture through the skin peripheral to the wound and bringing it out at the top of the conjunctival wound. The suturing is carried over-and-over until the margin is reached. A separate 5/0 silk suture is inserted exactly in the grey line on each side to give accurate approximation of the margin and if need be a similar suture is inserted at the lash line. These sutures are left about 1 inch (2·5 cm) long so that they can be held down onto the lid skin by a square of adhesive, and so kept away from the cornea. The skin and orbicularis oculi of the rest of the wound are closed in two layers. Except for the marginal ones, the skin sutures are removed in 5 days. The marginal suture or sutures, as well as the pull-out sutures, are removed after a week.

TARRANT

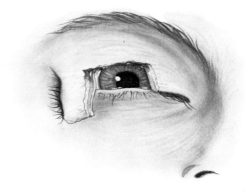

11a

Lacerated wounds

11a, b&c

There is a type of laceration of the eyelids which is caused by a blow on the lid directed away from the nose. If the force is strong enough the lid tears through at its weakest point. In the upper lid this is at first vertically through the large tarsal glands which run up in the tarsal plate. If the force continues, the tear then runs horizontally across the top of the tarsal plate through Müller's muscle and the levator aponeurosis producing an L-shaped wound. These wounds are closed in layers as already described, but separate continuous, pull-out sutures should be used for the horizontal and the vertical components of the tear.

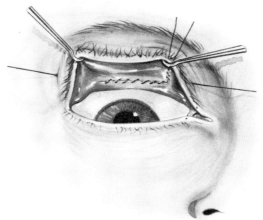

11b

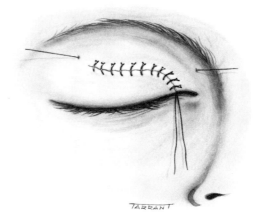

11c

12a

In the lower lid the weakest point is where the various heads of the orbicularis oculi are becoming small tendons, but have not yet united to form the strong medial canthal tendon. This is 1 or 2 mm medial to the punctum with the result that the lacrimal canaliculus is torn across.

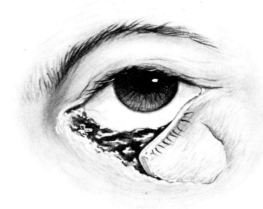

12a

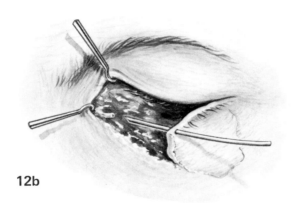

12b

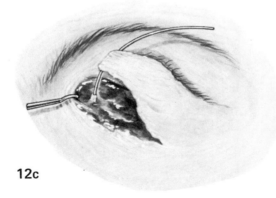

12c

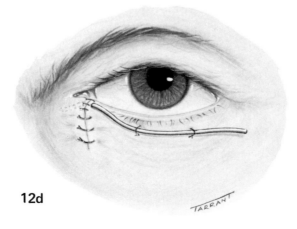

12d

12b,c & d

An attempt must be made at the time of injury to locate the medial divided end of the canaliculus, which usually shows up as a paler structure if normal saline is used to cleanse the wound. A 1 mm silicone tube is passed via the punctum and the peripheral part of the canaliculus into the medial opening, and thence into the lacrimal sac. The tube is lashed along the lid margin by sutures, and the conjunctiva is closed with 6/0 chromic catgut. A permanent suture of 5/0 Prolene or nylon is used to approximate the medial end of the tarsal plate to the medial canthal tendon. If this is not done, the powerful action of orbicularis oculi will drag the lid laterally and the scar will stretch considerably. Finally, the orbicularis muscle is closed with 6/0 chromic catgut, and the skin with 5/0 silk or Prolene. The tube is left in place for 2 weeks, and thereafter gentle probing weekly should help to ensure that at least about 60 per cent of these repaired canaliculi will remain patent. Even if the canaliculus does not remain patent, only a small proportion of patients will complain of troublesome epiphora, such as might call for more drastic surgery to produce a channel between the conjunctiva and the lacrimal sac.

Loss of tissue

Full-thickness loss of tissue involving an eyelid may on rare occasions result from an injury such as a bite, but is most often due to resection of an eyelid affected by cancer. A through-and-through defect is left which will require full-thickness reconstruction of the eyelid, a subject which is dealt with in full in the Plastic Surgery Volume.

13a - d

Scars

Full-thickness scars of the lids produce centrifugal contraction in all layers of the lid, which becomes notched and is not everted as with partial-thickness scars. It is unusual for the scars themselves to have to to be excised, and once an interval of 6—9 months has elapsed to allow all contraction of the scar to cease, a Z-plasty is carried out through *all* thicknesses of the lid. The various flaps are transposed and sutured in layers, using 6/0 pull-out Prolene to approximate as one layer the conjunctival and tarsal edges; these pull-out sutures are held under light tension by squares of adhesive tape. The orbicularis muscle and the skin are closed in layers as described previously. The skin sutures are removed on the fifth day, and the pull-out sutures on the seventh.

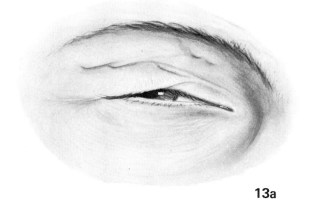

13a

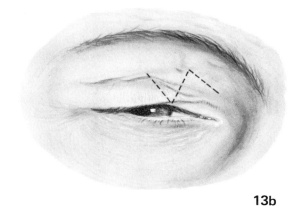

13b

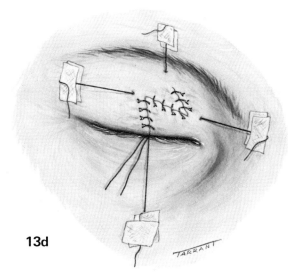

13d

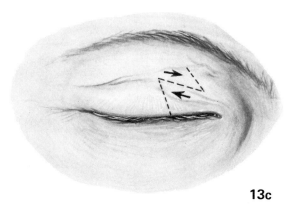

13c

[*The illustrations for this Chapter on Injuries of the Eyelids were drawn by Mr. T. Tarrant.*]

Management of Penetrating Wounds of the Root of the Neck

Archie Stein, F.C.S.(S.A.)
Baragwanath Hospital and University of Johannesburg, South Africa

INTRODUCTION

The problems in dealing with penetrating wounds of the root of the neck due to stab wounds or high- or low-velocity firearms are difficulty of access, the possibility of major or multiple. organ injury with inadequate localization of injuries owing to the urgency with which surgical intervention is often required. Arteriography, bronchoscopy, oesophagoscopy or Gastrografin swallow are not indicated when there is definite evidence of vascular or visceral injury or in the clinically unstable patient. The objective in treatment is to control bleeding by direct pressure or by a gauze pack and then to obtain first proximal and then distal control of the affected vessel by extending the incision, if necessary, before exposing the site of injury. The operative approach would depend on the suspected site and extent of the injury or injuries; the incision must be large to allow adequate display of injured viscera and to provide sufficient exposure for control of injured vessels and make provision for cervical, clavicular or axillary extension.

Emphasis is laid on gaining access because without adequate exposure, which may have to be achieved in a hurry, there can be no easy or safe repair. Techniques of repair are well accepted and can be found in other chapters but a matter of special importance is the risk of air embolism.

Injured blood vessels should be repaired when possible but ligation of major vessels, especially veins, may be expedient in certain circumstances. Tracheal and oesophageal injuries should be repaired primarily and the thoracic duct ligated if divided.

PRE - OPERATIVE

Indications for exploration

These are as follows.

All high velocity missile wounds. Continuing or renewed haemorrhage. Evidence of marked haemorrhage prior to admission, unexplained or persistent hypotension. A large or enlarging haematoma on clinical or radiological examination. A haemothorax not associated with a chest injury. Absent ipsilateral peripheral pulse. Air in the soft tissues of the neck or mediastinum on clinical and radiological examination. Widening of the mediastinum requires immediate exploration in the unstable patient, or arteriography if time permits. A history of dysphonia, dysphagia, coughing or vomiting of blood is an indication for exploration having first excluded injuries to the mouth and throat as a source of bleeding, or unless tracheal or oesophageal injuries have been excluded by contrast radiography or endoscopy.

Pre-operative preparation

Intravenous infusion should be administered via the contralateral limb or, in suspected mediastinal injuries, via the lower limbs. A large catheter is essential. An intercostal drain must be inserted before operation when a haemothorax or pneumothorax is present.

Position of patient

The patient is placed supine with a sandbag between the scapulae, with the arm abducted and the head rotated to the opposite side. The neck and chest should be cleaned and draped and instruments for sternotomy, thoracotomy and tracheostomy should be available.

172

THE OPERATION

THE INCISIONS

1

As a general rule, penetrating wounds lateral to the sternal head of the sternomastoid can be approached initially by a cervical incision and extended by a median sternotomy if required whereas medial wounds should be approached initially by median sternotomy, with cervical or clavicular extension when necessary. Median sternotomy is recommended if the nature of the injury is in doubt because it allows rapid access for proximal control of the major vessels and it can be extended into the neck with carotid or internal jugular injuries, laterally over the clavicle with sub-clavian vascular injuries, into the third or fifth inter-costal space with left subclavian or oesophageal injury, or, if required, a clavipectoral flap can be raised.

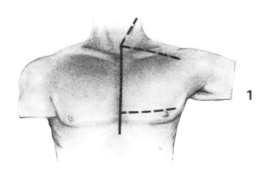

1

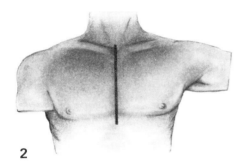

2

Median sternotomy

2

As adequate exposure is required, a full-length median sternotomy is performed with a Gigli saw. In those patients with a very long sternum the Roberts forceps may be too short to pass from the lower to the upper sternum and in these cases a sternotomy chisel or saw should be used.

3

The innominate vein and thymus may obscure the origin of the major arteries from the aortic arch and should be displaced upwards following division of some small veins. The subclavian artery is situated more laterally and posteriorly than is usually thought. The oesophagus should be approached from the right side after division of the azygos vein, with extension of the incision into the right fifth intercostal space following division of the internal mammary vessels if necessary. It may be necessary to divide the innominate vein to allow access to the injured vessels deep to it or repair of the trachea. This vein should be repaired if possible but it can be ligated with safety.

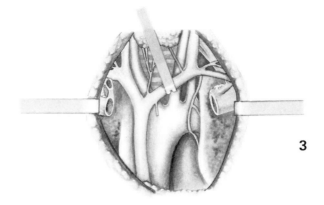

3

Cervical approach

4

The incision extends from 1 inch (2·5 cm) above the sternoclavicular joint and crosses the middle of the clavicle into the palpable deltopectoral groove. The platysma muscle and omohyoid fascia are then divided. The clavicular head of the sternomastoid muscle is divided, avoiding injury to the internal jugular vein and thoracic duct, which lie deep to it at its medial end. The clavicle is divided with a Gigli saw and the deltopectoral groove, in which the cephalic vein is situated, is widened and the underlying costocoracoid membrane is divided.

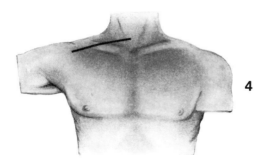

4

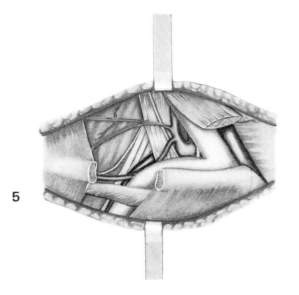

5

5

The subclavius muscle is divided, to allow retraction of the cut clavicle. The scalenus anterior muscle is divided at its lower border, avoiding injury to the phrenic nerve on its medial edge. The subclavian vein is anterior to the scalenus anterior muscle but deep to the clavicle. Injury of the thoracic duct should be excluded. The pectoralis minor muscle and tendon of the pectoralis major muscle should be divided if exposure of the axillary vessels is required.

6

Dividing the scalenus anterior and subclavius muscles exposes the full length of the subclavian and the first part of the axillary vessels. Proximal control of the first part of the subclavian artery on the left side and of the innominate artery on the right side can be obtained by blunt dissection for quite a distance into the mediastinum. Branches of the subclavian vessels may have to be divided to enhance mobility. If this approach does not allow adequate exposure of the subclavian vessels, particularly with venous injuries, the medial part of the clavicle can be excised subperiosteally; this causes little disability.

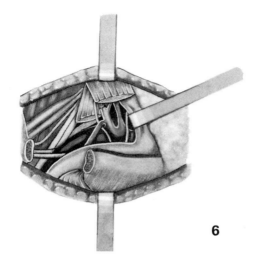

6

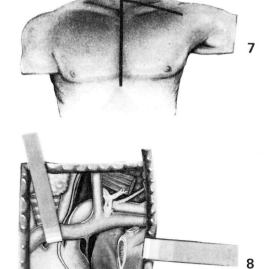

7

8

7 & 8

To extend median sternotomy into a thoracocervical incision or vice versa, it is necessary to divide the sternohyoid and sternothyroid muscles and the sternal head of the sternomastoid and ligate the anterior jugular veins as they run superficial to the sternohyoid and the sternothyroid muscles. Care should be taken to avoid injuring the internal jugular and vertebral veins and the recurrent laryngeal nerve as it crosses the first part of the subclavian artery.

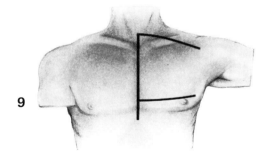

9

9

If a cervicothoracic approach is inadequate for dealing with the vascular, oesophageal, tracheal or pulmonary injuries that can occur with gunshot wounds, a clavipectoral flap should be raised.

10

The incision from the sternotomy is extended laterally into the third interspace and a flap consisting of upper portion of the sternum, sternoclavicular joint, clavicle and first three ribs attached to the pectoralis muscle is raised after subperiosteal division of the ribs. This allows very good exposure of all structures in the root of the neck as well as the lung and the pulmonary vessels.

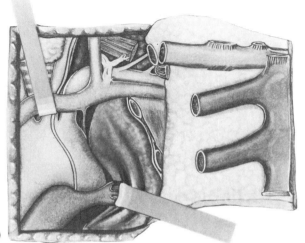

10

11

With injuries to the first part of the left subclavian artery which cannot be dealt with by a cervical approach, anterior thoracotomy in the left third interspace allows better access to the left subclavian artery than does median sternotomy.

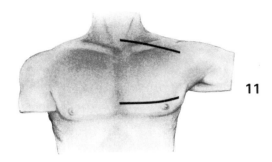

11

Carotid artery

Incisions

12

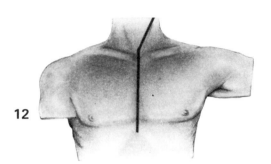

12

When distal control of the carotid artery or internal jugular vein is required after median sternotomy the incision is continued along the anterior border of the sternomastoid muscle, or vice versa if proximal control of the carotid or jugular vessels is required after a cervical approach.

13

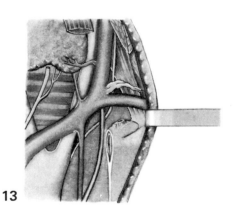

13

After dividing the platysma and deep cervical fascia and ligating the anterior jugular veins lying anterior to the sternohyoid and sternothyroid these muscles are divided. The sternomastoid muscle is retracted laterally and the thyroid gland medially. If necessary, the middle thyroid vein is divided before the carotid sheath is opened.

POSTOPERATIVE CARE

The mediastinal neck wounds should always be closed with drainage.

An intercostal drain should be inserted if the pleural cavity has been opened. Ischaemic changes must be looked for after arterial repair.

COMPLICATIONS

Wound infection.

Secondary haemorrhage.

An arteriovenous aneurysm may develop if careful exploration is not undertaken.

If division of the thoracic duct has gone unrecognized a chylous fistula occurs with metabolic disturbance; it requires re-exploration and ligation.

Tracheal or oesophageal injuries associated with a haemothorax inevitably lead to empyema thoracis.

Reference

Henry, A. K. (1957). *Extensile Exposure,* 2nd Edition. Edinburgh: Churchill Livingstone

[*The illustrations for this Chapter on Management of Penetrating Wounds of the Root of the Neck were drawn by Mr. C. P. Richards.*]

Tracheostomy and Laryngotomy

David Wright, F.R.C.S.
Consultant Ear, Nose and Throat Surgeon,
Royal Surrey County Hospital, Guildford

TRACHEOSTOMY

PRE-OPERATIVE

The operation of tracheostomy is best performed, whatever the indication, as an elective procedure under endotracheal anaesthesia in an adequately equipped operating theatre. If correctly anticipated an emergency tracheotomy will be avoided in most cases. Intubation with an endotracheal tube may provide an alternative interim procedure.

Indications

Respiratory obstruction

(*a*) *Trauma*: mandibular fractures complicated by oedema and haematoma. External or internal injury to larynx or cervical trachea.
(*b*) *Foreign body*: commonest in children.
(*c*) *Irritants, corrosives and burns*: causing damage to the mucous membrane of the mouth, larynx and trachea.
(*d*) *Infections*: acute laryngotracheobronchitis, acute epiglottitis.
(*e*) *Angioneurotic oedema* or drug sensitivity.

(*f*) *Bilateral recurrent laryngeal paralysis* or crico-arytenoid arthritis.
(*g*) *Malignant lesions, benign tumours and cysts* of the respiratory tract.

Tracheostomy may be required as a preliminary procedure to operations on the larynx and pharynx.

Secretory retention

Inadequate clearance of secretions from the tracheobronchial tree, producing hypoxia and hypercarbia

Respiratory insufficiency

Respiratory insufficiency caused by pulmonary, cardiovascular or muscular disease may need tracheostomy to enable intermittent positive pressure respiration which will reduce the air-flow resistance and the volume of the dead space. In some conditions it is desirable to produce respiratory paralysis by the use of drugs to provide controlled respiration.

Prevention of inhalation of fluids into the trachea

A cuffed tracheostomy tube may be required to prevent the inhalation of blood or the overspill of oral secretions and food when there is paralysis of the protective sphincter mechanism of the larynx.

178

Anaesthesia

An elective operation is best carried out under endo-tracheal anaesthesia. Drugs that might depress the respiratory system should not be given in the pre-operative period. Tracheostomy may be satisfactorily performed under local anaesthesia and this may be indicated in a patient with an obstructive lesion when general anaesthesia or intubation would prove difficult. Local anaesthesia is obtained by injection of the skin and subcutaneous tissues with 1 per cent procaine and 1 : 200,000 adrenaline. Before the trachea is opened 0·5 ml of 4 per cent cocaine should be injected into the tracheal lumen.

The patient should be warned that he may not be able to use his voice immediately following the operation.

Position of patient

A sandbag is placed under the patient's shoulders to give extension of the head and prominence of the trachea and larynx. If the patient has severe dyspnoea and the operation is to be carried out under local anaesthesia then a compromise position of extension will have to be found.

ELECTIVE TRACHEOSTOMY

1

The incision

A transverse incision approximately 5 cm in length is made 2 cm below the lower border of the cricoid cartilage through skin, subcutaneous fat and deep cervical fascia. Flaps are raised by undermining with blunt dissection for a short distance to expose the anterior jugular veins and infrahyoid muscles.

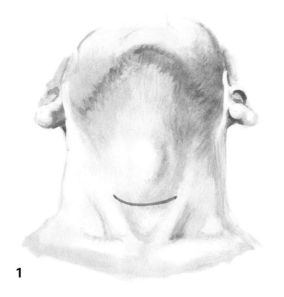

1

2

Separation of infrahyoid muscles

The fibrous median raphe in the interval between the right and left sternohyoid muscles is defined and separated with blunt dissection. The sternothyroid muscles on a deeper plane are identified and retracted laterally.

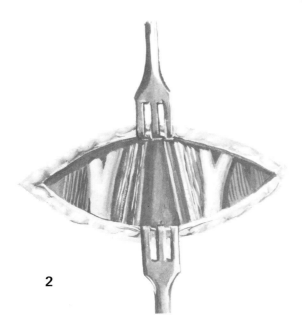

2

3

Identification of the thyroid isthmus

The thyroid gland and part of the trachea will then be visible. Anatomical variations in the size and position of the thyroid isthmus are to be expected. The thyroid isthmus may be small and not interfere with the approach to the trachea but in most patients it is of sufficient size to need dividing. A small horizontal incision is made through the pretracheal fascia over the lower border of the cricoid cartilage so that a small haemostat can be inserted into the incision and directed inferiorly behind the thyroid isthmus and its fibrous attachment to the anterior wall of the trachea. After determining the place of cleavage the thyroid isthmus can be completely separated from the trachea by blunt dissection.

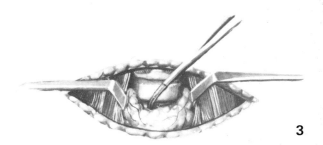

3

4

Division of the thyroid isthmus

A large haemostat is placed on each side of the thyroid isthmus, which is divided with a knife or diathermy. The cut surfaces of the thyroid are over-sewn or simply ligated on each side.

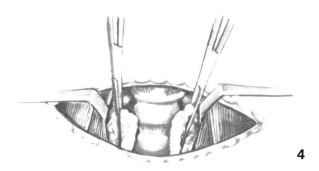

4

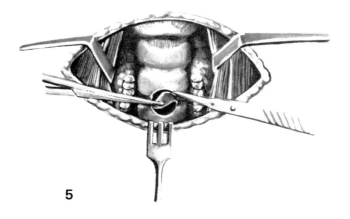

5

5

Opening of the trachea

Before the trachea is opened complete haemostasis must be obtained. A sucker with a catheter attached should be ready for aspiration of the trachea. At this stage sutures may be inserted into the skin edges in anticipation of closure of the lateral parts of the wound after the tube has been inserted. The trachea is retracted in an anterosuperior direction by inserting a tracheal hook below the cricoid cartilage. A transverse incision is made into the intercartilaginous membrane below the second or third ring and then converted into a circular opening by holding the upper and lower margins in turn with strong forceps and removing the cartilage with a knife. Alternatively a ring punch can be used. The first tracheal ring must on no account be disturbed.

6

Insertion of the tracheostomy tube

The type of tracheostomy tube which will be required in the immediate postoperative period should be selected. A cuffed portex tube will be needed if anaesthesia is to be continued and positive pressure ventilation required, or if the accumulation of secretions in the trachea from laryngeal overspill is to be prevented. If the operation is for simple airway obstruction a silver tracheostomy tube or a softer synthetic tube can be used. The latter tubes are provided with an obturator to help insertion through the fenestra in the anterior tracheal wall. The obturator is then removed and replaced by the inner tube.

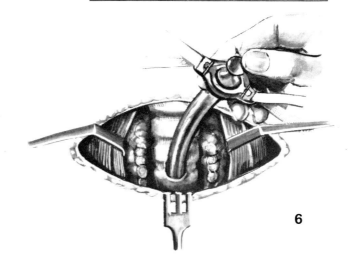

6

7

Fixation of the tube

When in position the tube is retained by tapes passed around the neck and secured by a reef knot on one side of the neck. It is important that the patient's head is well flexed when the ties are knotted otherwise the ties may become slack when the patient sits up in bed with the head forward, resulting in the possible displacement of the tube from the tracheal lumen when the patient coughs. A preformed sterile sponge tracheostomy dressing or antibiotic-impregnated Vaseline gauze is packed around the tube and the lateral margins of the wound loosely approximated with the skin sutures. There should be sufficient space remaining around the tube to minimize the danger of subcutaneous emphysema.

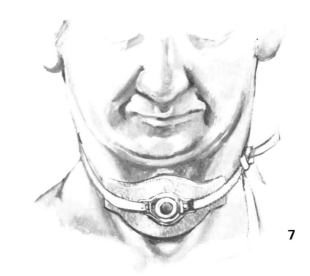

7

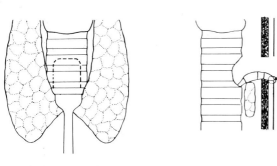

8a   8b

8a & b

Care of a tracheostome is made much easier if a flap of trachea is turned down and stitched to the skin. The flap should be cut to include the second ring of cartilage in the trachea and it should not remove more than about two-fifths of the circumference of the trachea. The stoma closes spontaneously, but this may take 2 or 3 weeks; there is no need to separate the flap from the skin.

EMERGENCY TRACHEOTOMY

An emergency tracheotomy is indicated when a patient's condition is rapidly deteriorating due to increasing hypoxia not affording the time for an elective tracheostomy and when the facilities of endotracheal intubation or the insertion of a broncho-scope are not available. The operation is not easy to perform on an infant whose trachea is soft and not easily palpable or in the short thick-necked adult, especially if there is disease at the site of the operation. The technique differs from the elective operation in the following ways.

(*1*) A vertical incision is made in the mid-line from the level of the cricothyroid membrane to the supra-sternal notch.

(*2*) The index finger of the left hand identifies the cricoid cartilage and, with the help of finger dissection, the thyroid isthmus is pushed inferiorly to expose the upper three tracheal rings.

(*3*) A mid-line vertical incision is made through the second and third tracheal rings. A tracheostomy dilator or haemostat is introduced into the incision while a suitable tube is inserted into the lumen. Once the air-way is established the procedure is followed by an elective tracheostomy.

LARYNGOTOMY (CRICOTHYROTOMY)

Laryngotomy is used for acute complete airway obstruction when endotracheal intubation is not possible. The opening into the airway is made through the cricothyroid membrane. The operation can be accomplished within 15 − 30 sec.

THE OPERATION

Position of patient

The patient's neck is placed in extension by a roll of clothing or towelling under the shoulders so that the thyroid notch becomes prominent. The forefinger should identify the carina of the thyroid in the mid-line and follow downwards to the prominence of the cricoid cartilage. The depression of the cricothyroid membrane is then identified and marked in the mid-line with the finger nail.

Incision

A vertical incision is made in the mid-line over the thyroid and cricoid cartilages. The subcutaneous tissues are retracted from the mid-line with the thumb and index finger. The wound is spread apart by finger dissection until the cricothyroid membrane is identified.

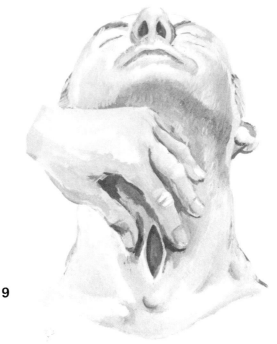

9

10

Incision of the cricothyroid membrane

The cricothyroid membrane is incised horizontally as close as possible to the cricoid cartilage to avoid the cricothyroid arteries, which run at a higher level across the membrane.

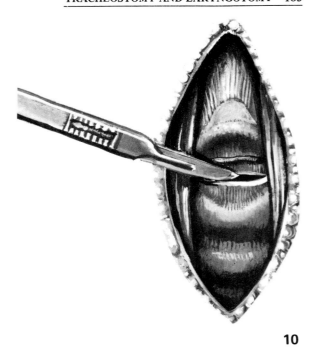

10

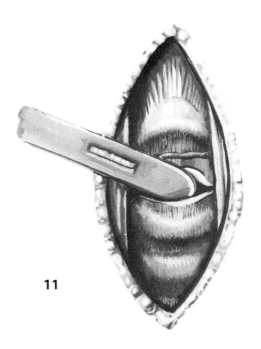

11

11

Establishment of an airway

The opening into the cricothyroid membrane is widened by insertion of the handle of the knife into the horizontal incision and rotating through 90°. A tracheostomy tube or similar tube if available can then be inserted. Once the airway is established, the procedure is followed as soon as is practicable by an elective tracheostomy.

Complications

Perichondritis, subglottic oedema and cicatricial stenosis may follow a prolonged thyrotomy.

POSTOPERATIVE CARE OF TRACHEOSTOMY

Prevention of tube displacement

Attention is required in maintaining the correct position of the tube within the trachea. The tension in the securing tapes must be regularly checked. If the tube has a tendency to displacement then the suitability of that tube must be suspected and a more satisfactorily shaped tube substituted. A soft tissue lateral x-ray of the neck will show the position of the tube within the tracheal lumen.

Care of the inner tube

The inner tube should be removed and cleaned every 2 or 3 hr during the first few days. The inner tube should be 2 or 3 mm longer than the outer tube so that secretions remain within the inner tube. If a cuffed tube is to be retained then a tube with a long cuff should be selected and inflated to produce an adequate air-tight seal. A short cuff or high pressure within the cuff should be avoided. If the pressure within the tube is correctly maintained periodic deflation of the cuff should not be required.

Humidification and prevention of crusting

Crusting may occur in the trachea unless the inspired air is adequately humidified. A constant room temperature of approximately 70°F should be maintained and humidification provided by a continuous thermostatically-controlled humidifier. Secretions should be removed from the trachea and bronchi with a soft sterile catheter. Suction should be applied only on withdrawal of the catheter. Prolonged or too frequent suction should be avoided.

Change of tube

The tube may be changed on the fourth day postoperatively. Changing the tube before that time may give rise to difficulty in re-insertion. Tracheal dilators and adequate illumination should always be available.

Voice

If after a few days it seems unlikely that surgical emphysema will occur due to resistance following expiration or coughing, an inner tube with an inspiratory valve may be used to allow the patient to speak.

COMPLICATIONS OF TRACHEOSTOMY

Apnoea and hypotension

An abrupt decrease in the carbon dioxide content of the blood may result in a loss of stimulus for breathing in patients with chronic laryngeal insufficiency, thus producing apnoea. The administration of 5 per cent carbon dioxide in oxygen may be necessary for some hours afterwards. The sudden decrease in carbon dioxide level may also lead to hypotension.

Displacement of the tube

Displacement of the tube may be prevented by the correct siting of the tracheostomy opening, the use of a correctly fitting tracheostomy tube and well adjusted and secured tapes around the neck. If these requirements are not fulfilled the tube may be displaced into the pretracheal space and this may not be quickly recognized.

Tube obstruction

The tube may become blocked by tenacious secretions. The risk of a blocked tube will be minimized by frequent changing of the inner tube, if present, adequate humidification and regular suction. If the tube cannot be cleaned adequately then it should be replaced by a new one.

Subcutaneous emphysema and pneumothorax

These complications are more likely to occur in children, especially if there is obstruction of the trachea or tracheostomy tube. Unnecessary dissection of tissue planes during the operation must be avoided and a clear airway maintained both before and after the operation. If the pleura is inadvertently incised, producing a pneumothorax during the operation, the incision should be closed.

Tracheal stenosis

Fibrous stricture in the subglottic region or around the tracheostome will be avoided by making the correct size of opening into the trachea below the level of the second tracheal ring and by avoiding an ill-fitting tube.

Difficult decannulation

Difficulty may occur in removing the tracheostomy tube in infants and small children due to the necessity to re-adjust the redirection of air through the larynx. The dependency on the tracheostomy may be decreased by gradually reducing the size of the tracheostomy tube in adults or partially corking the tube in children.

Failure of closure of the fistula after decannulation

If the edges of the fistula have become epithelialized in a patient who has maintained a tube for a long period the fistula should be allowed to contract for some weeks after the decannulation. The epithelialized tract can then be excised and the wound closed in layers. Keloid formation may follow an infected tracheostomy wound.

Pulmonary infection

Profuse bronchial secretions may occur due to irritation from the tracheostomy tube or to endotracheal aspiration and overspill. Atelectasis of the opposite lung may occur if the tip of the tracheostomy tube is too long and reaches the main stem bronchus. Pneumonia may be avoided by strict use of a sterile suction catheter.

Tracheitis siccus and crusting

Crusting may be reduced by adequate humidification and the careful removal of crusts until such a time as the upper part of the trachea has become adapted to directly receiving the inspired air.

Haemorrhage

Haemorrhage during the operation may be troublesome from the anterior jugular system, from the thyroid isthmus or from the tracheal wall. Haemostasis must be obtained before the trachea is opened. If secondary haemorrhage occurs blood may enter the trachea around the tracheostomy tube. A cuffed tube should be inserted as an immediate measure and the wound re-opened and the bleeding controlled. Fatal erosion of a large artery can occur from ulceration of the anterior wall of the trachea by the pressure of the tip of an incorrectly fitting tracheostomy tube. This underlines the importance of the careful selection of the size and shape of the tube for each individual patient.

[The illustrations for this Chapter on Tracheostomy and Laryngotomy were drawn by Miss M. Palmer.]

Drainage by Needle of Pleura and Pericardium

D. B. Clarke, F.R.C.S.
Consultant Cardiothoracic Surgeon,
The Queen Elizabeth Hospital, Birmingham

PLEURAL ASPIRATION

Aspiration of the pleura is indicated for the removal of long-standing collections of fluid within the chest. It is particularly applicable when these collections are loculated and exploration at several sites is required, or when a sample of pleural liquid is needed for diagnostic purposes. Needle drainage has little place in the urgent management of chest injury where rapid accumulations of blood and air must be speedily evacuated. An intercostal catheter is more efficient for this purpose.

1

Equipment

A 20 ml syringe with a three-way tap will be needed. Wide-bore needles (*A*) have the disadvantage that the point may tear the lung. If used, they should not be inserted deeply into the chest and should be held as nearly parallel to the chest wall as possible. The risk of injuring the lung is reduced if a fine trochar and cannula of the Martin pattern (*B*) is employed. A disposable plastic intravenous cannula makes a serviceable substitute.

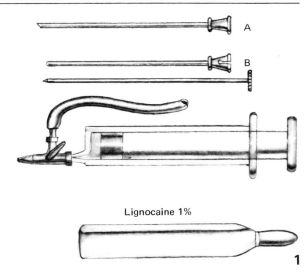

Lignocaine 1%

1

2

Position of patient

The usual reason for a 'dry tap' is that the pleural effusion has not been accurately located. Percussion and chest radiographs in the postero-anterior and lateral views will distinguish anterior collections of liquid from the more usual posterior collections.

The site of aspiration is infiltrated from the skin to the pleura with lignocaine 1 per cent.

Patients confined to bed will be most conveniently treated in the lateral position. The classical sitting position, leaning on a bed table, is uncomfortable for the patient and inconvenient for the surgeon.

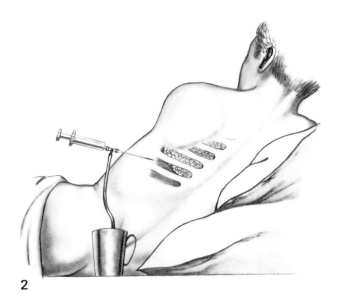

2

3

Withdrawal of liquid

The ambulant patient is conveniently seated astride a chair with his arms resting on a pillow laid on its back.

Every effort should be made to prevent air entering the chest. Connections between needle, tap and syringe must be firm. The needle is inserted one inter-costal space below the upper limit of dullness on percussion; a common mistake is to insert the needle too low.

Suction is applied as the pleura is entered. The appearance of liquid in the syringe confirms that the effusion has been reached.

As the liquid is withdrawn it is ejected into a container through the side arm of the three-way tap. The first sample may be injected into a sterile bottle for bacteriological studies. Intermittent withdrawal of the effusion on inspiration indicates that the pleural space is almost empty.

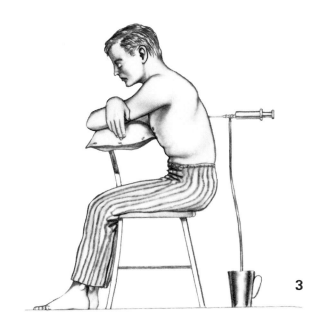

3

PERICARDIAL ASPIRATION

Collections of liquid within the pericardial sac compress the heart, restrict filling of its chambers and impair the cardiac output.

The clinical picture of a pale, hypotensive patient with distended neck veins, muffled heart sounds on auscultation and pulsus paradoxus suggests the diagnosis, which should always be considered when a penetrating injury in the chest or upper abdomen has been sustained.

Pericardial aspiration confirms the diagnosis and relieves the compression of the heart. This is a valuable temporizing measure while the theatre is being prepared for urgent thoracotomy but, except in the most experienced hands, it should not be used as definitive management for cardiac stab wounds.

4

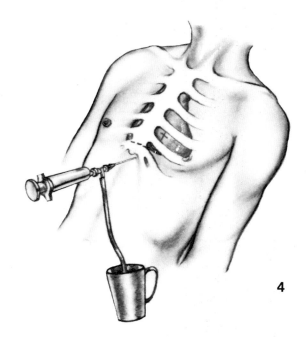

4

The preferred site for insertion of the needle is to the left of the xiphisternum. The alternative site to the left of the sternum has the disadvantage that the anterior border of the lung or the internal mammary artery may be injured.

The needle is inserted in an upwards and backwards direction at 45° to the anterior abdominal wall, maintaining suction until blood appears in the syringe. The principal difficulty lies in deciding whether this blood has been drawn from the pericardial sac or whether the heart has been pierced and blood is being aspirated from the right ventricle. It is unusual to sense the passage of the needle through the pericardium. Sometimes the heart will be felt to scratch on the end of the needle with each systole. If a unipolar electrocardiograph lead is clipped to the needle, an injury pattern will be traced whenever the heart is touched. Blood aspirated from the heart clots, that from the pericardium usually does not. If doubt remains it is helpful to aspirate about 50 ml. This small reduction in the circulating blood volume will have no effect on the patient's haemodynamic state if the needle lies within the heart, but if this amount is aspirated from the pericardium the transitory alleviation of cardiac tamponade will produce an immediate improvement in the blood pressure and aspiration can be continued with confidence.

[The illustrations for this Chapter on Drainage by Needle of Pleura and Pericardium were drawn by Mr. G. Lyth.]

Drainage of Pleural Space by Tube

D. B. Clarke, F.R.C.S.
Consultant Cardiothoracic Surgeon,
The Queen Elizabeth Hospital, Birmingham

INTRODUCTION

The introduction of a drainage tube into the pleural space is the most efficient method of evacuating large collections of air and liquid within the chest. Not only is full expansion of the lung achieved with rapidity, but the facility for continuous drainage ensures that further collections are removed as they accumulate. Blood lost from the pleural space is collected in the underwater seal bottle where it can be measured; this measurement provides a valuable guide to blood replacement by transfusion. Furthermore, continuous or severe haemorrhage will be apparent and the surgeon will readily judge which patients require urgent thoracotomy for the control of bleeding. None of these advantages is conferred by the laborious technique of needle aspiration of the pleura, which has a limited place in the early management of an injured chest.

1

Sites for insertion of intercostal tubes

Air collects in the apex of the chest and is best removed by a tube inserted through the second intercostal space two fingers' breadth from the edge of the sternum. The internal mammary artery will be severed if the tube is passed closer than this to the sternum.

Liquid collections are drained by a tube in the mid-axillary line, above the level of xiphisternum. Insertion below this level may result in penetration of the diaphragm and injury to the underlying spleen or liver.

Posteriorly situated tubes will be kinked where the patient lies on them.

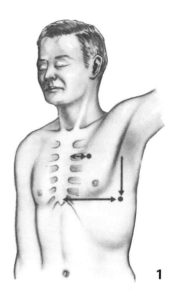

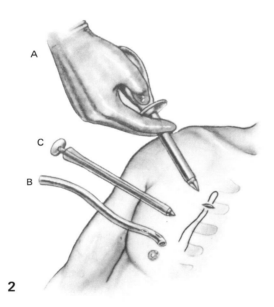

2

Generous infiltration of the skin and muscle layers down to the pleura is performed with lignocaine 1 per cent. A 1 cm incision is made in the skin and a mattress skin suture is inserted. This is left untied and is used to close the incision when the tube has been removed.

The tube is readily inserted with the aid of a large trochar and cannula (*A*).

A whistle-tip catheter (*B*) which fits snugly within the cannula is selected. Alternatively, an Argyle chest tube, which contains a pointed metal introducer within its lumen (*C*) can be used.

3

The trochar and cannula are inserted through the intercostal space into the pleural space. A firm twisting thrust is necessary. The trochar is withdrawn and a thumb is placed over the end of the cannula to prevent air from entering the chest.

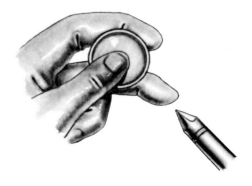

4

A pair of artery forceps is applied to the end of the whistle-tip catheter, which is rapidly threaded through the cannula into the pleural space.

5

The cannula is withdrawn by sliding it out along the catheter. The catheter is adjusted so that about 10 — 15 cm lie within the chest and is secured by a stout skin suture which is wrapped round several times before tying. The tube must not be transfixed. The artery forceps are re-applied close to the chest wall and the cannula removed. This sequence of actions reduces to a minimum the amount of air entering the pleural space.

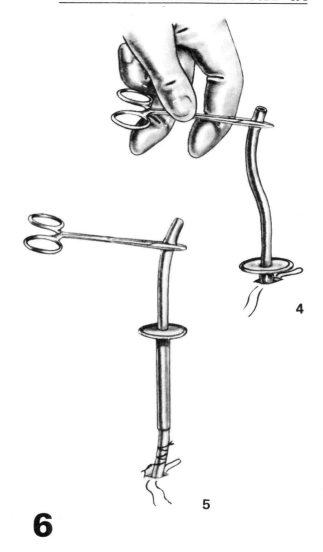

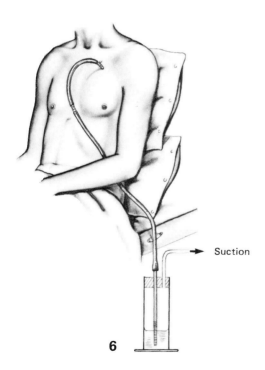

6

The catheter is connected to the calibrated drainage bottle with an underwater seal. Blood lost is recorded every 15 min. Replacement of blood is guided by this measurement together with observation of the central venous pressure and the clinical state of the patient. A chest radiograph will confirm that the tube has been correctly sited and that all liquid and air has been evacuated. Excessive air escaping from the lung will hinder re-expansion unless suction is applied to the waterseal bottle.

A suction motor capable of dealing with large volumes of air and sustaining a negative pressure of the order 5 — 10 mmHg in the system will be needed.

Intercostal catheters are removed when they no longer drain air or blood, or if disappearance of the respiratory swing of the liquid level in the tube indicates that the catheter has become blocked.

[*The illustrations for this Chapter on Drainage of the Pleural Space by Tube were drawn by Mr. G. Lyth.*]

Operative Fixation of Fractured Ribs

D. B. Clarke, F.R.C.S.
Consultant Cardiothoracic Surgeon,
The Queen Elizabeth Hospital, Birmingham

PRE - OPERATIVE

Indications

The introduction of mechanical ventilation of the lungs for the management of stove-in chests superseded the earlier techniques, which included operative fixation of fractured ribs and traction.

When crushing forces applied to the chest produce a double line of fractures, that section of the chest wall which has no longer any bony attachment to the thoracic skeleton moves paradoxically on respiration and this interferes profoundly with the mechanics of respiration. As soon as the patient is given a relaxant drug, intubated and ventilated, hypoxia is relieved and the loose segment is held in place on a cushion of expanded lung. This technique is widely employed and has been responsible for saving many lives. Because consolidation of the fractured ribs takes about 3 weeks, a tracheostomy must usually be performed. The recognized hazards of tracheostomy and mechanical ventilation have recently led some surgeons to re-appraise operative fixation as the method of choice in the management of this injury. Not only is early mobilization possible but the risk of pulmonary infection introduced through the tracheostomy is averted and the accurate reduction of fractures avoids late deformity and restriction of the size of the thorax caused by mal-union.

In some instances ventilation can be discontinued on the first postoperative day, but if not the period of artificial ventilation will at least be reduced in many patients and it is only when associated pulmonary contusion is present that prolonged ventilatory support will be necessary.

The association of injury of the chest wall with fracture of the clavicle is an indication for operative fixation of the fracture because the accessory muscles of respiration are thereby enabled to function more efficiently and a thoracoplasty deformity caused by the subsidence of the shoulder is prevented.

Pre-operative preparation

Primary treatment is directed to restoring the blood volume, passing an endotracheal tube and carrying out artificial ventilation while other injuries are treated. Operative fixation of the loose segment is performed as a planned procedure when the threat to life has been averted. Antibiotics are commenced and the electrocardiogram is recorded in order to give early warning of cardiac contusion, which should be treated by Digoxin and diuretics.

THE OPERATION

Choice of incision

1

This is determined by the position of the fractures. Anterior injury, commonly caused by the steering wheel in road accidents, may produce a line of fractures close to the costochondral junctions, sometimes with a second line of fractures in the axilla. This is best approached through incision *A*, which permits the pectoralis major to be detached and reflected from the chest wall.

Alternatively, the anterior ends of the ribs may be fractured on both sides, producing an anterior loose segment; the sternum is sometimes fractured as well. Incision *B* runs transversely just below the nipples and extends out to the anterior axillary line on either side. Skin flaps are reflected upwards and downwards to give access to the sternum and anterior chest wall.

More common than either of these injuries is the lateral pattern in which the ribs are fractured at their posterior ends and anteriorly, either in the axillary line or at the costochondral junctions. Access is gained by means of a posterolateral thoracotomy.

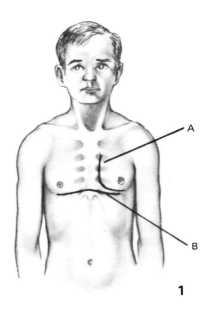

1

2

The patient is placed in the appropriate lateral position with the upper arm suitably supported. The skin incision runs from a point between the spine and the medial border of the scapula, curves below the angle of the scapula and extends to a point below and lateral to the nipple. Access to the first three ribs is obtained by extending the incision up towards the neck; additional exposure of the lowest ribs may be gained by a 'T' shaped extension to the incision as shown.

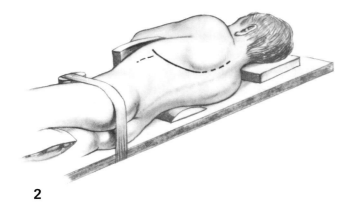

2

3

The latissimus dorsi and trapezius muscles are divided in the line of the skin incision with diathermy, care being taken to coagulate the many small arteries which are encountered. The fascia overlying the ribs often contains a large haematoma; this is evacuated and the serratus anterior muscle is divided from its insertion into the ribs. The scapula can now be lifted from the chest wall with a retractor, the extent of the injury determined and additional exposure obtained when necessary.

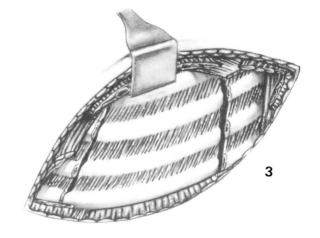

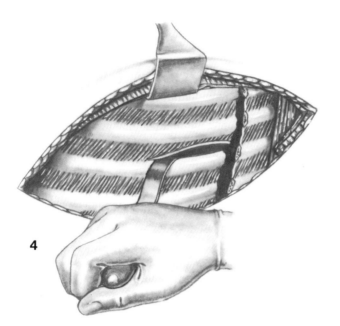

4

The pleural cavity is entered by stripping the periosteum from the upper border of the sixth rib. Alternatively, the rib can be excised.

5

Bleeding from intercostal or internal mammary arteries is controlled, blood and clot are evacuated from the pleural cavity and the surface of the lung is inspected for tears. Small tears can be left alone, larger ones may require closure with unabsorbable sutures after any severed pulmonary vessels or small bronchi have been ligated.

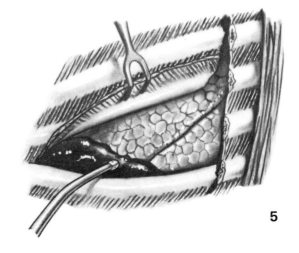

6

Two intercostal drainage tubes are inserted through separate incisions in an intact part of the chest wall. One passes to the apex of the chest, the other lies behind the lung in the lower part of the thorax.

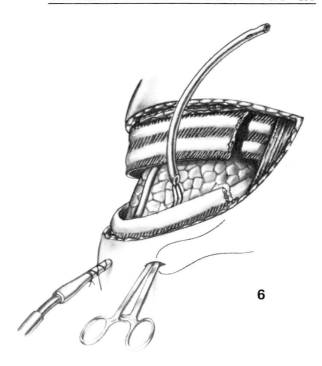

6

7

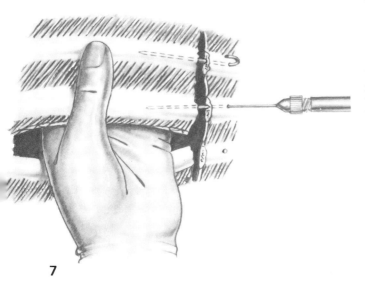

7

The loose segment is supported by a hand inside the pleural space. The outer cortex of the posterior ends of the ribs is drilled with an awl about 3 cm from the fractured ends. Lengths of Kirschner wire or short Rush nails are passed through these holes and along the medullary cavity, across the fracture sites and into the medullary cavity of the appropriate rib in the flail segment. The ends of Kirschner wires are bent over to prevent displacement. As many posterior fractures are pinned as can be reached conveniently. Access to anterior fractures is less easy, and although paradoxical movement will be relieved if the posterior fractures alone are fixed, undoubtedly better stabilization of the flail segment will be achieved if one or two anterior pins can also be inserted. If the ribs are fractured so close to the spine that there is insufficient length to obtain secure fixation of the pin, it is preferable to drill the ribs on either side of the fractures and secure them with stout wire sutures.

8

Additional security may be provided by stout sutures through the torn intercostal muscles.

The incision is closed by suturing the periosteum of the sixth rib to the muscle in the intercostal space below it.

The overlying muscles are closed in layers.

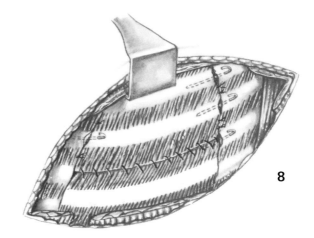

8

9

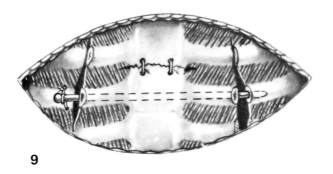

9

Anterior loose segments are immobilized by Abrams's bar, designed for the correction of pectus excavatum. A transverse incision as shown in *Illustration 1* is made. Fracture sites on either side of the sternum are exposed by splitting the fibres of the overlying pectoralis major muscles. The malleable bar is passed behind the sternum and its point is impacted into the medullary cavity of a rib. The other end is lashed to a rib with a braided wire suture. The bar is easily removed through a small incision some months later. Fractures of the sternum are reduced and immobilized by two stout wire sutures passed through drill holes.

POSTOPERATIVE CARE

Mechanical ventilation is stopped for a trial period on the first postoperative day. If the patient can breathe easily and the blood gas estimations are acceptable, the endotracheal tube is removed. If not, ventilation is resumed until subsequent trials demonstrate his ability to breathe adequately without assistance.

Reference

Moore, B. P. (1975). 'Operative stabilization of non-penetrating chest injuries.' *J. thorac. cardiovasc. Surg.* **70,** 619

[*The illustrations for this Chapter on Operative Fixation of Fractured Ribs were drawn by Mr. G. Lyth.*]

Median Sternotomy

R. H. F. Brain, F.R.C.S.
Consultant Thoracic Surgeon, Guy's Hospital, London

1

Position of patient

The patient should be in the full supine position with the left arm slung upwards for intravenous anaesthetic/medication and often for the administration of blood and other liquids.

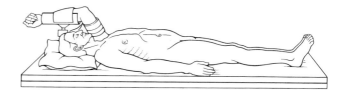

1

2

The incision

This is a simple vertical incision in the mid-line from the suprasternal notch to the tip of the xiphisternum.

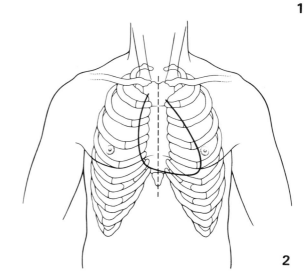

2

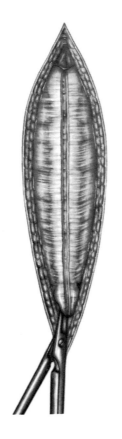

3a

The exposure

The skin is dissected back to approximately the edge of the sternum on either side. Above, the suprasternal notch is clearly defined to its posterior limit. Below, the central tendon of the diaphragm is divided at its attachment to the back of the sternum.

3a

3b,c&d

Division of the sternum

The periosteum over the sternum in line with the skin incision is incised and the bone divided with a pneumatic oscillating saw.

In the absence of this instrument a speedy entrance can be made using the Gigli saw introduced by a long Robert's type forceps that has previously been used to dissect the retrosternal tissues from the back of the sternum, using small gauze mops.

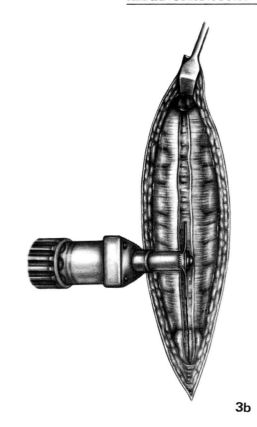

3b

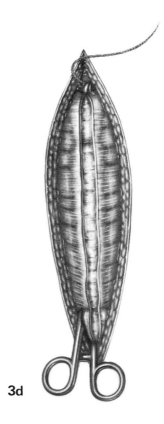

3d

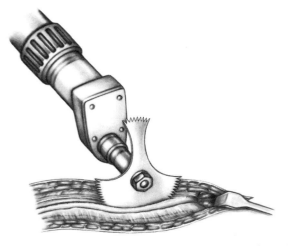

3c

4

Retraction of the sternum and exposure of the pericardium

Achieved by using a mechanical retractor of the Price-Thomas type after such overlying tissues as the edges of the pleural sacs laterally, and the thymus and the left innominate vein above have been dissected clear.

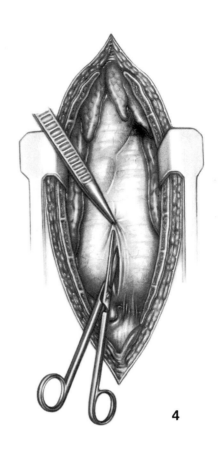

4

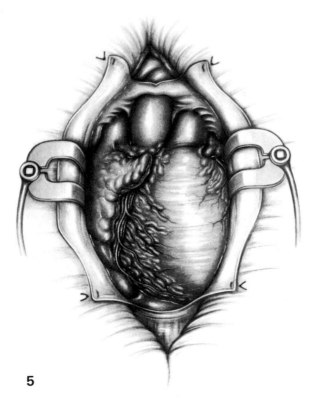

5

5

Exposure of the heart and great vessels

A vertical, or sometimes a cruciate, incision in the pericardium is made, the edges of which are sutured back to the wound.

Closure of the wound

6

The pericardium

Interrupted fine non-absorbable sutures are used over a drainage tube placed on the anterior surface of the heart.

7 & 8

The sternum

The sternum is closed by a series of trans-sternal monofilament, non-absorbable sutures over a second drainage tube placed in front of the pericardium.

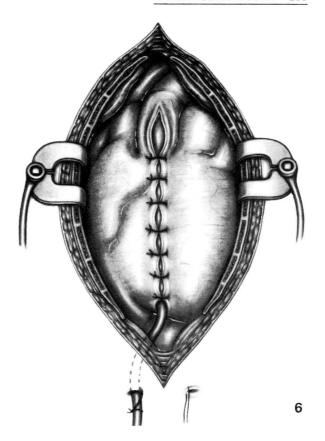

6

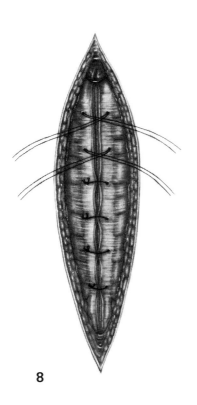

8

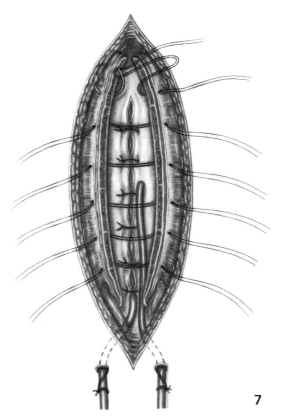

7

POSTOPERATIVE CARE

Patient monitoring

Essential to the management of cardiac operations are the continuous measurements of a variety of parameters, varying with individual surgeons, but the following are used frequently:

Venous pressure — catheter placed in the superior vena cava.

Arterial blood pressure.

Left atrial pressure — measured on those occasions when a low output and possible failure has been anticipated.

Continuous E.C.G. — fluorescent screen.

Urine secretion — volume, rate and osmolarity.

Peripheral temperature — limbs.

Ventilation/oxygenation/humidification — control.

Arterial blood gas, pH, bicarbonate measurements.

9

Chest drainage

All tubes are attached to separate underwater seal bottles, including those put into the pleural cavities should these have been opened. Accurate measurement is made of the rate of blood loss. Invariably suction is used.

Radiography

Regular daily, and sometimes more frequent, chest films are needed if concealed bleeding is suspected or there are difficulties with ventilation of the lungs.

Pain

This is often troublesome, especially so when ventilation is likely to be restricted by drugs affecting deep breathing and coughing. Mechanical ventilation, when used, abolishes these risks and enables a patient to be fully sedated safely. Physiotherapy at short intervals should be used.

Haemorrhage

This complication is rarely from bleeding chest wall vessels, but may be intrapericardial; when causing tamponade it requires thoracotomy, evacuation of the clot and arrest of the haemorrhage by suture.

Complications of the wound

These are rare but may include dehiscence, infection, osteomyelitis of the sternum and a late fibrous or non-union.

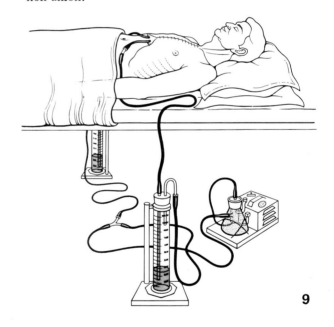

9

[The illustrations for this Chapter on Median Sternotomy were drawn by Miss P. Archer.]

Stab Wounds Entering the Thoracic Cavity

D. B. Clarke, F.R.C.S.
Consultant Cardiothoracic Surgeon,
The Queen Elizabeth Hospital, Birmingham

INTRODUCTION

The necessity for exploring all stab wounds of the neck and trunk when the clinical condition and chest radiograph give cause for concern cannot be emphasized too strongly. The direction and depth of the penetrating injury cannot be deduced from the slender evidence of the site of the entry wound and vital structures may be injured at some distance from this. The author has encountered knife thrusts which entered the abdomen in the region of the umbilicus, transfixed the liver and then passed through the diaphragm to enter the heart and lung. On other occasions wounds in the chest have been seen to pass through the diaphragm and involve the underlying spleen or kidney. Stab wounds at the root of the neck may injure the oesophagus, the aorta or its major branches. A tangential thrust has been observed to pass behind the sternum, sever the internal mammary artery and produce a massive haemothorax in the side of the chest opposite to the entry wound. Profuse bleeding is almost always due to injury of the major vessels in the mediastinum, the heart or arteries in the chest wall. Bleeding from the lung usually ceases spontaneously and bleeding points found at thoracotomy are simply under-run with interrupted atraumatic sutures or are ligated. Oesophageal wounds should be carefully explored because the mucosal tearing sometimes extends beyond the limits of the injury to the muscle coats. Repair is effected with interrupted non-absorbable sutures, the mediastinal pleura is closed loosely and the chest is closed with underwater seal drainage.

EMERGENCY THORACOTOMY FOR PENETRATING INJURY OF THE HEART

PRE-OPERATIVE

Indications

It is not unusual for patients to sustain a penetrating injury of the heart with a knife and to survive long enough to reach hospital. Such survival is unlikely if the injury is due to a high velocity missile which produces widespread damage and rapid death from haemorrhage. Rapid death from exsanguination usually follows a knife thrust which creates a wide breach in the pericardium. Only an immediate thoracotomy, perhaps on the floor of the receiving room without an anaesthetic, will save the patient. Few survivals from such heroic surgery have been described.

Fortunately, the usual penetrating wound makes a small hole in the pericardium which is soon sealed by clot. Blood which collects within the pericardial sac compresses the heart, impairs diastolic filling and often produces the clinical features of cardiac tamponade.

Any patient with a penetrating injury in the chest or upper abdomen who becomes pale and hypotensive with elevation of jugular venous pressure, muffled heart sounds and pulsus paradoxus should be considered to be suffering from cardiac tamponade. The clinical picture is not always typical; venous distension in the neck may be absent if the patient is hypovolaemic and pulsus paradoxus is not an easy physical sign to elicit with confidence. Enlargement of the cardiac shadow on a chest radiograph helps to confirm the diagnosis. If there is even a suspicion that the heart has been perforated it is wiser to proceed to thoracotomy than to temporize with this potentially fatal injury.

Pre-operative preparation

Speed is essential. Blood is taken for cross-matching and relief of tamponade may be achieved by pericardial aspiration, as described previously.

Some centres which are particularly experienced in dealing with cardiac injury, use pericardial aspiration as definitive management for tamponade but the surgeon who meets this emergency seldom is advised to proceed to urgent thoracotomy and to rely upon aspiration only as a means of sustaining his patient until he can be taken to the operating theatre.

Position of patient

There is, unfortunately, no surgical approach which gives equally good access to all aspects of the heart. The approach to be described has the advantage that no special instruments are needed, the position of the patient on the table does not require complicated supports and the anterior aspect of the heart, which is most commonly penetrated, is readily accessible.

THE OPERATION

1

The patient lies flat on his back. The left arm may be extended on an arm board, but this is not essential.

The left fourth intercostal space is defined by palpation and a curved skin incision is made over this space, running from the mid-line to the anterior axillary line.

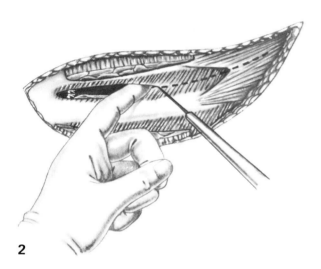

2

The intercostal space is exposed by dividing the overlying pectoralis major and serratus anterior muscles. The intercostal muscles are incised in the anterior part of the wound, keeping strictly halfway between the ribs. If the anaesthetist reduces the inflation pressure the lung will fall away as the pleural space is entered. As the incision is carried posteriorly the lung is further protected by a finger, as shown. Incision of the intercostal muscles proceeds cautiously as the sternum is approached and the internal mammary artery is defined and divided between ligatures. If greater access to the heart is needed, the sternum can be transected and the opposite intercostal space incised. Alternatively, the costal cartilages above and below the wound can be transected.

3

The wound edges are protected with large mops and a self-retaining retractor is used to separate the ribs. The pericardium is picked up with forceps or a dural hook and incised about 1 cm anterior to the phrenic nerve. An alarming quantity of blood will escape under pressure but when this is sucked away bleeding from the heart will usually be seen to be moderate and easily controlled. The lung is covered with a mop. Stay sutures are inserted into the pericardial edge and secured to the wound margins or the retractor so as to give maximal exposure of the heart.

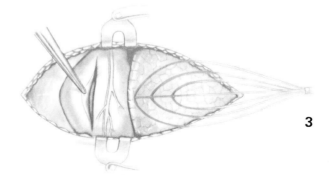

4

If the wound is not easily accessible, the heart is gently dislocated from the pericardium with one hand. Bleeding is controlled with a thumb or finger as shown, or the edges of the wound are pinched together. Displacement of the heart is usually well tolerated but if its action falters or the blood pressure falls the heart should be returned to the pericardium for a short time.

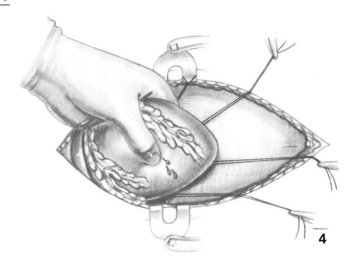

5

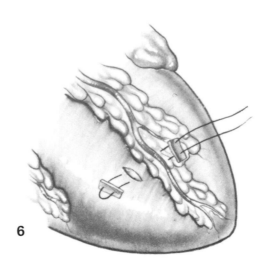

The anterior wall of the right ventricle is the usual site of penetration but transfixion of the heart with a posterior exit wound must be excluded. The wound is closed with interrupted unabsorbable sutures, preferably of the atraumatic type. Gentle finger pressure controls the bleeding. The finger is removed gradually, exposing the wound edges bit by bit as suturing proceeds.

Bites of the myocardium, about 1 cm across, are taken and sutures are inserted about 0·5 cm apart. Knots are tied firmly but not tightly or the cardiac muscle will be cut through.

6

Wounds close to coronary arteries are closed by mattress sutures which run under these vessels. They are buttressed by pledgets of Teflon felt, pericardium or muscle. This technique is valuable when simple sutures are found to cut through heart muscle. If a coronary artery is found to have been severed it should be ligated. Reconstruction procedures require specialist skills and are, in any case, unlikely to avert myocardial infarction.

7

Wounds of the atrium or its appendage are controlled by the application of an angled vascular clamp, which takes a side bite of the atrial wall. The same method is used to control haemorrhage from the great vessels, but it should never be employed for ventricular wounds. Wounds of the atria and great vessels may be closed with either an interrupted or continuous unabsorbable suture.

Injury to the interventricular septum or the heart's valves will require repair with cardiopulmonary bypass.

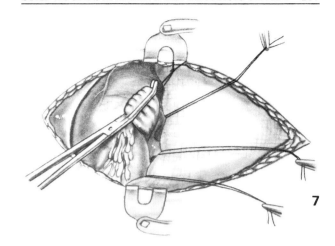

7

8

When haemostasis has been assured the pericardium is closed with a few interrupted sutures, leaving gaps for drainage. A drainage tube is inserted into the pleural cavity and connected to a bottle with an underwater seal. The rest of the incision is closed in layers. Because the intercostal muscles do not hold sutures well they should be supplemented by two or three wire pericostal sutures.

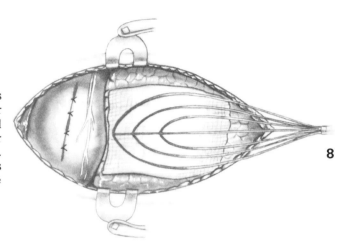

8

POSTOPERATIVE CARE

Blood pressure, pulse rate and the volume of blood drained from the chest are recorded at 15 min intervals for the first few hours after returning from theatre. The object of treatment is to maintain blood volume and ventilation at normal levels. Blood transfusion is guided by clinical observation and by the measurement of central venous pressure, systemic blood pressure and blood loss.

If there is any doubt about the patient's ability to breathe satisfactorily he should be managed with a mechanical ventilator. Ventilatory support usually can be discontinued about 12 hr after operation. The pleural tube is removed when drainage is very small in amount and the chest radiograph demonstrates that the lung is fully expanded.

[The illustrations for this Chapter on Stab Wounds Entering the Thoracic Cavity were drawn by Mr. G. Lyth.]

Traumatic Rupture of the Diaphragm

D. B. Clarke, F.R.C.S.
Consultant Cardiothoracic Surgeon,
The Queen Elizabeth Hospital, Birmingham

PRE-OPERATIVE

Diagnosis

Traumatic rupture of the diaphragm is usually produced by severe compression of the thorax and abdomen. Tearing is due to a sudden rise in intra-abdominal pressure and distortion of the rib cage. On the left side, which is the more commonly affected, the stomach, spleen and colon are displaced into the pleural space and on the right the liver is thrust into the chest. The clinical picture of lower thoracic and acromial pain that cuts short inspiration suggests the diagnosis, which is confirmed by radiographic studies. Opacity of the lower half of the hemithorax, perhaps with a liquid level in the fundus of the stomach, may be differentiated from haemopneumothorax by swallowing Gastrografin.

Associated injuries produced by the compression forces include fracture of the pelvis, rupture of the spleen, liver and fourth part of the duodenum and tears of the mesentery.

The signs of intra-abdominal bleeding may distract attention from the ruptured diaphragm, which will be overlooked unless chest radiographs are obtained routinely in all cases of thoraco-abdominal injury. Intraperitoneal bleeding is confirmed by tapping the abdomen.

Pre-operative preparation

Blood replacement by transfusion is commenced. Oxygen is given by mask, or if the patient is very distressed, an endotracheal tube is passed and the lungs are inflated by a mechanical ventilator. Manual inflation with a face mask is contra-indicated as gas will be driven down the oesophagus and distend the intrathoracic stomach.

A nasogastric tube is passed; aspiration of stomach contents relieves dyspnoea and facilitates reduction of the abdominal viscera at operation.

THE OPERATION

1

Choice of incision

Repair of the diaphragm is most easily performed through the chest. Posterolateral thoracotomy gives good access to the left upper quadrant of the abdomen, so that a ruptured spleen is readily excised, but it does not permit a thorough exploration of the peritoneal cavity. Mesenteric and duodenal injuries will therefore be difficult to recognize and repair. If there is clinical evidence of intra-abdominal injury an approach through a paramedian or mid-line abdominal incision would be more appropriate. The diaphragm is accessible for repair on the left but some difficulty may be encountered. A compromise thoraco-abdominal approach may be chosen or alternatively a thoracotomy can easily be extended across the costal margin into the upper abdomen if the operative findings dictate a wide exposure.

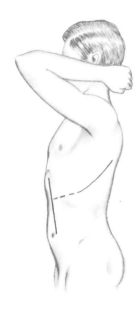

1

2

The incision

The patient lies on the uninjured side with the upper arm supported. The curved skin incision runs from a point halfway between the medial border of the scapula and the spine, passes two fingers' breadth below the tip of the scapula and extends as far forward as the nipple.

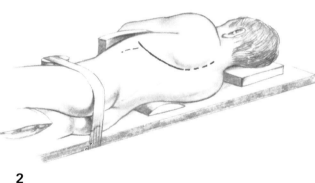

2

3

The latissimus dorsi and the serratus anterior muscles are divided in the line of the incision using diathermy. Numerous small arteries are severed and are coagulated. The eighth rib is identified and the periosteum is stripped from its upper border with a raspatory. The pleura is carefully nicked with a knife to allow air to enter the chest. It is then widely opened with scissors. The wound is covered with large mops and a self-retaining retractor is inserted.

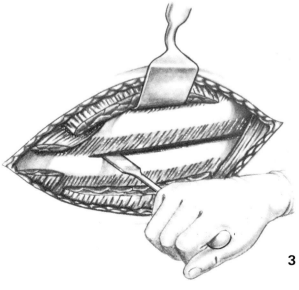

3

4

The lung is retracted to reveal the displaced abdominal viscera. These are examined carefully to exclude injury. If the spleen is torn, it is removed before the viscera are returned to the abdomen. The upper abdomen is explored. Any unexplained blood in the peritoneal cavity is an indication to extend the incision across the costal margin to the mid-line of the abdomen so that a more thorough examination can be carried out.

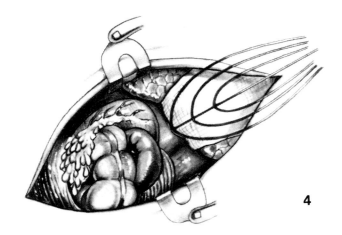

4

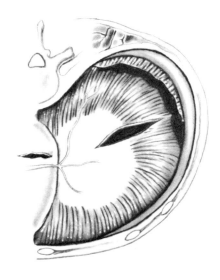

5

5

The diaphragm is now inspected. Often it has retracted so that there appears to be an alarming deficiency of tissue. This is seldom the case; direct repair by suture is always possible. The tear is commonly radial; sometimes there is a circumferential tear along the attachment of the diaphragm to the rib cage or both types of lesion may be present. In addition, the pericardium may be torn parallel to the phrenic nerve.

6

The abdominal organs are covered with a swab and protected by a large spatula.

The diaphragm is now repaired with multiple, interrupted 2/0 silk sutures. It is good practice to supplement the repair with a second layer of interrupted mattress sutures which invaginate the first line of stitches. Circumferential tears are closed by sutures which take bites of the diaphragm and the intercostal muscles. As access to the lesion is not easy it will be found helpful to insert all the sutures first, holding them on artery forceps before tying. A basal intercostal drain is inserted and the thoracotomy is closed in layers.

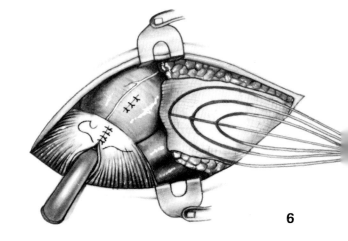

6

POSTOPERATIVE CARE

Deep breathing and coughing is encouraged by the physiotherapist. The intercostal drain is removed when drainage has almost ceased and the chest radiograph confirms that the lung is fully expanded.

[*The illustrations for this Chapter on Traumatic Rupture of the Diaphragm were drawn by Mr. G. Lyth.*]

Exploration of the Abdomen

Hugh Dudley, Ch.M., F.R.C.S., F.R.C.S.(Ed.), F.R.A.C.S.
Professor of Surgery, St. Mary's Hospital, London

INTRODUCTION

The *diagnosis* of abdominal injury will not be dealt with here. It is assumed that closed or penetrating injury is known to be present or is sufficiently suspect (perhaps as a consequence of peritoneal lavage) to warrant opening the abdominal cavity.

For *access* vertical mid-line or paramedian incisions are by far the best with the following exceptions.

(*1*) A penetrating wound is known, because of both exit and entry wounds, to have traversed only one quadrant. This is more usual in the upper half of the abdomen where the chest is also involved. A thoracotomy or thoracolaparotomy is then appropriate.

(*2*) In closed injury when diaphragmatic rupture has been diagnosed, particularly on the left side. Again, a thoracolaparotomy is indicated.

(*3*) In children below the age of 5 years (and either accidental trauma or deliberate battering brings such children to surgery) where a transverse incision just above the umbilicus carried well into the flanks gives good access and heals most satisfactorily.

THE OPERATION

1

If bleeding is massive its source is usually, though not inevitably, obvious. A large pack, deliberately and firmly applied, will nearly always arrest this and can be held in place by the assistant while the incision is appropriately lengthened or extended, say by a lateral cut through one or other rectus sheath.

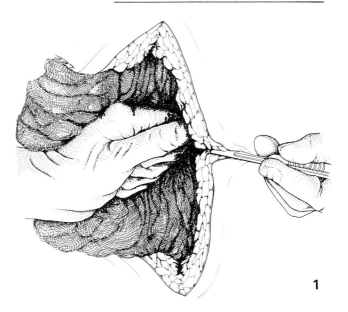

1

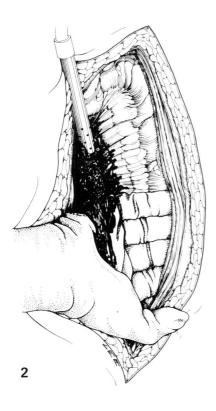

2

2

If bleeding is not catastrophic but if its source cannot be identified, the most effective way of clearing the abdomen before exploration is to cup the hand into the paracolic gutters or just medial to the colon if this is tightly bound down and insert a powerful sump sucker into the pool so formed. If coils of small bowel interfere the whole length of this may be eviscerated over the right margin of the wound, so exposing the left side of the pelvis. In most injuries the majority of blood gravitates there so it is a convenient place to apply suction and furthermore is a good point at which to begin the exploration.

3 & 4

Formal exploration follows. The author's pathway is illustrated, but circumstances of the injury and the individual surgeon's preference may alter this. However, whatever route is followed a systematic approach is vital if tiny but important or concealed injuries are not to be missed. To facilitate lower exploration the small bowel can again be removed from the abdomen and the left lower edge of a vertical wound raised. Intraperitoneal rectum, pelvic viscera and sigmoid descending colon are seen.

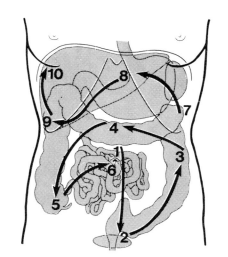

3

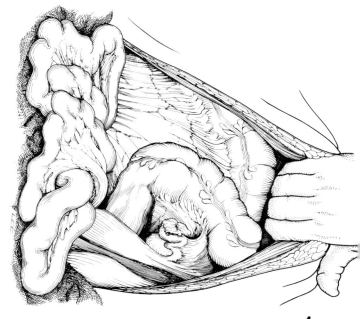

4

5

The small gut mesentery is then drawn downward and to the right either inside or outside the abdomen so as to expose the splenic flexure and transverse colon.

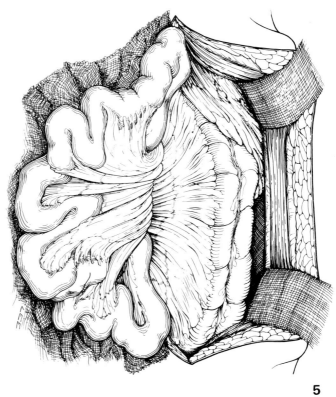

5

6

Working proximally and turning the small bowel to the left, the ascending colon and caecum are then seen.

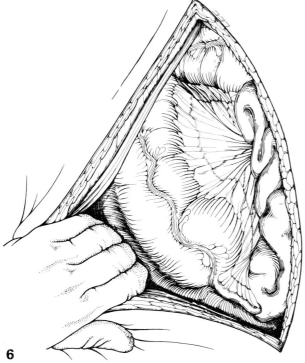

6

7

The small bowel is drawn systematically through the fingers from ileocaecal valve to ligament of Treitz and the retroperitoneum examined at this point for haematoma or staining by gut content (*see* Retroperitoneal rupture of the duodenum, page 217). If all is well the infracolic exploration is complete and the small bowel is finally returned to the abdomen.

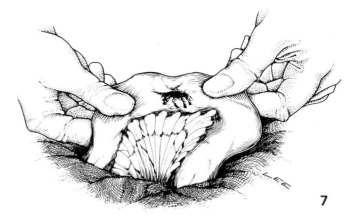

7

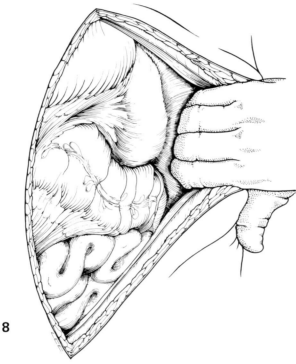

8

8

The supracolic compartment is then examined by raising the upper left corner of the wound and drawing the colon downward. Spleen, left hemidiaphragm and stomach are seen and felt.

9

Attention is turned to the right side to examine liver, porta hepatis, duodenum and right hemidiaphragm.

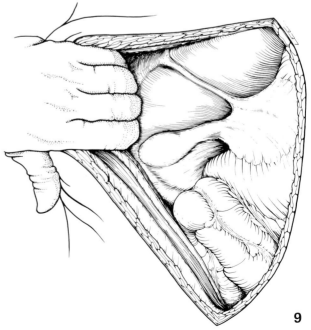

9

RETROPERITONEAL EXPLORATION

The indication for and techniques of mobilization of the duodenum are described on pages 291–295. Otherwise, surgical judgement must be used in relation to exploration. Small haematomas not closely associated with the gastro-intestinal tract, pancreas or bladder, and which are not expanding, can safely be left. Haematomas associated with a minor renal injury diagnosed pre-operatively or palpated at surgery, also do not constitute an indication to open the retroperitoneum.

10a&b

When access is required, long paracolic peritoneal incisions may be made on either side.

(*a*) On the right these will permit the duodenum and right colon to be swung off the great vessels exposing the right kidney and ureter, the vena cava and aorta (the latter less well).

Upward extension into the reflection of peritoneum off the posterior aspect of the right lobe of the liver permits access to the retrohepatic cava and if the liver is fully mobilized in the region of its bare area, to the right hepatic vein. Downward extension gives access to the common iliac vessels and intrapelvic right ureter.

(*b*) On the left, spleen, tail and body of pancreas and left colon may be mobilized in a similar way to expose left kidney and ureter and left common iliac vessels behind and to see the posterior aspect of the pancreas in front. In this way access can be gained to the aorta from the coeliac axis to its bifurcation.

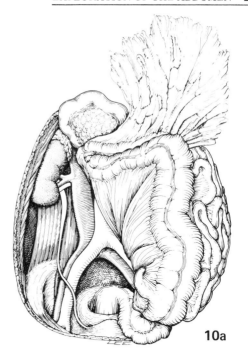

10a

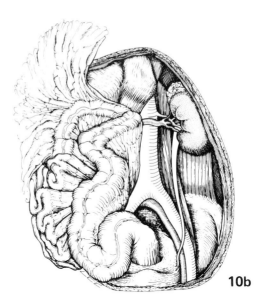

10b

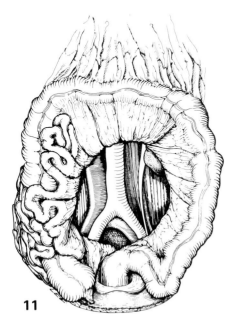

11

11

The infraduodenal great vessels can also be approached by incising the posterior parietal peritoneum in the midline as for an aortic aneurysm below the renal vessels. The duodenum is reflected proximally. Below, the peritoneum is incised down to the sacral promontory.

[The illustrations for this Chapter on Exploration of the Abdomen were drawn by Mrs. G. Lee.]

Techniques of Anastomosis in Gastro-intestinal Surgery

Thomas T. Irvin, M.B., Ph.D., Ch.M., F.R.C.S.(Ed.)
Senior Lecturer in Surgery, The University of Sheffield;
Honorary Consultant Surgeon, Sheffield Royal Infirmary

INTRODUCTION

A significant proportion of the operations on the gastro-intestinal tract involve the suture or anastomosis of the gut and it is this aspect of the surgery of the alimentary canal which is associated with dangerous complications. The breakdown of a suture line or anastomosis may result in peritonitis, faecal fistula and serious or fatal septic complications.

The immediate success or failure of a gastro-intestinal operation may thus depend to a large extent on the technical expertise of the surgeon in his performance of an intestinal anastomosis. This technical expertise is acquired with practice but a gastro-intestinal operation involves a series of exercises in surgical judgement, and it is only by attention to many details that safety is achieved.

In this chapter the general principles and techniques of anastomoses in gastro-intestinal surgery are described.

GENERAL PRINCIPLES

Several well-established general principles of surgical technique apply to the management of all sutured wounds, including gastro-intestinal anastomoses. Other aspects of wound management, such as suture technique, have special features in gastro-intestinal surgery, and several factors unrelated to surgical technique may affect the healing of intestinal anastomoses.

TECHNICAL PRINCIPLES

Access and exposure

Like most surgical procedures gastro-intestinal anastomoses become difficult if the surgical access and exposure are unsatisfactory. This may result from inadequate anaesthesia and muscle relaxation, poor assistance, an inappropriate surgical incision or one of inadequate length, and imperfect illumination of the operative field. Poor access for an anastomosis may also result from inadequate mobilization of the viscera, and this is prone to occur in the surgery of anatomically fixed and deeply-placed viscera such as the oesophagus, colon and rectum.

The surgeon should never have to struggle with an anastomosis because of limited access. When difficulty is encountered the problem should be carefully assessed and an attempt must be made to improve the exposure. If the difficulty seems insurmountable it may be prudent to consider an alternative procedure which avoids an anastomosis.

Blood supply

A poor blood supply is inimical to the healing of all wounds, and the preparation for an anastomosis must be meticulous to avoid disturbance of the blood supply to the cut ends of the gut. The only absolute criterion of an adequate blood supply is the presence of free arterial bleeding from the cut edges of the bowel. The absence of visible or palpable arterial pulsation in the mesenteric vessels is not necessarily of significance, but blanching or cyanosis of the cut edges of the bowel and the presence of a dark, venous type of bleeding are signs of an inadequate blood supply.

The blood supply to an anastomosis may be compromised in several ways: undue tension on the suture line resulting from inadequate mobilization of the viscera; devascularization of the bowel during mobilization or preparation for the anastomosis; strangulation of the tissues by tightly-knotted sutures; and the excessive use of diathermy coagulation in achieving haemostasis in the cut ends of the bowel.

Before commencing an anastomosis the surgeon should ensure that the ends of the bowel can be easily apposed, and if the ends can be made to overlap it can be safely assumed that there will be no undue tension on the suture line. Haemostasis in the cut edges of the bowel may be achieved either by the individual ligation of vessels or by the use of diathermy coagulation. The latter method has the disadvantage that it may result in a greater degree of tissue necrosis at the suture line but it is certainly a less tedious technique than the ligature of vessels and, in practice, little tissue damage will result if the use of diathermy is limited to controlling only the major bleeding points. Minor oozing should be ignored but serious arterial bleeding should be checked as there is a tendency for the bleeding vessels to retract within the tissues and produce unpleasant haematomas.

In performing an anastomosis some surgeons place non-crushing occlusion clamps across the bowel to avoid soiling of the operative field with intestinal contents. It is important, however, that these clamps are applied lightly, and never across the mesentery of the intestine for fear of damaging the blood supply to the anastomosis. The author avoids the use of these clamps in oesophageal anastomoses because the blood supply to the cut end of the oesophagus is entirely dependent on intramural blood flow, and this will be at least temporarily interrupted by occlusion clamps. Soiling of the operative field is seldom a problem in oesophageal anastomoses.

Suture technique

The basic principles of intestinal suture were established more than 100 years ago and have undergone little modification. Secure healing of an anastomosis is dependent on accurate apposition of the serosal or outer surfaces of the bowel, and this is achieved by the use of a suture technique which inverts the cut edges of the gut. The principle of inversion in gastro-intestinal anastomoses has been challenged by Ravitch *et al.* (1967), who claimed that everting techniques of suture gave satisfactory results in intestinal anastomoses in experimental animals. This has not been the experience of others, however, and clinical studies by Goligher *et al.* (1973) of everting anastomoses in the colon have shown that the everting method results in a high incidence of anastomotic dehiscence and that it is manifestly inferior to the traditional inverting technique.

The vast majority of surgeons use an open method of intestinal anastomosis. 'Aseptic' or closed techniques of anastomosis achieved some popularity in the earlier part of this century due to the belief that the breakdown of anastomoses resulted from the bacterial contamination of the peritoneum which occurred during the construction of the open type of anastomosis. Several ingenious techniques of 'aseptic' anastomosis were devised but they were not generally accompanied by a reduction in the incidence of anastomotic dehiscence and most surgeons now rely on the simpler, open methods of anastomosis.

One aspect of the technique of intestinal suture which remains the subject of some controversy is the use of one or two layers of sutures in anastomoses.

The two-layer inverting suture technique was devised by Czerny, and is the method used by the majority of surgeons. Halsted and Cushing recommended the use of one layer of sutures in intestinal anastomoses and it is alleged that the single layer of sutures results in less ischaemia and tissue necrosis, and less narrowing of the intestinal lumen than the two-layer method. In practice, however, narrowing of the bowel lumen is hardly ever a clinical problem with the two-layer inverting method of suture, and the author is not convinced that single-layer techniques have significant advantages in the majority of gastro-intestinal anastomoses. Studies in experimental animals have not established any consistent difference between one- and two-layer methods of suture (McAdams, Meikle and Taylor, 1970; Irvin and Edwards, 1973) and clinical observations have not suggested that there is a need to depart from the standard two-layer method of anastomosis (Irvin, Goligher and Johnston, 1973; Everett, 1975).

It appears, however, that the single-layer suture technique may be the method of choice in anastomoses involving the extraperitoneal rectum. Low rectal anastomoses made with the two-layer suture method have been associated with a high incidence of dehiscence and septic complications, and a recent clinical trial by Everett (1975) has suggested that single-layer suture technique has significant advantages in low colorectal anastomoses. Matheson has had a similar experience (Matheson and Irving, 1975). A single-layer suture technique is certainly a much simpler technical exercise than the two-layer method in very low rectal anastomoses, and the author recommends its use.

1a-d

Standard sutures

The standard two-layer anastomosis (*a*) consists of an inner layer of sutures incorporating the full thickness of the bowel wall and an outer layer of sutures inserted through all layers except mucosa. This second layer is frequently referred to as a sero-muscular stitch but it should in fact include the collagenous submucosal layer of the bowel since more superficial sutures have a tendency to cut out. Single-layer techniques of suture are shown in (*b*), (*c*) and (*d*). In (*b*) the suture is inserted from the mucosal aspect of the bowel through the full thickness of the bowel wall and inversion of the anastomosis results when the suture is tied. The Gambee stitch (*c*) is inserted through all layers of the bowel wall, and it is passed twice through the mucosa on each side of the anastomosis to secure mucosal inversion. The Gambee suture technique thus results in minimal inversion of the cut edges of the bowel, and it is a popular suture technique in the operation of Heineke-Mikulicz pyloroplasty. In (*d*) the suture is a submucosal stitch inserted from the serosal aspect of the bowel, as in the outer layer of a two-layer anastomosis.

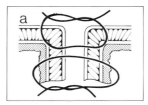 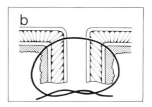
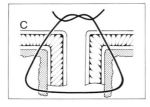 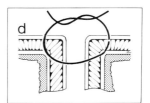

1

A variety of suture materials are used in the anastomosis of the intestine, and little is known of their relative merits. Recent experimental studies have suggested that anastomoses made with absorbable sutures are weaker than those made with non-absorbable materials during the early phase of healing but the difference is slight and probably of no clinical significance (Hastings *et al.,* 1975). In practice, two-layer anastomoses are made with an inner layer of absorbable sutures and an outer layer of non-absorbable sutures, and single-layer anastomoses are usually made with non-absorbable materials.

Chromic catgut is the most popular absorbable suture material, and there is no convincing evidence that other materials such as polyglycolic acid and polyglactin are superior to catgut for intestinal suture.

A variety of non-absorbable suture materials are used including silk, cotton, polypropylene and various synthetic polyesters. The presence of a non-absorbable suture material on the mucosal aspect of the gut provokes a significant foreign body reaction and granuloma formation is not uncommon. This is of little practical significance in anastomoses in the small and large intestine, but the presence of non-absorbable sutures in the gastric mucosa may result in ulceration and clinical symptoms. There are theoretical advantages in the use of monofilament non-absorbable materials such as stainless steel wire, nylon or polypropylene in that these materials result in little tissue reaction. However, the handling qualities of these sutures are poor and most surgeons prefer braided suture materials.

FACTORS AFFECTING THE HEALING OF ANASTOMOSES

Anastomoses of the stomach, duodenum and small intestine seldom give rise to complications and dehiscence is a danger chiefly in anastomoses involving the oesophagus, colon and rectum. Although technical factors may be implicated in the pathogenesis of many cases of anastomotic dehiscence it appears that other local and systemic factors also affect intestinal healing.

Local factors

Sepsis

There is evidence from clinical and experimental studies that peritoneal sepsis has an adverse effect on the healing of anastomoses (Schrock, Deveney and Dunphy, 1973). The problem of peritoneal sepsis arises chiefly in the surgery of the large intestine. A significant incidence of anastomotic dehiscence is encountered when a primary anastomosis of the colon is performed in the management of perforated diverticulitis or carcinoma, and injuries of the left colon. Experimental studies have shown that the synthesis of collagen in colonic anastomoses is impaired in the presence of peritoneal infection, probably as a result of excessive lysis of newly-formed collagen (Irvin, 1975).

The surgeon should avoid an anastomosis in the presence of established peritoneal sepsis and the bowel should be exteriorized as a colostomy or ileostomy. Alimentary continuity can be re-established later as an elective procedure.

Postoperative peritoneal sepsis and anastomotic complications may result when faecal contamination or soiling of the peritoneum occurs during operation. In some cases, such as advanced tumours of the large intestine, some soiling may be unavoidable but it should always be regarded as a serious complication. When gross faecal soiling occurs with other local factors which may propagate peritoneal infection, such as residual tumour, an extensive retroperitoneal dissection, or injuries of other viscera, it is often advisable to avoid an anastomosis and the bowel is exteriorized as a colostomy or ileostomy.

Mechanical state of the bowel

Faecal loading of the colon has an adverse effect on the healing of colonic or rectal anastomoses (Irvin and Goligher, 1973). The mechanical state of the bowel is a factor which may determine the success or failure of anastomoses in the left colon or rectum, and it is a major factor in the high incidence of dehiscence which follows primary anastomosis of the left colon in operations for acute obstruction.

Many surgeons also use antimicrobial agents before colonic operations in an attempt to reduce the infectivity of the colonic contents, but the role of such therapy in intestinal healing has yet to be established.

Drains

The use of peritoneal drains is regarded by many surgeons as a necessary feature of the management of anastomoses, particularly in the colon and rectum. Many advocates of the use of drains claim that when anastomotic dehiscence occurs drains safeguard the patient against anastomotic leakage by permitting the development of an enterocutaneous fistula rather than a diffusing faecal peritonitis. However, the value of drainage is by no means established, and experimental studies have suggested that peritoneal drains may actually increase the incidence of anastomotic dehiscence (Manz, La Tendresse and Sako, 1970).

The author uses peritoneal drains for the purpose of removing any blood or serum which may accumulate in the peritoneal cavity after operations involving extensive dissection and mobilization of the viscera, and in operations complicated by appreciable faecal contamination. The author does not deliberately place drains in the vicinity of anastomoses, and the drains are removed after 48 hr.

Faecal diversion

A proximal loop colostomy or a caecostomy may be used for the temporary protection of anastomoses in the left colon or rectum. These procedures are usually reserved for 'high-risk' anastomoses such as the very low colorectal anastomosis or an anastomosis made in the presence of unfavourable local conditions. There is no evidence that proximal faecal diversion prevents anastomotic dehiscence but it does appear that the septic complications of anastomotic dehiscence may be less serious when the faecal stream has been diverted (Goldstein and Duff, 1972).

Systemic factors

The precise role of systemic abnormalities in the pathogenesis of anastomotic dehiscence has not been clearly defined, and this is a subject of current interest.

THE ANASTOMOSES

Anastomoses may be made end to end, end to side, or side to side, but generally the method used in any operation is fairly standard. In this section, the indications for the use of the different types of anastomosis and the techniques of intestinal suture will be described.

END-TO-END ANASTOMOSIS

This is the method of choice for anastomosis of the small or large intestine following intestinal resection.

2a,b&c

Small bowel anastomosis

Insertion of posterior outer layer of sutures

The divided ends of the bowel are held in crushing clamps, and light occlusion clamps are applied across the bowel, with care to avoid the application of these clamps across the mesentery. The two-layer inverting anastomosis commences with the insertion of the outer layer of interrupted submucosal sutures on the posterior aspect of the anastomosis (*a* and *b*). Non-absorbable sutures of silk or other braided material are used, and they are inserted first at the mesenteric and antimesenteric borders of the intestine. The sutures are tied when this layer is complete, and the crushing clamps can then be amputated (*c*), thus opening the bowel lumen.

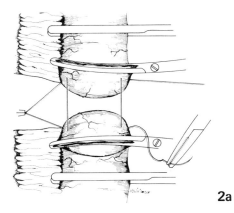

2a

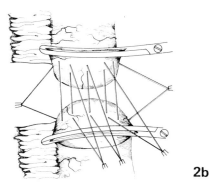

2b

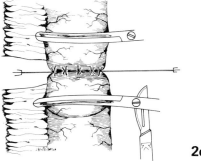

2c

3a-g

Inner layer of sutures

A continuous chromic catgut suture is used for the inner layer of the anastomosis, which begins at the antimesenteric end. The suture is inserted through all layers of the bowel wall, and tied on the serosal aspect (*a*). A forceps is applied to the short end of the suture which will be used again on completion of this layer. A continuous over-and-over suture technique is used for the posterior aspect of the anastomosis, care being taken to include all coats of the bowel wall (*b*). The mesenteric corner of the anastomosis is securely invaginated by the use of the Connell suture technique (*c*); inversion of the edges of the bowel is achieved when the suture is pulled tight (*d*). The anterior aspect of the inner layer of the anastomosis may be completed with an over-and-over suture technique, but a continuous Connell technique is generally preferred (*e*). The mucosa and edges of the bowel on the antimesenteric aspect are invaginated as the last Connell stitch is pulled tight (*f*), and the suture is tied to its other end (*g*).

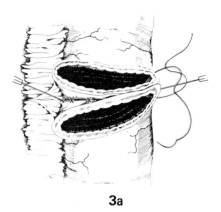

3a

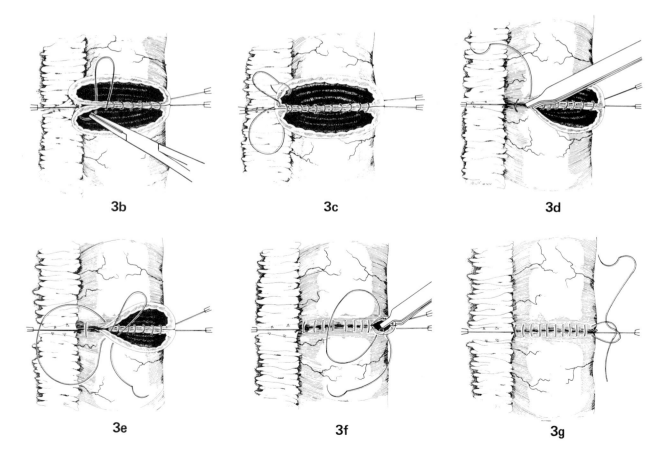

3b

3c

3d

3e

3f

3g

4a&b

Insertion of anterior outer layer of sutures

Interrupted, non-absorbable, submucosal sutures are then inserted on the anterior aspect of the bowel (*a*), and the anastomosis is completed (*b*).

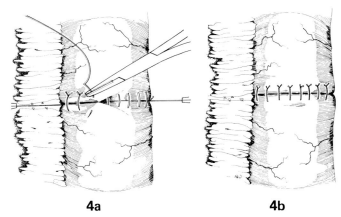

4a   **4b**

5a-d

Anastomosis commencing with inner layer of sutures

Some surgeons prefer to begin the two-layer anastomosis with the insertion of the inner layer of catgut (*a* and *b*). When this layer is complete, the outer layer of sutures is inserted on the anterior aspect of the anastomosis, and the anastomosis is then rotated (*c*), so that the outer layer can be completed on the posterior aspect (*d*). This method is apt to prove unsatisfactory in obese subjects when the mesentery is fat-laden because, after completion of the inner layer, insertion of the outer layer of sutures on the posterior aspect of the anastomosis is difficult to achieve with precision when the mesenteric fat encroaches on the bowel wall.

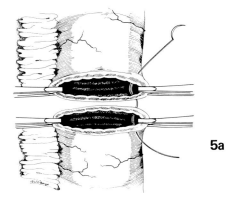

5a

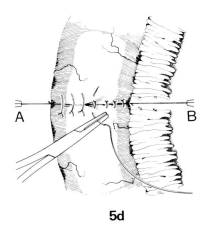

5d

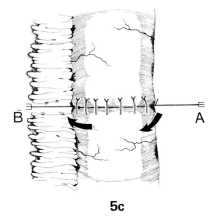

5c

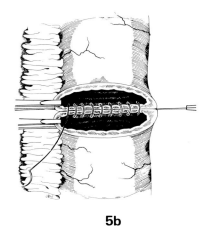

5b

Ileocolic anastomosis

6a-d

Correction for unequal ends of bowel

An end-to-end anastomosis is possible even when
there is considerable disparity in the size of the two
ends of bowel. This situation may arise in anastomosis
of the ileum to the colon after right hemicolectomy,
or in operations for small bowel obstruction (*a*).
The problem is solved by widening the orifice of the
smaller lumen: the outer layer of submucosal sutures
is inserted in an oblique fashion away from the cut
edge of the bowel on the antimesenteric aspect in
the end of smaller calibre (*b*); and the open end of
the bowel is widened by cutting along the antimesenteric border (*c* and *d*).

Most problems of disparity can be solved in this
way but some surgeons prefer to use an end-to-side
technique of anastomosis in these circumstances.

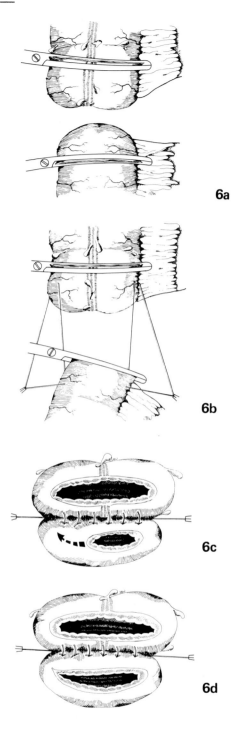

6a

6b

6c

6d

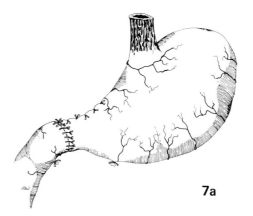

7a

7a,b&c

Gastroduodenal anastomosis

The most common end-to-end anastomosis involving
the stomach is the Billroth I gastroduodenal anastomosis (*a*). Care should be taken with regard to
haemostasis in this operation for the stomach is
endowed with a rich blood supply, and serious
postoperative bleeding from the suture line may occur
if haemostasis is not achieved. The Connell suture
technique is not haemostatic but a suitable method in
this operation is the 'loop on the serosa' technique
(*b* and *c*). This technique provides effective haemostasis, and adequate inversion of the cut edges of
the bowel.

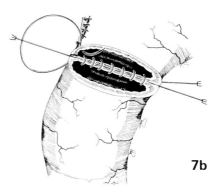

7b

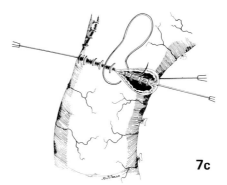

7c

Colorectal anastomosis

8a-d

Two-layer method

A modified suture technique is used in a two-layer anastomosis in the extraperitoneal rectum. In a low colorectal anastomosis, where access may be restricted, it is often simpler to insert the outer layer of submucosal sutures parallel to the cut edge of the rectum as horizontal mattress sutures (*a* and *b*). The use of this stitch in the extraperitoneal rectum is desirable also in that it is placed at right angles to the longitudinal muscle fibres, and there is less tendency for it to cut through the muscle tissue than a conventional vertical suture. The sutures are held in forceps until the outer layer is complete (*c*), and secure inversion of the suture line is achieved when these are tied (*d*).

A similar suture technique is recommended in two-layer oesophageal anastomoses.

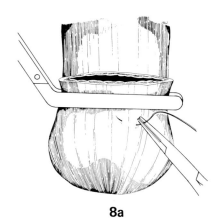

8a

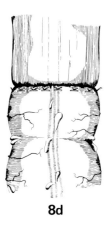

8d

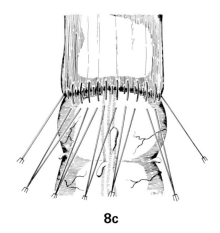

8c

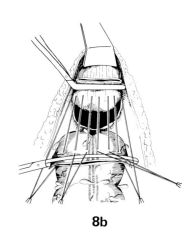

8b

9a-e

Single-layer method (see also pages 236–241)

A single-layer technique of anastomosis is the alternative, simpler and more satisfactory method for low rectal anastomoses. A braided suture material such as silk is used, and the anastomosis begins with the insertion of the mesenteric and antimesenteric sutures through all layers of the bowel wall (*a*). The posterior layer of the anastomosis consists of a series of through-and-through sutures incorporating all layers of the bowel wall. These sutures are held in forceps and tied when the layer is complete (*b*). The interval between each suture in the posterior layer should be relatively small otherwise there is a tendency for eversion of the mucosa to occur when the sutures are tied. The anterior layer of the anastomosis is made with a similar series of full-thickness sutures, knotted on the mucosa (*c*). A small gap in the suture line finally remains in the centre of the anterior layer, and this is closed with a submucosal suture inserted parallel to the edge of the suture line (*d*).

An alternative method of construction of the anterior layer is to use a series of submucosal mattress sutures (*e*), as in the outer layer of a two-layer rectal anastomosis.

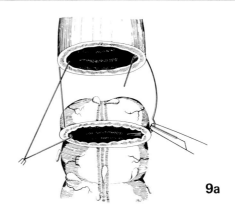

9a

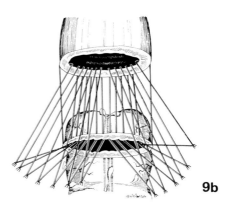

9b

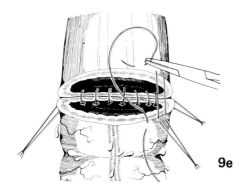

9e

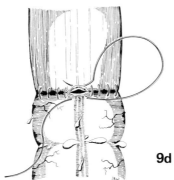

9d

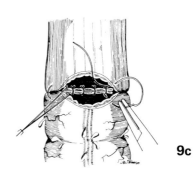

9c

12 a - d

Gastrojejunal anastomosis

After destructive injuries of the stomach (*a*), the gastric remnant may be anastomosed end-to-side to the jejunum. The construction of this anastomosis is simplified by the use of Lane's twin occlusion clamps (*b*). A two-layer inverting suture technique is used (*c* and *d*), and many surgeons use a double layer of continuous catgut in this anastomosis. Because of the rich blood supply of the stomach troublesome postoperative bleeding may occur from the suture line unless a haemostatic suture technique is used. For this reason a 'loop on the serosa' technique should be used for the inner layer of the anastomosis (*c*). The use of non-haemostatic suture technique, such as a Connell stitch, is permissible only if occlusion clamps are avoided, and the bleeding vessels in the suture line can be individually secured.

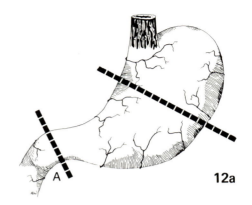

12a

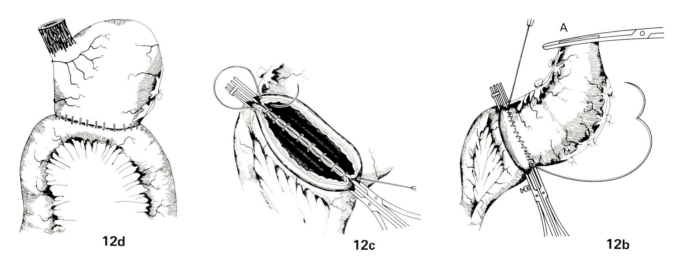

12d

12c

12b

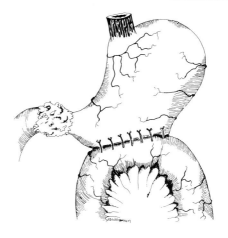

13a

13a,b&c

Bypass procedures

In the case of injuries of the region of the pancreas, duodenum and pylorus a gastrojejunostomy may have to be performed (*a*); anastomosis of the terminal ileum to the transverse colon is performed for obstructions of the right colon (*b*); and after damage to the common bile duct the fundus of the gall-bladder is anastomosed to a defunctioned loop of jejunum (*c*).

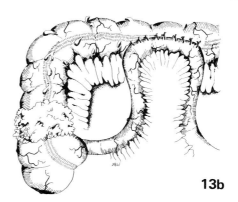

13b

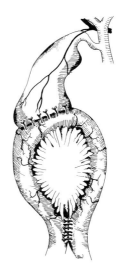

13c

POSTOPERATIVE CARE

The postoperative management of anastomoses in the gastro-intestinal tract is chiefly concerned with the restoration of normal alimentary function, and the early detection and control of complications.

A period of alimentary motor dysfunction inevitably follows anastomosis of the intestine and may or may not be apparent clinically. In some cases the early introduction of oral intake in the postoperative period is poorly tolerated. Vomiting may occur because of delayed gastric emptying; intestinal distension and vomiting may take place after anastomosis of the small or large intestine. Distension of the bowel at the suture line is undesirable on the theoretical grounds that it may cause ischaemia and an increased risk of anastomotic leakage, but there is little clinical evidence to support this thesis, and there is no standard programme for the postoperative management of oral intake.

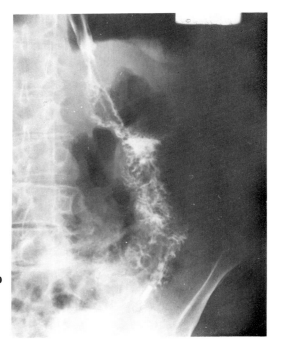

14a

14b

14a&b

The author does not routinely use nasogastric tubes but has a cautious attitude towards the introduction of oral intake after anastomosis of the intestine. After gastric resection, gastric emptying is assessed radiologically with Gastrografin on the first postoperative day, and oral intake is permitted only if satisfactory emptying is present (a). Oral intake after oesophagogastric resections is not permitted for at least 5 days, and then only after a Gastrografin swallow has shown that there is no leakage at the suture line (b). Oral intake after anastomosis of the small or large intestine is withheld until the patient has passed flatus, which usually occurs about the fourth postoperative day.

Intolerance of oral intake and ileus may indicate that anastomotic dehiscence has occurred. Other signs of dehiscence such as peritonitis, fistulation, and systemic evidence of sepsis depend on the site of the anastomosis, the extent of the dehiscence, and the nature of the intestinal contents. Dehiscence is a complication which occurs during the first few days after operation when the integrity and strength of the anastomosis are largely dependent on the intestinal sutures, and clinical features of dehiscence seldom arise *de novo* after the first postoperative week.

(a) *Gastrografin study showing gastric emptying on the first day after Billroth I gastrectomy*

(b) *Gastrografin swallow on the sixth day after total gastrectomy showing no leakage at the oesophagojejunal anastomosis*

References

Daly, J. M., Steiger, E., Vars, H. M. and Dudrick, S. J. (1974). *Ann. Surg.* **180,** 709
Everett, W. G. (1975). *Br. J. Surg.* **62,** 135
Goldstein, M. and Duff, J. H. (1972). *Surgery Gynec. Obstet.* **134,** 593
Goligher, J. C., Morris, C., McAdam, W. A. F., DeDombal, F. T. and Johnston, D. (1973). *Br. J. Surg.* **57,** 817
Hastings, J. C., Van Winkle, W., Barker, E., Hines, D. and Nichols, W. (1975). *Surgery Gynec. Obstet.* **140,** 701
Irvin, T. T. (1975). *Br. J. Surg.* **62,** 659
Irvin, T. T. and Edwards, J. P. (1973). *Br. J. Surg.* **60,** 453
Irvin, T. T. and Goligher, J. C. (1973). *Br. J. Surg.* **60,** 461
Irvin, T. T., Goligher, J. C. and Johnston, D. (1973). *Br. J. Surg.* **60,** 457
Matheson, N. A. and Irving, A. D. (1975). *Br. J. Surg.* **62,** 239
McAdams, A. J. Meikle, A. G. and Taylor, J. O. (1970). *Am. J. Surg.* **120,** 546
Manz, C. W., La Tendresse, C. and Sako, Y. (1970). *Dis. Colon Rectum* **13,** 17
Ravitch, M. M., Canalis, F., Weinshelbaum, A. and McCormack, J. (1967). *Ann. Surg.* **166,** 670

[*The illustrations for this Chapter on Techniques of Anastomosis in Gastro-intestinal Surgery were drawn by Mr. J. B. Williamson.*]

Single - layer Interrupted Serosubmucosal Anastomosis

N. A. Matheson, Ch. M., F.R.C.S.(Eng.), F.R.C.S.(Ed.)
Consultant Surgeon, Aberdeen General Hospitals

INTRODUCTION

Recently there has been a re-awakening of interest in single-layer techniques of intestinal anastomosis particularly because single-layer methods have been shown to give better results in the difficult area of colorectal anastomosis than conventional two-layer methods. Single-layer techniques almost always imply interrupted stitches, but vary according to the suture material used and whether the stitches incorporate all coats of the gut or exclude the mucosa.

Single-layer inverting anastomosis with interrupted non-absorbable seromuscular stitches was first advised by Halsted, but has not become popular despite the sound experimental work in animals upon which the technique is based. Nevertheless such a technique with minor modifications lends itself to the fashioning of anastomoses throughout the alimentary tract with the exception of the oesophagus and is appealing in its simplicity and safety. Lack of confidence in single-layer seromuscular anastomosis stems in part from apparent dependence on seromuscular sutures only, with exclusion of the submucosa which is accepted as the most important holding layer of the gut. However, it is emphasized that in the technique to be described the sutures are placed deeply with the intention of incorporating submucosa so that mucosa only is excluded. This technique may therefore be correctly termed interrupted single-layer serosubmucosal.

Materials

Braided nylon is less reactive than silk. It is also stronger and may be used in a finer gauge. Finally, braided nylon handles with a slight elasticity permitting a fine adjustment to knot tension particularly if the first throw is crossed and tension taken up on the second.

1

Anastomosis packets are prepared containing 24 16 mm fine gauge half circle needles threaded with 40 cm lengths of 2/0 braided nylon. For anastomosis after low anterior resection 75 cm lengths are used. During the course of an anastomosis one needle holder is used.

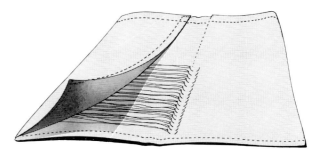

1

2

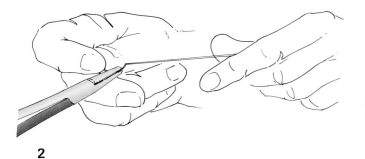

2

Each needle is drawn from the packet in turn by the theatre sister or nurse and is held as shown ready to be grasped by the needle holder. The nurse may steady the point of the needle holder with her right middle finger. Once each stitch has been placed the needle is discarded into a small gallipot and the next in the series taken from the sister's hold.

Anastomosis packets and the standard way in which they are used are common to all single-layer interrupted anastomoses, but modifications in the use of clamps and in suture placement are made according to site in the gut.

THE ANASTOMOSES

In small bowel anastomosis, Wangensteen's clamps are used and the technique is 'closed' throughout. 'Closed' or 'aseptic' intestinal anastomosis using Wangensteen's clamps is neat, clean, time-saving and technically satisfying. It is these attributes rather than a conviction that septic complications are diminished by its use that have led us to adopt the method wherever possible. Angle stitches are inserted in the transverse axis of the gut about 6–7 mm from the clamps and sufficiently deeply that mucosa only is excluded.

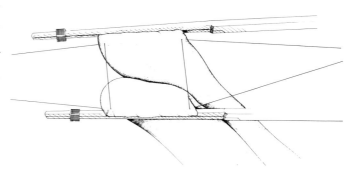

3

3&4

These stitches are held untied. The posterior stitches are then inserted longitudinally about 5 mm apart. A substantial bite of tissue is taken with each stitch so that all layers except mucosa are incorporated and entry and exit points of each needle are about 6 mm apart. Care is taken to ensure that at least 5 mm of bowel is spared between the stitches and the clamps so that these may be easily rotated. For the same reason the angle stitches are left untied while the posterior stitches are tied and cut. The clamps are now rotated, individual collars are slipped off and the double collar is pushed over the ends of both clamps to hold them firmly together.

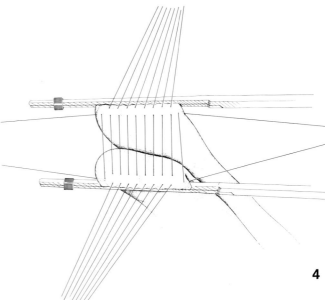

4

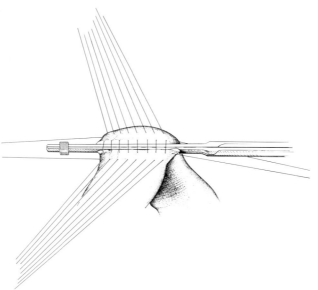

5

The anterior stitches are then inserted in a similar way to the posterior layer, except that they may be placed close to the clamps. Once in place, these stitches are held up taut by an assistant, the double collar is removed and the clamps are slipped out. Each angle stitch is tied and held, after which the anterior stitches are tied and cut.

5

6

Finally, the angle stitches are cut and patency of the anastomosis is established by breaking open the crushed bowel ends with pressure between finger and thumb. This last step must not be omitted.

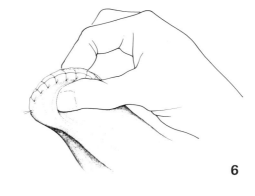

6

The same method may be used for ileotransverse anastomosis and for colonic anastomosis where the bowel ends are sufficiently accessible for Wangensteen's clamps to be applied. In practice the method is usually applicable unless the anastomosis is between colon and rectum.

When the single-layer serosubmucosal technique is used for gastroduodenal anastomosis it is modified to allow submucosal haemostasis and is therefore no longer 'closed' throughout. In making a gastroduodenal anastomosis after partial gastrectomy a new lesser curve is fashioned such that the distal stomach exceeds the duodenum by 1–1·5 cm in width.

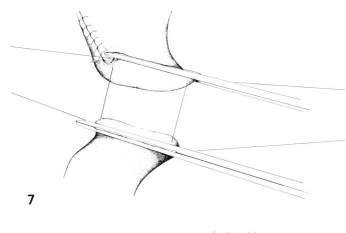

7

7&8

Schoemacker's clamps are applied to both stomach and duodenum and angle stitches are placed in the transverse axis of the gut about 5 mm from the clamps and sufficiently deeply that mucosa only is excluded. These stitches are held untied. The posterior stitches are then inserted longitudinally 2–3 mm from the clamps and about 5 mm apart. Entry and exit points of the needles are 6–7 mm apart and all layers except mucosa are incorporated. Once all have been placed the posterior stitches are tied and cut. The clamps are then removed and the angle stitches are tied and held. Residual submucosal haemorrhage is controlled using diathermy coagulation.

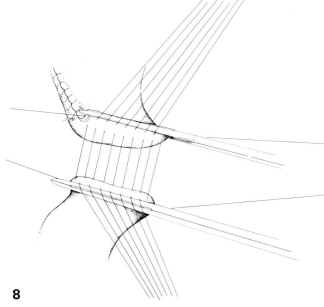

8

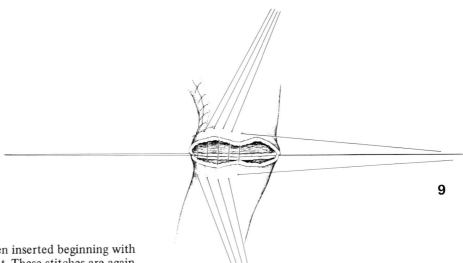

9

9 & 10

The anterior stitches are then inserted beginning with a stitch marking the mid-point. These stitches are again deeply placed so that only mucosa is avoided. Each needle is inserted approximately 7 mm from the cut edge of the stomach and emerges at the cut edge in the submucosal plane. It is re-inserted in the same plane at the cut edge of the duodenum to emerge 7 mm distally. Insertion and withdrawal of sutures in the submucosal plane, made possible by the absence of the clamps, makes for accurate placement and is apparently safe. The anterior stitches are tied and cut and finally the angle holding stitches are cut. This anastomotic technique results in minimal inversion of all coats posteriorly and in mucosal inversion only anteriorly, where the stitches are appositional.

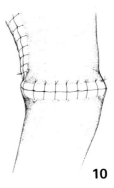

10

11-14

Colorectal anastomoses are also made open and clamps are avoided. Angle stitches are placed in the transverse axis of the gut about 5 mm from the cut edge and are held. The posterior stitches are then inserted at about 5 mm intervals close to the cut edge. If the muscular coat is substantial the stitches may be inserted and withdrawn in the submucosal plane at the cut edge of proximal and distal bowel as in the anterior layer of a gastroduodenal anastomosis and this type of stitch is now often used on both aspects of the anastomosis, but particularly on the anterior aspect. Whether such a variant is used or not a particular point of incorporating all layers except mucosa is again made and the entry and exit points of the needles, posteriorly and anteriorly, are some 8 mm apart. The posterior stitches are held up taut, the colon is slid down to the rectum, the stitches are tied and subsequently cut. The angle stitches are tied and held. The anterior stitches are inserted beginning with a mid-point marking stitch and are then tied and cut. The anastomosis is completed by cutting the angle stitches.

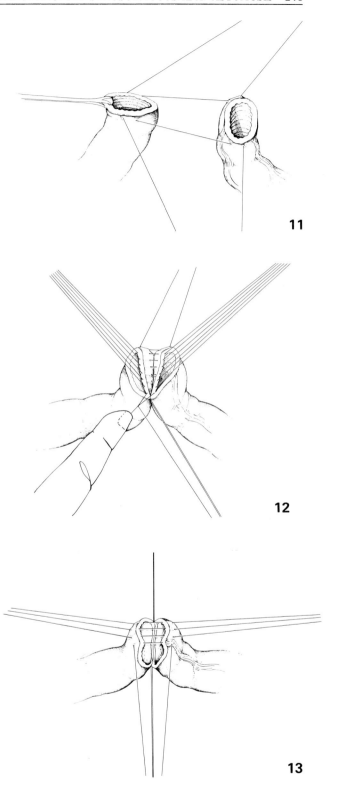

11

12

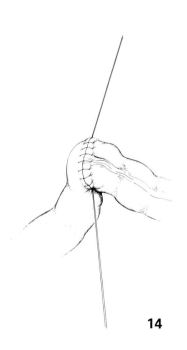

14

13

[*The illustrations for this Chapter on Single-layer Interrupted Serosubmucosal Anastomosis were drawn by Mr. N. Lucins.*]

Gunshot Wounds of the Abdomen

Colonel W. Cameron Moffat, O.B.E., M.B., F.R.C.S., L./R.A.M.C.
Senior Consultant Surgeon, British Military Hospital, Rinteln

GENERAL CONSIDERATIONS

Gunshot wounds of the abdomen sustained in war are almost always fatal unless treated by prompt and adequate surgery. The nature and extent of the injury may vary widely depending on the type and velocity of the missile and the track it follows into or through the body. A small regular missile of low velocity, such as a bullet fired from a hand gun, may penetrate or perforate a single viscus only and pose few problems in management. In contrast, high velocity rifle bullets or irregular bomb fragments are likely to produce alarming and disruptive multiple injuries in several internal organs.

The amount of damage inflicted by a missile is related to the kinetic energy transferred to static tissues by retardation on contact or penetration. The kinetic energy possessed by a missile is proportional to the product of its mass and the square of its velocity ($KE = \frac{1}{2} MV^2$) so that high speed missiles, even though small, may inflict an unexpec-tedly large injury because doubling the strike velocity quadruples the available energy.

Injury is caused in three main ways: by simple laceration; by cavitation caused by the violent outward acceleration of tissues away from the missile track, and by shock waves set up by missile impact. These shock waves travel at the speed of sound, almost 5000 feet/sec in aqueous solutions, and may inflict damage at a considerable distance from the missile track; this applies especially to thin-walled blood vessels and other liquid-containing structures such as the bile passages.

The amount of internal damage consequent on abdominal wounding by a missile is thus likely to be much greater and more widespread than expected and due allowance must always be made for this. In addition, the local damage in any one viscus may extend beyond that readily visible to the naked eye. This is of especial importance in relation to injury of the gut when it becomes necessary to decide whether to repair or resect damaged bowel.

1

There are two other factors of general importance. Missiles entering the shoulder, chest, back, perineum, buttocks or thighs may lead to an intra-abdominal injury which is not immediately apparent. The entry wounds themselves may be small or their presence may be obscured by more obvious wounding at other sites. Signs of intra-abdominal injury may be difficult to elicit in the presence of pain from a major limb injury or in an unconscious patient.

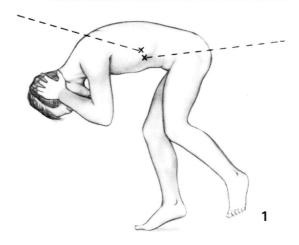

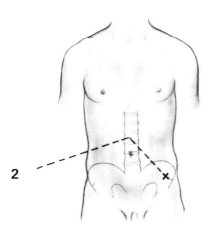

2

Missiles do not necessarily pass through the tissues in straight lines but may be widely diverted, especially if they strike bone. In that event a missile may break up, or may shatter bone, leading to the formation of many secondary missiles, all of which are capable of inflicting additional damage.

PRE - OPERATIVE

Assessment

It should be readily understood that pre-operative assessment in cases of gunshot wounds of the abdomen is by no means always easy. In the circumstances in which such wounds are likely to arise the question may not be whether or not to operate on a given patient but which of several patients should come to operation before others. There is a tendency to deal first with those who are most profoundly shocked and most seriously injured but it should be remembered that the surgery of abdominal injury is often difficult, demanding and time-consuming. Valuable time and energy may be wasted in an overambitious attempt to save a mortally wounded patient while others, less seriously injured, may miss the optimum time for operation.

The patient who has a wound which clearly penetrates the abdominal parietes clearly requires laparotomy. Where there is doubt about penetration the surgeon must maintain a high index of suspicion. The most useful general signs are those of skin colour and pulse rate. The presence or occurrence of profound pallor together with a rising pulse rate in the absence of overt bleeding should direct attention to the abdomen. The presence there of guarding, slight distension and tenderness, especially if increasing in degree or extent, calls for exploration. Absence of bowel sounds usually indicates intra-abdominal injury, but the reverse is not true. Tenderness in the recto-vesical pouch is a most useful sign and should always be sought by digital rectal examination. Plain x-ray films can be very helpful by demonstrating free gas in the abdomen or locating metallic foreign bodies and should, if possible, be obtained before the operation in all cases. Additional lateral or oblique views are usually required. Excretion pyelography may be helpful in the assessment of retroperitoneal injury but contrast radiography of the intestinal tract is not likely to be useful. In the absence of urethral injury, catheterization of the urinary bladder may reveal haematuria indicative of damage to the renal tract. Abdominal paracentesis by needle or fine catheter to demonstrate free blood in the peritoneal cavity is unlikely to add usefully to what is already known or suspected.

Preparation for operation

All patients coming to laparotomy should have at least one reliable intravenous infusion well established. An adequate quantity of compatible or group O rhesus negative whole blood should be available. A wide-bore nasogastric tube with a radio-opaque tip should be in place. The urinary bladder should be empty and an indwelling Foley catheter should be connected to a closed drainage bag. Antibiotics should be commenced intravenously. The choice of drug will vary with circumstances but a combination of ampicillin and cloxacillin is effective and safe.

Anaesthesia

Once a decision to operate has been taken pain should be relieved by an adequate dosage of a narcotic analgesic preferably given by the intravenous route. Additional premedication will depend on individual choice. General anaesthesia with a cuffed endotracheal tube and muscle relaxants is highly desirable. Preparation should be made for extending the operation into the chest. It should be remembered that seriously injured patients often exhibit low arterial oxygen levels even in the absence of severe perfusion disorder or overt pulmonary damage.

Position of patient and towelling

The standard supine operating position is usually satisfactory. A head-up or head-down tilt is helpful according to circumstance. If there is a wound of the back or limbs which requires immediate attention in the prone position it should be dealt with first to avoid the necessity to turn the patient after laparotomy, a manoeuvre which is sometimes associated with circulatory collapse.

A skin cleansing agent should be applied to the whole abdomen, including the flanks and the lower part of the chest and towels should be placed to allow generous wound extensions.

THE OPERATION

The incision

3

The placing of the incision will be to some extent guided by the pre-operative findings and should take account of the possible need to construct a stoma. A long right paramedian incision is usually preferable and it may be extended across the costal margin into either side of the chest.

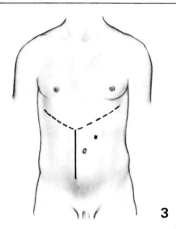

3

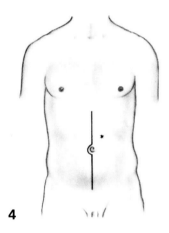

4

4

A mid-line incision may be used especially when speed in entering the abdomen is considered vital.

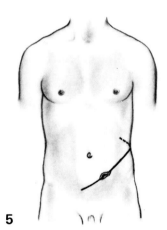

5

5

It is occasionally possible to incorporate the entry wound in the incision. As a general rule, however, excision of the missile wound is best left until the conclusion of intra-abdominal work. Transverse incisions rarely give adequate access to the entire abdomen and are not recommended.

Initial exploration

It is essential that a full and systematic examination of all intra-abdominal structures be made. The peritoneal cavity should first be cleared of blood or soiling contents by suction or mopping. Haemorrhage from solid organs should be temporarily controlled, by packing if possible, and other troublesome bleeding points ligated or under-run.

6 & 7

The transverse colon should be brought out with the omentum and turned upwards. The small bowel is then delivered, working carefully from duodeno-jejunal flexure to ileocaecal valve. Any injury to bowel or mesentery should be noted and marked with a tissue forceps or stitch as the evisceration proceeds. A moist warm pack is placed over the small gut, and the posterior abdominal wall, the left side of the abdomen and pelvis are carefully examined. Especial attention is given to the retroperitoneal colon. If there is suspicion of injury there the pelvic colon is drawn to the right, tensing the peritoneal reflection in the left iliac fossa and the peritoneum is incised from below upwards. The descending colon may then be rolled to the right and the posterior surface clearly seen.

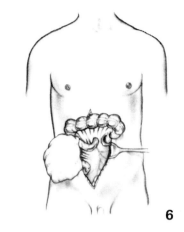

6

All injuries having been noted, the gut is returned to the abdomen and the exploration completed by examining the stomach, duodenum, biliary tract, right side of the colon and both colonic flexures. Again, care should be taken to exclude retroperitoneal injury (*see Illustrations 8, 9, 13 and 18*).

Individual repair should not be undertaken until exploration is complete and all injuries are assessed unless it is essential to control bleeding.

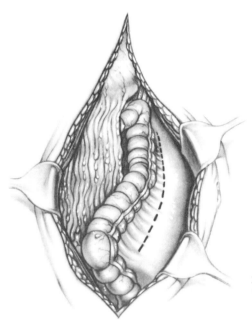

7

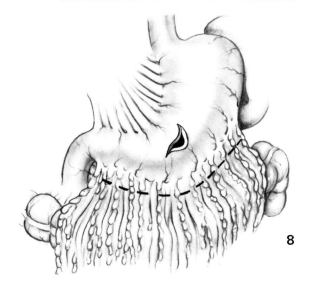

8

Stomach

8 & 9

Both surfaces of the stomach should be inspected by opening the lesser sac through the gastrocolic omentum. With the stomach turned upwards posterior injury is seen or excluded and the pancreas can be directly examined.

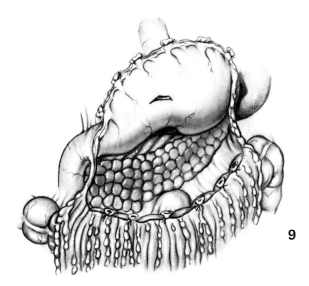

9

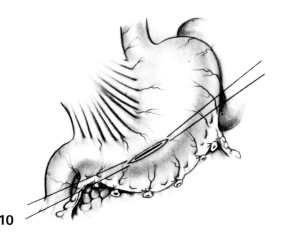

10

10

Wounds of the stomach should be excised to create clean, viable edges and even muscle and mucosal layers. Closure is assisted by using stay sutures or light tissue forceps to stretch the wound gently.

11

Closure should be in two layers. A continuous all-layers invaginating stitch of chromic catgut provides good initial closure and haemostasis. This should be re-inforced and 'water-proofed' by seromuscular stitches using fine linen thread or other unabsorbable material.

Some gastric injuries are clearly unsuitable for simple closure and require partial gastrectomy.

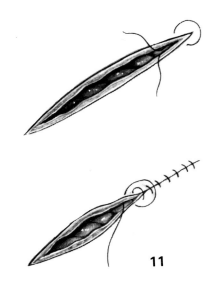

11

Duodenum

Severe duodenal injuries do not often come to operation because of the high early mortality associated with injury to related structures such as the liver, pancreas and vena cava. Survivors of such injury may require pancreaticoduodenectomy.

Lesser degrees of duodenal injury are relatively common and need careful assessment.

12

Any duodenal damage, even the presence of intra-mural bruising, points to the need for retroperitoneal inspection.

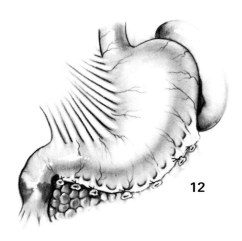

12

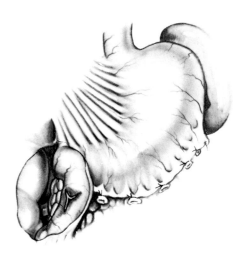

13

13

The peritoneum lateral to it should be incised so that the duodenum can be turned to the left. Lacerations should be closed transversely in two layers. The addition of gastrojejunostomy may sometimes be wise. The site of repair should always be drained through a separate stab wound in the right flank.

Small bowel

The injuries requiring attention are usually perforations or mesenteric tears. Perforations are commonly multiple but may be single due to tangential injury.

14

The mucosa tends to pout through the seromuscular coat and leakage of bowel content may be minimal. The detection of such lesions on the mesenteric border requires care.

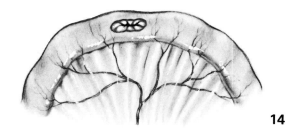

14

15

Isolated perforations should be closed transversely to avoid narrowing the lumen of the gut. Single-layer closure is safe if carefully done and it saves time if there are many scattered perforations.

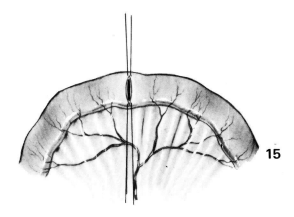

15

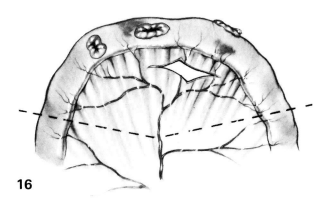

16

16

If perforations occur close together, or if there is a mesenteric injury which devitalizes or endangers bowel, resection is required. The line of section should be through clearly healthy bowel.

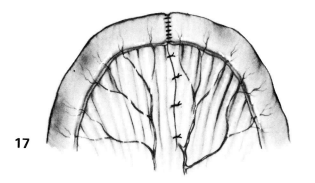

17

17

End-to-end anastomosis is the best method of restoring continuity and two-layer closure is advisable. The mesentery should be closed accurately, avoiding injury to blood vessels.

Large bowel

Right colon

18

An isolated wound of the caecum may be trimmed and converted to a caecostomy using a Foley catheter. The caecum itself should not be brought out of the abdomen.

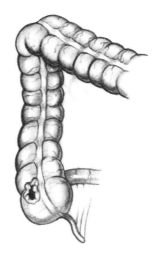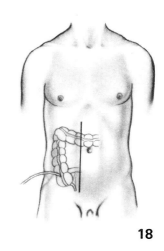

18

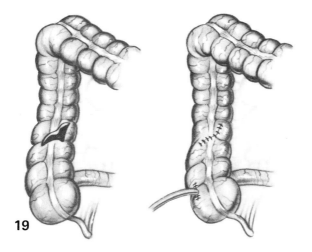

19

19

Single wounds of the ascending colon may be sutured in two layers provided that the retroperitoneal part of the colon is uninjured and a Foley catheter caecostomy is established. The paracolic gutter should be drained.

20

Any serious injury of the right side of the colon requires right hemicolectomy. Immediate ileotransverse anastomosis is unsafe, especially when other intra-abdominal injuries are present. A properly constructed terminal ileostomy should be made and the distal part of the colon brought out as a mucous fistula.

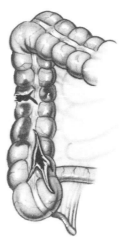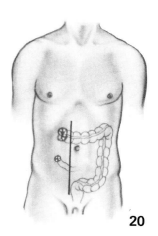

20

Transverse colon

21

An isolated lesion should be brought out without tension as a loop colostomy and held over a glass rod. The loop should be opened early by enlarging any wound to allow free egress of bowel content. Contamination of the laparotomy wound and the original missile wound should be avoided.

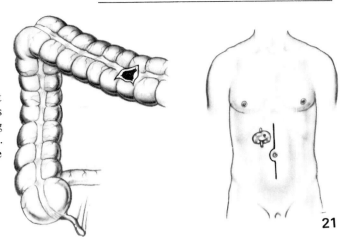

22

More serious damage to the transverse colon should be treated by resection with the construction of a right transverse end colostomy and distal mucous fistula.

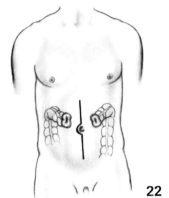

Left colon

Isolated wounds of the left side of the colon where the bowel is mobile or readily mobilized may be treated by exteriorization as for the transverse colon. It is in any event often essential to exclude retroperitoneal injury by mobilizing the descending colon.

23

Serious damage should be treated by resection with terminal colostomy and mucous fistula. When there has been faecal contamination drainage should be established through a separate stab wound in the left flank.

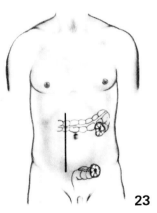

24

When the injury is in the pelvic colon and so low as to make it impossible to bring out a distal mucous fistula without tension the distal bowel should be closed in two layers and dropped back into the pelvis.

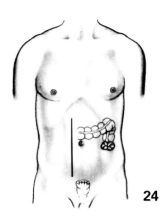

24

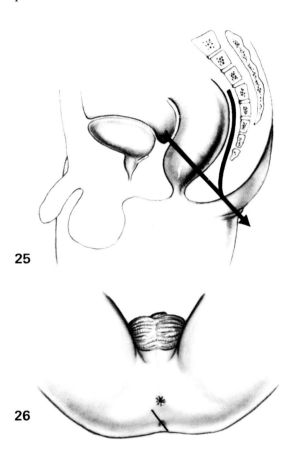

25

26

25 & 26

In that event the pararectal and presacral spaces should be developed from above to establish drainage via a near vertical, low incision in the natal cleft, excising the coccyx if necessary. This form of drainage is useful in any case when there is pelvic contamination or the likelihood of a pelvic collection.

27

In the event of rectal injury the faecal stream must be diverted using a pelvic end colostomy and separate distal mucous fistula. Proximal loop colostomy is not sufficient to divert faecal contamination effectively. Drainage of the pararectal and presacral space is required.

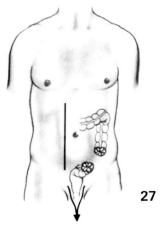

27

The missile wound

Wound excision should follow established principles (*see* Chapter on 'General Care of Gunshot Wounds', pages 19–25) but the peritoneum at least should be closed. If this cannot be done some soft tissue closure must be made if it can be accomplished without tension. In the rare event when the wound is so large that closure cannot be obtained the defect may be covered with moist packs. Any presenting abdominal contents will form granulations and split-skin grafts may be applied around the fifth day.

Laparotomy wound closure

The laparotomy wound should be carefully closed in layers using non-absorbable monofilament material for the rectus sheath or linea alba and placing an adequate number of deep tension sutures down to the peritoneal level. When the wound has been contaminated it should be irrigated with saline and a drain should be placed down to peritoneum. Spraying the wound with topical antibiotic or antiseptic such as povidone-iodine after peritoneal closure is helpful in the prevention of wound sepsis.

POSTOPERATIVE CARE

Intravenous infusion and nasogastric suction should continue until bowel function becomes re-established. Careful monitoring, recording and correction of water and electrolyte balance is essential. Dosage of sedatives and analgesics should be liberal to promote rest and facilitate nursing manoeuvres, deep breathing and coughing.

Antibiotics should be continued in high dosage by the intravenous route. The initial use of penicillin and cloxacillin with ampicillin or cephaloridine should not be continued for longer than 5 days unless laboratory confirmation of their continued effectiveness is obtained. Selection of antibiotics thereafter should be guided by the results of culture and sensitivity studies.

The haemoglobin level should be checked on the third postoperative day and if necessary restored at least above 11 g/100 ml by infusion of whole blood or packed red cells.

Patients who must be transported do badly if moved too early after operation. They should remain in the unit where they have received their initial surgical and nursing care until bowel function has been restored and the wounds are healing well. These conditions can rarely be met before the seventh postoperative day and it is thus unwise to move the patient, by any means of transport, in less than 1 week from operation.

[*The illustrations for this Chapter on Gunshot Wounds of the Abdomen were drawn by Mr. G. Lyth.*]

Colostomy

James P. S. Thomson, M.S., F.R.C.S.
Consultant Surgeon, St. Mark's Hospital, London

The construction of a colostomy is an essential part in the management of many patients with an injury to the large intestine. It may be used to exteriorize safely an injured segment of colon or to protect an injured part which has been repaired. Primary repair of tidy wounds of the right side of the colon may in rare circumstances be carried out without a protective colostomy, but this does not apply to injuries of the left side of the colon.

Types of colostomy

The four main types are: (*1*) loop colostomy (*2*) double-barrelled colostomy (*3*) divided colostomy (Devine) (*4*) terminal colostomy.

Loop colostomy

A loop colostomy is the most usually formed temporary colostomy. The site of the loop will depend on the place of the injury. However, the most common sites are in the transverse and sigmoid colon. In principle, a loop of colon is brought to the surface and held there by a glass rod or rubber tube. It is now usual for these colostomies to be opened at the time of operation and for a mucocutaneous suture to be performed.

Double-barrelled colostomy

A double-barrelled colostomy is used in the Paul-Mikulicz operation. A spur is constructed between the two limbs of the colostomy and can subsequently be crushed by the application of an enterotome. This type of colostomy should close spontaneously after the spur is crushed, but usually a formal closure is required.

Divided colostomy

A divided colostomy is constructed with a bridge of skin between the two limbs of the stoma. It was thought that this defunctioned the distal bowel more efficiently than a loop colostomy. However, this is not the case and because a loop colostomy is more satisfactory to close, a divided colostomy has little place in current surgical practice.

Terminal colostomy

A terminal colostomy is required when the rectum is so severely injured, as by crushing or explosion, that it has to be abandoned or removed. Such a colostomy may also be needed when a length of colon needs resection. An end-to-end anastomosis in the presence of unprepared bowel is contra-indicated and so the proximal opening may be brought to the surface as a terminal colostomy and the distal opening either over-sewn and returned to the abdominal cavity, or brought to the surface as a 'mucous fistula'.

The stoma is made by bringing the colon through an excised cylinder of anterior abdominal wall. At the conclusion of the operation a direct mucocutaneous suture is performed.

Anaesthesia

General anaesthesia is to be preferred as traction on the mesentery causes pain and nausea. However, it is possible to undertake this operation under local field anaesthesia.

THE OPERATION

LOOP COLOSTOMY

1

Incision

The sites of the incision for a transverse colostomy and a colostomy in the left iliac fossa are shown in the accompanying illustration. The ideal site for a transverse colostomy is in the right upper quadrant mid-way between the umbilicus and the costal margin, placed over the rectus abdominis muscle and running just lateral to the lateral border of the rectus abdominis muscle. It is usually 6 cm in length. The details may have to be varied depending on the injuries.

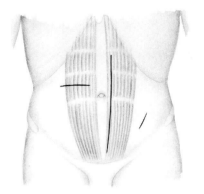

1

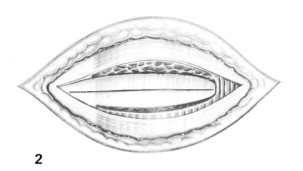

2

2

Division of rectus abdominis muscle

The incision is deepened through all the layers of the anterior abdominal wall and the muscle fibres of the rectus abdominis are divided as indicated.

3

Preparation of the colon

The colon must be prepared prior to delivery through the anterior abdominal wall, either, in the case of the transverse colon, by incising the greater omentum or by bringing it below the free border of the greater omentum, and in the case of the left colon by mobilizing it from the posterior abdominal wall. A small hole is made in the mesocolon by the edge of the bowel wall and a rubber tube placed through the hole to facilitate delivery of the colon through the anterior abdominal wall.

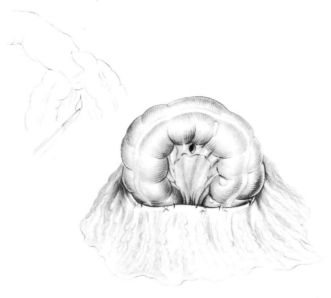

3

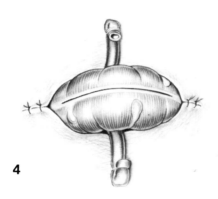

4

4

Securing the colostomy

Once the colon has been delivered through the anterior abdominal wall, it is held on the surface, with either the aid of a glass rod, or rubber tubing. This latter method allows easier application of the colostomy appliance. The colon may be opened longitudinally, as indicated, but some surgeons prefer to open the colon transversely as this damages fewer of the encircling vessels in the colonic wall.

5

Mucocutaneous suture

Once open, the mucosa is sutured to the skin using a chromic catgut suture. Tincture benzoin co. is then applied to the skin around the stoma and an appliance immediately fitted.

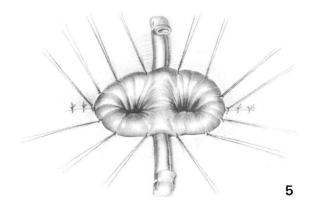

5

TERMINAL COLOSTOMY

6

Removal of skin disc

The exact site for the colostomy, whether it is to be made in the region of the left rectus muscle or the oblique muscles, should be selected to ensure that an appliance will fit satisfactorily away from the umbilicus and the anterior superior iliac spine. A disc of skin approximately 2 cm in diameter is excised. This may be done using a cruciate incision and excising the four pieces of skin with curved scissors.

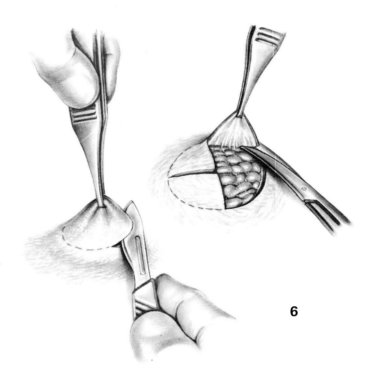

6

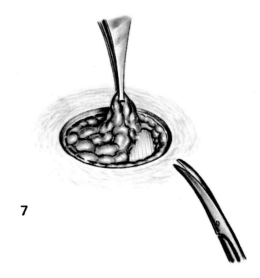

7

7

Removal of cylinder of superficial fascia

A cylinder of superficial fascia is removed, care being taken to obtain good haemostasis.

8 & 9

Division of muscle layers

A disc of the external oblique or anterior rectus sheath is excised in the line of the skin hole and the underlying muscle divided. The peritoneum is also divided. There is a potential space between the fibrous layer of the superficial fascia and the external oblique or anterior rectus sheath. It is in this space that the considerable bulge of a colostomy hernia occurs. This space may be obliterated by a series of sutures joining these two layers.

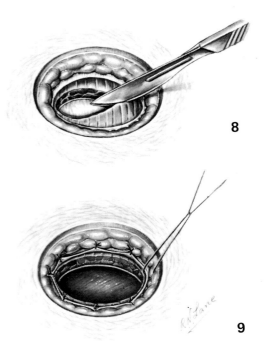

8

9

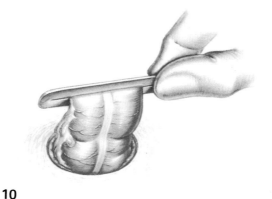

10

10

Delivery of colon through abdominal wall

The colon is delivered through the anterior abdominal wall. If it remains totally intraperitoneal it is desirable for the space between the mesocolon and the abdominal wall (the lateral space) to be closed using nonabsorbable sutures. This prevents the possible complication of internal herniation of the small intestine. Alternatively, the colon may be brought to the surface extraperitoneally.

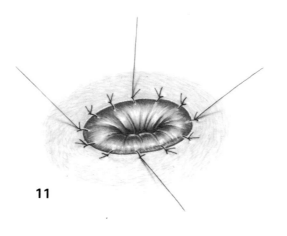

11

11

Mucocutaneous suture

Once the main abdominal incision has been sutured and dressed, the clamp on the distal colon is removed and a mucocutaneous suture performed. Before the main abdominal incision is closed it is important to ensure by adequate mobilization of the colon that there is no tension on this suture line.

POSTOPERATIVE CARE

General management

The general care of the patient will be largely determined by the indication for performing the colostomy and the other injuries sustained by the patient. It is generally wise for the patient to be maintained on intravenous liquids until the colostomy has discharged some flatus and the bowel sounds are well established.

It is important to examine the viability of the colostomy after the operation and also to make certain that the colostomy has not retracted.

Care of the colostomy

It is usual to apply an appliance as soon as the stoma has been fashioned. Because the effluent from a transverse colostomy is somewhat liquid some protection of the skin ought to be provided and Stomahesive or a Karaya gum washer is very useful in this respect because it can be shaped to the colostomy. If the colostomy effluent is very liquid, the oral administration of hydrophilic substances such as Isogel or codeine phosphate usually results in reduction in the colostomy activity.

COMPLICATIONS

Loss of viability

This occurs early after the operation if the blood supply to the colon has been compromised. The operation has to be repeated with viable colon.

Separation of the colostomy

Tension at the mucocutaneous junction is the cause and if this occurs the colostomy will have to be re-established. Partial separation may also occur all the way round either because of tension or infection and will usually heal spontaneously provided that less than half the circumference is involved.

Infection

Although established in a potentially septic field it is very rare for sepsis to complicate the construction of a colostomy. This does, however, occasionally happen with surrounding cellulitis and there may be some separation of the edge of the colostomy. An haematoma surrounding the stoma is a possible predisposing factor and emphasizes the importance of good haemostasis in the colostomy wound. Provided that there is adequate drainage the colostomy will heal but subsequent scarring may lead to some stenosis at the mucocutaneous junction.

Stenosis

Stenosis of a stoma usually occurs at the mucocutaneous level but, provided that there has been no sepsis, it is unusual when direct mucocutaneous suture has been performed. To correct this complication the colostomy needs to be refashioned after excising a disc of skin and any scar tissue that may be present. While this is best carried out under general anaesthesia it may be performed under local anaesthesia.

Hernia

Some degree of herniation is very common after a terminal colostomy. It usually takes the form of an interstitial bulge between the muscle layer and the superficial fascia. Occasionally it results from considerable widening of the hole in the muscle layer. The former is usually best treated initially by wearing a belt. If, however, it is large or the belt is unsatisfactory, the excess colon may be excised after mobilizing it at the stoma. The space between the muscle layer and the superficial fascia will also need to be closed.

The latter type of colostomy hernia is best treated by resiting the stoma and closing the defect by direct suture or by inserting a piece of synthetic material.

Prolapse

Prolapse may occur with either a transverse colostomy when it more commonly involves the distal limb, or a terminal colostomy. Because transverse colostomy is usually a temporary measure prolapse is relatively unimportant, although occasionally, if the viability of the prolapse is in question, re-operation may be needed. If prolapse of a terminal colostomy troubles the patient and causes dysfunction reconstruction, usually at a new site, is required.

[*The illustrations for this Chapter on Colostomy were drawn by Mr. R.N. Lane.*]

Splenectomy for Trauma

Hugh Dudley, Ch.M., F.R.C.S., F.R.C.S.(Ed.), F.R.A.C.S.
Professor of Surgery, St. Mary's Hospital, London

PRE - OPERATIVE

Splenectomy for trauma differs only in detail from routine splenectomy. At least in the Western World and increasingly elsewhere chronic inflammatory diseases are on the wane, the spleen is of normal size and technical difficulties are related more to blood loss and its control than to splenic mobilization.

There is little indication for a specialized incision such as a left subcostal. The laparotomy will have been undertaken because of the diagnosis — acute abdomen, query ruptured spleen — though specific features of the history of injury including the application of the force or the presence of a suggestive penetration may make the diagnosis almost certain. Thoraco-abdominal penetration, the presence of well marked clinical signs in the chest, or the observation of features of a ruptured diaphragm on chest x-ray films, are indications for primary thoracotomy, extending the incision across the costal margin into the abdomen as occasion demands.

THE OPERATION

1

If a median or left paramedian incision has been made, it is vital that it should be adequate in length. Retraction so that the lienorenal ligament can be seen requires an incision which goes well below the umbilicus.

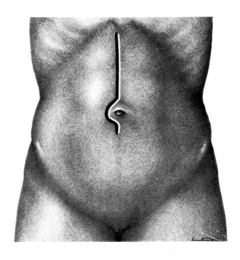

1

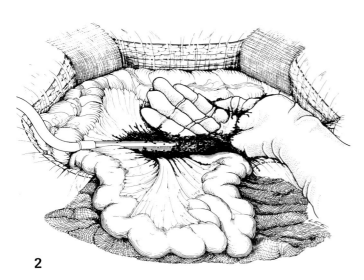

2

2

On opening the abdomen the injury to the spleen may at once be apparent. More commonly, there is blood, diffusely but chiefly in the left paracolic gutter. This is most conveniently removed (*a*) by scooping out clots with the hand and (*b*) aspirating liquid by making a cup with the hand into which the suction tip is then passed. Unless the situation is desperate (as it may be with a completely avulsed spleen), it is well to suck out all the blood that has passed up and down the paracolic gutter into the subdiaphragmatic area and the pelvis. If this is not done, blood constantly wells up into the operative field, making for an untidy procedure.

#

When bleeding is catastrophic or the patient exsanguinated to the point of death, the splenic pedicle should be grasped with the finger and thumb of the right hand. Provided that this is the only injury, transfusion can then be undertaken using either stored blood or that aspirated from the peritoneal cavity. There will be some back-bleeding from short gastric vessels, but this is usually minor and transfusion rapidly repletes the circulating volume, allowing the operation to proceed safely.

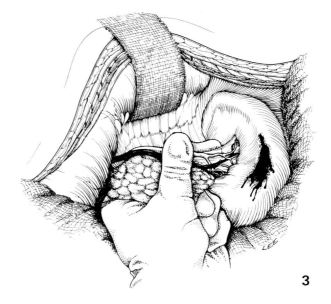

3

4

Alternatively, the lienorenal ligament may be divided (*see Illustration 5*) allowing a soft clamp to be placed across the pedicle, but if this is possible then the patient is usually in a condition to allow splenectomy to proceed.

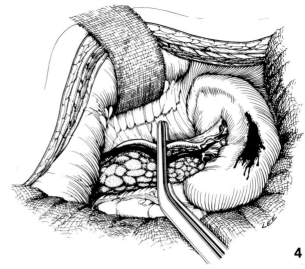

4

5

Division of the lienorenal ligament

A large pack is inserted into the left paracolic gutter and across the splenic flexure of the colon, so displacing the latter downwards. The peritoneum flowing backwards from the colon over the lower pole of the left kidney is then brought into view. Superiorly, this becomes continuous with the lienorenal ligament which is often short and poorly formed. The left hand displaces the spleen to the right, so stretching the ligament which is entered with scissors, displayed and split upwards to the diaphragm. There may be a few adhesions between the outer surface of the spleen and the under-surface of the diaphragm to be divided as well, preferably well clear of the splenic substance. At the upper pole of the spleen there is often very little depth to the ligament, the peritoneum turning forward to become continuous with the gastro-splenic ligament, which contains the uppermost short gastric vessels.

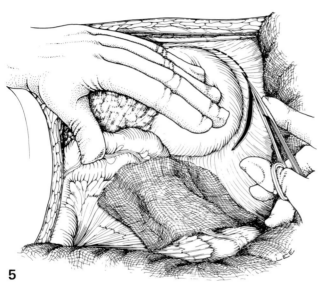

5

6

The spleen can then be boldly swung forward on its pedicle and a large pack at once inserted behind it over the raw area of the cut lienorenal ligament. Not only does this staunch any trifling bleeding from the dissection, it also maintains the spleen forward from under the left costal margin while its vascular attachments are dealt with.

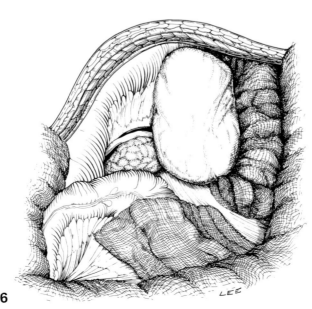

6

7

A small consistent strand of greater omentum is next dealt with at the lower pole. If this is not done it tends to tear away, giving rise to further troublesome bleeding.

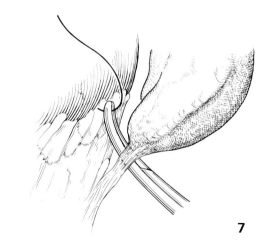

7

8

Provided that heavy bleeding is not occurring, the superior vessels are next ligated. The uppermost are usually attached to the greater curvature (short gastric vessels). Below this, as shown, they are branches of the splenic vessel. The serial procedure of passage of a ligature using opposed curved artery forceps is recommended. At all costs, avoid the accumulation of forceps in the field: they tend to obscure the view and are easily dislodged. Ligatures on both sides must be precisely applied, but this is more particularly true of the gastric aspect where it is possible to pick up the gastric wall and so produce a lateral gastric fistula.

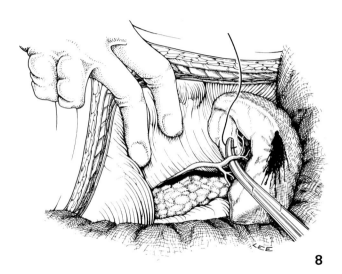

8

9

As the upper short gastric vessels are divided it is possible to insinuate a finger from above downwards behind the pedicle, so throwing it forward. This simple manoeuvre displays the splenic artery emerging from behind the tail of the pancreas, which, though it usually stops short of the splenic hilum, may be closely applied to it. It is essential accurately to display the pancreatic tail, for once again a carelessly applied ligature may lead to pancreatic necrosis, subphrenic cellulitis or a fistula.

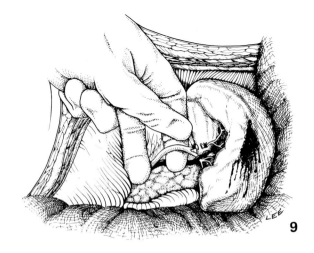

9

10

The splenic artery is ligated first, followed by the splenic vein. It is unusual to have to deal with other vessels below this point.

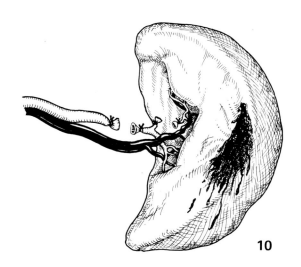

10

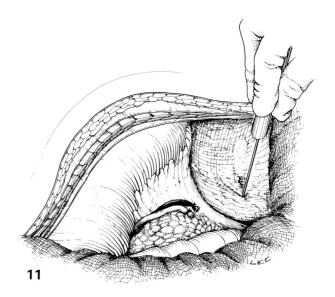

11

11

The raw area does not require to be covered by peritoneum. The splenic bed and cut aspect of the lienorenal ligament are inspected for bleeding and haemostasis obtained by diathermy. Drainage is *not* necessary.

[*The illustrations for this Chapter on Splenectomy for Trauma were drawn by Mrs. G. Lee.*]

Rupture of the Liver

E. Truman Mays, M.D., F.A.C.S.
Professor of Surgery, University of Kentucky School of Medicine

INTRODUCTION

Rupture of the human liver, considered universally fatal until the latter nineteenth century, continues with increasing frequency to challenge surgeons. Gunpowder, the combustion engine and modern high speed expressways are technological advances responsible for an increasing incidence of hepatic injury. About 50 per cent of the patients admitted to US hospitals for abdominal injuries have wounds of the liver.

The years since World War II have evidenced a remarkable reduction in death from injury to the liver. This decrease has resulted as much from learning what not to do as from the discovery of new methods of treatment. Much credit must be given to better methods of resuscitating injured victims, more rapid

Table 1
Detrimental Treatment

1. Packing
2. Absorbable haemostats
3. Suturing deep wounds
4. Clamping the porta
5. Choledochal tubes
6. Glucagon
7. Antibiotics

transport of the injured, a greater knowledge of shock, the increased availability of blood and blood components, and the more intensive care of patients in special facilities. There have also been important improvements in the surgical management of the injured liver. Despite a favourable decrease in overall mortality, a disheartening fact endures: since a reported mortality of 78 per cent in 1887 after hepatic rupture (Edler, 1887), there has been little reduction in death rates associated with this particular kind of injury. In a later series the mortality was 71 per cent (Mikesky, Howard and Debakey, 1956).

The greater number of survivors has occurred in patients with minor lacerations and stab wounds of the liver. When these patients are included in surveys along with hepatic rupture it reduces the overall mortality rate. But this is deceptive. Hepatic ruptures, once thought to be rare, are beginning to constitute the greater part of hepatic trauma.

Haemorrhage and sepsis are and have long remained the major cause of death when the human liver ruptures. Frequently accompanied by injuries to the central nervous system, hollow viscera, skeletal and renal systems, haemorrhage and sepsis related to the hepatic injury overshadow these associated injuries and are the main obstacles to survival. Haemorrhage must be stopped quickly and permanently and perihepatic collections obviated if death rates are to be further reduced. While it is true that there has been a significant reduction in death from all hepatic trauma, the mortality after severe rupture remains great.

To set about improving the treatment of patients with hepatic rupture, we must begin with the main cause of death: haemorrhage. If anyone wants to reduce death from hepatic rupture he must devise simpler, better and more rapid operative methods of stopping haemorrhage from the ruptured liver.

Conventional methods fail dismally to achieve hepatic haemostasis. Packing the wound with a patch of omentum or gauze not only failed to reduce death from bleeding but brought on new and serious complications, such as abscesses within the liver or in the perihepatic spaces. Hepatic necrosis was observed in areas that had been packed and peritonitis, hepatitis, fistulae and numerous other complications followed these methods. Disastrous secondary haemorrhage often followed removal of gauze packs. Such complications led to the abandonment of packing as the primary method of controlling haemorrhage from the liver. There followed an immediate reduction in death rate from 30 to 17 per cent (Madding, Lawrence and Kennedy, 1943).

The need for rapid haemostasis in a ruptured liver caused surgeons to suture the cracks and crevices of the ruptured liver in attempts to stop bleeding. After the failure of gauze and omental packs, suture repair rapidly became the most frequent method of treating wounds of the liver. With the advent of absorbable haemostatic agents, the combination of suture over an absorbable haemostatic agent was frequently used. Had suturing or suturing in combination with absorbable haemostatic agents been successful in controlling haemorrhage from the ruptured liver, we should be able to prove the efficacy of such treatment by a clear decrease in death from hepatic haemorrhage. But we cannot confirm it. All large groups of patients reported over the past 30 years have established haemorrhage as the leading cause of death in patients with hepatic rupture (Mikesky, Howard and DeBakey, 1956; Trunkey, Shires and McClelland, 1974).

Sepsis is the second most common cause of death in patients with liver injuries. The site of sepsis after hepatic rupture has been about evenly divided above and below the diaphragm; infection above the diaphragm is predominantly pneumonitis and/or pleural space infections. Below the diaphragm the incidence and degree of sepsis is clearly related to the inability of the surgeon to drain perihepatic spaces effectively. Subphrenic and subhepatic abscesses are the usual consequence of poor drainage of perihepatic spaces and antibiotics may have done the reverse of preventing infection.

The successful treatment of hepatic rupture has been learning what not to do as much as learning better methods of treatment: a list of 'detrimental factors' instructive (see Table 1).

HEPATIC ANATOMY

1

All operations to treat the ruptured liver require a fairly detailed knowledge of its anatomy.

The liver is irregularly shaped. It has an extensive smooth, convex surface separated from the diaphragm only by a potential space. This diaphragmatic surface has four parts: ventral, superior, dorsal and right. The other surfaces of the liver are concave and irregular and they are separated from the surrounding viscera by spaces that can fill with blood, bile or sequestered parenchyma which are difficult to drain.

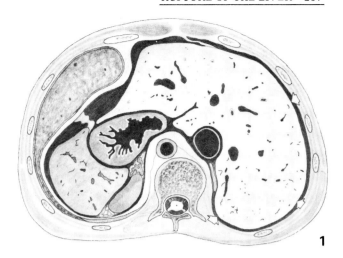

1

The liver is fixed to the undersurface of the diaphragm and to the ventral wall of the abdomen by five ligaments. Four are reflections of the parietal peritoneum; the fifth is the obliterated umbilical vein.

The supporting ligaments are important in the treatment of ruptured livers. Some require surgical division for mobilization and inspection of the liver, others may be needed for patching the raw surface of the liver, while still others may have to be divided to obtain drainage of the perihepatic spaces.

Traditionally, three of the five supporting ligaments (falciform ligament, round ligament and ligamentum venosum) mark the junction of the right and left lobes of the liver and many surgeons continue to accept this concept of the lobar fissure although this concept was disproved many years ago.

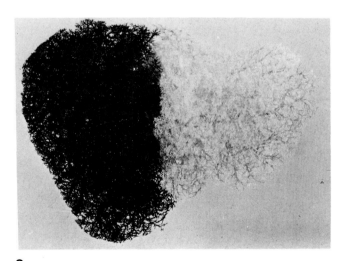

2

2

Cantlie (1897) found a relatively avascular fissure extending from the fundus of the gall-bladder to the exit of the major hepatic veins and proposed that this avascular plane was the true lobar fissure dividing the liver into right and left lobes and that division by the falciform ligament was unscientific, untrue, and untenable. Corrosion casts of the liver confirm this.

The lobar fissure described by Cantlie has no external identifying landmarks and it is not visible on the external surface of the liver but if the rami of the hepatic artery and portal vein are ligated this lobar fissure becomes clearly visible and allows anatomical lobectomy to be carried out.

3&4

Each lobe is further subdivided into two segments; the segmental division of the left lobe runs in a sagittal plane producing a lateral segment and medial segment whereas the segmental fissure of the right lobe lies in the coronal plane and forms an angle of about 15° with the coronal body plane. This cleavage divides the right lobe into anterior and posterior segments. These four segments of the liver are further divided into subsegments that are rarely a consideration in operations for rupture of the liver.

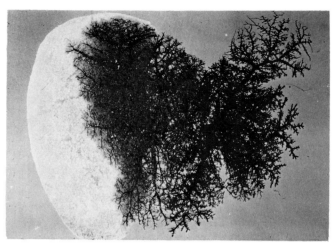

3

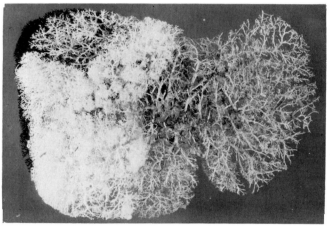

4

Because the segmental fissure of the right lobe lies in the coronal plane, any rupture on the right nearly always involves the two segments equally so that the treatment of a rupture on the right encompasses the lobe and not its subunits. On the left, the segmental fissure is in a sagittal plane and rupture of the left liver can and frequently does involve a single segment. The operative treatment of left lobe injuries can frequently be directed toward a single segment instead of an entire lobe.

There is a natural propensity of the liver to crack along its natural lobar fissures so that such ruptures often spare the separate lobes and the parenchyma of the lobes is not damaged. Consequently these lobar crevasses have a better chance of a successful outcome than a stellate rupture totally confined to the right or left lobe.

THE HEPATIC VEINS

5

The efferent venous drainage of the liver does not completely follow the lobar distribution established by the afferent blood supply. The main right hepatic vein drains the greatest part of the right lobe, but the major left hepatic vein drains only the lateral segment of the left lobe. The middle hepatic vein drains mainly the medial segment of the left lobe, but it crosses the lobar fissure and drains part of the anterior segment of the right lobe. This crossing of the main lobar fissure by the large middle hepatic vein means that when the liver ruptures along the main lobar fissure this vein is likely to be torn and cause severe and rapid bleeding.

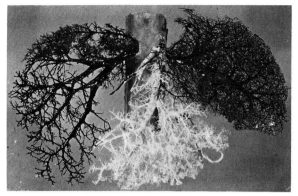

5

The main left and right hepatic veins empty directly into the inferior vena cava, as depicted by the corrosion cast in *Illustration 5*. The extrahepatic parts of these two major hepatic veins are very short, usually no more than 2–3 cm in length. The middle hepatic vein usually empties into the main left hepatic vein in its intrahepatic segment about 2·5 cm before the left hepatic vein drains into the inferior vena cava.

When this occurs, the middle hepatic vein and the left hepatic vein enter the inferior vena cava as a common channel. The extrahepatic part of this common channel can be dissected and isolated outside the hepatic capsule. Occasionally the middle hepatic vein will anastomose directly with the inferior vena cava by a separate orifice.

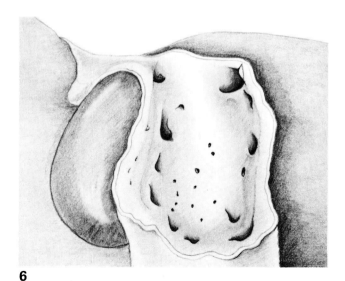

6

6

In addition to these three main hepatic veins there are between 12 and 20 smaller hepatic veins emptying into the retrohepatic vena cava so that this vein must therefore be considered an integral part of the liver.

7

THE PORTAL VEIN

The portal vein, hepatic artery and the bile form a scaffolding upon which the parenchyma of the liver is supported.

At the hilum of the liver the portal vein divides into right and left rami. The division is usually shaped like the letter 'Y' but occasionally it has more of a 'T' shape.

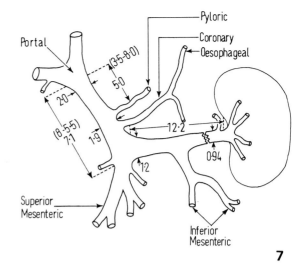

7

8

HEPATIC ARTERY

The common hepatic artery divides slightly to the left of the true lobar fissure. The quick division of the left hepatic artery makes its main trunk extremely short. In 40 per cent of patients the rami of the left hepatic artery follow the pattern of the hepatic ducts by dividing into a medial and a lateral segment artery. In 35 per cent of patients the left hepatic artery does not divide in this manner. Instead the left ramus divides quickly into superior and inferior subsegment arteries. In such instances the medial segment artery arises from either the lateral superior or the lateral inferior subsegment artery. This variation in the branching of the left hepatic artery always takes place well to the right of the segmental fissure on the left. In about 25 per cent of patients there is no left hepatic artery, in which case the medial and lateral segmental arteries arise directly from the common hepatic artery.

The right hepatic artery passed behind the hepatic duct in 87 per cent of specimens studied by Healey (1954) and by Healey *et al.* (1953). In 11 per cent of the specimens it coursed in front of the hepatic duct. The right hepatic artery terminates by dividing into anterior and posterior segmental arteries. This

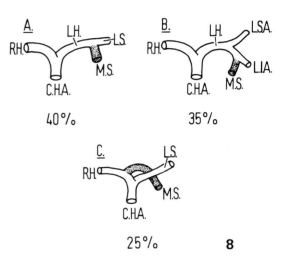

8

division of the right hepatic artery may occur within or outside the liver.

Since ruptures of the right lobe of the liver involve both segments equally, operations are usually conceived to treat both segments of the right lobe; dissection of the right hepatic artery into its two segmental branches is therefore not necessary.

HEPATIC DUCTS

The triad of duct, vein and artery is dispersed throughout the portal canals within the liver and is always enfolded by the fibrous capsule of Glisson so that within the liver, the triad of Glisson is treated as a unit for ligation or transection. It is only in their extrahepatic parts that they are treated as individual structures.

The extrahepatic segments of the two main hepatic ducts are extremely short and any operative manipulation of these structures must be done with great care. The right hepatic duct averages only about 9 mm in length. The left hepatic duct is usually a little longer. They unite to form the common hepatic duct, which varies in length from 1 to 5 cm. The hepatic duct passes to the right between the layers of omentum and at variable sites is jointed by the cystic duct to become the common bile duct.

The common bile duct (choledochus) is remarkably consistent in its course and anatomical relationships. It is about 1·5 cm long and descends in the free margin of the hepatoduodenal ligament until it passes dorsal to the superior part of the duodenum and ventral to the vena cava to the right of the portal vein. At its termination it is nearly completely embedded in the head of the pancreas and is closely associated with the terminal part of the pancreatic duct as it passes obliquely through the muscular and mucosal layers of the duodenum. About 60 per cent of the time the ducts unite for form a common channel.

It is uncommon for the extrahepatic bile ducts to be injured by blunt trauma. On rare occasions when they are avulsed or disrupted they must be repaired. If one third of the circumference of the choledochus or hepatic duct is uninjured reconstruction can usually be done over a T-tube. Complete transection of the extrahepatic ducts is best repaired by implanting the proximal end of the duct into the duodenum or into a loop of jejunum which has been isolated by the Roux-en-Y technique. It is important to know that the average width of the injured, but otherwise healthy common duct is about 3 mm so that commercially available T-tubes are much too large.

INCISIONS

When operating on critically injured patients there is only one acceptable incision because it must allow exposure and operative repair of all intra-abdominal injuries and not just the liver. A generous mid-line incision from the tip of the xiphoid to the caudal side of the umbilicus is best. It can be extended cranially when needed and if injuries of pelvic viscera are discovered the mid-line incision can be rapidly extended to the pubis and permits exposure of the extreme lateral parts of the abdominal cavities.

9a & b

A thoraco-abdominal incision is accomplished by extending the original abdominal incision into the chest cavity via the seventh or eighth intercostal space. After the costal cartilage is transected the diaphragm is sharply divided in a ventral to dorsal direction. This combined thoracic and abdominal incision always produces a large triangle of tissue containing the ribs, cartilages and upper abdominal wall which make it liable to slip from under a retractor and snap back into position.

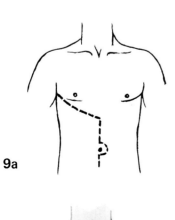

9a

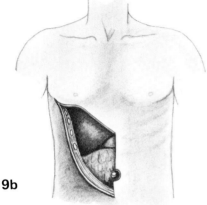

9b

For these reasons, the thoraco-abdominal incision is frustrating for the surgeon and it is also detrimental to the patient because of the risks of atelectasis and pneumonia of the right lung and a good deal of pain.

When access to the right chest is deemed necessary a sternal split is better than the classic thoraco-abdominal incision. Postoperative pain, atelectasis and other pulmonary complications are less after the median sternotomy than after a combined thoraco-abdominal incision. Median sternotomy is well tolerated by the patient, it is quick and safe, it is easy to close and it permits total exposure and vascular isolation of the liver.

Although nearly all operative procedures needed to treat the ruptured liver can be done through a simple mid-line abdominal incision, the patient's chest should always be scrubbed and prepared as well as the entire abdomen, both flanks and upper thighs. It is wise always to be prepared to extend the original upper abdominal mid-line incision in any direction. To stop in the middle of an operation, scrub and redrape the patient is awkward and not in the best interest of the patient.

STOPPING BLEEDING

Haemorrhage has always been the prime cause of death after rupture of the liver and the surgeon must take particular care when operating on a patient who has bled profusely.

Whatever the method the surgeon uses to stop bleeding from the liver, it must be quick and easily done in any operating room. A method that can be done only in large regional medical centres or special casualty hospitals defeats the prime aim of treatment: immediate control of haemorrhage. If patients with ruptured livers are allowed to continue bleeding while being transported to central hospitals for expert care, an increased incidence of renal failure, pulmonary insufficiency, sepsis and death can be expected.

Many methods of stopping hepatic bleeding have been used and some are now of historical interest only.

ARTERIAL BLEEDING

The most recalcitrant source of bleeding from the ruptured liver is arterial. Arterial defects deep within the interior of the liver do not lend themselves to control by suture techniques because they are usually beyond the reach of sutures; to burrow into the depths of the liver in search of bleeding vessels can increase bleeding and destroy more parenchymal tissue.

Experience with hepatic arterial ligation over the past 10 years shows it to be a quick, simple and highly effective means of stopping haemorrhage from the ruptured liver (Aaron, Fulton and Mays, 1975, Canty and Aaron, 1975; Mays, 1971, 1972, 1973).

The teachings about hepatic arteries must be re-examined in the light of new knowledge. Hepatic arteries are not end-arteries, as has been shown by selective catheterization of the hepatic artery (Mays and Wheeler, 1974). Furthermore portal bacteraemia is not present in healthy humans, which explains the difference between the effects of ligating the hepatic artery in man and dogs, cats and rabbits.

Hepatic artery ligation has proved extremely effective in stopping haemorrhage from ruptured livers and it can be done by a surgeon working alone with a nurse and an anaesthetist.

10

The abdomen is opened with a mid-line incision. If the liver is ruptured, the common hepatic artery should be identified in the hepatoduodenal ligament. When both lobes are involved or when there is a large deep crevasse along the lobar fissure, no further dissection is needed. The artery is interrupted by metal clips or ligature. If only the right lobe is injured additional dissection is required. The common hepatic artery is traced to its bifurcation from where the right branch is traced to where it enters the substance of the liver; the ligature or clip is applied there. If the injury is confined to the left lobe, the left hepatic artery is dissected and occluded with a ligature or metal clip.

After ligation of an hepatic artery, there are biochemical consequences, but if ligation has been done before there is blood loss requiring massive transfusions, the biochemical disturbances pass off within 7 to 14 days.

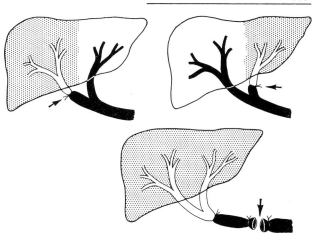

10

11

Blood flow in the intrahepatic arteries is restored by collaterals within 12 to 24 hr of ligating the hepatic artery. This can be displayed by selective hepatic arteriograms. Arteriograms are not necessary for the patient's care or treatment if he is recovering uneventfully, but if bleeding has not been stopped, arteriography is essential to determine whether the appropriate artery has been ligated.

After ligation of the hepatic artery the liver begins to extract additional oxygen from the portal vein blood (Tygstrup *et al*. 1962). This means that oxygenation and blood flow in the portal vein must be sustained throughout the operative and postoperative period, to which end the patient is kept fasting for 7–10 days after the artery has been interrupted. Portal venous flow is best assured by early and rapid replacement of blood volume. A critically injured hypovolaemic patient will do well as long as vascular volume is restored promptly, even if his blood has been diluted to an haematocrit of 25 or 30; balanced salt solutions should be used to restore the blood volume while waiting for stored blood to be typed and cross-matched.

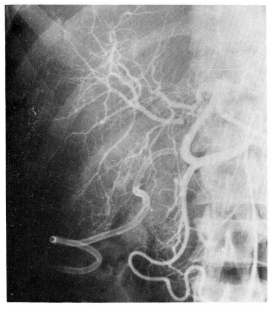

11

VENOUS BLEEDING

Haemorrhage from disrupted veins within the liver has not proved a great obstacle to recovery, but bleeding from the great veins outside Glisson's capsule is very dangerous. The tendency of venous bleeding inside the substance of the liver is to stop spontaneously. Gauze packs may be placed firmly against the surface of a ruptured liver while the surgeon attends to other operative necessities but after a few minutes they should be removed. If venous oozing from the interior of the liver continues, the appropriate hepatic artery may need to be ligated. An alternative method of stopping venous bleeding from the liver is manual compression of the ruptured organ between the hands but with central ruptures of the liver neither packs nor manual compression may succeed. The middle hepatic vein may have been torn and, if so, it requires clipping or ligating. Remember that the middle hepatic vein crosses the main lobar fissure to drain a small part of the anterior segment of the liver (*see Illustration 5*). Where it crosses the fissure it is about 2–4 cm from the surface of the liver and any split extending more than 2 cm along the lobar fissure probably will injure this vein. After ligating the hepatic artery and aspirating blood from the split, the two ends of the middle hepatic vein can usually be seen and ligated or occluded with metal clips.

Selective ligation of the hepatic artery also reduces the oozing from portal veins because the hepatic artery empties directly into the radicles of the portal vein before the latter empty into the sinusoids (Wakim and Mann, 1942). However, ligating the hepatic artery does nothing to control bleeding from hepatic veins; intrahepatic venous bleeding must be stopped by temporary gauze packing or manual compression as described above, but extrahepatic venous bleeding is an entirely different problem.

HEPATIC RESECTION

Surgical ablation of parts of the liver is not a new operation but there are two major problems in successfully using hepatic resection to treat patients with ruptured livers. First, there are no clear criteria for deciding which patients need this very formidable procedure. Recent reports from the United Kingdom and the United States indicate that such operations have become fashionable, but most authorities agree that out of the entire group of patients admitted to hospitals with injured livers, only 2–3 per cent need resection. However, several recent authors have said that they are using this method in 30–40 per cent of patients admitted to their hospitals. This practice needs discouraging because the mortality rate for major hepatic resections done in hypovolaemic, acutely injured patients is very high. Most university medical centres in the United States and the United Kingdom are reporting 43–59 per cent death rates. Occasionally an initial good report with a low mortality (20 per cent) (McClelland, Shires and Poulos, 1964) has had to be changed in a second report from the same institution to a greater death rate (Trunkey, Shires and McClelland, 1974).

12

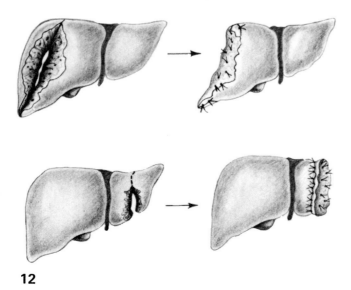

Lobectomy should not be done in acute injuries; the place for hepatic lobectomy is in treating complications of hepatic rupture which develop days after the acute injury. In these patients the mortality rate of an anatomical lobectomy is much less than while the patient is already in varying degrees of shock. In order to avoid confusion it should be stated that there are five different kinds of hepatic resections used to treat ruptured livers:

(*1*) resectional debridement;
(*2*) right lobectomy;
(*3*) left lobectomy;
(*4*) segmental (sublobar resections);
(*5*) trisegmentectomy (right hepatic lobectomy extended to include medial segment of the left lobe).

Of the five, resectional debridement is the only one to be used in the acutely injured patient, simply to remove the hepatic tissue already separated from the liver by the initial accident.

13

Resectional debridement certainly should not be used for central ruptures of the liver in which the crevasses pass through the lobar fissure. It is inappropriate in the large stellate shaped ruptures of the right lobe and large subcapsular haematomas with an underlying rupture of the liver. The operative technique of resectional debridement is straightforward. One simply uses the fracture line produced by the accident, and with the handle of a scalpel bluntly dissects through the remaining tissue, teasing out the vascular and biliary elements between the thumb and index finger. These structures are ligated or occluded with metal clips. Because resectional debridement is not an anatomical resection, it should always be accompanied by ligation of the hepatic artery supplying the injured lobe. Because it follows the line of fracture created by the accident and because it is not an anatomical technique, there are hazards. Random lines of dissection deprive unknown but possibly important parts of the liver of its vascular and biliary connections. Infarction, venous congestion and biliary obstruction can occur in such segments and delay recovery or cause death from sepsis.

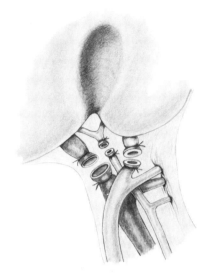

13

HEPATIC LOBECTOMY

This is a formidable procedure and should rarely be used as primary treatment. The justifications for doing hepatic lobectomies in acutely hypovolaemic patients are the reduction of a single lobe to complete pulp and to obtain exposure of the retrohepatic vena cava for repair of juxtahepatic venous injuries when exposure cannot be obtained by simpler methods. Beyond these two, there are no good reasons for carrying out a formidable procedure, which carries grave risks in acutely injured people. There are simpler and safer methods of preventing exsanguination.

The best use of hepatic lobectomy is for treating the late complications of rupture. The mortality rate of removing a lobe of the liver is greatly reduced in these patients because they can be brought to the operating theatre with normal blood volumes and better haemodynamic and respiratory conditions.

TECHNIQUE OF LOBECTOMY

14

The first step in removing either lobe of the liver is mobilization. This is rapidly done by incising the supporting ligaments of the lobe to be removed; the right triangular and right leaves of the coronary ligament are cut when the right lobe is to be removed; the left triangular ligament and the left leaves of the coronary are cut when the left lobe is to be removed. The falciform ligament is divided back to the junction of the hepatic veins with the vena cava regardless of which lobe is to be removed. The cutting of the ligaments must be carefully performed in the region of the two major hepatic veins. Accidental injury to one or both of these veins is a serious complication because air can rapidly enter the vena cava and cause cardiac arrest and death.

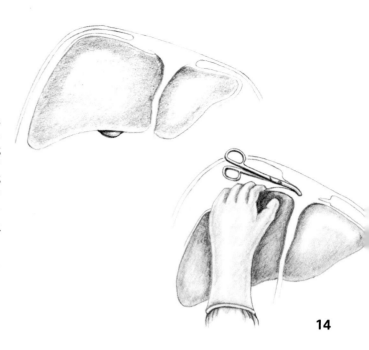

14

15

Mobilization of the lobe is completed by lifting the lobe up and away from the retrohepatic vena cava. The reflection of the fibrous capsule of Glisson is incised in the trough between the retrohepatic vena cava and the dorsal surface of the liver. The numerous smaller hepatic veins passing directly from the liver into the anterior surface of the vena cava are frequently injured while doing this manoeuvre. A little more time and care in dissecting such veins is expedient.

Catastrophe can occur during this stage of mobilizing the lobe for excision. Lifting up one lobe of the liver pushes dorsally on the retrohepatic vena cava and can completely occlude the return of blood to the heart. This sudden withdrawal of venous blood from the right side of the heart produces cardiac arrest in many patients and in others the anaesthetist will notice a sudden and severe drop in blood pressure. As soon as the surgeon lets go of the lobe and relieves the pressure on the vena cava, venous blood flow to the right heart resumes and cardiac output is immediately improved; the blood pressure rises.

15

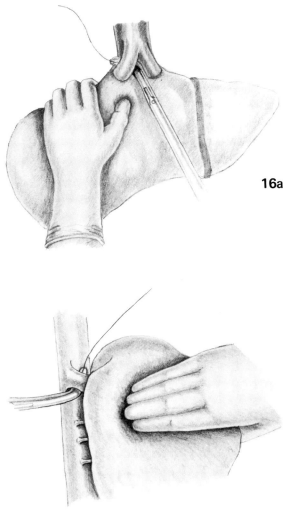

16a

16b

16a & b

After these steps to mobilize the lobe have been completed, hilar dissection is started. The gall-bladder is removed. The hepatoduodenal ligament is incised and the common duct and hepatic artery are uncovered. These structures are traced to their terminal divisions. The rami of the portal vein, hepatic artery and hepatic duct are divided after securely ligating each separately. Of these three, the bile duct is the most difficult to isolate and divide. To prevent mistakes, the author sometimes opens the common duct and passes rubber catheters or metal probes into the intrahepatic segments of the hepatic ducts. These assist as guidelines while chiselling out the hepatic duct and prevent accidental injury of the wrong duct.

Soon after completing the hilar dissection and ligation of the structures supplying the lobe to be removed, the lobar fissure becomes clearly visible on the external surface of the liver. The isolated lobe takes on a bluish appearance while the perfused normal lobe remains pink and healthy (Mays, 1971).

There are two ways of completing lobectomy. One is to start dividing the liver along the lobar fissure, leaving the isolation and division of the major hepatic vein to the very last. The other is uncovering the major hepatic vein at its junction with the inferior vena cava and ligating it securely. After control of the main hepatic vein, the lobe is cut off along the lobar fissure.

When possible, the author prefers the second method. A serious danger in lobectomy has been embolism by air and fat. By leaving the clamping and tying of the major hepatic vein until last the chances of air or fat entering the veins is greatly increased.

17-20

To tie off the major hepatic vein, the lobe is pulled caudally and the soft flimsy tissue in the bare area of the liver is unroofed. This process is continued until the hepatic vein can be seen leaving the surface of the liver and entering the anterior part of the vena cava. The supporting fascia around the vein is picked up with tissue forceps and carefully incised. The perivascular space is entered. Painstaking and gentle dissection in this space allows the hepatic vein to be completely encircled and a ligature passed. After securely ligating this large hepatic vein, the risk of air embolism is greatly reduced. The alternative method is to lift the lobe upwards (ventral) and approach the main hepatic vein from the dorsal surface of the liver.

With these steps completed the lobe is ready to be removed. This can be accomplished by several different methods. Special clamps have been devised to place across the liver (Storm and Longmire, 1971). These clamps compress the liver and the parenchyma can be divided in a nearly bloodless field. Before the clamp is removed the cut ends of the intrahepatic veins and vasculobiliary elements in the portal canals must be identified and ligated.

The parenchymal tissue may also be divided bluntly with the back of the knife handle or any other thin, blunt instrument. When this technique is used the vascular and biliary elements are ligated as they are chiselled out from the surrounding hepatic substance.

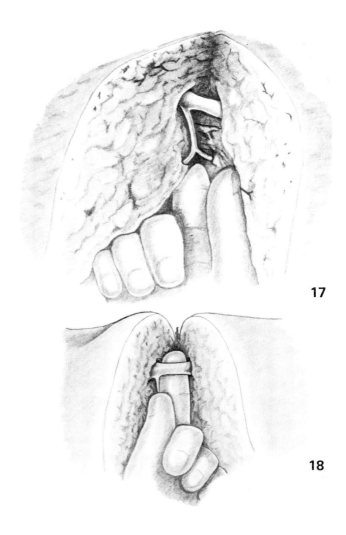

17

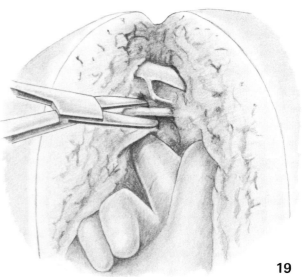

18

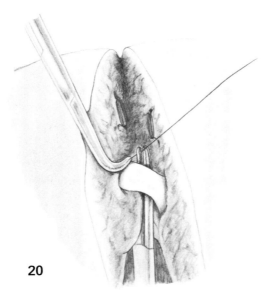

20

19

The preferred method of dividing the hepatic parenchyma is the 'finger-fracture' technique. After the vessels and bile duct have been divided in the hilus of the liver and the main hepatic vein ligated at the vena caval junction, an incision is made in Glisson's capsule following the line of demarcation between the two lobes. This lobar fissure usually runs in a slightly oblique direction from the gall-bladder fossa to a point mid-way between the junction of the hepatic veins with the inferior vena cava. Once Glisson's capsule has been cut with a knife along the line of demarcation, the thumb and index finger are inserted and the parenchymal tissue crushed. This process of crushing the parenchymal tissue of the liver between the thumb and index finger is continued deeper into the liver along the lobar fissure. By this method the hepatic veins and the structure in the portal canals are teased out with the thumb and index finger. Each structure is then occluded by metal clips or ligatures of silk, and cut between the ligatures. In this manner the entire thickness of the liver is traversed until the lobe is nearly free except for its dorsal attachments to the vena cava by the continuation of the fibrosa capsularis perivascularis (Glisson's capsule). Clamps are then placed along this remaining area and the lobe is cut off. After removing the lobe, a running-locking haemostatic stitch is placed along the dorsal surface of the liver, including the fibrosa capsularis in the stitch. This provides haemostasis in an extremely vascular region.

After completely removing the lobe, some surgeons try to cover the raw surface with various kinds of patches, omentum, fascia, or even other viscera. This practice can be hazardous because it prevents drainage of bile and sequestered parenchymal tissue. Also it fosters collections of blood and serum between the patch and the raw surface of the liver. The author prefers not to cover the raw surface of the liver. Whatever may drain from the raw surface is less hazardous to the patient if given freedom to drain outside the patient's body and anything that interferes with this complete, external drainage is not in the best interest of the patient's recovery.

If the common duct is 10 mm or greater, a T-tube is inserted and the choledochus closed around the T-tube with fine catgut sutures. The tube is brought out through a small stab wound in the right upper quadrant and connected to closed gravity drainage. While a T-tube is helpful after an anatomical hepatic lobectomy, it is hazardous to use routinely for all hepatic trauma.

Postoperative management

When looking at metabolic events after lobectomy it is essential to differentiate those due to shock, hypoxia and numerous blood transfusions from those alterations attributable to reduction in functioning hepatocyte mass. Those patients having an hepatic lobectomy as an emergency procedure for rupture of the liver have greater concentrations of serum hepatic enzymes and bilirubin values after surgery than those patients having an elective or planned procedure. Coagulation deficiencies are much greater in patients having emergency lobectomies than in patients having elective lobectomies. These findings indicate that many of the metabolic events reported to be due to lobectomy are in reality due to shock and multiple transfusions with stored blood.

The two most common consequences of hepatic lobectomy in animals are hypo-albuminaemia and hypoglycaemia. In humans the extent of such biochemical derangements cannot be studied. Exogenous supplementation of albumin and glucose is so critical to survival that omission of these substances would be unethical. Glucose and albumin must be started during the operation and continued into the postoperative period until such time as the residual lobe can once again assume the full responsibility, sustaining acceptable blood concentrations of glucose and albumin. Cholinesterase values can be used as a good indicator of the liver's ability to synthesize albumin. Patients with high cholinesterase activity show the most rapid return of albumin synthesis after lobectomy. Failure to support patients with glucose and albumin can be catastrophic. Patients with low serum albumin values have a greater incidence of severe pulmonary insufficiency and require mechanical ventilation for longer periods.

Hepatic lobectomy reduces prothrombin concentrations significantly, but usually causes no untoward clotting difficulties when the lobar fissure has been used to remove the lobe. Surgeons not using the lobar fissure as the line for transecting the liver have reported irksome problems with continued bleeding in the postoperative period. Their patients had reductions in coagulation factors V, VII, platelets and increased fibrinolytic activity.

While the liver manufactures coagulation factors II, V, VII and X, deficiencies in these substances are known to occur in the absence of lobectomy and can be observed after haemorrhage and shock from severe gastro-intestinal bleeding or other common causes of oligaemia. Such deficiencies should not be attributed to a reduction in hepatocyte mass by lobectomy. When these deficiencies occur they usually require specific replacement to prevent bleeding from the ruptured liver as well as other sites, but the best way to avoid these deficiencies is to stop bleeding from the liver quickly by hepatic arterial ligation and by replenishing circulating blood volume early.

Cholesterol synthesis is reduced after lobectomy but, as with protein synthesis, this is a transient effect. Regeneration of hepatocyte mass renews the capacity of the liver to manufacture cholesterol.

CHOLECYSTECTOMY

The gall-bladder should be removed in nearly all patients with ruptured livers. This is especially true if the hepatic artery has been ligated. Thirty-five per cent of Markowitz's dogs, who died after hepatic arterial ligation, died because of rupture of the gall-bladder and severe bile peritonitis. In a group of our patients treated with hepatic arterial ligation there were two who required second operations for complications related to the gall-bladder; one required cholecystectomy after 10 days for gangrenous cholecystitis and the other at 18 months for atrophic cholecystitis.

But severe rupture of the liver alone sets in motion a series of poorly understood events leading to stasis of bile flow, distension and inflammation of the gall-bladder. Such gall-bladders removed after 14—21 days have nearly always shown microscopic evidence of inflammation. The walls are thickened and oedematous and have lost their lustre and normal robin's egg blue hue. If this kind of gall-bladder is left *in situ* it hinders the smooth recovery of the patient. Sometimes post-operative fever is prolonged because of a smouldering inflammatory process in the gall-bladder. This produces localized subhepatic tenderness which cannot be differentiated from a subhepatic abscess except by laparotomy.

Most surgeons are reluctant to remove the gall-bladder during the first operation and the reasons are obvious. Immediately after rupture of the liver the gall-bladder is completely normal. To remove a healthy uninvolved organ purely for prophylaxis perturbs surgeons. Nevertheless the added time and risk of a cholecystectomy at the first operation are slight compared with those of a second laparotomy or the disadvantages of recovery prolonged by smouldering inflammation in the gall-bladder.

Occasionally when the liver ruptures the gall-bladder is torn from its bed. This avulsion of an intact gall-bladder from its hepatic fossa is usually caused by the forces of deceleration, which are sometimes forgotten and seldom discussed. Hass (1944) studied deceleration forces in aircraft accidents and stated 'whenever one part of the body is decelerated at a rate which is different from that of another part, the connection between the two parts is placed under stress'. With increased emphasis on speed and rapid transit, deceleration promises to be one of the most common injuring forces acting on the liver. Differences in rates of deceleration between the liver and gall-bladder are responsible for avulsing the gall-bladder from the hepatic fossa. The point of stress is the fascial anchor between the liver and gall-bladder and the reflection of Glisson's capsule from the liver onto the gall-bladder. When these anchors succumb to decelerative forces the liquid-filled gall-bladder literally pops out of its fossa. The treatment of this injury is cholecystectomy.

Forces of deceleration are also important in hepatic venous avulsions.

DETRIMENTAL TREATMENTS

Packing

Some patients in whom packs have been used as primary treatment have survived, but recovery has been delayed and survival has been in spite of and not because of packs.

Absorbable haemostatic agents

The gelatin sponges and fabrics prepared by the controlled oxidation of regenerated cellulose were hailed as providing means of overcoming the dangers of gauze packs. Because they could be dissolved and 'absorbed' by the body they did not have to be removed. This appeared to be a great advantage because many of the dangers of gauze packs arose when they were removed. Now products were available which did not have to be removed.

While in small amounts these synthetic materials are absorbed by human tissue, in the amounts required to control hepatic haemorrhage they are foreign bodies. Abscesses, biliary fistulae, haemobilia, intestinal obstruction from adhesions and erosion of the oxidized cellulose through the intestinal wall are serious complications attributed to using these synthetic foreign bodies for treating ruptures of the human liver.

Suturing splits

Suturing the ruptured liver is hazardous and frequently followed by haemobilia, traumatic sequestra, secondary haemorrhage and intrahepatic cavitation with subsequent sepsis and hepatic failure.

Bleeding into the biliary system after hepatic trauma was reported as early as 1848 by Owen. Sandblom suggested the term 'traumatic haemobilia' and elucidated the anatomical and pathological features (Sandblom, 1948). Others have linked haemobilia with primary suture of deep liver ruptures.

The treatment of these complications of suturing the liver is frustrating to the surgeon and dangerous to the patient.

Clamping the porta

In 1908 Pringle proposed arresting hepatic haemorrhage by cross-clamping the afferent blood supply in the hepatoduodenal ligament (Pringle, 1908). This method became instantly popular and widely used. Now referred to as the Pringle manoeuvre it is said to be safe for periods of 10–15 min in normothermic patients, but it is unreasonable to subject the entire liver to total anoxia, if only for 10–15 min, when only one lobe has ruptured. Any physiologically acceptable method of stopping haemorrhage from the injured lobe must ensure continued perfusion of the uninjured lobe.

Choledochal tubes

The insertion of a T-tube into the common duct, said Merendino and associates (Merendino, Dillard and Cammock, 1963), can decompress the intrahepatic bile collecting system and should reduce the incidence of biliary fistulae and decrease extravasation of bile after rupture of the liver. There were other theoretical advantages but such expected bonuses never materialized in prospective clinical trials conducted by Lucas (1971).

A rare indication for surgical decompression of the biliary tract occurs in the occasional patient with a large bile duct and an extensive rupture involving intrahepatic bile ducts. Routine drainage of the choledochus by T-tubes is hazardous and should be discarded from the common practice of treating burst livers.

JUXTAHEPATIC VEIN INJURY

Injuries to veins of either the portal or hepatic system within the interior of the liver are not usually troublesome. Bleeding from such venous injuries is at low pressure and can nearly always be controlled by manual compression or tamponade with temporary gauze packs. The structure of the liver works in favour of spontaneous haemostasis in veins inside the capsule of the liver. Even if one of the three major hepatic veins is torn, as long as it is within the capsule of the liver it usually can be clotted by packing and allowing several minutes to pass before the packs are removed. While the tampons are still in place the hepatic artery can be dissected and the artery supplying the injured lobe ligated. This supplements the haemostatic effects of the pressure packs because the arterial tree opens into the portal venules at several different sites. This interruption of the hepatic artery reduces the volume and flow within the terminal portal venules and in combination with temporary pressure packs will usually control haemorrhage from intrahepatic veins.

But injury of veins outside the liver capsule constitutes an entirely different problem. Profuse haemorrhage and profound shock are the usual consequences of juxtahepatic venous injuries. They require direct suture repair. But exposure to permit suture repair is, in most instances, extra-ordinarily difficult.

For purposes of reporting and describing patients with these injuries, a more standard terminology is needed. That part of the inferior vena cava passing dorsal to the liver is 9—10 cm in length and 3—4 cm in diameter. It is such an integral part of the liver that it must be considered as an hepatic organ. On its ventral surface it receives blood from 12—20 hepatic veins (*see Illustration 6*). Some call this part of the vena cava the intrahepatic vena cava, but as can be seen in *Illustration 1*, the dorsal part is not covered completely by the liver. It is free and receives no major veins. There are four parts of the inferior vena cava: (*1*) suprahepatic; (*2*) retrohepatic; (*3*) infrahepatic and (*4*) infrarenal.

Exposure and repair of three parts of the inferior vena cava need only corrective surgical technique usually applied throughout the field of vascular surgery, but the portal vein and the retrohepatic vena cava are so intimate with the liver they deserve our special attention. Together, these hepatic organs (portal vein and retrohepatic vena cava) comprise the juxtahepatic veins.

Patients with juxtahepatic vein injuries reaching hospital alive usually require immediate resuscitative laparotomy, which parallels blood volume replacement rather than following it.

24,25&26

The successful exposure of the retrohepatic vena cava depends upon proper surgical incisions. A generous mid-line incision from xiphoid to below the umbilicus is the quickest and most versatile method of entering the peritoneal cavity. This mid-line incision aids in quick exposure and subsequent control of overt haemorrhage either with a haemostat or the surgeon's finger. To treat some retrohepatic vena caval injuries, the mid-line abdominal incision must be extended cephalad as a median sternotomy. The diaphragm is incised in an anterior to posterior direction avoiding the phrenic nerve's insertion into the diaphragm. Such an incision in the diaphragm comes directly down onto the junction of the suprahepatic vena cava with the retrohepatic vena cava. It is here that the major right and left hepatic veins enter the retrohepatic vena cava. This sternolaparotomy allows easy access to the retrohepatic vena cava, the heart and particularly the right atrial appendage, which can be used to insert an intracaval shunt when needed. The many advantages of this mid-line incision over the customary right thoraco-abdominal incision have already been listed.

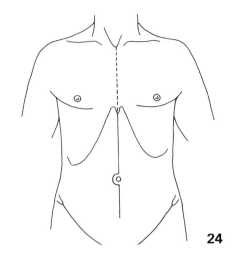

24

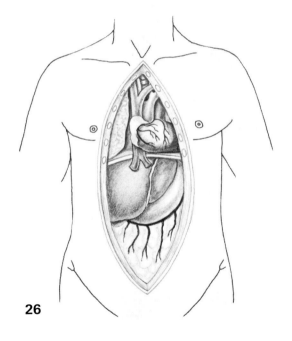

26

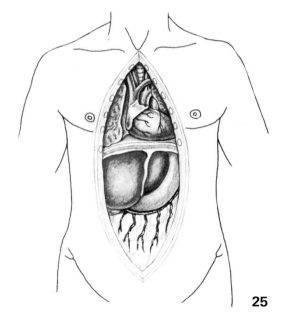

25

Acutely hypovolaemic patients do not tolerate the physiological and haemodynamic consequences of abruptly interrupting blood flow in the retrohepatic vena cava. Clamping above and below the liver has been advocated, but this abrupt stopping of blood from the kidneys and lower torso produces cardiac arrest in most patients and serious cardiac arrhythmias in others. The fact that clamping the infrahepatic and suprahepatic vena cava can be done safely in patients undergoing orthotopic liver transplants is not relevant to patients in shock with hypovolaemia and profuse bleeding from the retrohepatic vena cava. The few patients who survive complete clamping above and below the liver almost always have serious renal insufficiency in the postoperative period. This transiently reduced renal function is secondary to the renal venous hypertension resulting from cross-clamping the infrahepatic vena cava.

To prevent these two tragic complications of cross-clamping the intrahepatic and suprahepatic vena cava (Schrock, Blaisdell and Matherson, 1968) have suggested the insertion of an intracaval shunt. This allows continued flow of blood from the lower torso and kidneys, preventing both cardiac arrest and renal insufficiency. There are two methods for inserting such shunts; one uses the right atrial appendage. The other method is to insert the shunt directly into the vena cava either above or below the renal veins. Straight catheters do not achieve a completely dry operative field. There is continued oozing from the many retrohepatic veins. To prevent this, we have designed a balloon catheter to completely isolate the retrohepatic vena cava (Aaron and Mays, 1975).

Insertion of the balloon catheter is facilitated by using the readily accessible and expendable right atrial appendage. This saves a great deal of time compared to the time involved in dissecting the infrahepatic vena cava and getting proximal and distal control with encircling tapes to permit the insertion of the caval shunt. Haemorrhage from the retrohepatic vena cava is controlled quickly by balloon tamponade and simultaneous clamping of the hepatoduodenal ligament. The entire retrohepatic vena cava is isolated by the long balloon. Such isolation was tolerated by the experimental animals without the usual consequences of cardiac or renal malfunction.

The objectives in treating wounds of juxtahepatic venous injuries are: (1) rapid control of haemorrhage; (2) prevention of air embolism; (3) optimum venous filling of right heart and; (4) avoidance of renal venous hypertension. The specific treatment of each individual wound will vary greatly within these general guidelines. The operative technique proceeds in a step-wise manner because the entire procedure may not have to be done in every patient.

(1) Surgical preparation includes neck, chest, abdomen and upper parts of the thighs.

(2) The initial mid-line incision is xiphoid to umbilicus.

(3) If the source of haemorrhage is liver, ligate appropriate hepatic artery and apply pressure packs to perihepatic spaces.

(4) Attend to other operative necessities.

(5) Remove pressure packs from liver wounds and perihepatic spaces.

(6) If haemorrhage continues after ligating hepatic artery and removal of pressure packs, mobilize the liver. This is done by cutting the supporting ligaments of the liver.

(7) If there is simple avulsion or a linear tear in major hepatic vein, control haemorrhage with finger and repair defect with cardiovascular suture.

(8) When a complex injury of retrohepatic cava and juxtahepatic veins is detected, immediately replace pressure packs.

(9) Extend mid-line skin incision from xiphoid to suprasternal notch.

(10) Incise cervical fascia at sternal notch and gently dissect soft tissue from the superior segment of posterior sternum.

(11) Incise diaphragmatic attachments to xiphoid and inferior sternum.

(12) Separate the mediastinal structures and soft tissues from posterior sternum.

(13) Split sternum from sternal notch to xiphoid.

(14) Separate pleura and soft tissue from the posterior surface of the sternum and enter the right pleural cavity.

(15) Incise diaphragm in mid-line from anterior to posterior exposing juncture of inferior vena cava and major hepatic veins.

(16) Insert self-retaining chest retractor and spread halves of sternum.

(17) Control bleeding points from undersurface of sternum.

(18) Open pericardium.

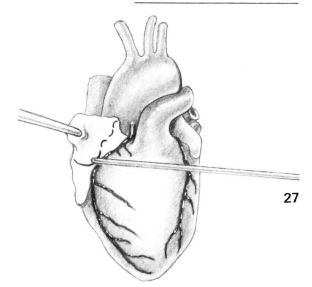

27

27 & 28

(*19*) Place 2/0 purse-string suture in right atrial appendage.
(*20*) Control atrium with appropriate vascular clamp and cut off atrial appendage.

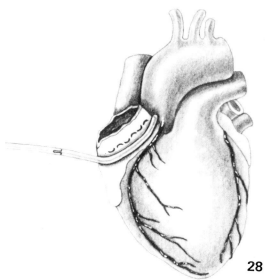

28

29

(*21*) Insert balloon catheter into right atrium and guide into position in vena cava behind liver.

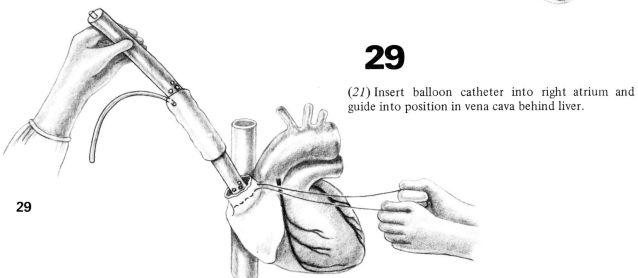

29

(*22*) Tie purse-string suture in atrial appendage.
(*23*) Connect infusion catheters proximal to catheter.
(*24*) Occlude afferent blood supply to liver.

30

(*25*) Inflate balloon catheter.

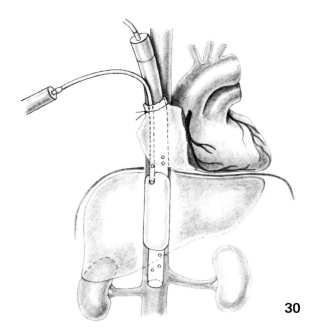

30

(*26*) Aspirate blood. Locate venous injury and repair with suture.

(*27*) If more than 15 min elapse, release occluding clamp on porta hepatis for several minutes before finishing repair.

(*28*) Deflate balloon, remove caval catheter and replace vascular clamp on atrium.

(*29*) Repair atrial appendage with vascular suture.

(*30*) Close the diaphragm and insert intercostal tube into right pleural space at mid-axillary line.

(*31*) Drain the perihepatic spaces extensively.

(*32*) Close the sternal and abdominal incisions.

Not all hepatic vein injuries require such extensive surgical procedures. Some can be treated through just the simple abdominal incision by mobilizing the liver and lifting it up and away from the retrohepatic vena cava. Minor holes or avulsions of a single hepatic vein can be controlled by finger pressure and direct suture repair. The liver is best mobilized by cutting the appropriate supporting ligaments of the liver and the fascia around the retrohepatic vena cava. Other hepatic vein avulsions or retrohepatic vena caval tears can be exposed by completing the removal of a part of the injured liver. Once the injured liver is out of the way, the lacerations in the juxtahepatic veins can be sutured directly. This is one of the few remaining indications for hepatic resection. The sternal incision and the intracaval shunt are not necessary for these kinds of wounds. Patients with these injuries treated with a shunt and without (clamping above and below the liver) have high morbidity and mortality rates regardless of which method is used.

THE PORTAL VEIN

Most injuries of the portal vein involve only part of the circumference of the vein. Haemorrhage can usually be controlled by finger pressure or vascular clamps. Dissection of the hepatoduodenal ligament can usually expose these minor tears and lacerations for direct suture repair (Burns and Britt, 1975). When there is avulsion of the portal vein with actual tissue loss, there are three methods of repair. The first is still experimental. It consists of replacing the injured portion of the vein with a vascular graft. The difficulty with this method is the lack of suitable prosthetics.

The second method of portal vein repair is ligation of the distal portal vein and construction of a portacaval shunt with the remnant of the proximal portal vein. The prospect of success of this technique depends upon the condition and length of the proximal portal vein.

The third method is simply to ligate both ends of the injured portal vein. While this may not be ideal, it is important for every surgeon operating on these patients to know that the portal vein can be ligated with survival of the patient. But if the hepatic artery has already been ligated to stop bleeding, the portal vein must not be ligated. Child *et al.* (1952) proved that man could survive acute and total occlusion of the portal vein. While this may not be ideal treatment, it is far better than allowing a patient to bleed to death on the operating table from a portal vein injury which cannot be repaired easily with sutures.

COMPLICATIONS OF HEPATIC RUPTURE

The most common complications of ruptured livers are pulmonary atelectasis, pleural effusions, pulmonary insufficiency, pneumonia, haemothorax, pneumothorax, and biliary pleural fistulae or effusions.

The next most common complication of hepatic rupture is infection.

The basic treatment of all abscesses is incision and drainage of the pus.

The third most common complication in patients with ruptured liver is fistula. These are nearly always bile fistulae draining to the outside but a biliary-pleural fistula is the most dangerous and the hardest to treat successfully.

Ironically, many complications are not the result of the original injury, but are due to the way the ruptured liver is treated. Almost all haemobilia has occurred in ruptured livers that have been packed with gauze or omentum or sutured. Hepatic sequestra have nearly always been related to closure of deep hepatic ruptures with stitches. Hepatic infarction due to intrahepatic haemorrhage is usually related to failures of techniques used to obtain hepatic haemostasis.

Other complications of hepatic rupture are listed in Table 2.

Table 2
Complications of Hepatic Rupture
(In order of decreasing frequency)

Thorax	Pulmonary insufficiency
	Pleural effusions
	Atelectasis
	Pneumonia
	Haemothorax
	Pneumothorax
Infection	Wound
	Respiratory
	Subphrenic abscess
	Subhepatic abscess
	Urinary tract
	Generalized sepsis
	Intra-abdominal
	Intrahepatic
Fistula	Biliary-cutaneous
	Biliary-pleural
	Colon
	Small bowel
	Pancreatic
	Gastric
Haemorrhage	Secondary hepatic
	Stress ulceration of stomach
	Haemobilia
	Intrahepatic haematoma
	Coagulation abnormalities
Other	Acute renal failure
	Phlebitis
	Transfusion reactions
	Wound dehiscence

POSTOPERATIVE CARE

The care of patients with ruptured livers does not differ from the standard care provided for all patients after operations except in a few specific instances.

Special postoperative care must be given to patients after selective ligation of the hepatic artery or after removing large amounts of hepatic tissue; the patient should be kept fasting for 7–10 days. Concentrated solutions of glucose are given to increase blood glucose above 100 mg/dl because this reverses the efflux of glucose from the ischaemic liver and protects against glycogen depletion. Serum albumin is given intravenously in 25–50 g increments daily to bolster the liver while its capacity to synthesize protein is reduced.

Early ambulation is important in all these patients; on the day after their operation they walk with the assistance of several nurses and strong orderlies.

Nasogastric decompression of the stomach is beneficial because of severe ileus occurring in most of these patients.

Indwelling urethral catheters are essential in postoperative care, especially for monitoring the flow of urine.

References

Aaron, W. S., Fulton, R. L. and Mays, E. T. (1975). 'Selective ligation of the hepatic artery.' *Surgery Gynec. Obstet.* **41**, 187
Burnś, R.P. and Britt, L.G. (1975). 'Massive venous injuries associated with penetrating wounds of the liver.' *J. Trauma* **15**, 757
Cantlie, J. (1897). 'On a new arrangement of the right and left lobes of the liver.' *Proc. Anat. Soc. Great Britain, Ireland* **32**, 4
Canty, T.G. and Aaron, W.S. (1975). 'Hepatic artery ligation for exsanguinating liver injuries in children.' *J. ped. Surg.* **10**, 693
Child, C.G., Holswade, G.R. *et al.* (1952). 'Pancreaticoduodenectomy with resection of the portal vein in the macaca mulatta monkey and in man.' *Surgery Gynec. Obstet.* **94**, 31
Edler, L. (1887). 'Die traumatischen Verletzungen der patenchymatosen Uferleigsorgane.' *Arch. Klin. Chir.* **34**, 343, 573, 738
Hass, G.H. (1944). 'Types of internal injuries of personnel involved in aircraft accidents.' *J. Aviation Med.* **15**, 77
Healey, J.E. (1954). 'Clinical anatomic aspects of radial hepatic surgery.' *J. Int. Coll. Surg.* **2**, 542
Healey, J. E., Schroy, P. C. and Sorensen, R. J. (1953). 'The intrahepatic distribution of the hepatic artery in man.' *J. Int. Coll. Surg.* **20**, 133
Lucas, C. E. (1971). 'Prospective clinical evaluation of biliary drainage in hepatic trauma.' *Ann. Surg.* **174**, 830
Madding, G.F., Lawrence, K.B. and Kennedy, P.A. (1943). 'Forward surgery of the severely injured.' *Second Aux Surgical Group* **1**, 307
Mays, E. T. (1966). 'Bursting injuries of the liver.' *Archs Surg.* **93**, 92
Mays, E.T. (1974). 'The hepatic artery.' *Surgery Gynec. Obstet.* **139**, 595
Mays, E.T. (1972). 'Lobectomy, sublobar resections and resectional debridement for severe liver injury.' *J. Trauma* **12**, 309
Mays, E.T. (1971). 'Hepatic lobectomy.' *Archs Surg.* **103**, 216
Mays, E.T. (1973). 'Hepatic trauma.' *New Engl. J. Med.* **288**, 402
Mays, E.T. (1972). 'Lobar dearterialization for exsanguinating wounds of the liver.' *J. Trauma* **12**, 397
Mays, E.T. (1971). 'Complex penetrating hepatic wounds.' *Ann. Surg.* **173**, 421
Mays, E.T. and Wheeler, C.S. (1974). 'Demonstration of collateral arterial flow after interruption of hepatic arteries in man.' *New Engl. J. Med.* **290**, 993
McClelland, R., Shires, T. and Poulos, E. (1964). 'Hepatic resection for massive trauma.' *J. Trauma* **4**, 282
Merendino, K.A., Dillard, D.H. and Cammock, E.C. (1963). 'The concept of surgical biliary decompression in the management of liver trauma.' *Surgery Gynec. Obstet.* **117**, 285
Mikesky, W. E., Howard, J. M. and DeBakey, M. E. (1956). 'Injuries of the liver in 300 consecutive patients.' *Surgery Gynec. Obstet.* **103**, 323
Pringle, J. H. (1908). 'Notes on the arrest of hepatic hemorrhage.' *Ann. Surg.* **48**, 541
Sandblom, P. (1948). 'Hemorrhage into the biliary tract following trauma – traumatic hemobilia.' *Surgery* **24**, 571
Schrock, T. F., Blaisdell, F. W. and Matherson, C. (1968). 'Management of blunt trauma to the liver and hepatic veins.' *Archs Surg.* **96**, 698
Storm, F. K. and Longmire, W. P., Jr. (1971). 'A simplified clamp for hepatic resection.' *Surgery Gynec. Obstet.* **133**, 103
Trunkey, D.D., Shires, G.T. and McClelland, R. (1974). 'Management of liver trauma in 811 consecutive patients.' *Ann. Surg.* **179**, 722
Tygstrup, N., Winkler, K., Mellemgaard, K. *et al.* (1962). 'Determination of the hepatic arterial blood flow and oxygen supply in man by clamping the hepatic artery during surgery.' *J. clin. Invest.* **41**, 447
Wakim, K.G. and Mann, F. (1942). 'The intrahepatic circulation of blood.' *Anat. Rec.* **82**, 233

[*The illustrations for this Chapter on Rupture of the Liver were drawn by Miss A. Barrett.*]

Duodenal Injuries

Hugh Dudley, Ch.M., F.R.C.S., F.R.C.S.(Ed.), F.R.A.C.S.
Professor of Surgery, St. Mary's Hospital, London

INTRODUCTION

Duodenal rupture is almost invariably retroperitoneal. The exceptions are penetrating anterior injuries. Concomitant injury to the neighbouring pancreatic head is not unusual and the force of injury — usually a violent blow from a blunt object or a deceleration injury against a seat belt — may cause other intra-abdominal injuries. Thus, wide laparotomy and exploration are essential.

The pathological mechanisms of closed rupture include the development of intramural haematoma. The progress of this condition may stop at such a point and furthermore, in young children resolution can be confidently expected. However, most adult haematomas produce continuing duodenal obstruction for which operation is required. More serious injury tends either to be an initial tear or progression to devitalization of the duodenal wall with breakdown over the next hours or a day or two, presumably aided by the digestive properties of duodenal content. This course accounts for two things — the sometimes insidious onset of the condition and the appearances at laparotomy or autopsy when the duodenal wall may be found to be friable and oedematous so that closure is difficult. Both factors contribute to a high mortality (about 20 per cent).

Diagnosis

Duodenal rupture must always be suspected when a blunt injury has occurred to the upper abdomen and minimal signs, often with considerable vomiting, persist. Diagnostic peritoneal lavage is less helpful with retroperitoneal than intraperitoneal lesions. Laparotomy should be undertaken on suspicion.

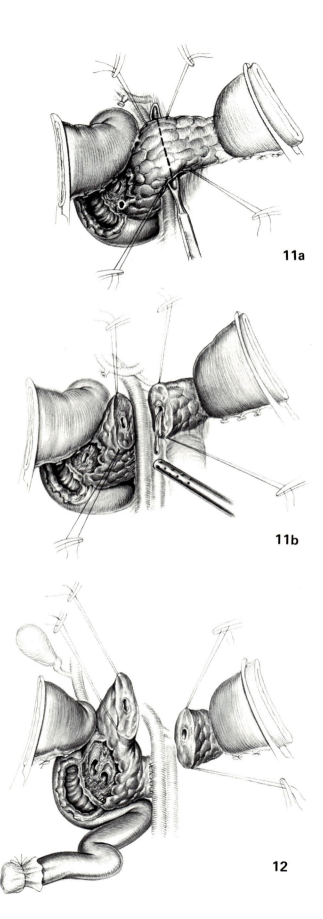

11a

11b

12

11a & b

A Kocher dissector is now passed beneath the mobilized neck of the pancreas and the gland is divided between stay sutures as shown. The common bile duct is then transected and the gastroduodenal artery ligated and divided.

12

Attention is now turned to the proposed distal line of section of bowel, which in most instances will be the third part of the duodenum. The bowel at this point is divided between clamps and the distal end closed as a blind stump. Severe damage to this area, however, will necessitate total duodenectomy and division of the jejunum just distal to the ligament of Treitz. As a first step in this dissection the transverse meso-colon is elevated, the duodenojejunal junction identified and the jejunum divided. Incision of the ligament of Treitz will allow the mobilized duodenum to be drawn through and to the right of the superior mesenteric vessels before removal.

13

At this stage of the operation the head of the pancreas remains attached to the superior mesenteric vessels by the short vessels passing to the uncinate process and by the inferior pancreaticoduodenal artery, which enters the groove between the pancreas and duodenum. Although the larger of these vessels may be ligated with ease the smaller, stouter veins are often difficult to control directly and it is advisable to leave a small portion of uncinate process *in situ* to protect the main vein.

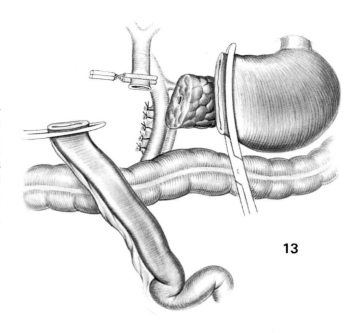

13

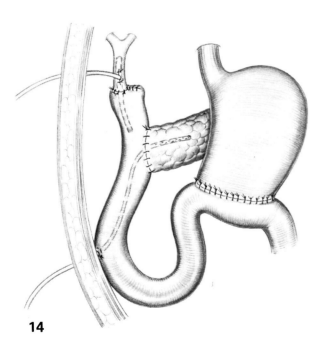

14

14

Reconstruction now begins. The free end of the jejunum (or jejunal Roux-en-Y if the third part of the duodenum has been transected) is brought into the upper abdomen through the mesocolon and the common bile duct, pancreas and stomach are anastomosed to the bowel as shown. A T-tube is placed in the common bile duct and a vacuum drain is passed from the pancreaticojejunal anastomosis, through the jejunal lumen and thence to the exterior.

POSTOPERATIVE CARE AND COMPLICATIONS

The intensity of postoperative observation and treatment will depend on the operation performed and the severity of associated injuries. Ideally, the patient should be transferred to an intensive care unit for careful recording of vital signs, water balance, central venous pressure, urine output, the blood picture and chemistry to detect at the earliest possible stage the development of complications. Intravenous infusion and nasogastric aspiration will be necessary during the early postoperative stage, with blood transfusion as required. Intravenous feeding through a central venous catheter may be instituted after 24 hr and continued until oral feeding has been re-established. Prophylactic antibiotics are desirable after extensive resections and penetrating wounds. Indwelling pancreatic and biliary drainage tubes should be attached to a low-pressure suction apparatus for 48 hr, after which gravity drainage into a collecting bag is satisfactory. On the tenth day after operation these tubes may be removed if free flow of bile or pancreatic juice into the bowel is demonstrated by pancreatography and cholangiography.

After operations for pancreatic injury complications are common and include postoperative haemorrhage, particularly from drainage sites, pancreatitis, pancreatic fisulae, intra-abdominal abscess, pseudocyst and diabetes if pancreatic resection has been extensive.

Pancreatic fistulae develop in about 25 per cent of these patients; they are usually transient and in the majority of instances close spontaneously within a few weeks. Occasionally leakage of pancreatic juice is more serious, resulting in rapid disturbance of electrolyte and water balance, with severe excoriation. For this condition continuous suction drainage of the fistula will protect the skin and at the same time allow accurate measurements of liquid lost. Persistence of a pancreatic fistula raises the possibility of obstruction of the pancreatic duct, a condition that is easily confirmed by fistulography. Resection of pancreas to the left of the fistulae or drainage of the main duct into jejunum or stomach may be required.

Pseudocysts which are enlarging or causing symptoms should be drained internally into the stomach or jejunum or, in a severely ill patient, it may be more appropriate to drain them externally.

[*The illustrations for this Chapter on Rupture of the Pancreas were drawn by Mr. R. N. Lane.*]

Surgical Exposure of the Kidney

G. F. Murnaghan, M.D., Ch.M., F.R.C.S.(Ed.), F.R.C.S., F.R.A.C.S.
Professor of Surgery, University of New South Wales;
Honorary Urological Surgeon to The Prince Henry,
The Prince of Wales and The Eastern Suburbs Hospitals, and
Honorary Consultant Urologist to The Royal South Sydney Hospital,
The Canterbury Hospital, Sydney, and The Royal Hospital for Women, Paddington, New South Wales

PRE - OPERATIVE

Pre-operative assessment and preparation

Careful assessment of the patient's respiratory and cardiovascular systems is required before surgical exposure of the kidney is undertaken. Retroperitoneal dissection, particularly through the loin, predisposes to respiratory complications and paralytic ileus. Smoking should be discontinued, physiotherapy should be used to ensure maximum ventilatory capacity and a control radiograph of the chest should be taken. Regular, adequate bowel action should be assured as part of the usual preparation for general anaesthesia; the level of haemoglobin should be recorded and at least two units of compatible blood should be available. The posture and range of lateral flexion in the dorsolumbar spine should be noted and skin prepared should extend from the nipple line to the pubis and almost out to the opposite flank on both the front and back of the trunk. Representative and up-to-date radiographs should be chosen from the urological studies and illuminated for easy reference in the operating theatre.

Choice of incision

Choice of incision is influenced by the size, site and mobility of both the lesion and the kidney, by the age and build of the patient, by spinal mobility or curvature and by the distance between the costal margin and the iliac crest in the mid-axillary line, which is where maximum width of the wound is usually obtained.

A standard approach through the loin using a subcostal incision will give adequate exposure of a mobile kidney which is not enlarged, provided that a plain radiograph of the renal region shows that the twelfth rib does not project below the mid-hilar level. The subcostal approach should be carefully considered whenever subsequent re-exposure of the kidney is likely to be required.

Exposure of a high, adherent or enlarged kidney can be improved by resection of the twelfth rib or the eleventh rib if the twelfth is underdeveloped. This transcostal approach is most useful when there has been previous exposure of the kidney by the subcostal route, or when a reconstructive operation is contemplated.

If there is a large or fixed kidney there is particular need for access to the upper polar region or pedicle and this can be obtained by an incision above the eleventh, or less commonly the twelfth, rib, which gives extrapleural and extraperitoneal exposure. Wide access may also be obtained through a Nagamatsu approach, which extends the posterior end of a subcostal incision upwards in a paravertebral line to the ninth intercostal space to allow for resection of 2·5 cm segments of the posterior ends of the lowest two or three ribs.

Similar wide exposure may be obtained by a transthoracic approach with a high transcostal or intercostal incision combined with an anterior abdominal extension of the wound to allow for simultaneous transperitoneal exploration and any necessary dissection of lymph nodes.

An anterior extraperitoneal approach to the kidney may be useful in infants and small children as a more commodious alternative to the exposure generally obtained through the lumbar incision in young patients. It provides direct but localized access to the lower renal pole, pelvi-ureteric junction and upper part of the ureter in all ages, but it is particularly useful for the exposure of one or both kidneys in patients with severe cardiorespiratory limitation or with immobilizing disabilities such as osteo-arthrosis of the spine, scoliosis or kyphosis. Simultaneous exposure of both kidneys is best obtained through an extensive transverse or curved, muscle cutting, upper abdominal approach with medial reflection of the organs and peritoneum overlying each kidney.

THE OPERATION

All illustrations show access to the right kidney; the posterior aspect of the wound is on the left.

1

The incisions

The lines of incision for approach by the subcostal, the transcostal (twelfth rib), supracostal (eleventh rib) and thoraco-abdominal (tenth space) routes of exposure are illustrated. Incisions relating to ribs should curve downwards slightly in their abdominal extension to avoid damage to the neurovascular bundle from the rib above. The foreshortened skin incision for the anterior extraperitoneal exposure of the kidney is shown as a dotted line.

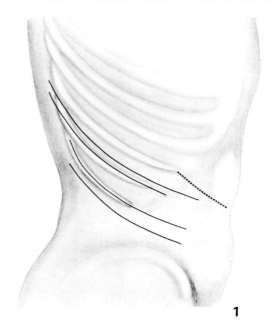

1

2

Positioning the patient

For any lateral approach the patient lies on the opposite side, somewhat nearer to the back edge of the operating table, with any segmented cushions replaced by a continuous sheet of thick sponge and with the kidney bridge just below the costal margin. The patient's back is kept vertical by flexing the lower knee and thigh while the upper knee remains straight and is supported on a pillow. The upper arm is supported horizontally by a rest and is convenient for venous cannulation and recording the blood pressure. The underneath arm is disposed in comfortable flexion with padded support. Rolling of the patient is then prevented by padded fixtures on the table and by a leather strap or broad band of adhesive strapping which crosses between the iliac crest and greater trochanter and is attached firmly beneath the table. Lateral flexion of the spine to open the costo-iliac space is obtained by a convenient combination or choice of sandbag in the opposite loin, elevation of the bridge and breaking of the table. The pelvis should be kept vertical and it should be ensured that there is no embarrassment to cardiorespiratory function, that there has been no undue angulation of the spine and that the buttocks remain on the table. An anterior approach to the kidney is facilitated by support for the lower, posterior part of the chest and loin on one or both sides of the supine patient.

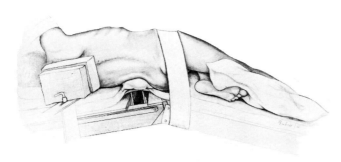

2

SUBCOSTAL APPROACH

3

The skin incision extends from the angle between the twelfth rib and the outer border of the erector spinae muscles and passes forwards about 1 cm below and parallel to the rib and then to a point about 2 cm above and anterior to the anterior superior iliac spine. With careful haemostasis the fat and deep fascia are divided to expose the external oblique muscle in the anterior portion of the wound, with latissimus dorsi muscle in the posterior portion. The next useful plane is entered by dividing latissimus dorsi in the line of the incision to expose the posterior edge of the external oblique muscle and adjacent lumbodorsal fascia.

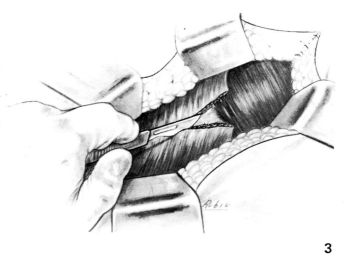

3

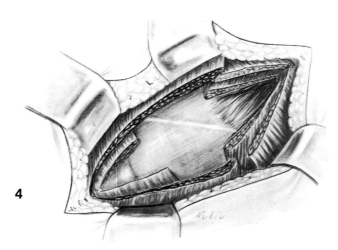

4

4

Division of superficial muscles

Posterior extension of the division of latissimus dorsi exposes the serratus posterior inferior, which is incised to expose the lateral edge of erector spinae beneath the lumbodorsal fascia. Division of the external oblique in the anterior portion of the wound allows for division of the internal oblique muscle from its posterior edge and forwards across the line of its fibres. Care must be taken to avoid the subcostal nerve which in thin patients may be seen crossing the wound beneath the lumbodorsal fascia, having left the twelfth rib about the junction between its middle and distal thirds.

5

Division of lumbodorsal fascia

An incision is made into the lumbodorsal fascia in a somewhat more vertical direction than the main line of the incision so that the subcostal nerve can be recognized and dissected clear as the opening in the fascia is extended backwards as far as erector spinae. Blunt dissection forwards beneath the lumbodorsal fascia should proceed carefully to separate the parietal peritoneum from the deep layer of the transversus abdominis muscle, the fibres of which will separate as the fascial incision extends forwards. Careful haemostasis should be obtained and the subcostal neurovascular bundle may be retracted forwards or backwards to obtain the best lie.

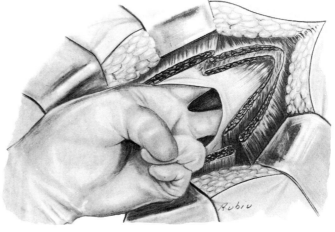

5

6

Exposure of the perinephric space

Retraction of the free edges of the lumbodorsal fascia allows deep digital exploration of the posterior end of the wound and a gentle gauze reflection forwards of the parietal peritoneum and extraperitoneal fatty tissue to expose the perirenal fascia. If the present exposure is considered to be inadequate, further upward retraction of the twelfth rib will be facilitated by posterior extension of the incision of the anterior layer of the lumbodorsal fascia to include the external arcuate ligament but any bleeding from subcostal vessels must be carefully controlled.

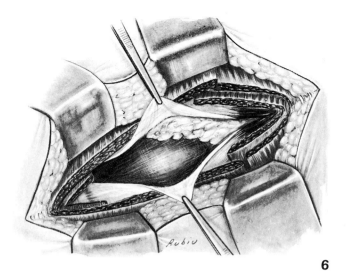

6

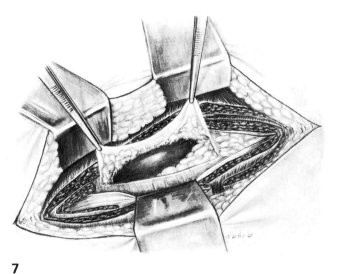

7

7

Incision of the perirenal fascia

A longitudinal cut is made with knife and then scissors through the perirenal fascia a short distance from and parallel to its reflection from the surface of the quadratus lumborum muscle. The anterior edge may be grasped in forceps and elevated to lift the perinephric fat to allow gentle dissection and exposure of the capsular surface of the kidney.

8

Exposure of the anterior surface and pedicle

Strong anterior retraction of the peritoneum will allow continued forward dissection and elevation of the perirenal fascia, with displacement of the overlying abdominal organs. Gentle lateral traction on the kidney aids blunt dissection through the flimsy fascia to expose the pedicle in the hilum. In the presence of adhesions the plane of the pedicle can more easily be entered after identification of the ureter, medial to the lower pole of the kidney, and by gentle upwards dissection in the plane of the ureter and renal pelvis but with care to avoid segmental renal vessels.

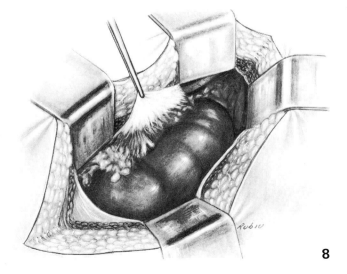

8

9

Exposure of the posterior aspect

Recognition of the ureter near to the lower pole of the kidney is a useful guide to the plane of the renal pelvis. Access is facilitated by delivering the lower pole of the kidney into the wound whilst the upper pole remains deep. Though the main pedicle usually lies anteriorly, all posterior dissection of the kidney should be careful and blunt without jeopardy to segmental renal vessels and ureteric blood supply.

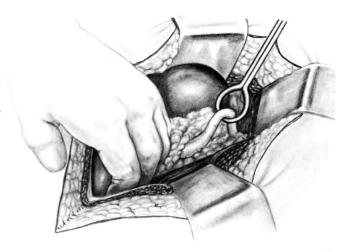

9

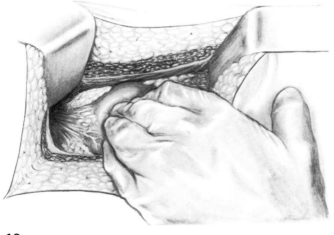

10

Exposure of the upper pole

Strong, deep retraction of the posterior third of the wound rather than the posterior end of the incision, combined with downward and deep displacement of the kidney will expose the upper renal pole and suprarenal gland. Strong fibrous bands intermingled with fat may adhere to the renal capsule and may contain quite large blood vessels.

10

TRANSCOSTAL APPROACH

11

Incision and exposure of rib

Accurate localization of the rib by palpation may be difficult until the skin, fat and superficial fascia have been divided. After subsequent identification a bold incision is made through the latissimus dorsi and serratus posterior inferior muscles onto the rib, which is steadied between finger tips placed in the eleventh intercostal space and beneath the twelfth rib. The incision should extend into the fascial attachments and periosteum of the outer surface of the rib with clearing of the external oblique muscle from the costal cartilage. Forward extension of the incision with division of the abdominal muscles is postponed until the rib has been resected.

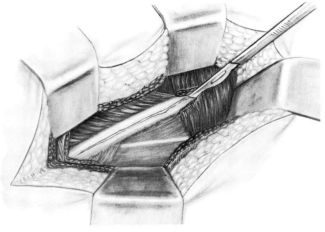

11

12

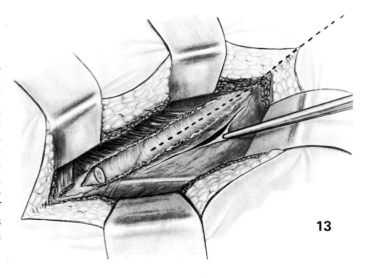

12

Excision of rib

The incised periosteum and its attachment on the outer surface of the rib are reflected to the upper and lower borders with a rugine or elevator. Safe and easy entry into the subperiosteal or extrapleural plane on the deep surface of the rib is obtained by careful passage of the rugine along the upper border of the rib from behind forwards and in the reverse direction along the lower rib border. This plane is carefully developed with a raspatory so that the rib is mobilized subperiosteally from the posterior angle to the costal cartilage. The posterior portion is divided with a costotome and the rib is elevated from its bed using a knife to divide the tip and margin of costal cartilage.

13

Division of abdominal muscles

The reflection of the pleura crosses deep to the periosteum of the rib bed. It may be difficult to identify and will restrict safe posterior extension of any incision through the rib bed into the extraperitoneal space. The subcostal neurovascular bundle should be identified as it leaves the lower margin of the rib bed beneath the lumbodorsal fascia. The fascia can be opened safely to avoid both the rib bed and the subcostal vessels and nerve, which can be dissected and displaced posteriorly to allow for easy access to the extraperitoneal space with forward extension of the incision into the abdominal wall muscles. This anterior dissection is similar to the subcostal approach as detailed in *Illustrations 4, 5* and *6*.

13

SUPRACOSTAL APPROACH

14

Mobilization of the rib

The skin incision extends along the whole length of the eleventh rib, it is deepened through the overlying muscle to expose but not incise the rib and it is carried through the abdominal wall muscles for a short distance beyond the tip of the rib. The intercostal muscle is detached from the upper surface of the rib with the diathermy knife to leave the periosteum bare. A fingertip is inserted into the extrapleural space to protect the deep tissues as the extrapleural plane is opened. The supracostal release must extend posteriorly to allow for division of the posterior supracostal ligament so that the rib is free to rotate downwards at the costovertebral articulation.

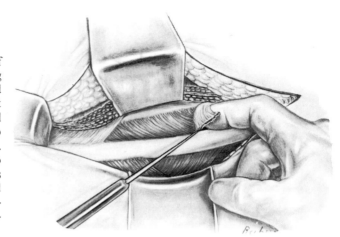

14

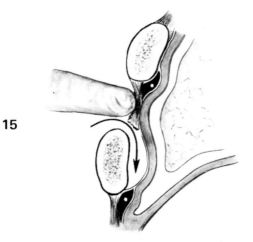

15

15

Release of the intercostal nerve

Incomplete division of the intercostal muscle leaves the innermost fibres intact so that they peel away from the rib with the extrapleural fascia as pressure is applied to the outside surface of the intercostal muscle. The extrapleural fascia splits along the lower border of the rib to enclose the intercostal nerve and the outer layer of fascia must be divided longitudinally with scissors in order to release the nerve and to allow for downward progression of the extrapleural dissection.

16

Division of the diaphragm

The diaphragm is divided as low down as possible to detach it from its origin but with preservation of its full length to facilitate closure. The eleventh rib should retract downwards and backwards quite easily to give wide access to the subdiaphragmatic and retroperitoneal space. The peritoneum may be reflected forwards with concomitant fat to expose the perirenal fascia and suprarenal gland.

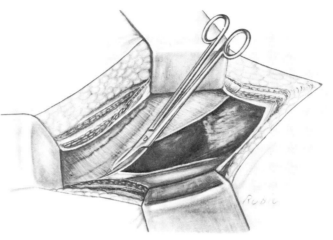

16

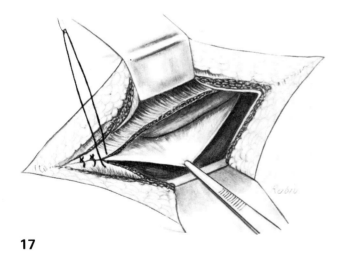

17

17

Closure of supracostal approach

The deeper closure with separation of the thoracic and abdominal compartments is accomplished by pulling the upper margin of the free edge of the incised diaphragm through the intercostal space so that it can be sutured to the intercostal muscles and to the muscles on the outer surface of the rib below, that is serratus posterior inferior posteriorly and latissimus dorsi anteriorly. Any pleural tear can also be approximated in these interrupted sutures after deliberate expansion of the lung by forced ventilation. The superficial muscles are closed in layers and any required drainage is effected through a separate stab incision below the subcostal nerve and twelfth rib.

THORACO-ABDOMINAL APPROACH

18

Thoracotomy

Wide exposure of the kidney with easy access to the pedicle may be obtained by a transpleural approach through the bed of either the tenth or eleventh ribs. The chosen rib is resected subperiosteally as described for the transcostal approach, with incision of overlying muscles including the latissimus dorsi, serratus posterior inferior posteriorly and some fibres of the external oblique muscle in the anterior portion of the wound. A similar exposure is afforded more easily by incision through the ninth or tenth intercostal space without rib resection. The superficial layers of muscle must be incised as far back as the lateral edge of the erector spinae.

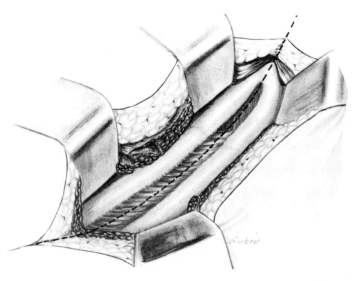

18

19

Exposure and incision of the diaphragm

Incision of the intercostal muscles, intercostal membrane, costal cartilage and underlying pleura exposes the lung, which collapses or is retracted to expose the diaphragm. The retroperitoneal space is then entered by division of the diaphragm and overlying pleura in the mid-portion of the wound. The diaphragmatic incision is then extended posteriorly towards the angle of the twelfth rib so that adherent peritoneum may be dissected free from the undersurface of the diaphragm to allow for forward extension of the incision through diaphragm and the transversus abdominis muscle, which interdigitate. The wound is then extended forwards by incision of the abdominal wall muscles in a manner similar to the description for the anterior extraperitoneal approach (*see Illustrations 20* and *21*). The perinephric fascia is exposed by forward displacement of the subdiaphragmatic peritoneum and fat. The peritoneum may be incised in conjunction with the anterior extension of the thoraco-abdominal approach to give extensive access to the abdomen.

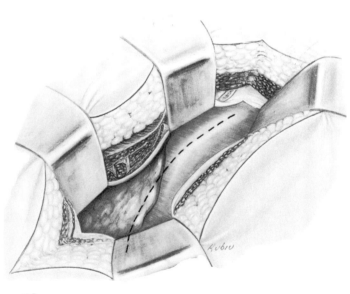

19

ANTERIOR EXTRAPERITONEAL APPROACH

20

Exposure of the peritoneum

The skin incision extends from the tip of the tenth rib to cross the lateral edge of the rectus abdominis muscle in the direction of the umbilicus. The external and internal oblique muscles are divided across the line of their fibres and the bundles of the transversus abdominis muscle are gently separated to enter the extraperitoneal plane. Finger or gauze dissection between the peritoneum and the transversalis fascia must be gentle but extensive. The peritoneum becomes more adherent to the posterior rectus sheath in the anterior portion of the wound. Both the anterior and posterior layers of the sheath of rectus abdominis can be incised over a short distance to improve access through this approach, which can also be combined with thoracotomy.

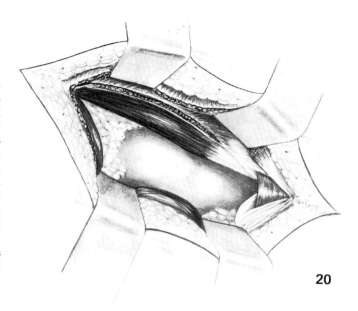

20

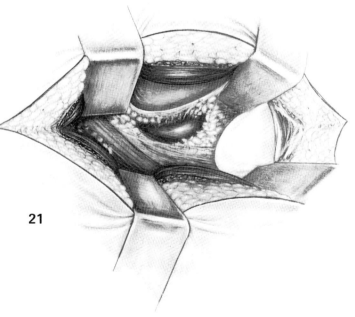

21

21

Retraction of the peritoneum

The extensive and lateral mobilization of the peritoneum allows it to be retracted medially so that the perinephric fascia is exposed on the stretch. The fascia is incised longitudinally, parallel to the renal axis and is mobilized medially with perinephric fat and peritoneum to expose the lower pole of the kidney, the pelvi-ureteric junction and the upper spindle of ureter.

RE-EXPOSURE OF THE KIDNEY

Most careful review of renal position and mobility and the nature of any previous renal surgery should precede the choice of incision for re-exposure. An alternative to the primary approach is usually desirable and the transcostal route is generally very much easier than approaching through the scar of a previous subcostal incision. Re-exploration is cautiously staged. Excessive tension in the parietes from lateral extension of the spine in the 'kidney position' must be avoided in order to prevent sudden splitting of any adherent kidney on the deep surface of the previous muscle closure as the incision is deepened and the wound edges separate. The extraperitoneal plane should be identified at a renal pole away from the main site of previous surgery. The peritoneum may be densely adherent on the lateral as well as the anterior aspects of the kidney and may be included in the scarring of previous drainage sites. Dissection may be started more easily around the upper part of the ureter and a safe plane may be developed proximally to isolate the renal pedicle.

CLOSURE OF WOUNDS AFTER EXPOSURE OF KIDNEY

Despite careful haemostasis there is a tendency for serosanguinous oozing and there is sometimes urinary leakage. Accordingly it is usually wise to drain the perinephric space, with loose approximation of the perinephric fat and fascia around the drain, using a few interrupted absorbable catgut sutures. Drains should be flexible and generally are more effective if corrugated rather than tubular. Gross drainage may be collected by surface applicator for measurement and analysis. Drains should be delivered in front of the mid-axillary line, where they can be included in muscular rather than fascial closure of the wound and will not cause added discomfort to the patient with change in lateral posture. Negligible drainage from the wound would encourage shortening of the drain by 2 – 3 cm each day and early removal from the retroperitoneal space discourages paralytic ileus.

When closing the wound care should be taken to avoid including intercostal or subcostal nerves in stitches. The deep closing sutures in the lumbodorsal fascia or rib bed should be placed first at the posterior end of any loin wound before the bridge is lowered to reduce lateral spinal flexion and so narrow the wound. Muscles should be closed layer by layer except when this is impracticable after re-exposure. Interrupted sutures of fine unabsorbable material are most dependable for the closure of clean wounds but this technique is time-consuming. Running sutures of 1/0 chromic catgut are satisfactory provided that independent interrupted sutures are placed on either side of any drain and in each muscle layer separately.

Diaphragmatic incision must be securely approximated by a re-inforced layer of interrupted horizontal mattress sutures of unabsorbable material other than silk. The parietal pleura and any periosteal bed of resected rib are carefully closed with a continuous suture of fine nylon before the parietal muscles are approximated with unabsorbable sutures. It is not necessary to approximate either the parietal pleura or the intercostal muscles in closing a thoracotomy through an intercostal space. The adjacent ribs are brought together and bound with interrupted ligatures of double 2/0 chromic catgut. The wound becomes airtight with approximation of the superficial muscles by a continuous suture of unabsorbable material In closing the chest cavity care must be taken to re-expand the underlying lung and a soft intercostal catheter of size 32 Ch is inserted through a stab incision in the eighth intercostal space in the mid-axillary line to provide for underwater sealed drainage.

The special technique for closure of the supracostal approach is shown in *Illustration 17*.

POSTOPERATIVE CARE

Approaches to the kidney through the loin, lower thorax and retroperitoneal space predispose to pulmonary complications, tympanites and paralytic ileus. If the retroperitoneal dissection has been extensive, and particularly in obese patients, food and drink should be replaced by intravenous infusion until the bowels become active again. Physiotherapy with early activity of the patient, supported by analgesics and comfortable wound dressings promote pulmonary expansion and avoid atelectasis.

References

Nagamatsu, G. R. (1950) 'Dorsolumbar approach to the kidney and adrenal with osteoplastic flap.' *J. Urol.* **63**, 569
Turner-Warwick, R. T. (1967). 'The supracostal approach to the renal area.' *Br. J. Urol.* **37**, 671

[*The illustrations for this Chapter on Surgical Exposure of the Kidney were drawn by Mrs. F. Rubiu.*]

Injuries to the Kidney

J. P. Mitchell, *T.D.,* M.S., F.R.C.S., F.R.C.S.(Ed.)
Professor of Surgery (Urology), University of Bristol;
Consultant Urologist, United Bristol Hospitals and Southmead General Hospital

The kidney may be injured by external violence or by a penetrating missile. Sport is still the commonest cause of renal trauma, in which case the injury may be limited to the kidney alone, whereas in road traffic accidents the injuries are often multiple, the kidney being probably only one of several damaged structures. The damage to the kidney is commonly the result of a heavy blow or crush injury to the loin, and is unaccompanied by an external wound (closed injuries).

1

In the majority of cases the blow is transmitted via the lower costal margin. Gunshot injuries or stabbings account for most penetrating wounds (open injuries).

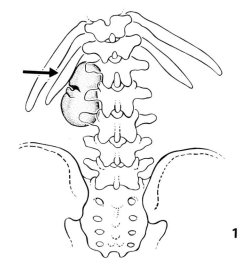

1

OPEN WOUNDS OF KIDNEY

In penetrating wounds, the renal lesion may be only one incident amongst other serious abdominal or chest injuries, which demand precedence in treatment. Exploration by intraperitoneal laparotomy will usually be demanded to exclude or identify damage to other viscera and to remove any fragment of clothing or other foreign body. There is much evidence that uncomplicated projectile injuries of the kidney heal well, and that a conservative policy regarding the removal of the injured organ is occasionally justified. Gross renal lesions, however, require primary nephrectomy, and it is wise to perform this operation when there is doubt about the viability of the kidney or the likelihood of further severe haemorrhage. When a penetrating wound of the kidney is associated with a laceration of the colon, nephrectomy is usually a prudent procedure so as to avoid the possibility of leakage of urine into the retroperitoneal space already contaminated by faeces.

CLOSED INJURIES OF KIDNEY

Renal lesions vary from mild contusions to gross lacerations of the renal parenchyma, which may involve the calyces and pelvis. The renal vessels may be partially or completely torn. Avulsion of the renal pedicle may still be compatible with life, despite the size of the renal artery and the volume of its circulation, because recoil of the intima can occasionally control the bleeding sufficiently for the patient to reach hospital. Rarely, the ureter is divided. The haematoma may be subcapsular and small, or it may leak extensively into the perirenal tissues via a tear in the renal capsule, resulting in a large retroperitoneal haematoma of the loin.

Urine can escape into the haematoma from a split in the renal parenchyma involving one of the minor calyces, or a leak may occur from a tear of a major calyx, or even of the renal pelvis.

Initial treatment and investigations

Ninety-six per cent of renal injuries resolve without operative interference (Slade, 1971). Unless there is evidence of concomitant abdominal injury, a watching policy should be pursued and observation directed to determining the severity and persistence of the haematuria and perirenal bleeding. However trivial the injury may appear, all these patients should be put to bed and sedated to ensure complete rest. The pulse and blood pressure are recorded quarter-hourly at first, and the degree of haematuria is checked at each act of urination, successive specimens being saved for comparison. A change from red to brown will precede any reduction in intensity of discolouration. In the early stages it is not possible to determine with accuracy the severity of the lesion, and to forecast the ultimate course.

Intravenous pyelography should be arranged at the earliest possible opportunity in order to ensure that the opposite kidney on the uninjured side is normal. Delay in this investigation may lose valuable time in assessing the degree of trauma, and can often result in poor definition of the kidneys because of accumulation of overlying gas in the bowel; a developing perirenal haematoma will obscure the psoas shadow; distortion of the calyceal pattern may be due either to tearing of the renal parenchyma or accumulation of blood clot within the pelvis. Extravasation of contrast medium may be seen beyond the renal outline, and often there will be a scoliosis with the concavity towards the side of the injury.

Although some centres have attempted selective renal angiography within 24 hr of injury, the value of this investigation in the acute phase is questionable, since the time involved in transporting the patient from the site of injury to the hospital, plus the time of investigation by pyelography followed by angiography, is unlikely to be less than the warm ischaemic time of devitalized renal tissue. Even if an immediate angiogram reveals impaired renal circulation, with an area of marked narrowing of the renal artery, suggestive of severe intimal damage, still a conservative approach can result in satisfactory function of the injured kidney (Mitchell, 1973). Nevertheless, an injured kidney that is functionless on intravenous pyelography, justifies selective renal angiography, if only to aid prognosis.

Cystoscopy and retrograde pyelography are rarely required to establish the diagnosis of renal injury. Furthermore, this investigation does carry with it the risk of infection and of aggravating renal bleeding.

Indications for operative treatment

Exploration of the damaged kidney is indicated: (1) when haematuria or perirenal bleeding persists, and threatens to endanger the patient's life, (2) when associated renal disorder is discovered on intravenous pyelography, (3) in the presence of uncontrollable renal or perirenal infection, which could give rise to recurrent severe haematuria and (4) when renal damage is associated with major injury to other viscera.

Antibiotic therapy

A large perirenal haematoma is an excellent culture medium for any organisms which may escape from the bowel, possibly via torn lymphatics. A broad-spectrum antibiotic is therefore justified as a prophylactic measure to be started as soon as the diagnosis is confirmed.

Even with an injury limited to a blow in the loin, without damage to other parts of the body, it is still possible that other structures, in addition to the kidney, may be injured. In left-sided abdominal injuries, the spleen may be ruptured; in right-sided abdominal injuries the liver is also likely to be involved. Renal injury is often associated with a fracture of one or two lower ribs as well as rupture of the diaphragm, and other possible intrathoracic damage.

EXPLORATION OF INJURED KIDNEY

Preparation

A central venous pressure gauge will have to be set up to help to assess the patient's circulatory state. At least 4 units of whole blood should be readily available. Rapid transfusion may be necessary in the event of severe haemorrhage during the operation.

Approach to the kidney

If a firm diagnosis of ruptured kidney, uncomplicated by other injuries, has been made, then the best approach is through the bed of the twelfth rib, which has to be resected subperiosteally. Haematoma may be found immediately the periosteal bed of the rib is incised. If, on the one hand, the haematoma is not extensive it may still be contained within the perirenal fascia or even beneath the renal capsule. The perirenal fascia, if still intact, is incised and blood clot is removed gently and with great care not to disturb any sealed vessels.

If, on the other hand, the abdomen is being explored for suspected intraperitoneal damage, and the kidney injury is only part of the patient's multiple trauma, then a transabdominal exploration is indicated. In these circumstances, a retroperitoneal haematoma will be found around the kidney area and a quick assessment should be made of the extent of this haematoma as soon as the abdomen is opened. By the time damage to other viscera has been inspected and repaired, it will be possible to re-assess the perirenal haematoma and decide whether it is increasing—in which case it must be explored. Transabdominal exploration of an injured kidney may be difficult and, if the haematoma appears to be extending during the period of the laparotomy, it is probably safer to close the abdomen and explore the kidney through the loin.

Assessment of renal damage

After mobilization of the kidney, lacerations of the cortex are noted, and any ischaemic area of the kidney is inspected. The pelvis and major calyces, as well as the upper ureter, are examined for any possible urinary leak and of course the renal vessels are checked for a good strong pulse.

Although a small tear in one of the renal vessels might conceivably be sutured, a major tear, a complete avulsion or a pulseless pedicle due to thrombosis, is a clear indication for nephrectomy, as the warm ischaemic time of the kidney will almost certainly have expired. If the vessels have been completely torn across, the kidney will remain attached only by its ureter, the proximal ends of the vessels may be lost in a mass of bloodstained fat and connective tissue, and these should be found and tied off. If the bleeding has stopped and the vessels are difficult to find after a reasonable search, it is then wiser to pack the wound with a roll of wide gauze.

Provided the surgeon is satisfied by preliminary intravenous pyelography that the contralateral kidney is healthy, then a severely lacerated kidney is probably better removed. When the contralateral kidney is small, diseased, poorly functioning or absent, then every effort at conservative surgery of the damaged kidney must be made.

Smaller lacerations of the cortex of the kidney can be sutured. An ischaemic lower pole of the kidney can be removed by a partial nephrectomy, and a leak in the renal pelvis or major calyces can be closed.

THE OPERATIONS

Nephrectomy

2

When the decision has been made to remove the kidney, the ureter is first divided between clamps, and the distal end ligated. The kidney and ureter are then gently raised to expose the renal pedicle. This area will be heavily infiltrated with blood, rendering identification of the individual vessels difficult. It is advisable to perform the minimum of manipulation and dissection, lest in so doing a damaged vessel is inadvertently torn, it may then retract and be difficult to retrieve amongst the bloodstained fat and connective tissue. It is preferable to ligate the artery and vein individually, but division of the pedicle as a whole may be the most expedient in circumstances of urgency, when the patient's general condition is giving rise to anxiety.

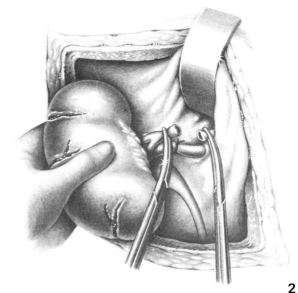

2

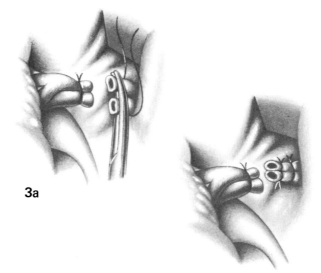

3a

3b

3a&b

Under no circumstances should a transfixion suture be used to tie off the pedicle, because of the risk of a traumatic aneurysm later. Even after placing a single ligature of 1/0 chromic catgut below a clamp on the whole pedicle, there may be sufficient renal artery and vein to put a more distal tie on each vessel independently. Any remaining bleeding points are ligated. When the control of bleeding is complete the wound can be closed without drainage. If there is slight venous oozing, or if the injury was due to a penetrating wound, or if there has been gross haematoma formation, the renal bed should be drained for 24 hr. A Redivac, a soft Penrose tube drain, or even a corrugated rubber drain may be used.

4

*Suture of lacerations of the renal parenchyma
or pelvicalyceal system*

To repair a ruptured kidney, it is essential to control
the bleeding and suture the lacerations. An attempt is
made to pick up bleeding vessels in the parenchyma
and ligate them with 4/0 plain catgut. If a simple
ligature fails to control the bleeding, it may be
necessary to under-run the vessel. Any pelvic or
calyceal tear seen, either in the hilum of the kidney
or in the depths of a tear, should be closed if possible
by suturing with 4/0 plain catgut. To help control the
bleeding and also to reduce the risk of the suture
cutting through the tissues, it may be advisable to
place a piece of crushed muscle or a strip of gelatin
foam in the wound and beneath the suture before
tying. The suture should be of 2/0 plain catgut and
must include the renal capsule. These sutures should
not be tied so tightly that the renal tissue enclosed is
ischaemic. As the renal pelvis or calcyes may have
been perforated, it is essential to drain the renal bed
for a few days.

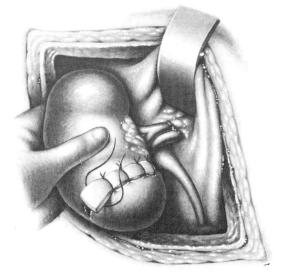

4

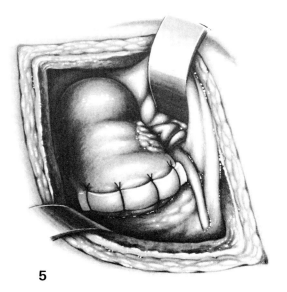

5

5

Partial nephrectomy

If the trauma is confined to one pole of a kidney
(usually the lower pole), partial nephrectomy may
be performed. The vessels running to the injured area
are picked up and divided at the hilum. The damaged
area will be clearly demarcated either by the laceration or the ischaemia; the edges of the laceration
should be trimmed and, if possible, converted into a
wedge excision. All ischaemic tissue should also be
removed. Bleeding points on the cut surface are then
ligated or under-run and any openings into calyces or
into the pelvis itself should be closed with 4/0 plain
catgut. Crushed muscle or gelatin foam can be
applied to the cut surface of the kidney and held in
place with 2/0 plain catgut sutures.

SPECIAL POSTOPERATIVE CARE AND COMPLICATIONS

Following operation, any blood lost should be restored by transfusion. To control infection a broad-spectrum antibiotic should be administered for at least 10 days. If a drain has been placed in the wound, it should not be removed until all urinary or sanguinous discharge has ceased—usually about the third or fourth day.

When the antibiotics are discontinued, a weekly culture of the urine should be carried out and, if positive, further appropriate antibiotics or chemotherapeutic agents are given. It is advisable to repeat these cultures up to 6 weeks after the injury. At the end of 3–4 months, the function of the injured kidney is assessed by another intravenous pyelogram. If the kidney has not returned to normal anatomy then a third intravenous pyelogram is advisable at the end of 12 months. Otherwise a straight x-ray film of the abdomen is sufficient to show whether any calcification is occurring. A final record of the blood pressure will exclude hypertension following the injury.

Paralytic ileus

Retroperitoneal haematomas are frequently accompanied by some degree of paralytic ileus, which may demand gastric suction, nothing to drink, and administration of intravenous liquids and electrolytes.

Secondary haemorrhage and sepsis

Following the repair of an injured kidney some haematuria may persist for a few days and slight perinephric bleeding may occur. If the bleeding increases or suddenly recurs 7–14 days after the operation, sepsis in the wound must be suspected. With correct antibiotic cover this should be rare, but occasionally recurrent haematuria may demand a later nephrectomy as a life-saving procedure. Similarly, infection of a perinephric haematoma following trauma is likely to end in nephrectomy for secondary haemorrhage, and simple drainage of the perinephric abscess is unlikely to be sufficient, unless it already has been sterilized by antibiotics.

Urinary fistula

When a wound involving the pelvis or calyces has continued to leak, drainage may be necessary. Unless there has been complete transection of the renal pelvis or ureter the leak rarely continues for more than 3 weeks. If the peritoneum has been torn, or deliberately opened for exploration at the time of operation on the kidney, urine may leak into the peritoneal cavity and a mild peritoneal irritation will develop. Provided that the tear in the renal pelvis is small, the urine may ultimately be restored to its normal channel spontaneously and with complete healing of the pelvic wall.

References

Badenoch, A. W. (1950). 'Injuries of the kidney.' *Med. Ill.* **4**, 53
Cheetham, J. G. (1941). 'The clinical management of renal trauma.' *Int. Abstr. Surg.* **72**, 573
Ferrier, P. A. and Knigge, W. (1943). 'Ruptured kidney.' *J. Urol.* **49**, 457
Lowsley, O. S. and Menning, J. H. (1941). 'Treatment of rupture of the kidney.' *J. Urol.* **45**, 253
Mitchell, J. P. (1973). 'Current concepts, trauma to the urinary tract.' *New Eng. J. Med.* **288**, 90
Poole-Wilson, D. S. (1950). *Br. J. Surg.,* war Supplement No. 3, p. 472
Slade, N. (1971). 'Management of closed renal injuries.' *Br. J. Urol.* **43**, 639
Swan, R. H. (1940). 'Injuries of the kidney.' *Br. J. Urol.* **12**, 161

[*The illustrations for this Chapter on Injuries to the Kidney were drawn by Mr. M. J. Courtney.*]

Partial Nephrectomy and Heminephrectomy

J. C. Christoffersen, M.D., M.A.
Professor of Surgery and Director of Urology, Bispebjerg Hospital, Copenhagen

PRE-OPERATIVE

In the present context partial nephrectomy is the operation by which a segment is excised from an anatomically normal kidney while heminephrectomy is the method by which one half of a double kidney is removed or more rarely, one half of a horseshoe kidney. The two types of surgery differ in that the vascular supply must be more carefully assessed prior to partial nephrectomy in order to preserve the supply to the remaining part of the kidney, whereas such assessment is less important in the case of heminephrectomy since the two renal elements are in the main individually supplied and are in addition provided with two renal pelves which never communicate.

Indications

The main indication for partial nephrectomy is the presence of calculi in the lower pole of the kidney especially if the lower calyces are dilated; the operation may also be of benefit in other cases of nephrolithiasis for instance in the presence of multiple stone or minor coralliform calculi. A localized, infective focus whether specific (tuberculous) or unspecific (carbuncle) may be an indication, though not as often since antibiotic control has become more efficient. Tumour formation in a solitary kidney is a rare but definite indication. Cysts may be managed by partial nephrectomy, but excision of the cyst will usually be sufficient.

Partial nephrectomy may be indicated in cases of renal rupture and it should be noted that in conservative treatment of large hydronephroses it is often useful to remove a dilated, poorly functioning lower pole of the kidney.

Heminephrectomy is indicated in the presence of tumour formation, hydronephrosis, infection, or stone in one part of the double kidney; furthermore, it is indicated in the presence of an ectopically ending ureter from a double kidney manifesting itself as incontinence.

Diffuse pyelonephritic change affecting the entire kidney is a specific contra-indication.

Special investigations and equipment

Renal angiography may occasionally be of value though it is rarely essential except in the case of a tumour in a solitary kidney.

If the intrarenal intervention is expected to be of long duration it may be of value to have equipment by which the kidney can be cooled while a clamp is employed for compression of the renal pedicle.

THE OPERATION

1

Exposure

The approach is from the loin as for nephrectomy (page 307). Through a wide incision the kidney is mobilized and the pedicle dissected free. The ureter is disengaged and marked. The hilar vessels, and also the vessels to the segment to be excised, are dissected free. By compression of these vessels and on the basis of the line of demarcation which appears it will be possible to determine the scope of the resection to be done. The vessels are then ligated. A soft clamp is applied to the remaining part of the pedicle so that it will be possible to accomplish the resection without bleeding. Manual compression of the parenchyma at a site above the line of resection will occasionally be sufficient. If the intrarenal procedure is expected to last more than 10—12 min, the clamp may be slackened or the compression discontinued for a short time while the kidney is perfused with blood.

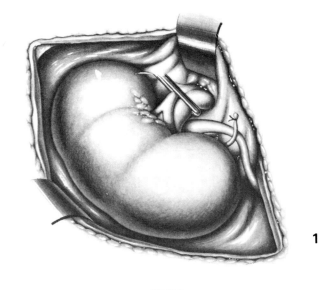

1

2

Incision

Partial nephrectomy can be performed with either a wedge-shaped or a transverse excision. The former method is preferred since it facilitates haemostasis and the closure of the cut surfaces. In this way the fibrous capsule need not be disengaged. A sharp incision into the parenchyma is made immediately above the line of demarcation or occasionally at a site indicated by the pathological process or by the findings obtained by pre-operative investigation. If a transverse incision is to be used, the renal capsule should first be opened over the pole and reflected from the segment to be excised.

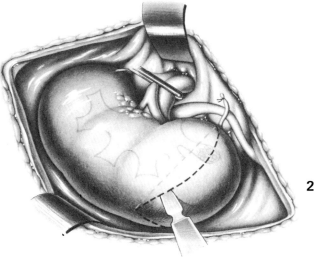

2

3

Excision

When the incision measures a few millimetres, traction is exerted on the circumcised renal segment and blunt or sharp dissection is then continued obliquely towards the neck of the calyx, which should be the last structure to be cut. Then the renal pelvis should be opened to the extent required.

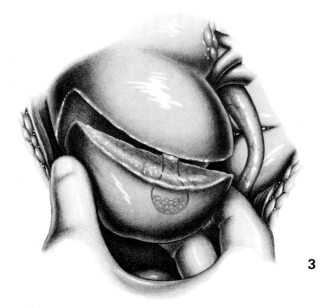

3

4

Haemostasis

After completion of the intrarenal intervention, compression of the pedicle or parenchyma is discontinued and definitive haemostasis established by ligation or stitching of the arteries and veins using 3/0 catgut. If major branches of the artery or vein have been accidentally cut tangentially during the procedure they must be sutured while compression is re-established for a short time. Oozing is of minor importance since it stops as soon as the cut surfaces are closed.

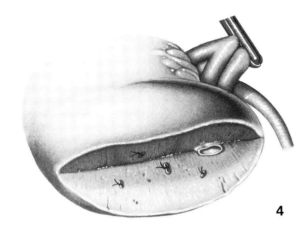

4

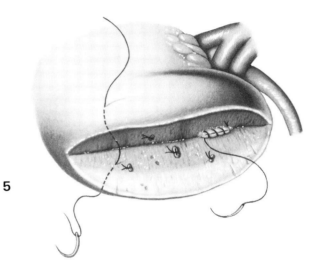

5

5

Closure of the pelvis

The neck of the calyx, and incisions, if any, extending into the pelvis are closed by continuous catgut 3/0 suture on an atraumatic needle.

6

Closure of the parenchyma

The cut surfaces are closed by deep sutures, using 2/0 catgut. Co-aption of the surfaces is usually easy and mattress sutures should be avoided as they give rise to marginal necrosis. If a transverse guillotine cut has been used for the incision, fat or muscle tissue may be sutured to the surfaces of the resection before the latter is covered by the fibrous capsule which was previously everted from the pole of the kidney.

The kidney is then replaced in the fossa. If it is very mobile it may be stabilized by tightening the fatty capsule into the form of a cushion below the resected pole and if necessary by attaching it to the fascia of the psoas muscle. Drainage is accomplished by means of a corrugated rubber drain.

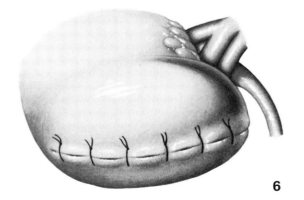

6

OTHER TYPES OF PARTIAL NEPHRECTOMY

7

Resection of the upper pole

This requires that the vessels are dissected free more carefully than otherwise necessary in the case of the lower pole. A blind cut may involve an injury to the descending branch of the posterior segmental artery which may thus compromise the vascular supply of large parts of the kidney to be preserved.

Resection of the middle part of the kidney is rarely indicated and most authors advise against it. Preliminary ligature of the segmental arterial branches is hardly ever possible and there is a large venous plexus in the hilum. Both these factors complicate the establishment of haemostasis and deep controlling sutures may compromise the vascular supply to the adjacent segment.

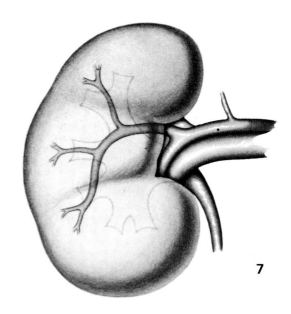

7

8

Heminephrectomy

This operation is generally easier to perform than partial nephrectomy as the pelves of the two renal segments are always separated and they usually have separate vascular supplies. Furthermore, the transition between the two segments is often evident from the pathological process affecting one of them. If not, the line of demarcation will at least become more distinct as soon as the vessels have been ligated. The connecting bridge of tissue where the incision is made should not contain the calyx from either pelvis.

During isolation and cutting the ureter from the affected segment, care must be taken that the vessels to the unaffected segment are not injured. Delicate dissection may be necessary at this point.

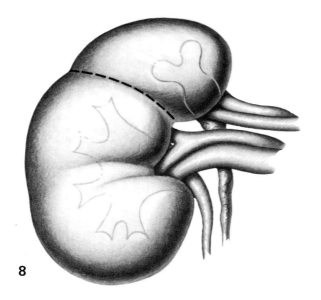

8

POSTOPERATIVE CARE AND COMPLICATIONS

The drain can be removed on the third day if there is no urinary leakage or bleeding. Leakage practically always stops after a few days. Secondary haemorrhage may be serious enough to demand intervention, and if it is necessary, a re-resection at a higher level will be the operation of choice. If this is not possible, nephrectomy may be inevitable.

[The illustrations for this Chapter on Partial Nephrectomy and Heminephrectomy were drawn by Mr. M. J. Courtney.]

Injuries to the Ureter

J. P. Mitchell, *T.D.,* M.S., F.R.C.S., F.R.C.S.(Ed.)
Professor of Surgery (Urology), University of Bristol;
Consultant Urologist, United Bristol Hospitals and Southmead General Hospital

CLOSED INJURIES

Non-penetrating injuries of the ureter are extremely rare owing to the small size, mobility and deep position of the ureter on the posterior abdominal wall.

PENETRATING WOUNDS

Gunshot and stab wounds of the ureter will almost certainly involve other organs, which are much more likely to provide the symptoms and signs indicating the need for surgical exploration. Injury of the ureter will only be suspected from (*1*) evidence of leak of urine and (*2*) the direction of entry of the missile, and the depth of penetration as assessed on x-ray.

SURGICAL INJURIES OF THE URETER

The ureter may be tied, divided, burnt with diathermy, or its blood supply severely damaged by extensive mobilization or it can be compressed by a postoperative haematoma sufficient to occlude its lumen.

Recognition of the injury

A surgical injury may be noticed at the time of operation, or may reveal itself at a later date by the onset of one or more of the following conditions: (*1*) anuria; (*2*) peritonitis or pelvic cellulitis; (*3*) renal pain; (*4*) leakage of urine from an abdominal or vaginal wound; or (*5*) an intra-abdominal (extraperitoneal) swelling due to extravasation of urine.

Exposure of the ureter

When the ureteric injury is recognized during the course of a pelvic operation, reparative procedures may be carried out through the peritoneal opening in the floor of the pelvis. At the close of the operation a drain is placed in the extraperitoneal tissues down to the ureteric anastomosis. Every effort should be made to close the peritoneum in the base of the pelvis.

Treatment

The aim of treatment must be, first, to identify the exact site of obstruction or leakage and, secondly, to conserve the function of the kidney corresponding to the damaged ureter, by restoration of its continuity with the bladder.

TREATMENT OF INJURIES RECOGNIZED AT OPERATION

The ureter may be damaged by being caught in a ligature or haemostatic forceps, or it may be partially or totally divided.

Ligation of the ureter

If the ligature has been loosely tied, there may be little or no visible damage to the wall of the ureter, and uneventful recovery may occur. However, the degree of damage may be extremely difficult to assess and, if in doubt, it is probably advisable to re-implant the ureter into the bladder. To assess the degree of damage, a small linear incision may be made into the ureter a short distance above the damaged area, and a bougie passed down. This will demonstrate patency of the ureter and, provided that the mucosa has not been torn or devitalized, there is a reasonable chance that it will heal without stricture. If the ligature has been drawn tightly around the ureter, late stricture is almost inevitable and the damaged area should be excised.

Ureter crushed by haemostatic clamp

A closed haemostatic clamp causes gross damage to the wall of the ureter and a fistula or late stricture will probably occur. The damaged area should therefore be excised.

Partial section of ureter

Only a simple longitudinal tear can be closed with confidence that it will not stricture in the future. 4/0 Plain catgut sutures should be passed through the wall of the ureter and just the edge of the mucosal lining.

Any tear in the ureter which is partially circumferential should be extended both upwards and downwards so that, when this is sutured transversely, the lumen at the site of the suture line is considerably wider than the lumen of the rest of the ureter. The area of the injury is drained by a Redivac or corrugated drain placed extraperitoneally. A T-tube (size 8 Ch) can be used to splint the ureter, with the lower limb of the T passing across the site of injury.

Complete division of the ureter

When the ureter is completely divided, the function of the corresponding kidney may be preserved by: (1) re-anastomosis of the divided ends of the ureter; (2) re-implantation of the proximal end of the ureter into the bladder (ureterocystostomy); (3) re-implantation of the ureter into a tube flap from the bladder; (4) substitution of a segment of ileum for the lower end of the ureter; or (5) the ureter may be brought across to the other side of the abdomen and anastomosed end to side to the healthy ureter of the opposite side; (6) as a temporary measure, some form of cutaneous ureterostomy may be considered.

The choice of time and indication for temporary drainage

It is preferable to repair the ureter immediately, if the injury is recognized at the time of operation. For the repair to be watertight in the immediate post-operative stage and also to reduce the risk of subsequent stricture it must be performed with care and in a clean field with no risk of spilling infective material. Immediate repair can add many minutes to an operation which, in itself, is probably of major severity, and extending the time of operation may actually endanger the patient's life. In no circumstance should the patient's life. Under no circumstances should the ureter be tied off. It is a relatively simple procedure to drain the upper end of the ureter by means of a fine tube of about 8 Ch size passed up to the pelvis. The most suitable drain is a plastic oesophageal catheter, which is soft and pliable and has a convenient nozzle at the distal end for connecting to drainage tube or drainage bag.

THE OPERATIONS

1

Alternatively, a T-tube can be used, one limb being passed upwards towards the kidney, the other limb being passed down the distal cut end of the ureter towards the bladder.

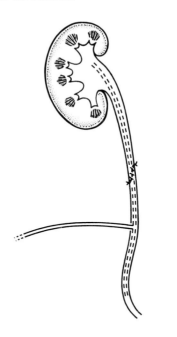

1

The oesophageal tubes are made of plastic and can be left in with safety for 2 or 3 weeks. T-tubes may also be available in plastic, but a latex T-tube should not be used because it will soon be obstructed with phosphatic encrustation. The added advantage of using one of these forms of drainage, is that the two cut ends of the ureter are located more easily at the second stage.

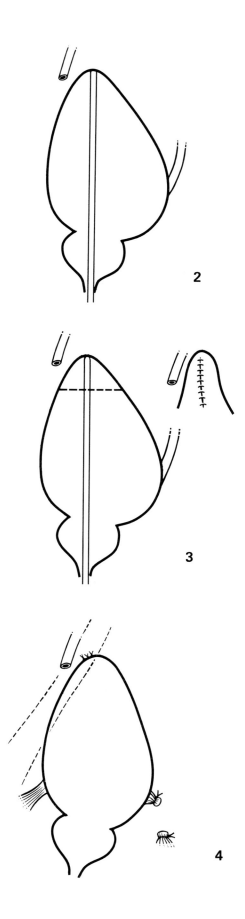

Re-implantation into the bladder

Re-implantation of the proximal end of the ureter into the bladder gives the most certain results, but can only be performed when there is sufficient ureter to reach the bladder without tension. Preferably there should be 2 cm more than the minimum length, so as to have sufficient ureter to create an antireflux implantation.

2,3&4

In order to locate the highest point to which the bladder can be elevated on the side of the cut ureter, a rigid instrument, such as a urethral dilator, or a pair of Nelson Roberts forceps, is passed up *per urethram,* so that the wall of the bladder can be tented up towards the brim of the pelvis.

Additional height may be achieved by making a transverse cut at right angles to the instrument in the bladder. When this cut in the bladder wall is sutured longitudinally it can give as much as an additional 2 cm of bladder wall. Turner-Warwick has suggested cutting the vesical pedicle on the side opposite to the ureteric injury, which he claims gives additional mobility to the bladder. Finally, a flap of bladder wall can be cut to make a tube (Boari procedure). Alternatively, an isolated loop of ileum can be used to re-form the lower end of the ureter, but such a measure is rarely applicable for an emergency repair.

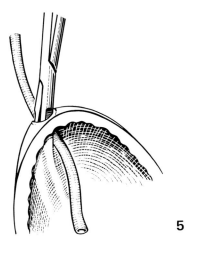

5

5, 6 & 7

The implanted end of the ureter should pass through the muscle wall of the bladder at the highest point to which the bladder can be elevated by the urethral dilator, or Nelson Roberts forceps, which has been passed *per urethram*. A tunnel is then constructed between the mucosa and muscle layer of the bladder wall and the ureter to be implanted is drawn through this tunnel, giving a submucosal length of approximately 2 cm. The end of the ureter is then fishtailed. The bladder mucosa below the end of the tunnel is split to make a bed 1·5 cm long for implanting the end of the ureter, the margin of which is then sutured around this bed, the suture knots being buried.

At the end of the operation the ureter should lie extraperitoneally and the bladder wall should be hitched to the posterior abdominal wall or lateral wall of the pelvis ('the psoas hitch'), so that there is no tension on the ureterovesical anastomosis. The bladder should be drained by an indwelling urethral catheter for a minimum of 5 days. For additional security a fine catheter (size 8 Ch) is left in the ureter. This catheter may be brought out onto the surface, either via the urethra, in which case it can be strapped alongside the urethral catheter, or it can be brought out independently through the anterior wall of the bladder suprapubically.

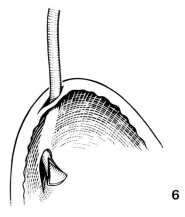

6

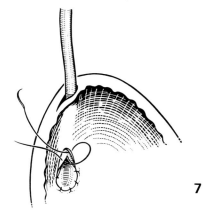

7

End-to-end anastomosis

When the division of ureteric wall is too high to consider re-implantation into the bladder, then re-anastomosis of the cut ends should be considered. This anastomosis should be performed over an indwelling splint catheter of plastic or silicone (8 Ch).

8

In order to increase the length of the suture line, a longitudinal cut is made to enlarge each end of the cut ureter. This operation has earned the reputation for giving rise to stricture. Fibrosis at the line of union inevitably causes some narrowing of a re-anastomosis of ureter but if the anastomosis is constructed obliquely and if fibrosis is reduced to a minimum by careful suturing of the ureteric margins, the resulting stenosis need not diminish the calibre of the original ureter. Suturing the margins in eversion may also lessen the tendency to stenosis.

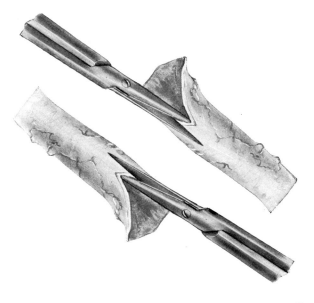

8

9 & 10

The ends of the ureters are then brought together by two 4/0 plain catgut or polyglycolic acid (P.G.A.) stitches, each of which passes through the centre of the broad flap of one ureteric end and through the tissue at the apex of the vertical incision of the other. These two stitches are tied and used as stay sutures. The everted ureteric margins are then carefully united with a series of interrupted 4/0 plain catgut or polyglycolic acid (P.G.A.) stitches, which pass through the full thickness of the ureteric wall. The united ureter should be free from tension and the anastomosis practically watertight.

The site of the anastomosis should be splinted by either a T-tube inserted into the ureteric wall below the site of the anastomosis, so that the upper limb of the T splints the anastomosis (the T-tube being of inert material such as polythene or silicone rubber). Alternatively, a straight tube of silicone rubber is passed up the proximal end of the ureter to the kidney and down the distal end of the ureter to the bladder before finally closing the anastomosis. The lower end of the splinting tube is then passed down the urethra, this manipulation being carried out through a hole made in the anterior wall of the bladder. The tube is then anchored to an indwelling urethral Foley type catheter. Whichever type of splint drain is used, the reason for the drain is to avoid adhesion of the apposing sides of the anastomosis of the ureter, and the splint should be left *in situ* for 10 days.

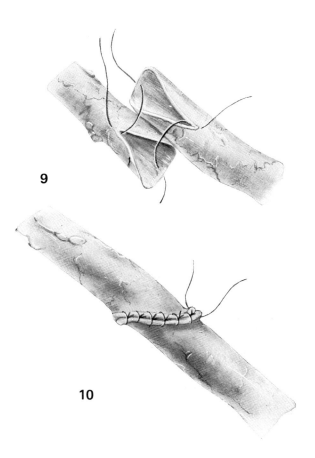

9

10

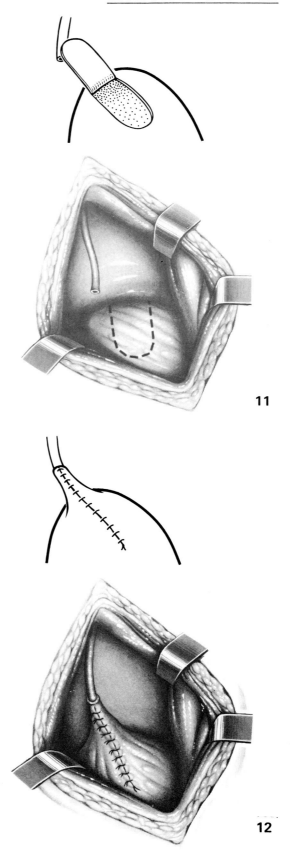

Re-implantation of the ureter into the bladder

Every effort should be made to construct a submucosal tunnel for the ureter so as to reduce the risk of vesico-ureteric reflux. If the damage to the ureter is at its lower end it should be possible to mobilize sufficient ureter to carry out such an anastomosis without mobilizing the bladder.

If the damage to the ureter is high in the pelvis, or at the pelvic brim, then some mobilization of the bladder will be necessary to bring the vault of the bladder high enough to construct the anastomosis.

When preparing the drapes before such an operation, access to the external meatus must be possible, and a screen towel can be placed across the lower part of the operation area to avoid contamination from the perineum. At the beginning of the operation a urethral dilator or long curved instrument, such as a Nelson Roberts forceps, is inserted via the urethra and left in the bladder. The surgeon can then, after handling the perineum, change his gloves.

11 & 12

Another procedure is to construct a Boari flap. This flap is cut diagonally across the anterior surface of the bladder; it should begin on the opposite side of the anterior wall of the bladder near the bladder neck, and can be taken across the whole of the anterior wall to the highest point already determined by the instrument passed *per urethram*. The flap should be approximately 3 cm wide, and is then made into a tube and the anterior wall of the bladder is repaired. Such a flap, using a bladder of normal capacity, can even be made to reach the renal pelvis.

11

12

Anastomosis of the ureter to the bladder should be constructed with a submucosal tunnel (*see* page 331) to avoid reflux. The implant can then be constructed through the cystotomy wound, performed for elevating the highest point of the bladder. A small opening is made in the bladder wall at the highest point and the ureter is drawn through. From this point downwards towards the internal urinary meatus, a tunnel is constructed approximately 2 cm long between the mucosa and the muscle of the bladder. This tunnel separates easily by blunt dissection, using the tips of a pair of McIndoes' scissors. The ureter is then drawn through this tunnel and anchored to the wall of the bladder approximately 1 cm beyond the lower end of the tunnel. The highest point of the bladder, where the ureter passes through, is then hitched to the psoas muscle. The point of anchorage of the cut end of the ureter is then completed by a mucosa-to-mucosa suture inside the bladder, using plain 4/0 catgut or polyglycolic acid. A polythene or silicone rubber splint drain can then be inserted up the ureter to the kidney, the lower end of the tube being brought out either via the urethra or via a suprapubic wound.

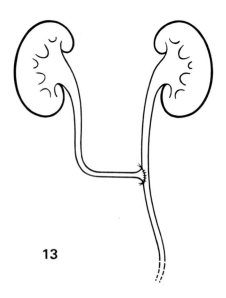

13

13

Transuretero-ureteric anastomosis

When direct anastomosis is impossible and the upper end of the divided ureter and the bladder cannot be mobilized sufficiently to make an adequate ureterovesical anastomosis, and when the bladder wall is too thick to construct a Boari flap, the upper end of the divided ureter can be brought across the abdomen and anastomosed to the opposite side. Such a procedure can be very successful provided that neither upper urinary tract is infected. Theoretically, dilatation of one ureter could cause stasis and a risk of pyelonephritis from uretero-ureteric reflux, but in practice this has not proved so, provided that there is no infection.

References

Badenoch, A. W. (1959). 'Injuries of the ureter.' *Proc. R. Soc. Med.* **52**, 101
Blandy, J. P. (1975). 'Injuries of the ureter in the male.' *Injury* **7**, 77
Davalos, A. (1947). 'Ureteral anastomosis: experimental studies.' *J. Urol.* **58**, 22
Graham, S. W. and Goligher, J. C. (1954). 'The management of accidental injuries and deliberate resections of the ureter during excision of the rectum.' *Br. J. Surg.* **42**, 151
Khashu, B. L., Seery, W. H., Smulewicz, J. J. and Rothfield, S. H. (1975). 'Gunshot injuries to ureter.' *J. Urol.* **114**, 182
Mitchell, J. P. (1971). 'Trauma to the urinary tract.' *Br. med. J.* **2**, 567
Orkin, L. A. (1952). 'Spontaneous or non-traumatic extravasation from the ureter.' *J. Urol.* **67**, 272
Pyrah, L. N. and Raper, F. P. (1955). 'Some uses of an isolated loop of ileum in genito-urinary surgery.' *Br. J. Surg.* **42**, 337
Smith, I. (1969). 'Trans-uretero-ureterostomy.' *Br. J. Urol.* **41**, 14

[The illustrations for this Chapter on Injuries to the Ureter were drawn by Miss J. Perry and Mr. M. J. Courtney.]

Injuries to the Bladder

J. P. Mitchell, *T.D.,* M.S., F.R.C.S., F.R.C.S.(Ed.)
Professor of Surgery (Urology), University of Bristol;
Consultant Urologist, United Bristol Hospitals and Southmead General Hospital

PRINCIPLES OF TREATMENT

Treatment of a ruptured bladder is not a matter of extreme urgency for the first 12—24 hr after injury. Urine is normally sterile and, therefore, is unlikely to cause any serious complications from extravasation provided that this is recognized, drained and evacuated within 36 hr. Even when urine escapes into the peritoneal cavity, the irritation produced is only moderate in the early stages. Neither leakage of urine from the bladder, nor stagnation of urine in the tissues should be allowed to continue after 36 hr. Finally, and most important of all, every precaution should be taken to avoid the introduction of infection into the traumatized area where haematoma, damage to tissues, extravasated urine and also, probably, broken bone ends, will form a perfect nidus for the culture of any organisms.

MODE OF PRESENTATION OF RUPTURE OF BLADDER

Injuries of the bladder may be closed or open injuries. Closed injuries usually occur following a heavy blow in the lower abdomen, or in association with a fracture of the pelvis. Open wounds result from penetration of the lower abdomen by stabbing or gunshot wounds. The penetration by the missile may be suprapubically or via the perineum. Injuries occurring from falling astride a spike or stake which can pass up through the perineum or even via the anus and rectum to enter the bladder.

For the bladder to rupture it must, of necessity, have been full at the time of the accident. A blow in the lower abdomen can then cause disruption of the wall of the bladder from sudden increase in intravesical pressure, giving rise to an explosive disruption of the viscus. The unsupported part of the bladder wall, namely the vault, gives way and results in an intraperitoneal rupture. The tear in the bladder wall is then usually a large hole, even perhaps complete bivalving of the bladder.

When associated with a fracture of the pelvis, the rupture may be either penetration of the anterior wall by a spicule of bone from the pubic ramus, or the bladder rupture may be caused by the same blow in the lower abdomen which fractured the pelvis. In other words, an extraperitoneal rupture of the anterior bladder wall is the commonest lesion associated with a fractured pelvis, but intraperitoneal disruption of the bladder may occasionally be seen.

335

Associated injuries

Rupture of the bladder may be associated with a rupture of the posterior urethra in cases of fractured pelvis.

Many bladder injuries may be due to road traffic accidents, where other multiple injuries are sustained and some of these, if severe, may take priority over the bladder injury in their urgency for treatment.

Following any severe blow in the abdomen or a serious multiple injury, the possibility of other intraperitoneal lesions must be considered. Even damage to the upper (kidney) as well as the lower urinary tract (bladder) have been known to occur at the same time and in the same patient.

Pre-operative investigations

The diagnosis of an extraperitoneal rupture of the bladder can be made during the first 24 hr, when the patient will produce no urine, will develop no signs of a distended bladder, and will gradually show some deterioration in his general condition with increasing suprapubic pain. Intraperitoneal rupture of the bladder will present with slowly developing peritoneal irritation, an increasing amount of free fluid in the abdomen, as indicated by steady increase in girth measurement, and also possibly by needle aspiration or peritoneal lavage; the tentative diagnosis will be some intraperitoneal lesion.

The passage of a catheter *per urethram* is unwise, because it may introduce infection and may be misleading in the diagnosis. Furthermore, there is a 10—15 per cent risk of a double injury of bladder and urethra when, again, the diagnostic catheter would be unwise and even dangerous (*see* Chapter on 'Injuries to the Urethra', pages 341—347). In an extraperitoneal rupture due to a spicule of bone from one pubic ramus, the hole in the bladder wall may be very small and the bladder could still hold as much as 200 ml of urine. The patient with a small puncture wound of the bladder wall has even been known to pass urine spontaneously, usually with at least a trace of blood.

A penetrating wound or gunshot wound which could involve the bladder, or a perineal injury from falling onto a spike, where penetration of the bladder base is possible, must all be explored without delay. The track of the missile must be identified and injury to the bladder excluded.

If there is no blood at the external meatus, rupture of the urethra is unlikely. A urethrogram and a cystogram may be helpful in confirming the diagnosis, but the more valuable procedure is to carry out an intravenous pyelogram to ensure the integrity of the upper urinary tract. With good concentration of contrast medium, extravasation may be seen even from the bladder. The bladder base may also be seen to be elevated and compressed laterally by a haematoma and extravasated urine (the 'pear drop' bladder).

Endoscopy should be carried out only just prior to operation; first to ensure that the urethra is intact, and, secondly, to observe the bladder wall. A tear in the bladder wall may be difficult to identify if there is any bleeding. Furthermore, having seen the tear in the mucosa, this does not necessarily indicate that the rupture is through the entire wall of the bladder. Finally, if there is a hole of any size, the bladder cannot be distended and no view will be obtained by cystoscopy.

EXPLORATORY OPERATION

Indications

With a closed injury of the bladder, exploration may be indicated by a failure to pass urine without the development of a distended bladder within 24 hr of injury, by which time there will be some evidence of deterioration of the patient's condition and increased suprapubic tenderness. There may be a fracture of the pelvis, with a spicule of bone seen on x-ray, which, by virtue of its position and direction, could have penetrated the anterior wall of the bladder.

Alternatively, the patient's condition may suggest an intraperitoneal lesion, and the only indication that this might be due to a ruptured bladder is the failure to produce any urine. On the other hand, the patient may be going to the theatre for another important operation, and the bladder injury is merely suspected at that stage.

All penetrating wounds that may have damaged the bladder must be explored without delay in order to identify the track of the missile, to carry out a urinary or bowel diversion as necessary, to remove any foreign body, such as clothing carried into the wound, and to drain the wound freely.

Preparation and anaesthesia

No particular preparation is required other than cleansing the skin of the lower abdomen and perineum. The patient should be invited to try to pass water just before going to the theatre. General anaesthesia is indicated.

The incision

The peritoneum and prevesical area are explored by a mid-line suprapubic incision. This can then be extended upwards if any intraperitoneal lesion is suspected.

INTRAPERITONEAL RUPTURE

The peritoneal cavity is opened and free urine and blood is removed by suction and mopping. Full examination of the abdominal viscera should be made, including the liver and spleen. Following a blow in the abdomen, the stomach and full length of the intestine should be examined, as well as the mesenteries. The retroperitoneal area should be inspected for haematoma. An intraperitoneal tear following a blow in the abdomen is usually at least 4 or 5 cm long and will allow inspection of the interior of the bladder, both with a finger and subsequently by visual inspection. The rupture is closed with a continuous layer of 0/0 gauge plain catgut, or polyglycolic acid (P.G.A.). The outer layer of muscle and serosa are then closed with continuous 0/0 gauge chromic catgut. The peritoneal cavity is closed without drainage, but a small drain should be placed in the prevesical (retropubic) space. Provided there has been no blood at the external meatus, which is unlikely if the intraperitoneal rupture has been due to a blow on the abdominal wall, then the bladder can be drained by an indwelling urethral catheter. If there is any suspicion of damage to the urethra at the time of injury, as may be indicated by blood at the external meatus on the patient's admission to hospital, then a urethral catheter is best avoided, and the bladder should be drained by a suprapubic catheter (26 Ch Foley type).

EXTRAPERITONEAL RUPTURE

Extraperitoneal rupture is usually associated with a fracture of the pelvis, the anterior wall of the bladder being penetrated by a spicule of bone. The hole in the bladder wall is likely to be much smaller than in the case of intraperitoneal rupture and it may even be difficult to find. Urine and blood will well up from behind the symphysis pubis and the anterior wall of the bladder may be suffused with blood and difficult to identify. Under no circumstances should an instrument be passed *per urethram*, because there may be an associated lesion of the posterior urethra. In view of the difficulty in locating the tear in the bladder wall, it is advisable to make a formal cystotomy in order to identify the site of the rupture from inside the bladder. At the same time the bladder neck, anterior surface of the prostate, and position of the fractured pubic ramus in relation to the prostate and bladder can be decided. Usually, there is no need to trim the rupture of the bladder wall, because it is relatively small.

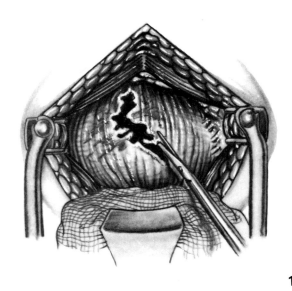

1

1&2

Repair of the rupture

The rent in the bladder wall is then sutured in two layers, 0/0 gauge plain catgut is used to suture the mucosa and adjacent muscle layer, 0/0 gauge chromic catgut is used for the outer muscle layer. If there was blood at the external meatus at the time of admission, indicating probable rupture of the urethra, then the bladder should be drained by a suprapubic cystostomy for about 2 weeks until the urethra can be inspected by means of a panendoscope. If there was no blood at the external meatus at the time of admission, then rupture of the urethra is unlikely and a catheter can be passed with reasonable safety *per urethram* and left indwelling for 4—5 days until the bladder wall has united adequately. The retropubic space is drained with a corrugated rubber drain, or a Redivac, or a Penrose tube drain.

2

POSTOPERATIVE CARE

Bladder lavage

At the close of the operation, the bladder is washed out thoroughly via the indwelling urethral or suprapubic catheter, so as to ensure that all blood clot has been removed. The catheter is connected to a closed drainage system, which need not have irrigation incorporated.

In view of the extent of soft tissue damage, the haematoma, and the extravasated urine, it is advisable to put the patient on to a broad-spectrum antibiotic for the next 10 days.

Removal of drains

The prevesical (retropubic) drain can usually be removed at 2—3 days, unless oozing of serum persists. The indwelling urethral catheter can be removed at 5 days, after which the patient should be able to pass urine normally. If a suprapubic drain has been left in, this should be retained until the urethra can be inspected by panendocystoscopy, which is usually between 10 and 21 days after the injury.

PENETRATING INJURIES

The bladder may be damaged by a gunshot wound or a stabbing injury. The perforation of the bladder may be only one of many severe lesions, depending on the direction of the missile, which may also have penetrated the peritoneal cavity, or perforated the rectum, or shattered portions of the pelvic girdle. The amount of damage to the bladder is very variable. A bullet may traverse the bladder leaving only a minute entry and exit wound, whilst a fragment of shell or bomb may tear a large opening and destroy much of the bladder muscle.

Examination of superficial wounds

Examination and toilet of the superficial wounds are undertaken. When entrance and exit wounds are present, they provide a valuable guide to the course of the missile and to the possible structures damaged. A urethrogram can be carried out under strictly sterile precautions and will help to show whether the urethra is damaged as well as the bladder. The wound is already potentially infected and, therefore, the passage of a urethral catheter is not contra-indicated on grounds of risk of introducing infection. Nevertheless, the diagnostic value of the urethral catheter is still very questionable, because a ruptured bladder may have only two small perforations from a high velocity missile, and can still retain some urine; hence withdrawing urine from the bladder does not exclude injury to the bladder wall. On the other hand, a dry tap with the catheter could mean: (*1*) a damaged urethra, (*2*) anuria, or (*3*) a ruptured bladder. The passage of a urethral catheter may, therefore, not be a helpful diagnostic procedure.

After starting treatment for shock, the abdomen is explored through a mid-line suprapubic incision, the peritoneal cavity is opened and any free blood and urine are removed. All intra-abdominal viscera are searched for injury, with particular reference to the small and large intestine and their mesenteries. If an intraperitoneal perforation of the bladder is present, the margins are excised and the wound closed in two layers. When there is evidence of either intraperitoneal or extraperitoneal injury to the rectum, a left iliac colostomy is established at this stage. The peritoneum is then closed without drainage. The bladder is next exposed in the suprapubic region and, if there is no evidence of an extraperitoneal wound, it is opened anteriorly

between stay sutures. A careful search is made for injuries, and any foreign bodies or loose fragments of bone are removed.

The subsequent course depends on the degree of vesical damage. Whenever possible the vesical wounds are excised and sutured. In civilian life, many missile perforations of the bladder may be treated by complete closure of the bladder wall, drainage of the retropubic space and an indwelling urethral catheter to drain the bladder itself. In war, meticulous after-care may be lacking and long-distance evacuation necessary so that, in such circumstances, an indwelling urethral catheter is better replaced by suprapubic drainage of the bladder, using a Foley balloon catheter (26 Ch) which is brought out at the top of the bladder incision and as high in the suprapubic wound as possible. The retropubic drain may be a Redivac, a Penrose tube drain, or simply a strip of corrugated rubber drain.

Wounds of the vault

Wounds of the vault of the bladder usually present no difficulty to close. The bladder wall is freely mobile and the margins may be easily approximated even after wide excision.

Wounds of the anterior and lateral walls

Injuries to the upper portions of the anterior and lateral walls may be easily closed. Difficulties may arise when the bladder wound is low down and is accompanied by shattering of the pelvis and an open wound in the pubic or groin regions. A considerable area of bladder wall may be destroyed and contusion of the tissues may make identification of the limits of the vesical wound difficult. The base of the bladder is also relatively fixed and difficulty may be experienced in bringing the wound margins together. In such circumstances, a tense suture line may break down and allow urine, probably infected, to drain into the perivesical tissues and into the pubic fractures, causing chronic osteomyelitis. The margins of the vesical wall become adherent to the pelvic wall and if the superficial wound has given way, a permanent urinary fistula is established.

To avoid such troubles, every effort must be made to close the bladder as satisfactorily as possible and to drain the urine from the bladder as rapidly as it is secreted.

ARRANGEMENTS FOR DRAINAGE

3

A Foley catheter (20 Ch—5 ml bag) is passed up the urethra to drain the base of the bladder. Suprapubic drainage is also established by passing a Foley catheter (26 or 28 Ch) into the bladder either through the upper portion of the wound when it is large or, more commonly, through the exploratory incision in the anterior wall of the bladder. The bladder wounds are then closed as completely as possible and the pre-vesical tissues drained.

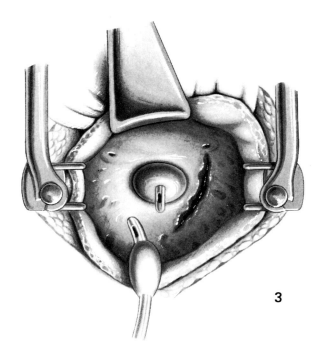

3

Suction drainage

By attaching a low power suction apparatus to the Foley catheter the urine may be continuously removed. The Roberts electric pump is suitable for this purpose. When suction is being employed, it is an advantage to arrange the suprapubic tube so that it may act as an inlet vent for air. The bladder suction is then continuous and the mucosa of the bladder wall is not drawn into the eyes of the catheter by the negative intravesical pressure.

Wounds of the base of the bladder

Owing to the fixity of the tissues it is usually impossible to suture wounds of the base of the bladder satisfactorily and more harm than good may result from attempting to do so. Provided a colostomy has been established a very high proportion of rectovesical fistulae will heal spontaneously. When a ureteric orifice has been damaged it is usually unwise to attempt any wide exposure of the ureter with re-implantation into the bladder. A catheter (polythene oesophageal catheter size 8 or 10 Ch) can be passed from the bladder up the ureter, to act as both drain and splint. This catheter is then brought out, either through the suprapubic wound or via the urethra. If any ureteric obstruction ensues a formal exploration and re-implantation may be performed later.

References

Cass, A. S. and Ireland, G. W. (1973). 'Bladder trauma associated with pelvic fractures in severely injured patients.' *J. Trauma* **13**, 205

Culp, O. S. (1942). 'Treatment of ruptured bladder and urethra.' *J. Urol.* **48**, 266

Gordon-Taylor, G. (1950). *Br. J. Surg.* War Supplement No. 3, p. 468

Macalpine, J. B. (1940). 'Wounds of the bladder.' In *Surgery of Modern Warfare*. Edited by H. Bailey, Vol. 2, p. 247. Edinburgh: Livingstone

Mitchell, J. P. (1973). 'Current concepts: trauma to the urinary tract.' *New Engl. J. Med.* **288**, 90

Poole-Wilson, D. S. (1950). *Br. J. Surg.*, War Supplement No. 3., p. 475

Poole-Wilson, D. S. (1954). 'The treatment of injuries of the urethra and bladder.' In *Surgical Progress*, Edited by Sir Ernest Rock Carling and Sir James Patterson Ross, p. 17. London: Butterworths

Ross, J. C. (1944). 'Injuries of the urinary bladder.' *Br. J. Surg.* **32**, 44

[The illustrations for this Chapter on Injuries to the Bladder were drawn by Mr. M. J. Courtney and Mr. G. Lyth.]

Injuries to the Urethra

J. P. Mitchell, *T.D.,* M.S., F.R.C.S., F.R.C.S.(Ed.)
Professor of Surgery (Urology), University of Bristol;
Consultant Urologist, United Bristol Hospitals and Southmead General Hospital

INTRODUCTION

1

For the purposes of diagnosis and treatment, trauma to the urethra must be divided into open and closed injuries, into those involving males or females and, lastly, into the various sites of injury in the male, for example penile (D), bulbar (C), at the level of the triangular ligament (B), and, finally, ruptures of the posterior urethra (A), which are usually associated with a fracture of the pelvis.

The commonest cause of urethral injuries is road traffic accident, in which many other structures and systems may be involved. Also, it should be remembered that 10–15 per cent of injuries of the posterior urethra may also have a ruptured bladder. Furthermore, double injuries of upper and lower urinary tract have been reported.

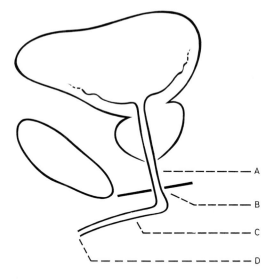

1

2

Injuries of both anterior and posterior urethra are frequently partial ruptures (B), that is to say part of the wall of the urethra is torn, but the whole circumference of the urethra is not transected. Occasionally the damage to the urethral wall is only a contusion (C). Injuries at the level of the triangular ligament, however, are usually complete transections (A). The most important principle in the management of urethral injuries is to ensure that no additional damage is done to the remaining strand or bridge of tissue, which may exist between the two torn ends of urethra. This bridge of tissue should be preserved at all costs, as it can make all the difference between a successful repair and a severe stricture.

Extravasation of urine is, in fact, unlikely to occur as the bladder neck usually goes into spasm and the patient is unable to pass urine, ultimately developing a distended bladder. Even if extravasation does occur, by far the majority of patients will have sterile urine which can cause little harm within the first 24 hr. It is, therefore, safe in closed injuries of the urinary tract to give priority to the treatment of other major injuries.

OPEN INJURIES OF URINARY TRACT

Gunshot wounds, penetration of the perineum by sharp objects, such as falling astride a spike, or broken glass, any trauma to the penile urethra, which may be caught in machinery or involved in some sexual misadventure, must all be treated by exploration without delay. The wound of entry must be explored, if necessary the urethra can be examined by panendoscopy and the damage repaired by immediate suture over an indwelling silicone catheter, 14 or 16 Ch. The patient should be given a broad-spectrum antibiotic, because infection will have been carried into the wound on the penetrating missile, and there is bound to be a fairly extensive haematoma, which forms a perfect nidus for organisms to multiply.

CLOSED INJURIES OF URETHRA

Injuries of the perineal part of the urethra (principally bulbous urethra), transections of the urethra at the urogenital diaphragm, and closed injuries of the posterior urethra associated with a fracture of the

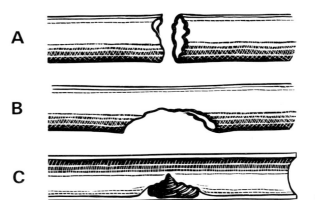

pelvis require careful management to assess the degree of damage and the localization.

Diagnosis depends on the presence of blood at the external meatus, when the patient is first seen in casualty, the inability of the patient to pass any urine and the ultimate development of a distended bladder, easily palpable above the haematoma which rises out of the pelvis. If a distended bladder is not palpable within 24 hr of admission to hospital, the possibility of an associated bladder rupture should be considered.

If an urgent diagnostic answer is required because the patient will be going to the operating theatre for other major trauma, a urethrogram using an aqueous opaque medium will readily demonstrate the site and extent of the urethral rupture. If it is necessary to go to the theatre so urgently that a urethrogram cannot be performed because the patient's condition is too critical, then a suprapubic diversion of the urine is a wise precaution, even if the only physical sign is blood at the external meatus.

Under no circumstances should a diagnostic catheter be passed *per urethram,* as the information obtained can be unreliable; there is a serious risk of contaminating the haematoma at the site of injury by carrying organisms on the catheter from the external meatus, and an appreciable risk of inflicting further damage on the slender bridge of tissue that may constitute only a partial rupture of the urethra. If the diagnostic catheter draws no urine it may mean the catheter has passed out of the urethra through the rupture, it may have passed into an empty bladder, it may have been obstructed at the bladder neck, or the bladder itself may have been ruptured. If, on the other hand, the catheter draws some urine, this does not exclude a partial rupture of the urethra, nor does it exclude a small puncture hole in the anterior wall of the bladder.

OPERATION FOR RUPTURE OF THE BULBOUS AND PERINEAL URETHRA

3&4

With the patient in the lithotomy position, the extensive haematoma in the perineum is opened. Identification of the urethra will be difficult, as the tissues will be so discoloured by blood. The bladder is then opened suprapubically by a vertical mid-line incision and a Harris catheter, 22 Ch in adults (and correspondingly smaller in children) is passed down the posterior urethra from the internal meatus to present in the wound. The tip of this catheter will then identify the proximal end of the ruptured urethra. A smaller sized Foley catheter, preferably silicone (16 Ch) is then passed from the external urinary meatus (after instillation of chlorhexidine in glycerine as lubricant and antiseptic), so that this second catheter also presents in the wound and identifies the distal end of the torn urethra. The dorsal aspect of the two torn ends of urethra can then be approximated by a few sutures of 4/0 plain catgut (or polyglycolic acid). These sutures will also help to control bleeding from the corpus spongiosum. There should be no attempt at mobilizing either end of urethra, which should come together easily.

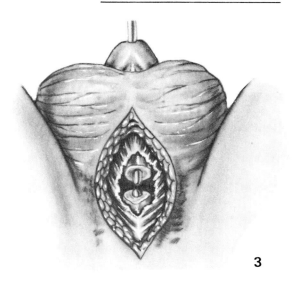

3

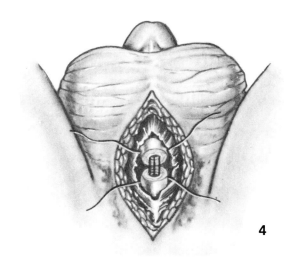

4

5&6

The tip of the larger catheter is then cut off, leaving the catheter still with at least one of its eyes intact, the distal smaller catheter is then passed into the lumen of the larger catheter so that a thread tie can be passed through the eyes of both catheters to secure them together. The larger catheter is then withdrawn into the bladder, bringing the tip of the smaller catheter within it. As the catheters are being withdrawn, the proximal end of the ruptured urethra should be watched to ensure that it is not drawn upwards by the retreating catheter. When the smaller gauge Foley catheter has reached the bladder, the balloon is distended in order to anchor it; the bladder is then closed leaving a suprapubic Foley catheter (22 Ch) draining the bladder by suprapubic cystostomy. The urethra is then closed in layers with a perineal drain.

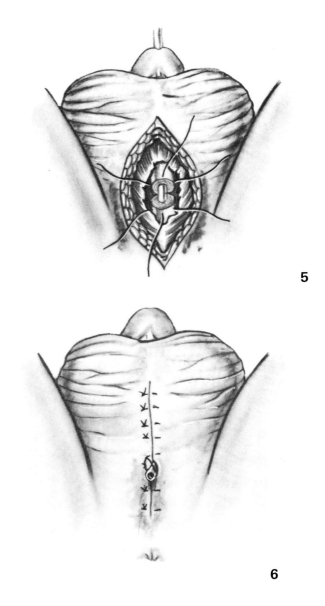

5

6

This patient is almost certain to develop a stricture in due course and should be referred to a department of urology at the earliest possible opportunity. Silicone is a completely inert material and the catheter can, therefore, be left indwelling for 2, 3 or 4 weeks. The patient should be treated with a broad-spectrum antibiotic, and the external urinary meatus should be cleansed by meatal toilet twice a day.

When the patient reaches the urology department, the urethra will be inspected by panendoscopy and urethrography and treated initially by intermittent dilatation of the stricture. Ultimately his stricture will be repaired by some form of urethroplasty (*see* Urology volume of this series).

RUPTURE OF THE URETHRA AT THE UROGENITAL DIAPHRAGM

This type of injury is usually due to a blow in the perineum. There may be associated damage to the anus, with tearing of the perineal skin, converting the injury into an open injury.

Although injury to the urethra at this site is uncommon, it is nearly always a total transection and both torn ends of urethra retract above and below the urogenital diaphragm respectively.

Immediate repair is difficult, the proximal catheter will present in the pelvis and will then have to be threaded through the triangular ligament. If it finds its way through the triangular ligament, it does not readily carry the proximal end of the urethra with it. Stricture is inevitable, and will almost certainly require some form of urethroplasty for repair. In this type of injury definitive posterior urethroplasty should be performed as soon as the local tissue reaction following the trauma has subsided, i.e. 2—3 months.

RUPTURE OF THE POSTERIOR URETHRA

This injury is almost always associated with a fracture of the pelvis and in 10—15 per cent there is, in addition, a rupture of the bladder.

The patient is placed on the table in the supine position and draped with towels so that there is access to the external meatus, as well as to the lower abdomen. A vertical mid-line suprapubic incision is made and the extravesical space is opened. Blood and urine are aspirated or mopped gently from the prevesical space. It will be difficult to determine the exact site of the lesion because of the blood-stained effusion. If the bladder is distended, the lesion must be situated below the internal vesical sphincter. Often the haemorrhage from the depths of the pelvis can be stopped only with packing. The bladder is then identified by the direction of its muscle fibres, which may be discoloured by suffused blood. With a finger inside the bladder the damage to the bony pelvis can be felt and it may be possible to move a central mobile fragment into position. The finger in the bladder then feels for the internal urinary meatus and the prostate gland to assess whether this has been grossly displaced. If the prostate gland is lying high in the pelvis, then there is almost certainly a total transection of the membranous urethra and immediate repair should be performed. If the prostate does not appear to be grossly displaced, then there is a high chance of a partial rupture of the posterior urethra, in which case it is only necessary to leave a suprapubic drain (Foley catheter 26 Ch).

7,8&9

Immediate repair

If the prostate is lying high in the pelvis and there is no likelihood of any bridge of tissue remaining between the two torn ends of urethra. in other words this must be a total transection of the urethra, then a Harris catheter (22 Ch) is passed from the bladder via the internal urinary meatus to present in the pelvis. This catheter should be of very soft material and should be passed with great gentleness, so as not to damage any other structures. After inserting 5 ml of chlorhexidine in glycerine into the external urinary meatus, a silicone catheter (16 Ch) is passed up the urethra and will also present in the depths of the pelvis. The tip of the Harris catheter is then cut off and the tip of the silicone Foley catheter is inserted into the cut end of the Harris catheter. A stitch through both catheters will ensure that they hold together. The proximal Harris catheter is then withdrawn, watching very carefully to see that the proximal torn end of urethra does not retract as the catheter recedes into the bladder. As the silicone Foley catheter enters the bladder its balloon is inflated.

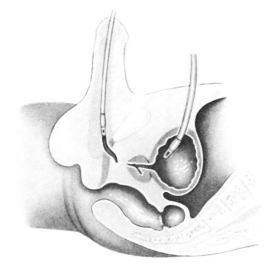

7

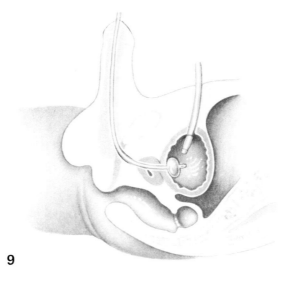

9

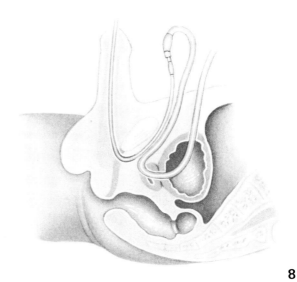

8

Suturing of the urethra is unlikely to be successful as absorbable sutures will disintegrate too soon, and non-absorbable sutures incur the risk of stone formation ultimately. Similarly, traction on the balloon catheter is unlikely to hold the prostate down.

Many of these patients will ultimately develop a stricture of the membranous urethra and will require a posterior urethroplasty, but the inert material of the silicone catheter will probably reduce the severity of the stricture formation. These patients should be referred to a department of urology for assessment by endoscopy and urethrography, with a view to urethroplasty.

Delayed repair

If, at the time of the initial suprapubic cystotomy, the prostate is found to be almost in its normal position, indicating the probability of the rupture being only partial urethral damage, then a suprapubic catheter, size 22 Ch, is left to drain the bladder via the suprapubic wound. A catheter is not passed via the urethra. After 10–20 days, depending on the patient's general condition, he is returned to the operating theatre and the urethra is inspected by panendoscopy. This should be carried out by an experienced endoscopist, who will probably be able to find his way through, past the partial rupture, guided by the intact bridge of mucosa into the bladder. After clearing the blood clot, a soft silicone Foley catheter is then passed via the urethra into the bladder and left indwelling for approximately 7–10 days. During that time the suprapubic catheter can be removed.

If endoscopy fails to find a route through, then the urethra must be explored suprapubically, as for immediate repair.

RUPTURED URETHRA IN THE FEMALE

Damage to the female urethra is much less common than damage to the male posterior urethra. It is usually associated with fracture of the pelvis, but may also be damaged by penetrating wounds in the perineum, or by a blow in the perineum. Injuries of the female urethra usually involve also the anterior wall of the vagina and will ultimately develop a urethrovaginal fistula. Repair of a high urethrovaginal fistula can be very difficult, owing to extensive and firm adhesions to the posterior part of the symphysis pubis. Such cases are best treated by the combined approach of the urologist from the suprapubic area and the gynaecologist from the perineum. Repair of the fistula in layers over a silicone Foley catheter will restore continuity, but still may leave the patient with limited control.

RUPTURED URETHRA IN CHILDREN

Under 10 years of age, rupture of the urethra can be a very severe injury in both the male and female child. In the male child the prostate has not yet developed and rupture is liable to occur just below the neck of the bladder and above the level of the external sphincter. In this event, blood may not be seen at the external urinary meatus, even though the urethra has been torn.

In the female child, rupture of the urethra and anterior wall of the vagina seems to be more common than in adults, when compared with the overall incidence of ruptured urethra. Bleeding from the urethra and vagina can be so severe that the patient may have to be taken to the theatre as an emergency to pack the vagina in order to control the bleeding.

Total transection of the urethra is more common in the child than in the adult, and therefore severe stricturing of the urethra is much more likely to occur in children. Whether the patient is treated by immediate repair or delayed repair does not seem to reduce the incidence of stricture.

References

Blandy, J. P. (1975). 'Injuries of the urethra in the male.' *Injury* 7, 77
Clarke, B. G. and Leadbetter, W. F. (1952). 'Management of wounds and injuries of genito-urinary tract.' *J. Urol.* 67, 719
Hunt, A. H. and Morgan, C. (1942). 'Complete rupture of the membranous urethra.' *Lancet* 2, 330
Hunt, A. H. and Morgan, C. (1949). 'Complete rupture of the membranous urethra.' *Lancet* 1, 601
Kidd, F. (1921). 'The end-results of treatments of injuries of the urethra.' *Rapport de la Societe Internationale d'Urologie*, Paris: Libraire Octave Doin.
Mitchell, J. P. (1968). 'Injuries to the urethra'. *Br. J. Urol.* 40, 649
Morehouse, D. D., Belitsky, P. and MacKinnon, K. (1972). 'Rupture of the posterior urethra.' *J. Urol.* 107, 255
Pasteau, D. and Iselin, A. (1906). *Ann. Mal. Org. gen.-urin.* 24, No. 2, 1601
Poole-Wilson, D. S. (1947). 'Injuries of the urethra.' *Proc. R. Soc. Med.,* 40, 798
Poole-Wilson, D. S. (1949). 'Missile injuries of the urethra.' *Br. J. Surg.* 36, 364
Poole-Wilson, D. S. (1954). 'The treatment of injuries of the urethra and bladder.' In *Surgical Progress*, p. 17. Edited by Sir Ernest Rock-Carling and Sir James Patterson Ross. London: Butterworths
Simpson-Smith, A. (1936). 'Traumatic rupture of the urethra.' *Br. J. Surg.* 24, 309.
Young, H. H. (1929). 'Treatment of complete rupture of the posterior urethra, recent or ancient, by anastomosis.' *J. Urol.* 21, 417

[The illustrations for this Chapter on Injuries to the Urethra were drawn by Mr. M. J. Courtney and Mr. G. Lyth.]

Injuries of the Spine

Terence McSweeney, M.Ch. (N.U.I.), M.Ch.(Orth.), F.R.C.S.(Eng.)
Senior Consultant Orthopaedic Surgeon and Surgeon in Charge, Spinal Injury Unit,
The Robert Jones and Agnes Hunt Orthopaedic Hospital, Oswestry;
Consultant Traumatic and Orthopaedic Surgeon,
Leighton Hospital, Crewe and South Cheshire Hospitals

INTRODUCTION

This chapter is primarily concerned with those injuries to the spine which are complicated by cord or nerve root damage. Similar principles apply to vertebral injuries without neurological involvement.

The philosophy of conservative management and the principles of postural reduction owe much to the pioneer work of Guttmann (1953, 1973) and Munro (1943), and are supported by Bedbrook (1976) and others. Cloward (1961) and Norrell (1971) advocate early surgery for cervical injuries, while Kallio (1963), Flesch et al. (1977) and Riska (1977) favour a more direct surgical approach for dorsolumbar injuries.

Two matters are important when deciding on the need for operative intervention on the injured spine. Firstly, the type of bony or ligamentous injury and its probable outcome should be considered. Secondly, it is generally accepted that most of the neural damage occurs as a result of the injuring forces and is greatest at the time of injury, or within a few hours. An obvious qualification of this statement is that inept handling of the patient may increase the neurological deficit.

Most injuries of the spine can be treated conservatively with a satisfactory outcome, and operative intervention is rarely indicated. Only a small number are associated with damage to the spinal cord or emerging nerve roots, but the potential for neurological deterioration must be the paramount concern of all who handle the patient until the critical period of transportation has been passed and a definite diagnosis has been made.

The distinction between stable and unstable injuries has been emphasized by Holdsworth (1970), Holdsworth and Hardy (1953), Nicoll (1949) and others and is fundamental to an understanding of these injuries. A stable fracture is one without ligamentous disruption and usually follows flexion forces. There is wedge compression of the vertebral body and neural damage is rare. In bursting fractures the mechanism is one of axial loading, and while the ligaments are intact these injuries may be associated with neural damage.

Unstable fractures, fracture-dislocations, dislocations and subluxations usually result from forces of greater magnitude in which torsion predominates. They are associated with a varying amount of damage to the posterior ligamentous complex and with a characteristic x-ray appearance. There is obvious soft tissue swelling and ecchymosis (except in subluxation) and a gap may be felt between the spinous processes when the injury is in the thoracic or the lumbar region. The neural damage may be mild or severe. As a general rule, fractures of the vertebral bodies are stable and most fracture-dislocations when adequately protected tend to stabilize in the fullness of time. Pure dislocations, subluxations and certain fractures (notably the slice fracture) behave in a less certain manner and often fail to achieve stability even after adequate immobilization.

In spinal injury centres most unstable injuries of the thoracic and lumbar spine can be re-aligned by postural methods, and the correction maintained without internal fixation until stability has been restored. Similar remarks apply to the cervical spine, where reduction is achieved by graduated skull traction, or reposition under endotracheal anaesthesia and with muscular relaxation.

The second important consideration is that in lesions with continuity of the spinal cord the essential damage is to the central grey matter.

In the more severe injuries there is a primary disruption of the long tracts by direct bruising, stretching or tearing in addition to the areas of central haemorrhagic necrosis.

There is now sufficient experimental evidence (quite apart from clinical experience) to put so-called decompressive laminectomy in a singularly untenable position. The long-abandoned procedure of mid-line myelotomy may yet have a place in the treatment of certain cord injuries, but pharmacological measures to control the curious histochemical changes will almost certainly prove to be a more fruitful field of research and therapeutic endeavour.

Initial evaluation

The examination should include a careful history of the accident and an assessment of associated injuries (McSweeney, 1968; Meinecke, 1976).

With uncomplicated vertebral injuries, apart from the management of the bony or ligamentous damage, no special problems arise.

Following severe damage to the spinal cord there is the well recognized sensory and motor paralysis and in addition there is an altered general response to injury. This is reflected in abnormal upper respiratory and vasomotor reflexes and in an exaggerated metabolic response (Dolfuss and Frankel, 1965; Cheshire, 1964; Cheshire and Coates, 1966). The physiological alterations are greater in more proximal and complete cord lesions, and have a direct significance in the timing of surgical intervention.

General pre-operative measures

These include respiratory care, gastro-intestinal suction and management of the bladder, with particular emphasis on the paralysed patient. Two hourly turning by a well disciplined team is essential in the prevention of pressure sores, but mechanical turning beds have a useful place in the nursing of these patients.

Tracheostomy is seldom necessary, and respiratory complications are few when continual physiotherapy is available. A nasogastric tube should be passed in anticipation of paralytic ileus.

The introduction of aseptic, 8 hourly, intermittent catheterization has revolutionized the management of the paralysed bladder.

The danger of overloading the circulation in acute tetraplegia cannot be over-emphasized. There is marked retention of sodium and water and a negative potassium balance. These facts, combined with the labile cardiovascular state, quickly lead to pulmonary oedema unless the administration of intravenous fluids is carefully controlled.

CERVICAL INJURIES

Skull traction

It is assumed that halter traction or a sorbo rubber collar will be used during transportation.

Most of the serious injuries of the cervical spine will require the application of skull calipers as an initial measure. The exceptions are hyperextension injuries in the elderly and minor compression fractures of the vertebral bodies.

A careful neurological and radiological examination is carried out before definitive treatment is instituted.

A variety of calipers is available. Crutchfield's are suitable for most cases, but if there are wounds over the top of the head Gardner's or Vinke's calipers are more appropriate.

1

Method

The nature of the procedure is explained to the patient. The head is shaved and a sagittal line is drawn on the scalp with a skin pencil or Bonney's blue. A second line connects the anterior edges of the mastoid processes. Local anaesthesia is used.

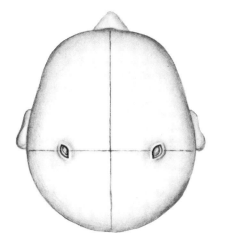

1

2

Crutchfield's calipers

The points are opened almost to the full extent and are used to mark the scalp. The apparatus should be inserted symmetrically. A 1 inch (2·5 cm) incision (centred over each mark) is made in the scalp down to the bone. The outer table of the skull is penetrated using a hand drill (3—4 mm depth, *see* inset). The points of the calipers are inserted and the area sealed with ribbon dressings. The locking nuts are firmly secured. Appropriate weights are attached to a pulley system and the head end of the bed is raised.

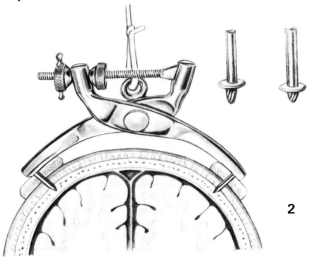

2

3

Blackburn's calipers

Blackburn's calipers are inserted at a lower level, above and behind the ears. They are heavier and less convenient than Cone's calipers and the long transverse bar makes the turning of the patient more difficult.

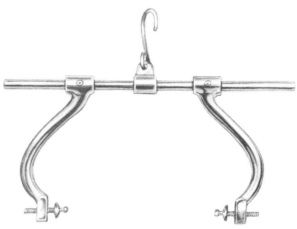

3

4

Cone's calipers

Small drills which have a preset depth are used to penetrate the outer table.

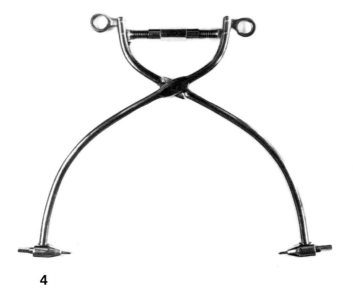

4

5

Vinke's calipers

A special undercutting tool is used to prepare the diploic space.

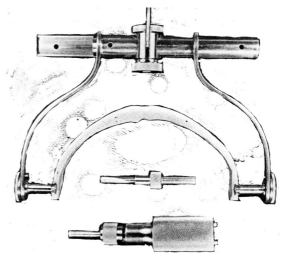

5

6

Gardner-Wells's

One of the points is spring-loaded so that when the device is in position each of the points induces a localized pressure atrophy of the outer table; thus no drilling is required. The traction tong is applied under local anaesthesia. After initial setting each of the points advances slightly and stability is achieved in 24 hr. No incision is necessary and the head need not be shaved. It is well tolerated by children.

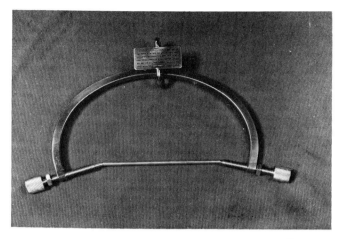

6

7

Sustained traction

Once the calipers are securely in position a small pillow is placed under the patient's neck, and the head end of the bed is raised.

The pulley system is inspected.

Hyperextension injuries in young patients are uncommon. Only gentle traction is required, the neck must not be allowed to extend and the pull is arranged towards flexion.

In treating compression injuries it is usual to start with 2 kg and more than 10 kg is seldom needed. Faulty posturing and distraction are checked with x-rays.

Flexion-rotation injuries usually show unilateral or bilateral locking of facets, often complicated by vertebral fractures. The duration of traction and the amount of sedation are regulated by the age and muscular development of the patient. Dislocations near the cervicothoracic junction are difficult to correct by closed methods. The traction is rapidly increased over 3 − 6 hr up to 12 kg. The pulleys are arranged so that the initial effect is towards flexion of the neck. When radiographs show the facets commencing to unlock, traction is continued in the horizontal plane with a small increase in the traction weight. The neck is allowed to extend when lateral x-ray films show that the facets are clear or have been edge-to-edge for an hour or so. Subject to satisfactory x-ray appearances a soft pillow is placed under the shoulders and the weights are gradually reduced to a maintenance pull of 5 kg or less. This method relies on appropriate sedation and good quality portable x-ray equipment.

If satisfactory correction is not achieved in 12 hr manipulation under general anaesthesia is favoured. Other surgeons are prepared to continue traction for longer periods.

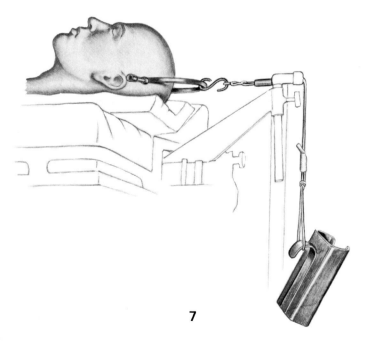

7

Manipulation

Endotracheal anaesthesia augmented by a muscle relaxant is essential for this manoeuvre. Reposition is a more appropriate description than manipulation as great care and gentleness are essential. The procedure is greatly facilitated by the use of an x-ray image intensifier.

Traction on the head is often sufficient to reduce bilateral dislocation of the articular facets.

In case of unilateral locking, slight rotation and lateral flexion away from the side of dislocation effects reduction.

Many experienced surgeons now favour manipulation, rather than sustained traction, as the initial management.

Aftercare

Following successful replacement of the joints the traction is reduced to 4 — 5 kg and the neck is held in the neutral position or in slight extension for 6 weeks. The calipers are then removed and a suitable collar is worn for 6 months.

During this time x-ray films are exposed at 4 weekly intervals. The early appearance of anterior bony bridging is a favourable sign.

Certain injuries are known to be habitually and inherently unstable. These include dislocation and subluxation in the upper part of the cervical spine, certain anterior subluxations in the middle and lower cervical parts of the spine (Cheshire, 1969; Evans, 1976; Webb et al., 1976), and a small number of bilateral dislocations of the facets. In these cases an early decision on the need for operative fusion should be made.

In the more usual case stability is assessed at 3 months. Lateral x-ray films made in flexion and extension may show abnormal mobility and will usually indicate the patients that are most likely to require fusion. For this purpose the image intensifier or video-tape recordings of neck movements are helpful.

OPEN REDUCTION OF DISLOCATIONS AND FRACTURE-DISLOCATION OF CERVICAL SPINE

This may be necessary after failure of closed methods to secure or maintain correction or acceptable alignment.

Lifting the patient to and from the operating table should be supervised by the surgeon.

8

The patient lies prone with the head in a horseshoe shaped rubber rest, or an adjustable cerebellar rest. Skull calipers are in position and facilities for lateral radiographs are available.

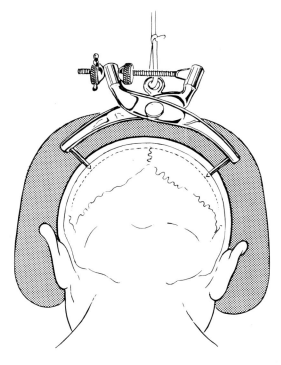

8

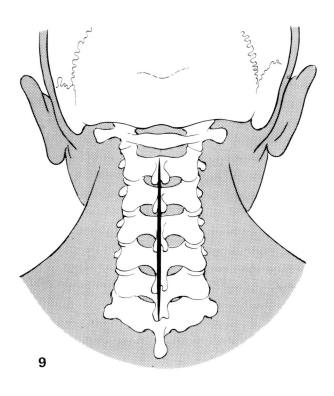

9

THE OPERATION

9

The incision

The skin incision keeps strictly to the mid-line between the second and the seventh spinous process but it may be extended as necessary. Infiltration of the sub-cutaneous tissues and muscles with 1:500,000 adrenaline-saline solution is a useful measure in this, as in other operations on the cervical spine.

Bleeding points are secured using curved artery forceps, and self-retaining retractors are inserted to spread the superficial tissues.

10

Exposure

The ligamentum nuchae is easily recognized if the tissues are kept stretched. It affords attachment to the neck muscles by means of a sinuous flexible band (the median raphe) which passes from the deep surface of the nuchal ligament to the interspinous ligaments. This is the key to reaching the interval between the tips of the spinous processes with the least loss of blood.

Cutting diathermy is useful in dividing the median raphe and the point of the instrument should not be permitted to wander into the muscles.

As the incision is deepened the bifid spinous processes are readily felt and the first stage of the exposure should finish in the interval between the bifid spines.

Using a wide fishtail osteotome (*see* inset) the muscles are stripped subperiosteally. The osteotome is inserted along the sides of the spinous processes and the muscles eased outwards from the mid-line, working from below upwards. The procedure is facilitated by nibbling off the overhang of each protuberance. The muscles are stripped laterally as far as the facets. Swabs are packed in between the muscles and the bone. When stripping and packing has been completed the swabs are removed and deep self-retaining retractors are inserted. Localization is checked radiologically after inserting a stout needle into an exposed spinous process.

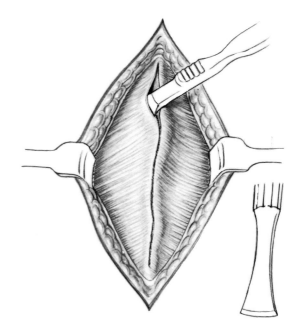

10

11

Correction of deformity

The site of dislocation is inspected, and an assistant applies traction to the head. As traction and gentle lateral flexion are applied it may be possible to replace the dislocation using fine, curved elevators hooked under the proximal facet. Only slight flexion to the neck should be permitted.

If correction cannot be accomplished, the superior surface of the distal facet should be carefully trimmed using a fine-pointed bone nibbler. Bilateral facetectomy is rarely required.

Fixation

Because the reduction is usually unstable it is wise to secure the spinous process of the dislocated vertebra to a distal spinous process. A hole is made near the base of the spinous process using an angled drill. Another hole is made near the mid-point of a more distal spinous process, usually the seventh. An aneur-

11

ysm needle carrying a 6 mm nylon ribbon (or 22 – 28 S.W.G. stainless steel wire) is passed through the holes and firmly tied. It is usual to augment the ribbon fixation with a bone grafting procedure (*see* pages 355–356). A second strand of nylon ribbon may be used to secure twin iliac grafts which span the laminae of the dislocated vertebra and those immediately above and below.

Token skull traction is continued for 6 weeks. A plastic or plaster collar is worn until fusion is achieved, usually in 3 months.

UPPER CERVICAL SPINE. OCCIPITOCERVICAL FUSION

The indications for this operation are instability of the upper cervical spine, often with progressive neurological signs. It has the advantage of dispensing with internal fixation, and is particularly suitable for cases in which the arch of the atlas is suppressed or otherwise deficient because of previous fractures or congenital anomalies. It is suitable in rheumatoid patients in whom ligamentous and bony softening is a feature. It is obligatory when bone has been removed as a result of neurosurgical procedures, and when a satisfactory pre-operative correction cannot be obtained. In the latter instance the interval between the odon-toid peg and the arch of the atlas is so reduced as to make passage of an instrument (aneurysm needle) extremely dangerous. In general it is reserved for stabilizing a very mobile segment.

Position of patient

The patient lies prone with the head firmly held in a head rest. The plaster bed technique is a useful alternative. Skull traction is applied, and endotracheal anaesthesia is favoured.

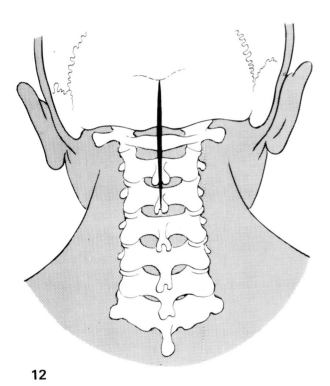

12

THE OPERATION

12

The incision

A long mid-line incision is made from just above the external occipital protuberance to the spinous process of the third cervical vertebra. Cushing's cross-bow incision is reserved for more difficult cases.

Exposure

The incision is deepened down to bone and the muscles are stripped subperiosteally, commencing at the spinous process of the axis. Only the central inch (2·5 cm) or so of the arch of the atlas needs preparation — thus avoiding injury to the vertebral vessels.

The muscles are erased from the under-surface of the occiput from near the foramen magnum almost to the superior nuchal line. An area of approximately 12 cm^2 is cleared.

13

Preparation of bone surfaces

The occipital area is roughened by gently raising slivers of bone using a light hammer and a sharp chisel. A power drill and burrs are used to decorticate the spinous process and laminae of the axis. Only minimal decortication of the central 2·5 cm or so of the atlas is required. Use of a chisel on the atlas is not recommended.

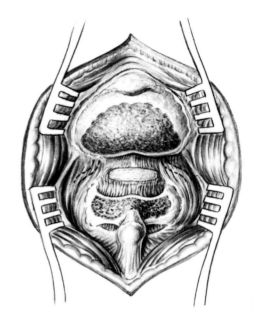

13

14

Bone grafting

Corticocancellous slivers are taken from the iliac crest with a quantity of cancellous bone. This latter is placed over the prepared area and followed by the bone slivers. The muscles and skin are sutured and a suction drain inserted.

Aftercare

Traction (2–4 kg) is continued for 4 weeks after the operation. When a plaster bed is used the patient remains recumbent for 3 months, and wears a plaster jacket or well-fitting polythene collar for the final 3 months. Fusion is usually complete in 6 months.

In older patients, or when a long period of recumbency is contra-indicated, a high-fitting plaster collar may be used in the postoperative period.

When applying the plaster collar, a cast is taken from which a collar of polythene or other suitable material can be made for later use. It is important that the collar should maintain the relationship between the head and neck which ensures the normal horizontal line of vision. Alternatively, the halo-body cast may be used.

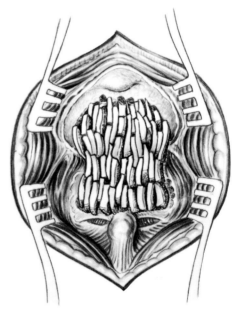

14

UPPER CERVICAL SPINE. POSTERIOR ATLANTO-AXIAL FUSION

Fusion of the atlas to the axis is required for conditions leading to manifest instability of the atlanto-axial joint. These include ununited fractures of the odontoid process and dislocations after which the ligaments often fail to heal despite adequate immobilization. Mild degrees of subluxation following injury are not uncommon, and there is often a difference of opinion on the necessity for fusion. When the distance between the anterior arch of the atlas and the intact odontoid process exceeds 3 mm in adults and 5 mm in children fusion is generally advised.

Instability often follows minor injuries in rheumatoid arthritis and other inflammatory conditions, as well as in congenital anomalies.

Pain and progressive neurological manifestations demand early intervention, but the operation is seldom an emergency one. Skull calipers are inserted a few days before operation, and dislocation is corrected as completely as possible, and appropriate x-ray films are made. The position of the patient and the general routine is similar to that already described for open reduction of cervical dislocations.

Alternative procedures

(*1*) Except in elderly patients, the use of a plaster bed has much to commend it. An anterior shell is made for use during the operation.

(*2*) Surgeons familiar with the use of the halo-body cast may prefer to use this method.

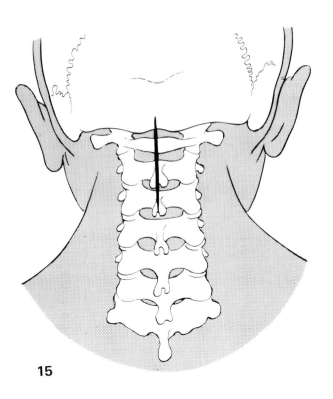

15

THE OPERATION

15

The incision

A mid-line longitudinal incision is made from just below the external occipital protuberance (inion) as low as is necessary to give adequate access. After dividing the skin and thick subcutaneous tissue the margins are firmly separated by self-retaining retractors. The median raphe is divided from near the base of the skull to just below the spinous process of the axis.

16

Exposure

Subperiosteal dissection of the suboccipital muscles exposes the laminae of the axis and atlas; Kocher's forceps are used to steady the spinous process of the axis. Great care is essential in exposing the arch of the atlas. The possibility of a mid-line defect should be kept in mind and the dissection should not be carried so far laterally as to endanger the vertebral artery. Only the central inch (2·5 cm) of the atlas should be exposed. Extra caution is advised in separating the suboccipital muscles from the thin atlanto-occipital and atlanto-axial membranes.

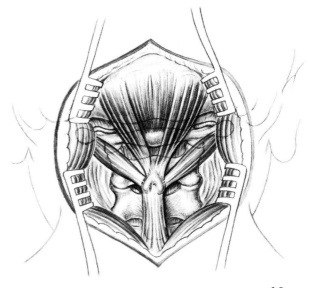

16

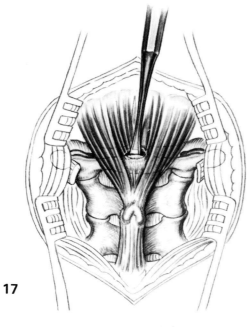

17

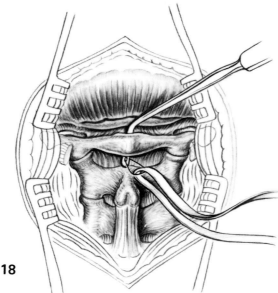

18

17&18

A fine curved periosteal elevator is useful at this stage and in the next one of separating the posterior atlanto-occipital membrane from the deep surface of the atlas near its mid-point. A long loop of nylon ribbon (6 mm × 30 cm) is attached to an aneurysm needle which, suitably bent, is passed deep to the arch of the atlas. The loop is retrieved as the aneurysm needle is withdrawn. For additional strength the manoeuvre may be repeated using a second loop, but again keeping strictly to the mid-line.

The loop is now severed and each band is passed deep to the strong spinous process of the axis on the same side. It is then passed over and around the spinous process of the opposite side to emerge on the original side. The security of each loop is tested. As a rule the bifid spinous process of the axis is sufficiently strong to accept small notches which will prevent the nylon from slipping.

Fixation of the graft

The laminae and spinous process of the axis are prepared using suitable burrs on a power drill. The cortical bone is denuded to expose bleeding points. Only minimal decortication of the atlas is advised.

19

A block of bone and a small quantity of cancellous slivers are removed from the iliac crest. The bone block is fixed in a vice and a prism-shaped graft is fashioned using an oscillating saw. The graft is bisected and the cancellous surface of each prism is placed over the prepared bone. The ribbons are loosely tied over the grafts, and at this stage a lateral x-ray film is advised. When a snug fit has been obtained, notches are cut before the knots are finally secured over the grafts.

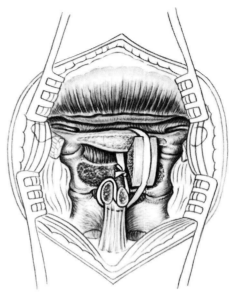

19

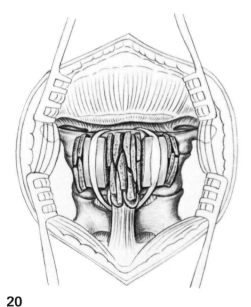

20

20

Closure

Cancellous slivers are placed over and around the grafts, but should not extend more proximally than the arch of the atlas. The muscles and ligamentum nuchae are sutured over the grafts before closure of the skin.

A sealed suction drain is maintained for 48 hr.

Aftercare

This is similar to that described on page 356.

MIDDLE AND LOWER PARTS OF CERVICAL SPINE. POSTERIOR FUSION

Spontaneous bony fusion probably occurs in the majority of compression injuries and in at least half of the fracture-dislocations. For these reasons posterior fusion of the middle and lower parts of the cervical spine is rarely necessary (McSweeney, 1971). This is in contrast to the upper cervical spine.

Indications for operation

(1) The presence of gross instability 3 months after injury.

(2) Progressive deformity associated with late pain and increasing neurological impairment.

(3) Certain injuries in the group of anterior subluxations (Cheshire, 1969; Evans, 1976; Webb *et al.*, 1976) would lead to an earlier decision on the need for fusion.

Pre-operative

The plaster bed method is safe, and especially applicable when there is no neurological deficit. An anterior shell is made and a suitable face piece removed to give the anaesthetist access. The shell is used during the operation and as a turning case.

The halo apparatus attached to an outrigger on a

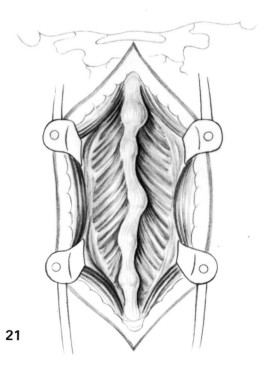

21

body cast has recently become popular, but its complications should be recognized (O'Brien, 1975).

When there is serious sensory impairment a well-fitting, removable plastic collar should be made available before the operation. In these patients the plaster bed should not be used, and the halo-body cast requires careful attention if pressure sores are to be avoided.

THE OPERATION

Incision

The patient lies prone on the anterior plaster shell, in the halo-body cast or with the head on a suitable head rest. When there is great instability halter traction or skull calipers are already in position.

Endotracheal anaesthesia, augmented by infiltration with 1:500,000 adrenaline-saline solution is satisfactory. A mid-line skin incision is made from the spinous process of the axis to the vertebra prominens.

The skin and dense subcutaneous tissues are retracted to expose the ligamentum nuchae in the mid-line. Small curved artery forceps are used to secure haemostasis. Self-retaining retractors are inserted.

21

Procedure

The spinous processes are identified and the ligamentum nuchae is incised in the mid-line. Keeping strictly to the median raphe is a tedious process. The surgeon should be familiar with the fact that this ribbon-like interval runs a sinuous course between the spinous processes. When the intervals between the tips of the spinous processes have been exposed by sharp dissection it should be possible to identify the vertebra involved. The interspinous ligaments should be examined as more than one may be damaged. A needle or Kocher's forceps is used to mark the suspect spinous process and a lateral x-ray film is exposed.

The fusion should include the vertebra above the site of maximal damage and two vertebrae below. More localized fusions lose sight of the possibility that the ligamentous damage is often more extensive than radiographs suggest.

Preparation of bone

The muscles are stripped subperiosteally, commencing at the most distal spinous process. Cautious use of the diathermy reduces bleeding. A fish-tailed osteotome is inserted along the side of each spinous process, which is steadied by Kocher's forceps. As the muscles are swept laterally, swabs are packed between the bone and the separated muscle to control haemorrhage.

Having completed the subperiosteal stripping the swabs are removed, and the muscles are parted with deep self-retaining retractors. Suction is useful for maintaining a dry field.

Decortication of the spinous process and posterior aspect of the laminae proceeds until freely oozing cancellous bone is exposed. A power drill carrying a large burr is useful, and the area is kept moist with saline. Fine nibbling forceps augment the removal of the cortex. The spinous processes to which the grafts will be tied need not be decorticated so extensively.

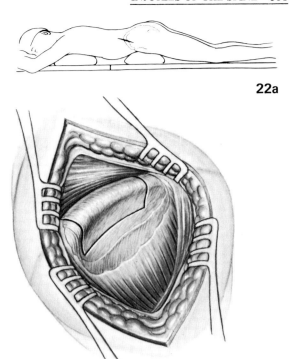

22a

22b

22a&b

At this stage an assistant removes the graft and a quantity of cancellous bone from the posterior part of the iliac crest.

23a&b

Drilling the spinous process

A hole is made with a right-angled power drill at the base of the spinous process. This is not easy because there is very little room between the retracted muscles and the spinous process, which is too hard to be pierced by a towel clip, but, once made the hole is enlarged with a towel clip, Lewin's forceps or a right-angled trocar. Sufficient margin of bone surrounds the hole to prevent weakening of the spinous process. Only the proximal and distal spinous processes should be drilled.

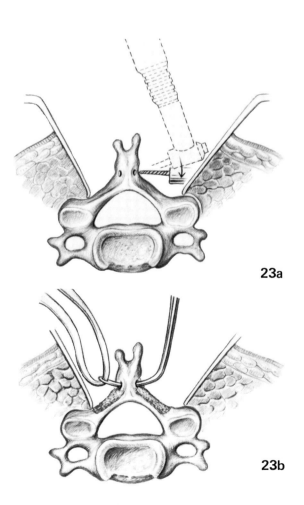

23a

23b

24

The curved iliac graft is now prepared. The graft is divided in its long axis and each half is laid in the paraspinous gutter with the cancellous surface facing medially. The curvature of the grafts fit conveniently in relation to the normal cervical lordosis.

Holes are drilled in the grafts to coincide with those in the spinous processes and 6 mm nylon ribbon is used to fix the grafts. An aneurysm needle to which the ribbon is attached facilitates the manoeuvre of tying the grafts to the spinous processes. Alternatively, a 22 – 26 S.W.G. stainless steel wire can be passed through the spinous processes and over or through the iliac grafts.

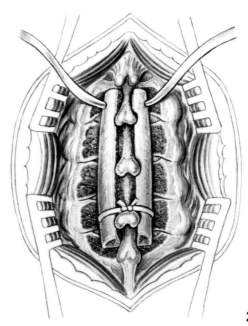

24

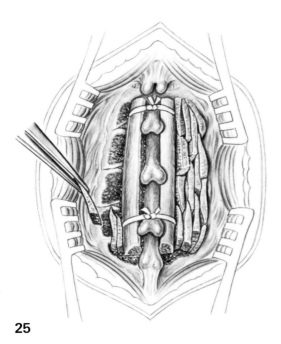

25

25

Before closing the muscle layers, slivers of iliac bone are placed around the grafts.

Vacuum sealed drainage is arranged before suture of the ligamentum nuchae and closure of the skin.

Postoperative care

Token traction of 2 kg is maintained for 6 weeks or so. A well-fitting collar is then applied and worn until there is radiographic evidence of fusion — usually in 4 – 6 months.

ANTERIOR FUSION OF CERVICAL SPINE

The early mobility permitted by anterior fusion for cervical spondylosis and other non-traumatic conditions has helped to popularize this method.

The approach is applicable where the damage has been to the vertebral bodies, discs or anterior longitudinal ligaments, rather than to the posterior ligamentous complex. It has a useful place when fusion is required in older patients and when a long period of recumbency must be avoided.

Early physical and psychological rehabilitation are cited as an additional advantage of anterior fusion, but in the early stages of serious cord injury, to be sat out of bed before autonomic reflexes have recovered may hinder rather than hasten the general rehabilitation programme. The concept still requires evaluation in tetraplegic patients. In the author's opinion the case for emergency anterior decompression and fusion is not supported by contemporary reports.

The patient is draped as for a thyroid operation. When the procedure is carried out in the later stage of injury, halter traction is in position, otherwise skull calipers are used.

The right-handed surgeon will usually find that the operation is more conveniently carried out from that side, but it should be remembered that the recurrent laryngeal nerve crosses the field near the level of the seventh cervical vertebra and is more vulnerable than when the exposure is from the left side.

THE OPERATION

26

The incision

The head is turned to the left and a rolled towel or inflatable neck rest is in position. The fifth cervical disc is at the level of the cricoid cartilage and the adjacent discs lie 1 cm above or below. A transverse incision is made two or three fingers' breadth above the clavicle, depending on the level of the proposed fusion. The incision extends from just lateral to the anterior border of the sternomastoid muscle to the mid-line of the neck. For exposing the third cervical disc the incision is at a higher level and should extend across the mid-line (*see* dotted line). For stabilizing injuries above the third cervical vertebra the author's preference is for a posterior approach.

Exposure

Skin flaps are raised to expose the platysma muscle, which is divided vertically in the line of its fibres. The underlying superficial jugular vein and the medial part of the platysma are retracted to the mid-line.

The anterior border of the sternomastoid muscle is cleared of areolar tissue and the carotid pulsation is then felt.

Using curved scissors, the pretracheal fascia is divided longitudinally to expose the strap muscles. Self-retaining retractors are inserted.

The interval between the carotid sheath and the oesophagus is developed by blunt dissection, using the fingers, gauze and scissors-spreading. The sternomastoid muscle and the carotid sheath are retracted laterally, and the thyroid gland, trachea and oesophagus are freed with the finger and displaced medially.

The omohyoid muscle, identified by its diagonal course, is cleaned and retracted downwards, or divided to afford better exposure.

The middle thyroid vein may require ligation at this stage. In exposing the seventh cervical vertebra care should be taken not to injure Sibson's fascia (dome of the pleura), and the inferior thyroid vessels should be ligated, having identified the recurrent laryngeal nerve.

Particular attention should be exercised in identifying the oesophagus and in separating it from the prevertebral areolar tissue. An assistant retracts the oesophagus, trachea and thyroid gland, alternating finger retraction with a suitably bent, well-padded, malleable retractor.

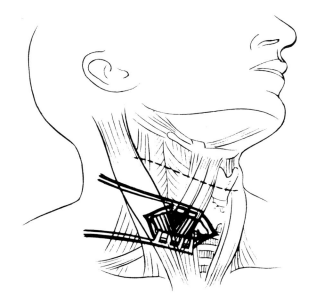

27

Keeping strictly to the mid-line, the anterior longitudinal ligament and the parallel medial margins of the longus colli muscles are identified. The interval between the longus colli muscles is an important landmark and as the muscles are separated considerable bleeding is often encountered. Diathermy and the use of Surgicel packs are recommended at this stage. A well-curved periosteal elevator completes the exposure of the front of the vertebral column. Malleable retractors are re-inserted to spread the longus colli muscles. Alternatively, Cloward's special tooth-bladed self-retaining retractors may be used. As a rule the site is identified by a step at the suspect level, but localization should be checked with a lateral x-ray film.

When the longitudinal ligament is well developed it is often feasible to raise a rectangular flap over the suspect disc, otherwise the ligament is divided in the mid-line.

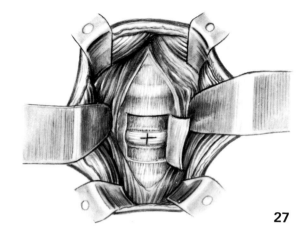

27

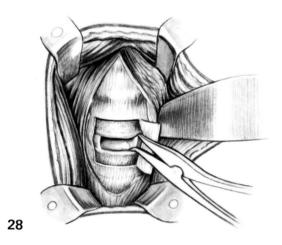

28

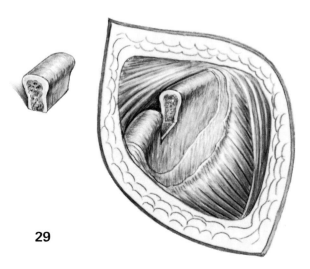

29

Procedure

The annulus is incised using a narrow pointed scalpel and the front half of the disc is removed with a rongeur. The overhang of cortical bone on the front margin of the vertebrae can often be preserved, but the lateral parts of the disc should be excised.

28

Head traction is now applied and a vertebral spreader is inserted into the disc space. The spreader is moved from side to side to facilitate clearance. The cartilaginous plates and remaining disc material are removed using a narrow periosteal elevator and curette.

The cortical bony plates should not be removed; at most they may be drilled through into the cancellous bone of the vertebral bodies. There is no need to display the posterior longitudinal ligament. It is important to recognize the normal obliquity of the disc and to remove an equal amount of bone from the adjacent vertebral bodies.

The aim is to excavate a rectangular space which will accept a horse-shoe shaped block of bone approximately 8 mm in height, 16 mm wide and 15 mm deep. In practice the space should be slightly smaller than the graft.

29

The graft is taken from the iliac crest with a small quantity of cancellous bone. It should include the full thickness of the crest and exceed the dimensions of the intervertebral space. Held in a vice it can be properly shaped, measured and cleared of soft tissues.

30a&b

Insertion of graft

The vertebral spreader is removed and the neck is slightly extended as the anaesthetist applies firm traction to the head. The neck is kept on full stretch while the bone block is inserted and firmly tapped into position using a punch and light mallet. The graft is countersunk with the cortical surface facing anteriorly, and any 'dead space' is packed with cancellous bone.

As the neck is brought to neutral position and the traction released, the block should be securely wedged between the vertebrae.

Closure

The flap of longitudinal ligament is sutured over the graft to the adjacent longus colli muscle or, when this is not practicable, the longus colli muscles are approximated over the graft. The strap muscles fall into position and the retractors are removed.

Suction drainage is advised.

The platysma is carefully sutured before closure of the skin incision.

Aftercare

Difficulty in swallowing and hoarseness quickly pass. The patient should be sat up as soon as possible. A sorbo rubber collar designed to prevent rotation of the head is worn for a few weeks. The position of the graft is checked by x-ray. Consolidation is usually complete in 4 months.

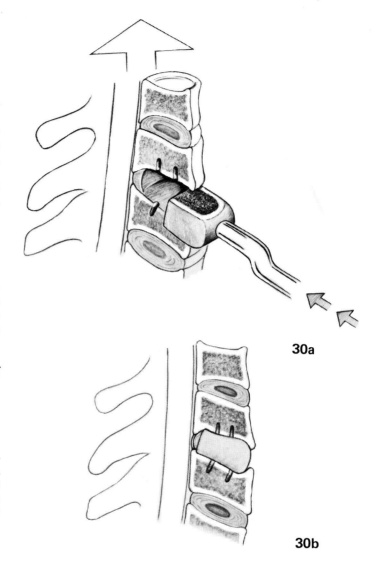

30a

30b

THORACIC SPINE

The splinting effect of the thoracic cage is such that operations on the thoracic spine following injury are rarely indicated. Even when there is severe displacement and comminution of bone, stability is rapidly achieved, provided that the patient is suitably postured and kept strictly recumbent for 8 – 10 weeks.

Crush fractures of the vertebral bodies are stable. They heal quickly and require bed rest on suitably placed pillows until the pain has abated. Extension exercises are most important, and spinal braces are seldom indicated.

It should be recognized that, when the patient is rendered paraplegic, the cord injury is complete in about 90 per cent of cases.

Operation may be needed when there is gross disruption of the thorax with serious vertebral damage. Thus fractures of the sternum, dislocations of the manubriosternal joint and multiple fractures at the costovertebral angles associated with a severe vertebral injury are often followed by increasing kyphosis or kyphoscoliosis.

The spinal injury is classically at the fourth thoracic level but more proximal injuries, including fracture-dislocation, also occur.

The key to the solution of the problem is early fixation of the chest.

31

To this end costal injuries require early fixation and sternal injuries can be stabilized with a Sillar's plate.

If radiographs then reveal a kyphosis of over 40°, or if there is further increase in the deformity while the patient remains recumbent, posterior fixation with twin Harrington's rods (or Knodt's rods) in distraction should be considered.

There is difficulty in securing good hook purchase above the third thoracic vertebra. For this reason these unusual injuries above the fourth thoracic vertebra (with severe deformity) are better managed by a delayed anterior approach.

Open correction and rod fixation is sometimes required at lower levels in the dorsal spine for gross fracture-dislocations which cannot be controlled by postural methods (Harrington, 1967, 1972).

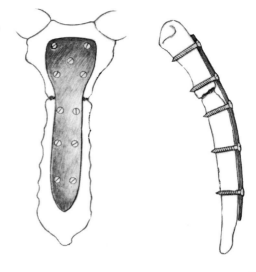

31

REPLACEMENT AND FIXATION OF FRACTURE-DISLOCATIONS OF MID-THORACIC SPINE

The patient is placed prone on pillows which are so arranged that the abdomen is not resting on the table. The site of dislocation should be directly over a hinged segment of the table. Facilities for radiography should be available.

THE OPERATION

The incision

The skin and subcutaneous tissues are infiltrated with 1:500,000 adrenaline-saline solution. A straight incision is made which should be sufficiently long to expose two vertebrae above and below the dislocation.

Procedure

The incision is carried down to the deep fascia. Self-retaining retractors are inserted. The site of the dislocation is readily identified by the haematoma and ligamentous defect.

The two distal spinous processes are exposed by sharp dissection. The subperiosteal muscle stripping commences at the lowermost spinous process. A large periosteal elevator (Cobb's) is used, keeping the spatula-like blade in the line of the spinous process and close to the bone. The two proximal spinous processes are similarly cleared. Deep self-retaining retractors are inserted at each extremity of the wound. Swabs are firmly packed between the muscle and bone as each interspace is prepared. In the thoracic spine the short laminae and the imbrication of the spinous processes should be noted. The subperiosteal dissection should be carried laterally to expose the facets.

Correction

The posterior elements of the dislocated vertebra are now exposed. The spinous process may be fractured, and leverage is better applied to the intact processes near the site of injury.

Re-alignment is secured by applying traction to the lower limbs and breaking the table at the level of the dislocation. At the same time bone levers are used to elevate the displaced vertebral body.

The table is then brought to the horizontal position and the replacement is confirmed by inspection and lateral x-ray films. If the position is satisfactory a notch is cut in the lower margin of the posterior joint two levels above the dislocation. The distraction hook is tilted into position and then driven into its purchase site so that the shoe abuts securely against the pedicle. The second hook is similarly placed on the opposite side. The inferior hooks are sited in notches cut into the upper surface of each lamina two interspaces below the site of injury. It might be thought that by distracting the back of the spine in this way the displacement would be restored but the appliance lengthens the spine without bending it.

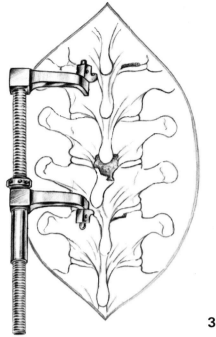

32,33&34

If correction proves difficult the Harrington outrigger may be used. As the distraction force is applied to the outrigger the resistance of the intact anterior longitudinal ligament should be encountered. The outrigger has a useful place in affording temporary stability while the distraction rod on the opposite side is locked into position. It is then removed and the second rod is clinched into position.

32

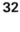

Bone grafting

In the thoracic as distinct from the lumbar spine, it is wise to complete the fixation with a bone grafting procedure. The exposed spinous processes and laminae are decorticated and strips of iliac bone are packed into the lateral gutters.

More formal excision of the facetal joints is seldom necessary.

Closed suction drainage is advised.

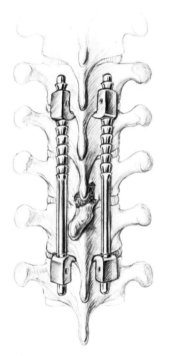

Aftercare

The patient may be sat up out of bed after 2 weeks and for the unparalysed patient walking is encouraged a few days later.

A light body cast is worn for 3 months.

33

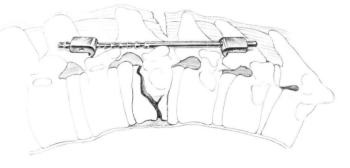

34

THORACOLUMBAR INJURIES

The place for operative correction after injuries from the tenth thoracic to the second lumbar vertebra will remain a debating point between surgeons of comparable experience.

It must be appreciated that while there are variations in the normal anatomy, the cord ends at the lower border of the first lumbar vertebra in at least 50 per cent of cases. The first and second sacral segments and all the lumbar roots normally cross the disc between the last thoracic and the first lumbar vertebrae.

Injuries at the thoracolumbar junction may damage the cord (conus), which is incapable of regeneration. The damaged lumbar roots are more tolerant of injury, and if not avulsed may in certain circumstances show evidence of recovery. This led Holdsworth and others to advocate anatomical correction and internal fixation (Holdsworth and Hardy, 1953; Ransohoff, 1970; Kelly and Whiteside, 1968).

The controversy continues, but the author's personal belief is that internal fixation does not materially influence the neurological outcome (McSweeney, 1976).

Indications

Internal fixation as an aid to nursing management has much to commend it. The conservative policy is satisfactory when the facilities of a specialized unit are available. In other circumstances the surgeon may decide that internal fixation is in the patient's best interest but second-rate surgery does not compensate for second-rate nursing. The injury must be inherently unstable, amenable to good internal fixation and the surgical facilities must be beyond reproach.

The absolute indication for operative correction is failure to secure or maintain acceptable alignment. This may arise when there is really gross displacement with interposition of soft tissues. In such cases x-rays often show persistent lateral angulation despite adequate posturing, or forward displacement of more than half the vertebral body.

Unexplained and significant progression of motor or sensory paralysis may be a valid indication for surgical exploration. It is a rare occurrence, and the possibility of two separate bony injuries or extending vascular thrombosis should be kept in mind.

When there is locking of intact facets, with little bony damage, attempts at postural correction may increase the deformity. Such injuries are rare at the thoracolumbar junction but not uncommon below the second lumbar vertebra. Zadik's clamp is particularly suitable as a fixation device following operation in such cases.

Rupture of the diaphragm with herniation of the abdominal contents into the chest may present as acute respiratory embarrassment. After repair of the diaphragm internal fixation of the vertebral injury is advised.

The presence of associated intra-abdominal or intra-pelvic injuries is an occasional indication for internal fixation of the spine.

General considerations

Following open correction it is usual to stabilize the fracture-dislocation. A number of methods are available, and two are in common use. Fixation by twin plates bolted through the spinous processes (Williams, 1963) should be regarded as a temporary measure and an aid to nursing.

Harrington's rods in distraction offer better stability. Alternatively, long Knodt's rods may be used. Some surgeons advise complementary bone grafting at the same time. The author regards this as unnecessary and a disadvantage to the wheelchair patient, who requires mobility in the lumbar region.

35

Twin-plate fixation

Lateral x-ray films should demonstrate that at least two spinous processes above and below the site of injury are intact. The patient is prone on the operating table with pillows under the pelvis and upper part of the chest and is placed so that the site of dislocation is level with the main hinge of the table.

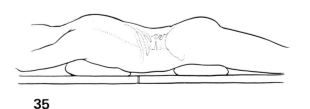

35

THE OPERATIONS

The incision

A straight mid-line incision is made over the gap between spinous processes. The forces of injury have usually stripped the muscles near the site and the spinous process of the dislocated vertebra is often broken at its base. Infiltration with 1:500,000 solution of adrenaline in saline and cutting diathermy help to limit bleeding.

Procedure

Subperiosteal exposure commences at the spinous process two levels below the site of injury and proceeds proximally to expose two spinous processes above. A large subperiosteal elevator is advised.

The dissection should proceed laterally to permit the use of instruments. The use of packs and suction ensures a dry field.

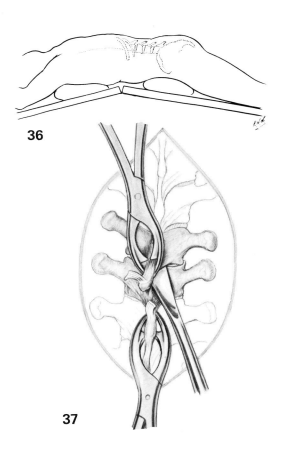

36

37

36 & 37

Deep retractors are inserted and the site of injury inspected. Traction on the lower limbs and lowering the foot end of the table will often improve the alignment.

The intact spinous processes are held in lion forceps and pulled backwards while the operator gently levers the displaced vertebra into line. The table is brought back to the horizontal position. Lateral x-ray films at this stage may indicate that a position of slight hyperextension is desirable and this is achieved by raising the head end of the operating table. The dura is not opened, but large tears should be sutured.

38

Fixation

The solidity of the spinous processes above and below the site of injury should be established.

The slotted plates are placed in position with the serrated edges facing laterally. The plates are adjusted so that the spinous processes can be drilled through the slots. This is a tedious process, and one which requires careful adjustment of the plates. An angled power drill is recommended, and the holes made in the spinous processes are then enlarged, using a right-angled trocar.

The special bolts are pointed to facilitate threading the serrated nuts, which are tightened with a ratchet spanner (*see* inset).

Closure

The muscles and skin are sutured after insertion of a vacuum drain.

Postoperative care

Two hourly turning and other measures appropriate to a paralysed patient continue. At 6 weeks x-rays usually show progress towards consolidation and at this time the patient can be sat up out of bed.

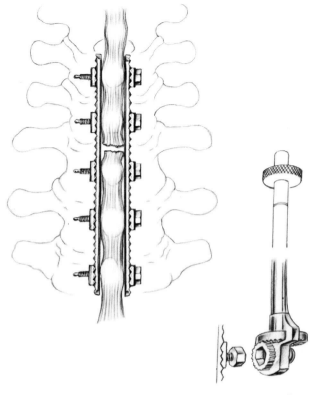

38

39

Fixation with Harrington's rods

The exposure is the same as that outlined above and the principles are similar to fixation of the mid-thoracic spine. Since the rods are used in distraction this method should not be employed in hyperextension injuries.

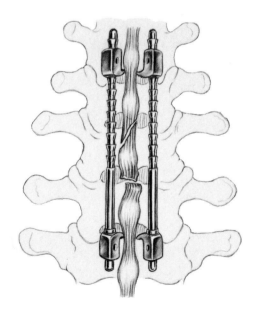

39

INJURIES BELOW THE SECOND LUMBAR VERTEBRA

These injuries are uncommon and apart from compression fractures seldom follow a definite pattern.

Compression fractures usually heal without difficulty. When there is serious ligamentous disruption, leading to subluxation or dislocation, internal fixation should be considered. In some instances the posterior joints are intact or the bony injury is minimal. At least one variety of lap seat belt injury falls into this category. Healing in such injuries is seldom satisfactory, late deformity may occur, and persistent pain is often a feature. For these reasons early fixation using Zadik's clamp or Knodt's distraction rods is advised.

40

Clamp fixation

The apparatus consists of two L-shaped rods threaded at the top ends, which interlock on the horizontal arms (Zadik, 1959). It is designed to grip on the spinous processes at the site of injury and replace the strong interspinous ligament.

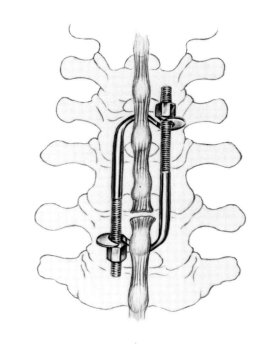

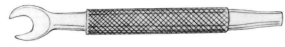

40

THE OPERATIONS

The incision and exposure

This is similar to that already described for the thoracolumbar junction and need not be so extensive.

Procedure

Deformity is corrected by breaking the table at the site of injury, thus flexing the spine, and by applying traction to the legs. The spinous processes are held with lion forceps and as the table is returned to the horizontal the displaced vertebra is guided into place. Correction is complete when the distance between the spinous processes is normal and is confirmed by lateral x-ray films.

Each half of the appliance is separately placed by pushing the shorter arm through the intact interspinous ligament in the space above and below the site of injury. The spinous processes may be notched to increase the purchase. The two halves are locked together and the nuts are tightened.

The muscles, deep fascia and skin are closed in the normal way.

Aftercare

The patient may be sat out of bed after 1 month. The appliance may be used for thoracolumbar injuries when the bony damage is not severe, but a longer postoperative period of recumbency is advised.

Fixation with twin distraction rods (Knodt)

The indications and exposure are similar to those described in connection with Zadik's apparatus. It is assumed that the vertebral body is intact or has suffered only minor injury.

41

The initial distraction is not maintained, but the degree of fixation due to the presence of the superincumbent body weight is greater than with Zadik's clamp. The appliance consists of a threaded rod mounted with two hooks facing away from each other (Knodt and Larrick, 1964). The device utilizes the screw jack principle and the rods are always used in pairs.

Procedure

The laminae are cleared of muscle. The uppermost hooks are inserted under the laminae at the site of injury or immediately above. Breaking the table to permit slight flexion helps in siting the hooks, for which an offset tamper is used. The lower hooks are seated over the laminae below the site of injury and as far laterally as possible. The central nut is turned with a spanner or tempered steel nerve hook. Working on the turnbuckle principle the hooks separate, and distraction can be measured by observing the spinous processes.

Depending on the severity of the ligamentous damage a localized fusion may be carried out using cancellous bone.

Aftercare

Early walking or sitting out of bed in a wheelchair (depending on the neurological state) is encouraged.

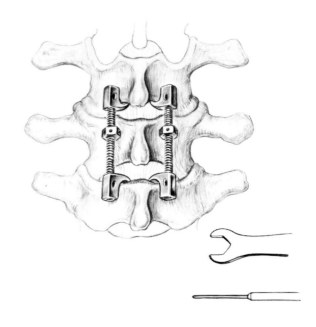

41

CONCLUSIONS

In ideal circumstances the long-term care of the tetraplegic or paraplegic patient is best carried out in a specialized spinal unit. Immediate and continuing medical supervision, physical, social and vocational rehabilitation demand the expert attention of many consultants and allied health workers.

Operations are not often required in the acute stages of injury. The plea that early surgery hastens the rehabilitation process still requires critical evaluation and must be measured against the disastrous results of injudicious intervention.

It is likely that the real advance in treatment will come from the work of biological scientists, aided by more efficient methods of internal fixation.

References

Bedbrook, G. M. (1976). 'Injuries of the spine and spinal cord.' In *Handbook of Clinical Neurology,* Vol 25, page 437. Edited by P. J. Vinken and G. W. Brun. Amsterdam: North Holland Publishing Co

Cheshire, D. J. E. (1964). 'Respiratory management in acute traumatic paraplegia.' *Paraplegia* **1,** 252

Cheshire, D. J. E. and Coates, D. A. (1966). 'Respiratory and metabolic management in acute tetraplegia.' *Paraplegia* **4,** 1

Cheshire, D. J. E. (1969). 'The stability of the cervical spine following the conservative treatment of fractures and fracture-dislocations.' *Paraplegia* **7,** 193

Cloward, R. B. (1961). 'Treatment of acute fractures and fracture-dislocations of the cervical spine by vertebral body fusion.' *J. Neurosurg.* **18,** 201

Dolfuss, P. and Frankel, H. L. (1965). 'Cardio-vascular reflexes in tracheostomised tetraplegics.' *Paraplegia* **2,** 227

Evans, D. K. (1976). 'Anterior cervical subluxation.' *J. Bone Jt Surg.* **58B,** 318

Flesch, J. R., Leiden, L. L., Erickson, D. L., Chou, S. N. and Bradford, D. S. (1977). 'Harrington instrumentation and spine fusion for unstable fractures and fracture-dislocations of the thoracic and lumbar spine.' *J. Bone Jt Surg.* **59A,** 143

Guttmann, L. (1953). 'The treatment and rehabilitation of patients with injuries to the spinal cord.' In *British Medical History of World War II,* pages 422–516. London, H. M. Stationery Office

Guttmann, L. (1973) *Spinal Cord Injuries.* London: Blackwell

Harrington, P. R. (1967). 'Instrumentation in spine instability other than scoliosis.' *South Afr. J. Surg.* **5,** 7

Harrington, P. R. (1972). 'Technical details in relation to the successful use of intruments in scoliosis.' *Orthop. Clins N. Am.* **3,** 49

Holdsworth, F. W. (1970). 'Fractures, dislocations, and fracture-dislocations of the spine.' *J. Bone Jt Surg.* **52A,** 1534

Holdsworth, F. W. and Hardy, A. G. (1953). 'Early treatment of paraplegia from fractures of the thoraco-lumbar spine.' *J. Bone Jt Surg.* **35B,** 540

Kallio, E. (1963). 'Injuries of the thoraco-lumbar spine with paraplegia.' *Acta Orthop. Scand. Suppl.* page 60

Kelly, R. P. and Whiteside, T. E. (1968). 'Treatment of lumbo-dorsal fracture-dislocations.' *Ann. Surg.* **167,** 705

Knodt, H. and Larrick, R. B. (1964). 'Distraction fusion of the spine.' *Ohio State med. J.* **60,** 1140

Kopits, S. E. and Steingrass, M. H. (1970). 'Experience with the halo-case in small children.' *Surg. Clins N. Am.* **50,** 4

McSweeney, T. (1968). 'The early management of associated injuries in the presence of co-incident damage to the spinal cord.' *Paraplegia* **5,** 189

McSweeney, T. (1971). 'Stability of the cervical spine following injury accompanied by grave neurological damage.' *Proceedings of the Eighteenth Veterans Administration Spinal Cord Injury Conference, Boston,* pages 61–65

McSweeney, T. (1976). 'Fractures of the thoraco-lumbar spine.' *Proceedings of the Third Mediterranean and Middle Eastern Orthopaedic Surgery and Traumatology Congress, Athens.* Edited by E. Vayanos and G. Hartofilakidis

McSweeney, T. (1976). 'Deformities of the spine following injuries to the cord.' In *Handbook of Clinical Neurology.* Vol 26, pages 159–174. Edited by P. J. Vinken and G. W. Brun. Amsterdam: North Holland Publishing Co

Meinecke, F. W. (1976). 'Initial clinical appraisal of spinal cord injuries and associated injuries.' In *Handbook of Clinical Neurology,* Vol. 26, pages 185–242. Edited by P. J. Vinken and G. W. Brun. Amsterdam: North Holland Publishing Co

Munro, D. (1943). 'Thoracic and lumbo-sacral cord injuries.' *J. Am. med. Ass.* **122,** 1055

Nicoll, E. A. (1949). 'Fractures of the dorso-lumbar spine.' *J. Bone Jt Surg.* **31B,** 376

Norrell, H. (1971). 'The role of vertebral body replacement in the treatment of certain cervical spine fractures.' *Proceedings of the Eighteenth Veterans Administration Spinal Cord Injury Conference, Boston,* pages 35–39

O'Brien, J. P. (1975). 'The halo-pelvic apparatus.' *Acta Orthop. Scand. Suppl.* page 163

Ransohoff, J. (1970). 'Lesions of the cauda equina.' *Clin. Neurosurg.* **17,** 331

Riska, E. B. (1977). 'Antero-lateral decompression as a treatment of paraplegia following vertebral fracture in the thoraco-lumbar spine.' *Int. Orthop. (SICOT)* **1,** 22

Webb, J. K., Broughton, R. B. K., McSweeney, T. and Park, W. M. (1976). 'Hidden flexion injury of the cervical spine.' *J. Bone Jt Surg.* **58B,** 322

Williams, E. W. M. (1963). 'Traumatic paraplegia.' In *Recent Advances in the Surgery of Trauma,* Edited by D. N. Mathews. London: Churchill

Zadik, F. R. (1959). 'Fracture dislocation of the thoraco-lumbar spine. A new method of internal fixation.' *J. Bone Jt Surg.* **41B,** 772

[*The illustrations for this Chapter on Injuries of the Spine were drawn by Mr. R. N. Lane.*]

Exposure and Fixation of Disrupted Pubic Symphysis

E. Letournel, M.D.
Professor of Orthopaedic Surgery and Traumatology,
Centre Medico-Chirurgical de la Porte de Choisy, Paris

PRE - OPERATIVE

Indications

It is often worthwhile attempting to restore the shape and stability of a fractured pelvis; even though there may appear to be merely disruption or overlapping of the symphysis pubis there is usually sacro-iliac damage as well, but this can be corrected if the pubis is fixed in place.

Operation is advisable: (*1*) when the pubic bones overlap; (*2*) when the pubic interval is greater than 1 cm; thus, only very small disruptions are treated conservatively.

Furthermore, this surgical treatment avoids all kinds of postoperative immobilization and allows walking with crutches sometimes only 10 days after operation.

Time of operation

This is not an emergency and delay of a few days allows: (*1*) the spontaneous arrest of bleeding from pelvic veins disrupted at the time of injury and (*2*) preparing the skin for incision through the pubic hair.

Anaesthesia

General anaesthesia is used.

The urinary bladder has to be evacuated either spontaneously or by catheter.

Position of patient

The patient may be placed upon an ordinary operating table, but an orthopaedic table may be useful to facilitate the reduction of the more severe disruptions by allowing asymmetrical traction on the limbs and internal rotation of both hips. The patient should be so placed that the hips can be hyperextended by suitable adjustment of the table.

1

The apparatus

There is no special device. One can use a vitallium modified Sherman plate with equidistant holes. If it is to be applied on the superior aspect of the pubic bones it has to be bent along its long axis in two directions, posteriorly and superiorly.

A plate of four or six holes is used. Thick and wide plates are not suitable; Sherman's are adequate as they can be shaped so as to lie perfectly on the bone.

To give the plate its posterior concavity one can use any bending apparatus, but two strong forceps grasping the plate on either part of the mid-line and taking hold of short screws inserted into the outer holes allow one to obtain the desired amount of posterior curvature.

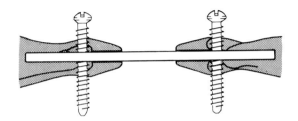
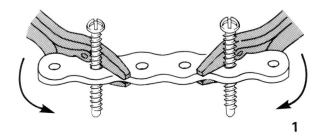

1

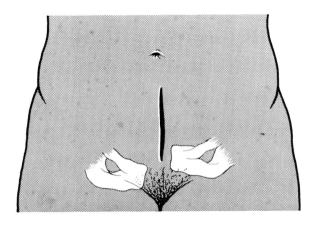
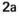

2a

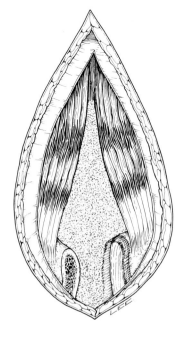

2b

THE OPERATION

2a&b

The exposure

In a case of simple disruption of the pubic symphysis, a vertical median incision is adequate. It should be 10–12 cm long and extend distally to the level of the superior border of the symphysis, i.e. crossing the pubic hair area.

The recti abdominis are separated along the linea alba.

Retzius's space is opened, the bladder is pushed back, and the posterior surfaces of the pubes are exposed.

The tear of a pubic symphysis is always asymmetrical.

On one side the bone has been cleared of all its muscular and ligamentous insertions, and the rectus itself is attached only to the prepubic soft parts. On the other side the rectus is normally attached, and the capsule and the cartilage remain attached to the bone; the anterior and inferior symphysis ligaments are torn in all cases.

3a&b

In some cases, a disrupted symphysis is associated with a vertical fracture through one obturator foramen that also crosses the pubic and ischiopubic rami. If this fracture is displaced it is necessary to reduce the displacement and plate it at the same time as the symphysis. In this case a vertical incision is not suitable and a horizontal approach such as a Pfannenstiel incision is more appropriate. If necessary, one rectus abdominis is cut transversely near its pubic insertion and repaired later on.

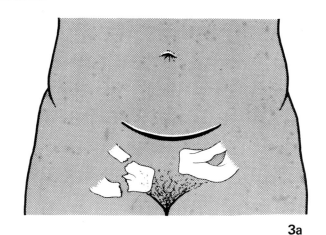

3a

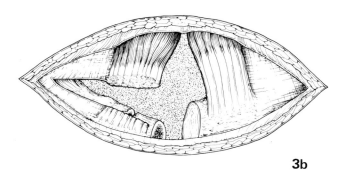

3b

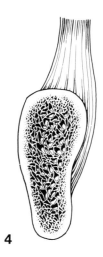 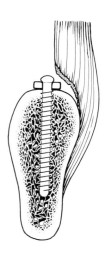

4

4

In any case it is necessary to free the superior aspect of the pubic rami where the plate will be inserted. As a rule, one side is already freed by the injuring force; on the other side the superior aspect has to be cleared from back to front, but the rectus must remain attached to the anterior border of that surface.

Removing the cartilage makes it easier to obtain a perfect correction of the displacement.

5a & b

The reduction

Internal rotation of both lower limbs, axial traction
and hyperextension of the hip, allowed by the
orthopaedic table, facilitate the reduction but a direct
action on the pubic bones is always necessary. The
author uses Faraboeuf's forceps, whose jaws take hold
of the anterior aspect of the pubic angle, or, better,
are inserted into the obturator foramina (*see Illustration 6a*).

Often the reduction is not achieved in one stage;
when several stages are needed allow a few minutes
between successive stages.

The symphysis must fit in all directions and not
only its superior aspect; a possible twist of the ilium
has to be corrected to align the posterior aspects of
the pubic bones correctly.

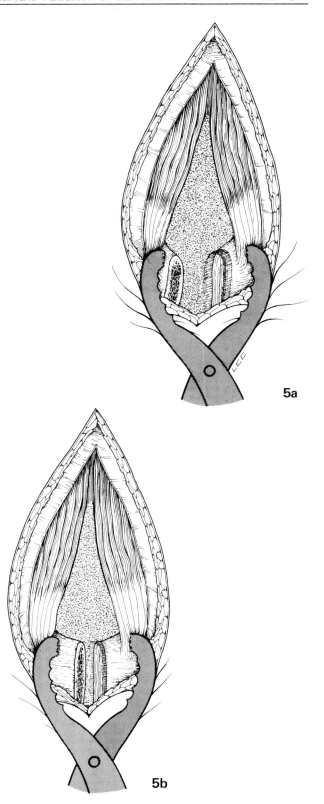

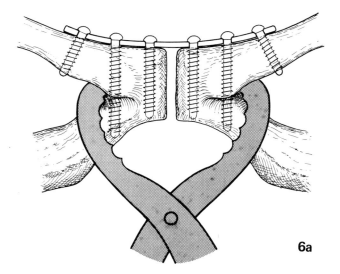

6a

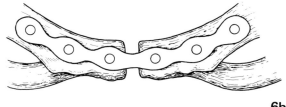

6b

The fixation

6a&b

As the reduction is achieved a four or six hole plate is shaped to lie perfectly on the superior aspect of each pubic ramus.

Two screws can be inserted in the body of each pubis. These screws should be parallel to the posterior surface of the pubis, that is to say directed obliquely backwards and downwards. From in front they look vertical and parallel or slightly divergent. Thirty-five or forty-five millimetre screws should be used.

If a six hole plate is used, the outer screws will be inserted into the superior pubic rami; they have to be shorter and must avoid the obturator vessels, but being screwed into two cortices they have a firm grasp.

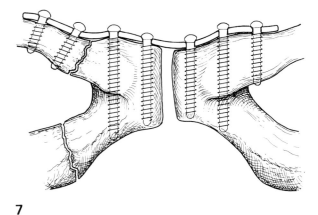

7

7

If it is necessary to span a disrupted symphysis and a fracture into the obturator foramen, the problem is more difficult and it is more important to understand the objective than to describe the procedure in detail. It may be best to start by fitting the symphysis accurately together, sometimes one should start with the fracture and hold it with a single screw. A long enough plate must be used to allow each fragment to be gripped by two screws and it must be made to fit all fragments accurately while they are accurately in place.

Closure of the wound

One or two suction drains are inserted, one in front, one behind the repaired symphysis.

If the rectus has been cut across it is repaired carefully.

The linea alba is sutured.

The skin incision is closed.

POSTOPERATIVE CARE

Prophylactic antibiotics may be used as the pubic hair area has been cut through.
    Suction drains are removed after 4—6 days.
    The patient remains in bed without any type of immobilization.
    Walking with partial weight-bearing and crutches is allowed after 14 days.
    Full weight-bearing is allowed after 6 weeks.

[The illustrations for this Chapter on Exposure and Fixation of Disrupted Pubic Symphysis were drawn by Mrs. G. Lee.]

Display, Correction and Fixation of Stove-in Hip Joints

E. Letournel, M.D.
Professor of Orthopaedic Surgery and Traumatology,
Centre Medico-Chirurgical de la Porte de Choisy, Paris

PRE-OPERATIVE

A stove-in hip is associated with different types of acetabular fracture.

To give the hip its original appearance and arrangement the central dislocation of the head has first to be corrected and then to be prevented by reconstructing the acetabulum, restoring perfect articular congruency and stability gives the patient the best chance of avoiding post-traumatic osteo-arthrosis.

1a,b&c

In order to gain a clear understanding of the fracture lines disrupting the iliac bone, four radiographic views are essential:

(*1*) the anteroposterior view of the whole pelvis in case there are fractures on both sides;

(*2*) the standard anteroposterior radiograph of the injured hip;

(*3*) the obturator oblique view, with the patient supine but rolled 45° away from the side of the injury;

(*4*) the iliac wing oblique view with the patient supine but rolled 45° *towards* the affected site.

The typical landmarks are studied carefully in each view.

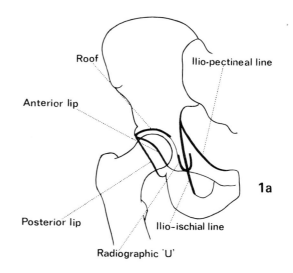

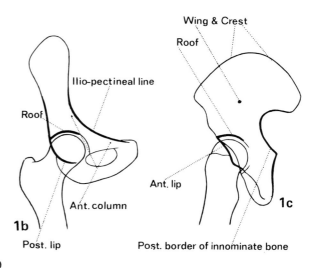

Indications for surgery

All the displaced fractures of the innominate bone resulting in a stove-in hip should be treated surgically. This applies whether the incongruity is shown by three, two or only one x-ray view. Even if the head can be reduced under a remaining part of the roof, surgical fixation offers the only possibility of restoring complete articular congruency.

One exception can be accepted: in some cases, among the most complex fractures, the different parts of the articular crescent are shown, by all three x-ray views, to be congruent with the centrally displaced head. In these cases bed rest and active exercises may lead to a good result, but the hip is never perfect and it remains displaced. Thus, if there is no contra-indication, operation is advised in order to restore a congruent hip in its normal place. The choice must depend on the surgeon, who must be confident of restoring an accurately fitting and correctly placed hip.

Time of operation

It is never an emergency, and the operation is perhaps easier when performed after 3–5 or 6 days when bleeding from pelvic veins disrupted at the time of injury has stopped.

The approach

This depends on the type of acetabular fracture associated with the stove-in hip.

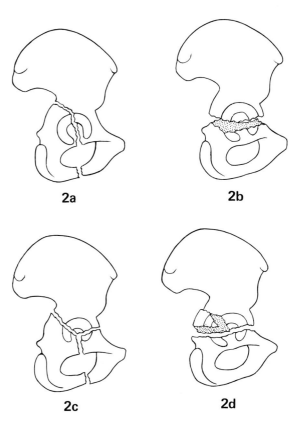

2a **2b** **2c** **2d**

2a-d

(a) If the centrally dislocated head is associated with:
(i) a posterior column fracture (a);
(ii) or any type of transverse fracture (b);
(iii) or a T-shaped fracture (c);
(iv) or an associated transverse and posterior fracture (d), good access is gained through a posterior or Kocher-Langenbeck type of incision.

3a,b&c

(*b*) If the associated fracture is either

(*i*) an anterior wall (*a*) or an anterior column fracture (*b*);

(*ii*) or a combination of anterior and transverse fractures (*c*), the ilio-inguinal, anterior approach has to be used.

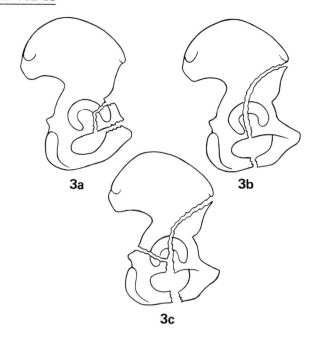

3a   **3b**

3c

4a&b

(*c*) If the fracture affects the whole of both columns, the whole articular crescent of the acetabulum is detached in several pieces, so that only the back part of the ilium remains connected to the sacrum.

A posterior approach may be used if the uppermost fracture-line extends to the anterior edge of the iliac bone (*a*), but when, as most often happens, the uppermost fracture-line reaches the crest (*b*), the ilio-inguinal anterior incision has to be used.

Some cases require the two approaches for the one operation. A more recently described lateral approach may be advisable in some cases.

Anaesthesia

Any form of general anaesthesia can be used, but good relaxation is particularly useful during an anterior approach.

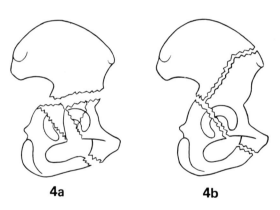

4a   **4b**

The equipment

5

Screws

Cortical screws from 22 to 120 mm long are most useful, but cancellous bone screws and Venable screws are needed from time to time.

Plates

Straight Sherman's vitallium plates, with equidistant holes, or Letournel's vitallium curved acetabulum plates with 6 to 12 holes are used.

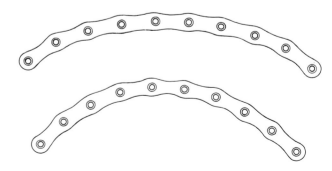

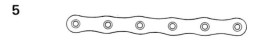

5

THE OPERATION

POSTERIOR APPROACH

The position of the patient, the equipment and the Kocher-Langenbeck approach are described in the Chapter on 'Replacement and Fixation of the Posterior Lip of the Acetabulum', pages 574–579.

Because the fracture lines divide the posterior column the hip's capsule is more or less torn and gives access to the inside of the joint. This access may be improved by a capsulotomy along either the posterior wall or the lateral lip of the roof, depending on the existing damage. The joint is cleared of clots and loose fragments, so that the intra-articular track of the fracture lines can be identified.

REDUCTION AND FIXATION

Principles

The centrally dislocated head is extracted with the aid of traction allowed by the orthopaedic table and supplemented by a big hook placed around the femur just under the neck.

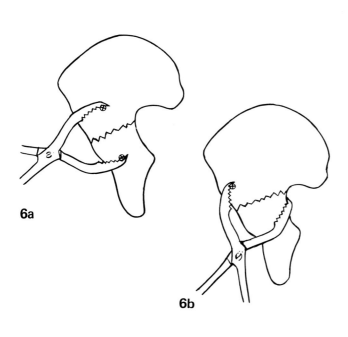

6a

6b

6a&b

The fragments are then set in place by direct manipulation, taking care to disturb their soft tissue attachments as little as possible. Replacement is sometimes difficult to achieve or to maintain and it may be advisable to use forceps to grip one or two temporary screws, which must be inserted away from the intended site of the plate.

The procedure adopted depends on whether or not part of the roof of the acetabulum remains intact and undisplaced.

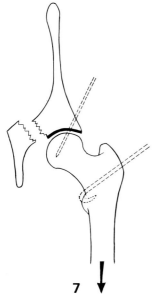

7

If part of the roof remains undisturbed under the blade of the ilium the head is replaced under it, taking care to get a perfect fit. The head is kept in place by traction or in some cases by temporary transfixion.

The means of reduction and fixation of the fragments depend on the type of the fracture.

7

8

Posterior column fracture

The big fragment is manipulated by forceps with one jaw inside the greater sciatic notch, the other taking hold of the outer aspect of the ilium or on a temporary screw. A plate is shaped so as to lie perfectly on the posterior aspect of the column from the upper pole of the ischial tuberosity up to the blade of the ilium, with at least three screws above the fracture-line. One must be careful to avoid leaving the column twisted out of line; this is done by control exercised from inside the pelvis, working through the greater sciatic notch.

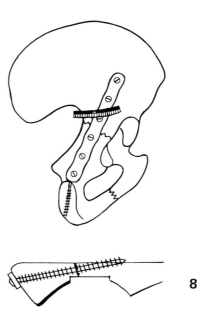

8

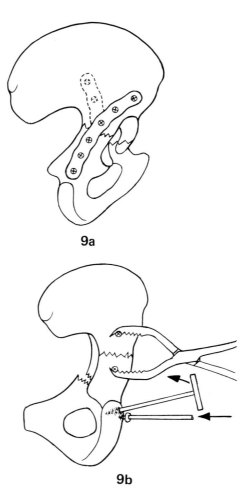

9a

9b

9a & b

Transverse fracture

The inferior part of the innominate bone is manipulated and plated as above, but there is often difficulty in dealing with the anterior part of the fracture at the level of the iliopectineal line. A finger introduced through the greater sciatic notch helps the manipulation, which can be further aided either by pushing the ischial tuberosity inwards or by inserting a femoral head extractor into it to act as a temporary handle. A 10—12 cm screw may be driven across the fracture-line to reach the superior aspect of the iliopectineal line.

10a & b

Associated transverse and posterior acetabular fractures

The transverse component is dealt with as above and fixed by a plate which is placed near the greater sciatic notch and passes under the gluteal muscles to be screwed into the posterior part of the ilium.

A large posterior acetabular fragment is fixed by isolated screws or, more safely, by a curved plate, as already described for this fracture on its own (*see Illustration 9a and b*).

11a & b

T-fractures

The head is placed and held under the roof and the fragment of the posterior column is set in place and plated as above, but one must avoid long screws which could reach the still displaced fragment of the anterior column.

Working through the greater sciatic notch, it may be possible to replace the anterior column and then to fix it with at least two long screws inserted from behind. If this is not possible this component must be approached from in front, using the appropriate incision (*see Illustration 11b*).

12

If none of the roof of the acetabulum remains attached to any part of the ilium that is still connected to the sacrum the operation is more difficult. This is the pattern that affects the whole of both columns.

First the head is extracted from the pelvis and maintained by traction in a position which allows the surgeon to reduce the posterior column fragment.

The placement of the posterior column fragment must be perfect and should be controlled both from inside the pelvis and on the outer aspect of the bone because if one accepts a small imperfection at this stage, it will be impossible to deal accurately with the other fracture-lines and the error will increase from step to step. The posterior column fracture is plated as if it were an isolated fracture of this part but avoiding screws long enough to reach and fix the displaced anterior column before it has been correctly replaced.

Then by freeing the inferior part of the ilium, up to its anterior border if necessary, the upper part of the anterior column fragment is replaced either by using forceps to take hold of a temporary screw or by a lever introduced into the fracture-line.

A curved acetabular plate fixes the upper part of the anterior column to the posterior one; it should, if possible, cross the inferior angle of the iliac fracture-line.

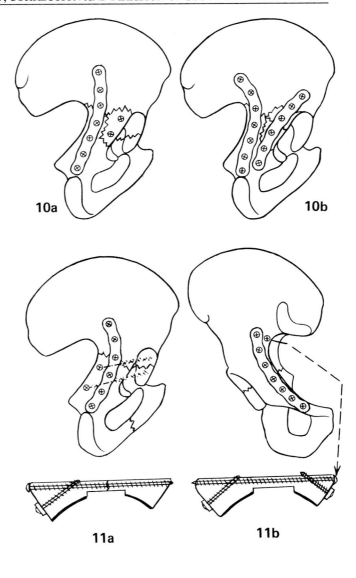

10a   10b

11a   11b

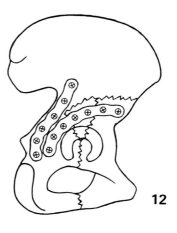

12

ILIO-INGUINAL APPROACH

Position of patient

The patient is supine on an orthopaedic table, unless there is a vertical anterior fracture-line of the opposite innominate bone, in which case traction would push upwards the two pubes and would prevent complete replacement.

13a & b

Towelling

The operative field has to extend: (*a*) upwards for three fingers' breadth above the iliac crest; (*b*) inwards for three to four fingers' breadth beyond the mid-line; (*c*) inferiorly from the level of the superior border of the symphysis, sideways to the femoral vessels and then obliquely to the greater trochanter; and (*d*) laterally to just behind the line of the femur.

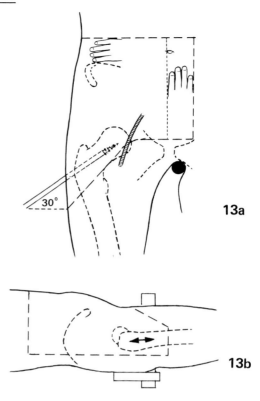

13a

13b

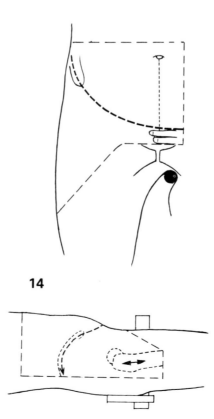

14

The approach

14 & 15

An incision is made along the anterior two-thirds of the iliac crest and then from its anterior superior spine towards the mid-line two fingers' breadth above the pubic symphysis.

Along the iliac crest the anterior abdominal muscles are detached and stripped in continuity with the iliacus from the inner aspect of the iliac wing. Beyond the fracture the rugine reaches the brim of the true pelvis. The iliac fossa is packed with a large swab.

The external oblique aponeurosis is incised 2 cm above the superficial inguinal ring and the inguinal canal is opened; the spermatic cord is then isolated and a tape is passed round it.

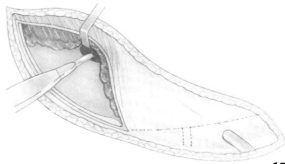

15

16

The short tendinous fibres of the origin of the internal oblique and transversus abdominis from the inguinal ligament are identified and cleaned. The scalpel divides either the tendinous fibres or the inguinal ligament itself, leaving above it enough fibrous tissue for the later repair. It enters the sheath of the iliopsoas muscle, where the femoral nerve must be located and safeguarded.

Near the anterior superior iliac spine the incision into the origin of internal oblique and transversus abdominis muscles is performed with great care, and further dissection in this region reveals and safeguards the lateral cutaneous nerve of the thigh, whose position is a little variable.

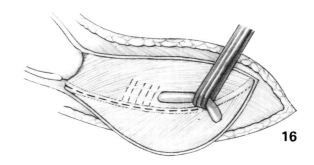

16

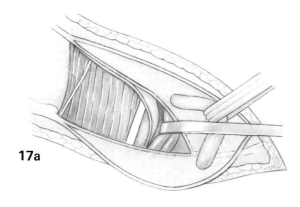

17a

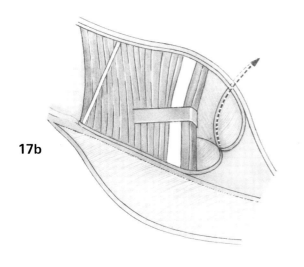

17b

17 a & b

A normal thickening (*1*) of the psoas fascia between the inguinal ligament and the anterior border of the iliac bone (*2*) is then isolated by sharp dissection, and cut carefully because it separates the femoral nerve from the external iliac artery. This step is essential and has to be followed by the detachment of the iliac fascia along the brim of the true pelvis (*3*), so as to provide wide access to that cavity.

The iliopsoas muscle, the femoral nerve, and the lateral cutaneous nerve of the thigh are encircled with another tape.

18

Medial to the femoral vessels the conjoint tendon and the transversalis fascia are divided and the retropubic space is entered and packed with a swab.

The vessels are mobilized gently with the finger in order not to damage lymphatics unnecessarily. The great vessels are encircled with a third tape.

When necessary, the tendon of the rectus abdominis can be divided about 1 cm from the pubis.

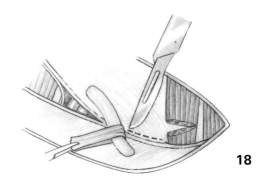

18

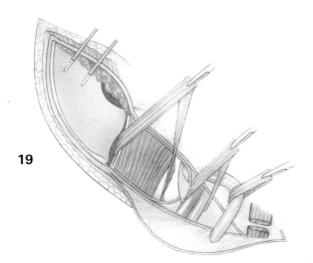

19

19

One or two Steinmann pins are driven into the sacro-iliac region to act as abdominal retractors.

By manipulating the tapes one can gain access to different parts of the pelvis: (a) medial to the spermatic cord one can reach the inner part of the pubic ramus and the pubic symphysis; (b) between the cord and the vessels, the outer part of the pubic ramus and the obturator vessels and nerve are accessible; and (c) between the vessels and the iliopsoas the middle part of the iliopectineal line can be reached and deep to this the quadrilateral surface that extends to the greater sciatic notch. Finally, lateral to the iliopsoas, the iliac fossa is widely exposed, the sacro-iliac joint can be reached and the anterior aspect of the sacrum can also be freed.

20

In most cases it is not difficult to extract the head from the pelvis but the best way to keep it steady while assembly and fixation of the fragments are performed is to apply lateral traction. This can be done by making a small cut over the ridge between the gluteus medius and vastus lateralis and fixing a femoral head extractor into the bone here; it should be inserted, and pulled on, in the line of the neck of the femur and traction is maintained by an assistant or a device attached to the table.

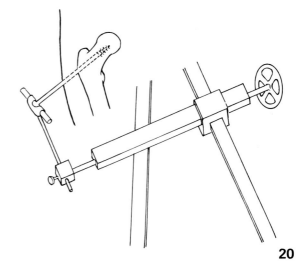

20

Replacement and fixation of fracture

If there is still a part of the articular crescent in its right place and attached to the wing it consists of the whole or a part of the posterior wall and a more or less important part of the roof, the fracture is of the anterior column type, either isolated or associated with a transverse fracture of the posterior column.

The head is replaced against the remaining part of the articular crescent, aided by both longitudinal and lateral traction.

21a, b & c

The fragments of the anterior column are then manipulated by means of forceps, or pushed directly into their normal position; a lever inserted in a fracture-line may facilitate this. A large fragment of the anterior column may be seized by a forceps astride either the crest of the ilium or the anterior border of the ilium between the anterior spines.

The correction achieved, a few screws are inserted from the anterior fragments to the intact posterior part of the roof or to the posterior column. Then the plates must be shaped. The anterior column may be fixed by one or more plates screwed along the superior or inner aspect of the iliac crest, in the iliac fossa, or along the superior aspect of the iliopectineal line from the sacro-iliac joint to the pubic symphysis if necessary.

If a fracture-line divides the posterior column, the reduction of its inferior fragment is achieved by direct manipulation of the fragment deep to the brim of the true pelvis, between the vessels and the iliopsoas muscle. Two 90—110 mm long screws are used to fix the fragment; they run parallel to the inner aspect of the bone and they may be used without a plate or to hole one of the plates in place.

If the whole articular crescent is broken and detached from the wing the fracture is a combination of both the anterior and posterior column types.

Combined lateral and longitudinal traction extracts the stove-in hip and keeps the head in approximately the right place; slight over-traction does not matter.

Then the fragments of the anterior column must be assembled as in the case just described.

Very often replacement is achieved by gripping the anterior column with forceps and using a lever in the fracture-line to restore the displaced pieces of bone to their proper relationship.

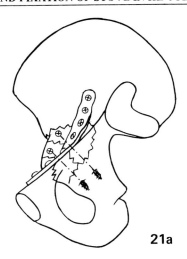

21a

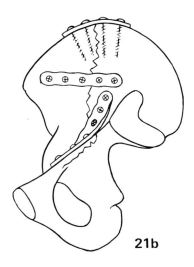

21b

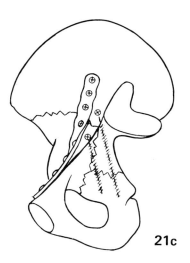

21c

22

The first steps in fixation are achieved by isolated screws, but it is nearly always necessary to use plates as well. One must at this stage take care not to insert screws that can reach the still displaced posterior column and so hold it out of place. When traction is released the head should be in perfect contact with the reconstructed anterior column and the roof.

When this is done, in most cases the posterior column remains displaced but its displacement has been lessened and, by working either between vessels and muscle or between vessels and cord, the posterior column can be pushed outwards and downwards and set perfectly or nearly perfectly in place. Screws to fix the posterior column can be inserted through the plate or apart from it. They need to be 90–120 mm long from the iliac fossa or the pubic ramus either parallel to the inner aspect of the bone, reaching the posterior aspect of the posterior column, or obliquely, to reach the quadrilateral surface.

By moving the hip before closure one can ensure that there are no screws in the joint.

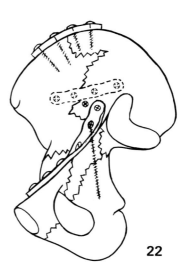

22

If a satisfactory position of the posterior column is impossible to achieve, the anterior incision is closed. The patient must then be placed prone, but this must not be done until the circulation has been stabilized by the replacement of any lost blood. The posterior column is then exposed and fixed from behind in the way that has already been described.

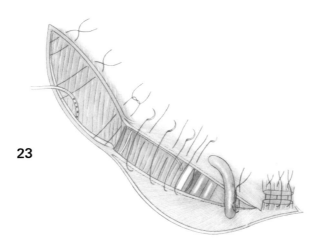

23

23

Closure of the ilio-inguinal incision is anatomical and straightforward, but it must be done with care. Suction drains are inserted into the retropubic space and into the iliac fossa. The abdominal muscles are re-attached. If divided, the anterior sheath of rectus abdominis, the conjoint tendon and the transversalis fascia are sutured. The tapes are removed, and one must see that the artery still pulsates and that the nerves are undamaged. The origins of the internal oblique and transversus abdominis are sutured to the inguinal ligament, using a fish hook type of needle. The spermatic cord is put in place and the external oblique repaired. The inguinal canal, which has been so widely opened is thus securely repaired.

THE LATERAL APPROACH

24

This is performed with the patient on his side on an orthopaedic table. The pelvic support inserted between the thighs of the patient can be moved downwards and upwards and this adjustment, combined with longitudinal traction, allows one to extract the head from the pelvis and keep it in the right position while rebuilding the acetabulum.

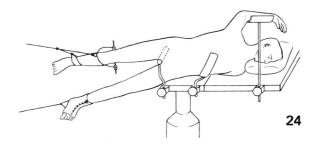

24

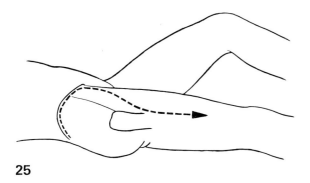

25

25

The skin incision is J-shaped and runs along the whole length of the iliac crest from the posterior superior spine and then downwards from the anterior superior spine to the middle of the thigh in the direction of the lateral side of the patella.

26

The gluteus muscles and the tensor fasciae latae are stripped from the outer aspect of the ilium, but from the anterior superior spine one should work within the sheath of the tensor, along the anterior border of the muscle, in order to avoid most of the branches of the lateral cutaneous nerve of the thigh. The fascia lata is split down to the end of the incision.

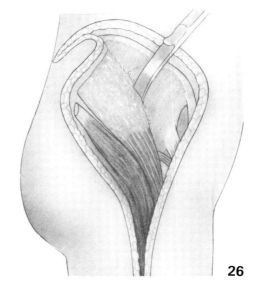

26

27

As the stripping of the gluteus muscles from the ilium progresses the articular capsule is reached along its anterior and superior aspects; these are also stripped, giving access to the anterior border of the greater trochanter. The tendon of gluteus minimus is then cut close to the greater trochanter, followed by the tendon of gluteus medius, which is cut close to the lateral aspect of the greater trochanter. This makes a large, thick flap containing the three gluteus muscles, the tensor fasciae latae, their blood and nerve supplies. The flap is retracted backwards to give access to the posterior part of the hip joint, which is covered by the external rotators. Piriformis and obturator internus are cut and marked by a stitch, as in a posterior approach, and the special retractor can then be inserted into either sciatic notch.

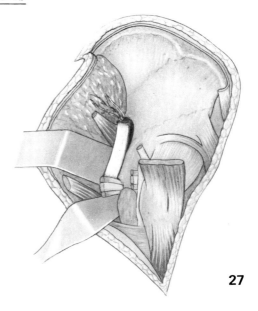

27

28

This approach gives access to the entire blade of the ilium, the whole posterior column up to the upper pole of the ischial tuberosity and to the anterior column, but not beyond the body of the pubis. One can strip the iliacus and gain access to the iliac fossa up to the iliopectineal line, but it is not easy to work there.

The approach is advisable for:

(1) transverse fracture passing through the roof of the acetabulum;

(2) transverse fractures associated with fractures of the anterior column and;

(3) some fractures of both anterior and posterior columns.

It is particularly useful in mal-united cases when it is decided not to rebuild the inferior part of the anterior column.

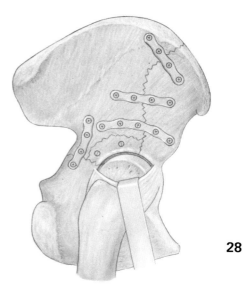

28

Closure

The wound is closed by re-attaching the gluteal muscles and two or three suction drains should be used.

POSTOPERATIVE CARE

The patient stays in bed for 10—15 days.

Passive exercises of the reconstructed hip begin on the third day.

Antibiotics are given for 2 days before and 8 days after an ilio-inguinal approach.

Anticoagulants are used in all cases.

Walking without weight-bearing is allowed from the fifteenth day.

The return to full weight-bearing usually requires 75—90 days according to x-ray appearances.

[*The illustrations for this Chapter on Display, Correction and Fixation of Stove-in Hip Joints were drawn by Mr. F. Price.*]

Fractures of the Shafts of the Long Bones

P. S. London, M.B.E., F.R.C.S.
Surgeon, Birmingham Accident Hospital

The methods of fixing fractures are dealt with in the Chapters on 'General Techniques of Internal Fixation of Fractures', pages 400–420 and 'Closed Intramedullary Nailing of the Femur and Tibia', pages 603–611. It remains to indicate the approaches that can be used when applying these methods to fractures of the shafts of the humerus, radius and ulna, femur and tibia.

FRACTURES WITH WOUNDS AND OTHER SKIN DAMAGE

This is no place to argue the case for or against internal fixation, suffice to say that if it is to be carried out there are some useful rules.

These remarks apply to both limbs, but particularly to the tibia, where skin is often seriously and extensively damaged as well as being very close to bone.

15 & 16

The surgeon should try to add as little damage as possible to skin that has already been injured; in other words, a wound, grazed skin and skin from which the fat has been torn should, whenever possible, be included in the incision. What may seem to be a much safer policy of keeping one's incision away from grazed and crushed skin carries the danger that it will cut off the blood supply to intervening skin. The surgeon will therefore be well advised to examine the skin carefully before deciding where to cut it.

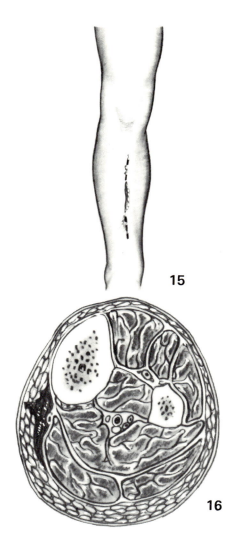

15

16

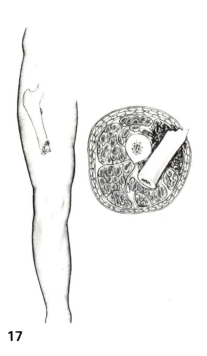

17

17

Puncture wounds

These should be probed with an instrument or even a finger in order to determine their direction or the extent of undermining and to find out whether the subcutaneous fat has been crushed: such crushing can be looked upon as the deep part of an incision to expose the fracture. If a small puncture wound is not to be included in a surgical incision, the surgeon may be well advised not to excise its edges because he may then find that, though still small, the wound cannot easily or safely be closed with stitches whereas an untouched puncture often heals uneventfully, if slowly.

18

Bruising

Bruising often thickens the skin and the soft tissues beneath it, but it can also be accompanied by disruption of the soft tissues, as by a fragment of bone that has not quite breached the skin. Such a bruise has a palpably soft centre and if the surgeon cuts through it he will find himself in a blood filled cavity with the fracture in its depths. It offers him as sure an approach as if he had gone through the wound of an open fracture. If he is daunted by the fact that such an approach will be from an unfamiliar and otherwise hazardous direction he can be re-assured by the thought that if a bone propelled blindly and by great force has done no damage to nerves and blood vessels the surgeon who uses the clearing made by the bone should do no damage either.

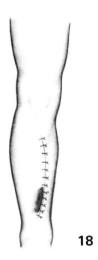

18

Grazed or crushed skin

This may die but if it remains dry and healthy there is no particular need to cut it out. Thus, the surgeon can justifiably cut through such skin and be prepared to leave the stitches for much longer than usual if there is any delay in healing.

It should not need emphasizing that sound decisions in these difficult cases require judgement based upon experience and enhanced by an understanding of how best to preserve the healing power of that most valuable wrapping for fractures — the skin.

Reference

Henry A. K. (1957). *Extensile Exposure,* 2nd Edition. Edinburgh and London: Livingstone

[*The illustrations for this Chapter on Fractures of the Shafts of the Long Bones were drawn by Mr. G. Lyth.*]

General Techniques of Internal Fixation of Fractures

R. L. Batten, F.R.C.S.
Consultant Orthopaedic Surgeon, General Hospital, Birmingham
and Royal Orthopaedic Hospital, Birmingham

PRE-OPERATIVE

Indications

One important indication for internal fixation of a fracture is to enable a patient to get out of bed soon and so to avoid the complications of long recumbency; this is especially indicated with fractures of the neck of the femur in the elderly. A second important indication is a fracture that enters or is near to a joint; it is then desirable to restore the shape of the articular surfaces in an attempt to reduce the degree of degenerative change. A third indication is that more than one segment of the same limb is involved and a fourth occurs with multiple injuries, when it is important to neutralize as many fractures of long bones as possible so as to make nursing easier. Internal fixation also plays a major part in the management of non-union, whether this has followed conservatively treated fractures or those which have been operated upon primarily. Other indications are pathological fractures and the restoration of the shape of bones where this is necessary for the sake of function or appearance, as for example, in the face, the forearm of adults, the hand and the foot and the protection of soft tissues that need repair. The ultimate example of this is the re-attachment of a severed part, but there are many severe injuries for which the risks of internal fixation are less than those of leaving fractures movable.

In general, the techniques of internal fixation require the use of wires, nails and screws either independently or in combination with metal plates. None of these implants should be used unless the conditions for internal fixation are all right. These conditions include satisfactory sterility of the theatre, the instruments and the implants themselves. The surgeon must make sure that he has the full complement of equipment necessary to undertake this sort of work and he should also possess the necessary judgement and skill. *Internal fixation of fractures is a potentially dangerous procedure and can produce very bad results unless high standards of aseptic technique can be ensured.*

Although a sterile air enclosure in the operating theatre may reduce the dangers of infection, these expensive devices are not widely available; safe operations can be carried on in normal theatres, as long as they are not also used for treating surgically dirty cases of any kind. The preparation of the patient's skin and the surgeon's hands is most safely done by the application of 0·5 per cent chlorhexidine in 95 per cent alcohol with 2 minutes' rubbing of the surgeon's hands, and rubbing this solution into the patient's skin with the gloved hand as a separate procedure (Lowbury and Lilley, 1975). It is important to isolate the area of operation as far as possible from the anaesthetist and the rest of the patient's body and the movement of persons inside the operating theatre should be reduced to a minimum. Whenever possible, it is desirable to use a bloodless field by applying a pneumatic tourniquet above the site of operation; it is probably better not to exsanguinate the limb, but simply to elevate it before the tourniquet is inflated.

KÜNTSCHER NAILING

The open method of Küntscher nailing is preferred by many surgeons on the grounds that a really accurate reduction of the fracture is more quickly and easily achieved, and one can be sure that no soft tissue is present between the bone ends. The other advantages are that x-ray control is not necessary during the operation, and that the large haematoma which is always present at the site of a fracture of the shaft of the femur can be evacuated and suction drains inserted.

Before engaging in medullary fixation, the full armamentarium must be available. There must be a full set of nails of all diameters and lengths, and each nail should be sharpened and slotted at both ends. A full set of reamers should be provided and the best are those in which there is a hole in the handle of the same diameter as the cutting end. This will ensure that the nail will not be too wide for the reamed-out channel.

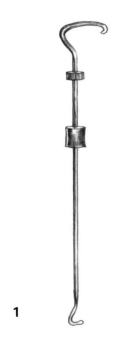

1

1 & 2

Extractors are long rods with a hook at the end and the best design has a sliding cylindrical hammer on the rod. It is important to have two of these, lest the hook break off one. To avoid the predicament in which a nail becomes jammed because of an error in technique, it is wise to have a blacksmith's hacksaw with a high-speed steel blade in the operating set, so that the nail may be sawn off short if it cannot be driven down fully.

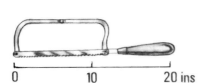

0   10   20 ins

2

TECHNIQUE FOR THE FEMUR

It is seldom possible to employ this method of treatment on the femur with the help of a tourniquet, so it is important to have enough blood available and an intravenous infusion running before beginning the operation. Diathermy and suction apparatus must also be arranged.

3, 4 & 5

The patient should be lying on the unaffected side with the injured thigh extended and separated from the underlying flexed limb by a macintosh-covered pillow. The limb should be securely towelled distal to the fracture so that it can be manipulated to help in the reduction of the fracture. A lateral longitudinal incision is made and the fascia lata is divided in the line of the incision. Using rake retractors the vastus lateralis is then split and retracted backwards and forwards to expose the shaft of the femur and the fracture. A number of perforating vessels must be picked up and coagulated, and good haemostasis must be secured before the fracture is approached.

The lower end of the upper fragment is caught with a bone clamp and brought out into the wound, care being taken not to retract or damage the periosteum around its end. A hook should not be used for this purpose because if, as is not unusual, there are cracks leading away from the main fracture, the hook may pull off another piece of bone.

6

Haematoma and small bone fragments are removed before a reamer is passed into the open end of the upper fragment. The size of the reamer is judged according to the appearance on the x-ray films and should be the largest size that will be accommodated by the narrowest part of the medullary canal.

The canal is reamed up to the greater trochanter and the cortex perforated here, after which the reamer can be removed. If it passes very easily, the next size of nail should be chosen, because it must be the thickest that can be firmly gripped in the medullary canal. The reamer is then withdrawn and a guide wire passed proximally through the hole in the trochanter and out through the skin of the buttock. This guide wire must not be too thick for the size of the nail that has been chosen for the fixation. A transverse incision 1·25 inches long is made over the buttock at the point of exit of the guide wire, and the chosen nail is passed into the femur along the guide wire. The

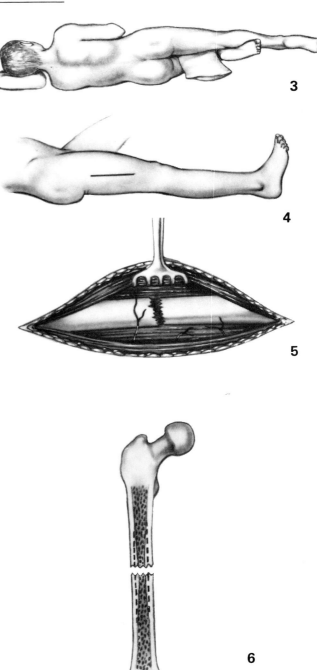

length of nail may be estimated by passing a guide wire down to the knee from the fracture and measuring the length of this segment, as well as passing the same guide wire up to the trochanter and measuring that length. The sum of the two lengths with an addition of 0·5 inches is the right length to choose for the fixation of a straightforward transverse or short oblique fracture.

7, 8 & 9

However, if the shaft of the femur is more than slightly bowed, a nail of this length may jam or it may perforate the cortex. It is desirable that whenever possible the nail should be long enough to get a purchase in the firm cancellous bone above the intercondylar notch. The nail is hammered down the medullary canal, directed by the guide wire, until it projects about 0·5 inches from the lower end of the upper fragment. The guide wire should then be removed, and using suitable bone-holding forceps of the Hey Groves type, the bone ends can be manipulated so that the lower end of the nail is engaged in the distal fragment. This may be most easily effected by flexing the femur so that the fragments are edge to edge and the projecting end of the nail engages in the open end of the lower fragment, after which the femur can be straightened again and the position held while the nail is driven finally home. When the upper end of the nail reaches the skin of the buttock, a cylindrical punch must be applied to it, so as to drive it down to the trochanter while protecting the skin. Half an inch of the nail should be left projecting because this has the slot that facilitates removal of the nail. At this point it is sensible to have an anteroposterior x-ray film taken of the knee to ensure that the nail is far enough down and not too far. A nail which ends 4 inches short of the knee joint gets an indifferent hold in the lower fragment, and the required degree of rigidity cannot be obtained. If the x-ray appearance is satisfactory, it must now be decided whether the fracture itself has enough resistance to rotational displacement to be left, or whether an additional antirotational measure is needed.

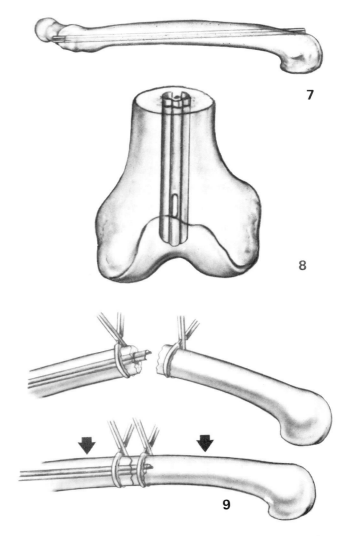

7

8

9

Supplementary fixation. Plating

10

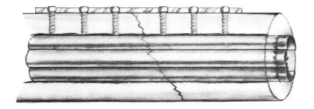

10

If there are strong bony teeth on a fracture of the shaft of the femur these can prevent rotation at the fracture but with oblique fractures and smooth transverse ones a simple medullary nail cannot be expected to do this. In this case it is a useful practice to apply a short stainless steel plate on the lateral side of the femur to span the fracture, and the A.O. (Arbeitsgemeinschaft für Osteosynthesefragen) dynamic compression plate is admirably suited to this. It does not require any further division of muscles to apply it, and being of a self-compressing type, the fracture gap itself can be snugly closed by its use. Single-cortex screws are adequate if they are of the A.O. type, for which the thread is tapped, using the appropriate tap before they are inserted. It is important not to damage the nail with either the drill or the tap while inserting this plate.

11 & 12

In a fracture with a third fragment or of a long oblique type, it may still be possible to get adequate fixation with a medullary nail, but an additional step will be required. This can be either to apply one or two cerclage wires, or to include the third fragment under the antirotation plate applied laterally. Cerclage wires are best passed subperiosteally, using a special curved tubular wire-passer. Having passed this device round the shaft of the bone, a length of stainless steel wire of 1·2 mm diameter can be inserted into the open end of the tube. When the device is removed it leaves the wire encircling the bone. It is often better to pass this same wire round a second time, using the same device and then to twist the ends up firmly with one of the several forms of wire-twister which are available.

The wire should then be cut off short, leaving two or three turns at the most, bent over and hammered home with a punch so that the movement of muscle over it is not disturbed. It may be necessary to put two separate cerclage wires round to hold a long oblique fracture. There is no place for Parham bands, which are often made of indifferent metal and certainly disturb the periosteal blood supply quite markedly.

Before closing the wound, haemostasis must be secured as far as possible, a suction drain should be inserted down to the fracture, and except in very thin young subjects, it is wise to insert another one in the

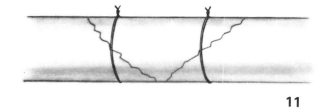

11

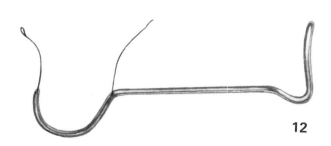

12

subcutaneous layer. The wound is then closed in layers with careful suturing of the skin and it is good practice, especially in females, to use a subcuticular prolene stitch in the skin. It is important to secure the exit points of the drains with a small length of strapping lest they become displaced while the patient is turned and lifted on to the trolley.

Postoperative care

13

The injured leg should be placed on a specially high Braun's frame with the knee well flexed for at least 48 hr.

The intravenous infusion can be taken down when it is certain that the blood lost has been fully replaced, though it must be expected that some loss from the suction drains will continue for 10 hr or so. To make sure that the drains are working efficiently, they should be withdrawn 0·5 inches in each hour because otherwise they may be blocked by soft tissue sucked into the holes. When each tube has been shortened so that the holes appear at the skin, the drains can be removed. Active exercises of the knee and foot can begin on the second postoperative day and the patient is often able to leave hospital within a week, walking on the good leg with crutches, and swinging the injured one. Comminuted fractures of the femur at whatever level are seldom suitable for medullary nailing and are better treated by applying a dynamic compression plate of suitable size.

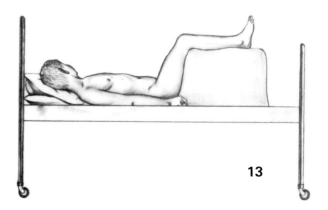

13

TIBIA

14 & 15

Medullary nailing has a place with fractures of the tibia, but it is not so often indicated as in the femur. Here again, the selection of the case is important and nailing should be considered for transverse or short oblique fractures of the shaft without comminution; the open method is the safest. The first step is to arrange the leg so that the knee is flexed with the foot held on the table by a sandbag to provide resistance to the hammering when the nail is driven home. A vertical incision is made alongside the patellar tendon and then in the mid-line through the tendon to reach the anterior edge of the upper end of the tibia, just in front of the articular surface. The medullary canal is then entered with a special triangular-pointed awl, opening up a hole wide enough for the passage of the appropriate guide wire. The fracture is then exposed by a longitudinal incision over the tibial crest and the guide wire passed down and directed into the lower fragment, holding the position either with a bone clamp alone or with a small plate held to each fragment with a pair of clamps. The guide wire is passed down until it reaches the level of the medial malleolus, when it is safer to confirm its position by a radiograph. A nail of this length is selected.

The medullary nail for the tibia has a curve at the upper end adapted to the shape of the tibia, and it is driven down the guide wire by gentle blows of the hammer, making sure that it goes across the fracture and does not impinge on the cortex of the lower fragment. When it is completely home, it should be almost flush with the cortex in the upper end but a small length must be left projecting to facilitate its removal.

Both incisions are then closed using suction drains. Active movements can be begun on the first day after operation. With a transverse fracture and good alignment is often possible to allow weight-bearing within the first 6 or 8 weeks.

A.O. advocate reaming out the medullary canal of both tibia and femur to a wide enough diameter to allow the passage of a very large nail to give full rigidity. This technique needs special instruments, including a flexible, powered reamer with increasing diameters of cutting head, and it gives excellent results in their hands. Although the endosteal blood supply is cut off by this technique, enough blood supply travels longitudinally in the cortex to maintain the nutrition, and there is no doubt that the extra rigidity allows rapid and uneventful healing in most cases. It

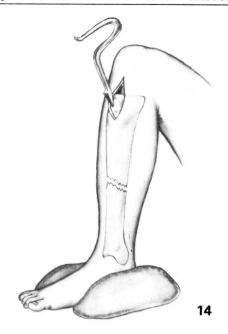

14

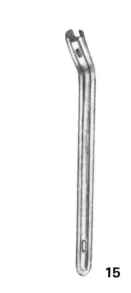

15

must, however, be admitted that much experience is needed to make this procedure safe, and it has no place in segmental fractures nor when there is much comminution. It is quite possible with a segmental fracture for the reamer to spin the middle fragment round, destroying all its soft tissue attachment and therefore killing it.

22a, b & c

A.O. cortex screws have threads designed for cortical bone, which extend from the neck of the screw to its tip. Cancellous screws have wider threads which only extend for part of the screw length from the tip, the remaining length being smooth. All these screws apply interfragmentary compression. Malleolar screws have a drill point so that they can be driven in without a drill hole after the cortex has been perforated.

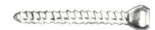

22a

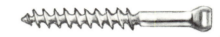

22b

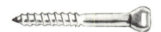

22c

23a & b

Compression plates are often used in combination with independent screws which are not passed through the plate, but pull together independent fragments of bone using the so-called lag principle. The 'lag' screw is inserted so that its tip can obtain a purchase on the cortex of the bone farther from its point of insertion. The threads of the screw nearest to the head must not bite into the bone if compression is to be achieved. Therefore, a hole is drilled in this first cortex wider than the outside diameter of the screw threads. The drill bit is changed to one which matches the core diameter of the screw and this is used to make the hole in the far cortex. This hole is then tapped with the appropriate tap. When the screw is inserted, the threads furthest from the screw head will engage the far cortex and as the screw is tightened, compression will be achieved. This is particularly true with 'butterfly' fragments of the tibia and with comminuted fractures of the upper and lower end of the femur.

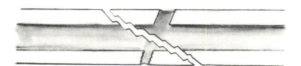

23a

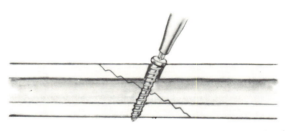

23b

With a single long spiral fracture of the lowest third of the tibia especially, screws may be used by themselves without the addition of a plate. The screws are then inserted to give compression and as the fracture is spiral they will lie in a spiral pattern themselves. With a butterfly fragment, however, a combination of independent screws and a plate with its own screws is necessary.

In a typical case the operation proceeds as follows.

An incision is made longitudinally just lateral to the crest of the tibia so that the suture line does not lie over the plate. It is important to make a long enough incision to avoid the need for vigorous retraction, and a long straight incision is better than a curved or S-shaped incision. The fracture is exposed, and taking care not to disturb soft tissue attachments, the broken

surfaces are cleaned of haematoma and any interposed soft tissue. It is determined to which main fragment the butterfly fragment has its major contact and this part of the fracture is then set and fixed with one or more compressing screws. Only one fracture line now remains and this fracture is set and held with bone clamps or a single temporary cerclage wire while the screws are inserted, again to provide compression. It is now important to add a plate to prevent disruptive stresses from falling on the screws themselves. The plate may be one with conical holes, but it is better to use the dynamic compression plate. This plate is applied under slight tension, which gives more rigidity, although the transverse screws are already applying interfragmentary compression. A plate under tension is stronger than an unstressed plate.

24, 25 & 26

Another good indication for fixation by plate and screws is a segmental fracture of a long bone. After exposure and setting of the fracture and temporary fixation with clamps and a loose plate, the definitive plate is applied to the middle segment first and screwed in place. Compression can then be applied at each end to bring both the upper and lower fragments into rigid contact with the intervening fragment. When there is an oblique fracture it is important finally to apply a screw near the middle of the plate to pass obliquely from one fragment to the other. This screw should also be applied so as to exert compression though all the other screws are inserted in the ordinary way, with threads biting in both cortices.

In the femur especially, a segmental fracture may have the two fracture lines so far apart that a single plate cannot span them both. It is then better to apply two plates, the upper one joining the uppermost fragment to the middle fragment, and the lower plate the middle to the distal fragment. Note that as the distances between all the screw holes in the A.O. plates are equal, it is possible to arrange that the screws inter-digitate and do not abut against each other when using two plates that overlap.

Positions of plates and contouring

In the case of the tibia, a plate applied to the proximal third or distal third will need to be bent to produce the correct alignment and, because the subcutaneous surface of the tibia, which is where plates are most often applied, has a twist at both ends, the plates used there must be appropriately contoured. A straight plate applied to the lower part of the femur will have to be contoured, but it is often better to apply a

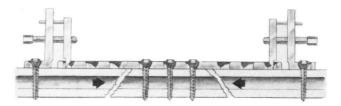

24

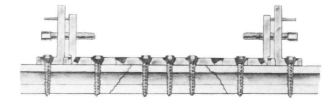

25

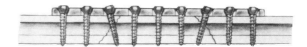

26

condylar plate, of which the 95° angle between blade and plate usually fits well without further bending. It is important to contour plates accurately with a power-full plate-bender, so that the bend can be placed between screw holes, and not, as is usual with the ordinary manual plate-benders, through the screw holes themselves. This is not so important with the dynamic compression plate because the spherical geometry of the screw/plate interface allows some alteration without disturbing the purchase obtainable by the screw head.

27-30

It must always be determined on which surface the plate will have its main effect and, when applying a plate under tension, it is necessary to discover which is the tension surface of the bone. This may be altered by the fracture shape, but in general the tension surface is on the anterior surface of the tibia and on the lateral surface of the femur. In the case of the tibia a compromise solution is to apply a plate on the medial surface, because the crest is unsuitable. A fracture at the middle of the shaft of either of these bones can usually be fixed with a straight plate which does not need contouring to make it fit. However, when it is applied under compression the effect will be to open up the fracture line on the far side of the bone, unless a precautionary step is taken. This involves bending the plate at its mid-point so that it stands 2 – 3 mm proud of the bone at this point when the bone is straight. When the first two compressing screws are applied adjoining the fracture, the bone is drawn towards the plate, which unbends to fit the bone, and a compressive force is then exerted on the cortex on the far side of the bone as well as under the plate itself. This is a most important step because it is very harmful to apply powerful compression on the cortex just deep to the plate while having a gap which may be of 1 or 2 mm in the cortex on the far side.

There are special needs for modifying the ordinary technique of plating a tibia when the bone is abnormally soft or when the plate has to be applied to the upper or lower end of the bone. To get adequate purchase it may then be necessary to use cancellous screws, which have a special thread to obtain a powerful grip on soft cancellous bone. All A.O. plates are provided with threads in the two holes at each end of the plate to take the wide threads of the cancellous screws. With the dynamic compression plate, cancellous screws can be inserted through any of the holes. Should a normal cortex screw fail to get a purchase on the far cortex, it can be replaced by a screw 2 mm longer, and a small special nut applied to its end, so that a good grip can be obtained beyond the far cortex.

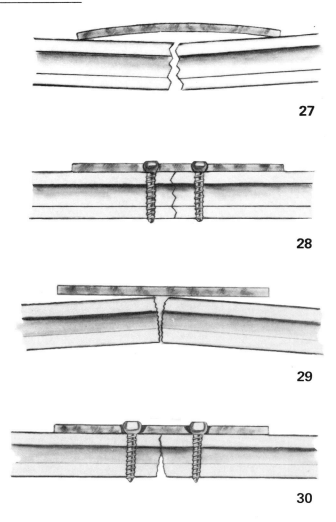

27

28

29

30

Postoperative care

It must be understood that rigid fixation with compression does not allow earlier weight-bearing than any other form of fixation and this must be explained to the patient, preferably both before operation and afterwards.

FRACTURES OF THE UPPER LIMB

These are also amenable to rigid fixation by the application of appropriate compression plates. Tibial plates are adequate for the forearm, and in normal sized adults it is wise to fix any fracture of the shaft of the radius or ulna with a six-hole plate to make sure that there are at least five cortices held on each fragment. It is here that the dynamic compression plate has a special advantage because there is no need for the extra exposure to allow the compression device for an ordinary A.O. plate to be applied. The incision depends on the shape of the fracture but most cases are better exposed using the posterior incision of Henry for the ulna and the anterolateral exposure for the radius. The most important indications for rigid fixation of forearm fractures are the Monteggia fracture for which the ulna must be fixed and the Galeazzi fracture, for which the radius must be fixed.

TIMING OF THE OPERATION

The forearm

Though there is some discussion about the usefulness of delaying internal fixation of many fractures of long bones, it is hard to justify delay with a Galeazzi or Monteggia fracture because of the difficulty of maintaining alignment and length of forearm bones by any other means. A comminuted fracture extending into the wrist joint may need to have a transverse screw applied as well as a dorsal plate.

The humerus

For the shaft of the humerus, when internal fixation is indicated, as with an unstable fracture when there are accompanying major injuries elsewhere, or when an earlier return to work is for some special reason necessary, a compression plate is justified. In an adult it is better to use the femoral DCP for the management of this fracture and it is wise to use the posterior Henry approach for fractures of the shaft of the bone. Fractures of the neck of the humerus are usually managed

without operation, but when there are other fractures in the same limb or multiple injuries, it may be necessary to fix this fracture internally.

31

The special T-plate designed for this particular area is then ideal. It is inserted either via a deltoid-splitting incision or an approach through the deltopectoral groove, depending on the shape and type of the fracture. It is particularly helpful for fracture-dislocation of the humeral head. The upper cancellous screws get a good purchase in the head and the compression is applied distally, using the compressor on the shaft of the bone, because the T-plate for this use has not yet been provided with oval holes.

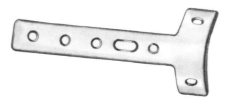

31

It is important to use one drain in the deep layers and one subcutaneously. Closure is in layers, restoring the muscles and nerves to their anatomical positions which may mean, in an upper third fracture, sliding the radial nerve back over the plate when this has been screwed home. There are some situations where the radial nerve is in jeopardy if a plate has to be applied near it, and it is then helpful to transplant the nerve through the fracture line to lie on the opposite surface of the bone so that the plate can be comfortably screwed home.

Postoperative care of upper limb fractures consists of elevating the limb for the first 24 hr and then encouraging active exercises.

APPLICATION OF COMPRESSION TO FRACTURES NEAR TO AND INVOLVING JOINTS

32-35

Lower end of the humerus

With T, Y or other comminuted fractures of the lower end of the humerus, compression techniques play an important part. The patient is first anaesthetized and placed prone on the operating table with the arm supported on an arm board, and the forearm hanging down and securely draped. It is then convenient if there is no fracture in this area to expose the lower end of the humerus by osteotomy of the olecranon, and turning it and the attached triceps upwards. The re-attachment of the olecranon is made easier by first drilling a longitudinal hole through it and into the shaft of the ulna, and tapping this for the cancellous screw that will be inserted finally. The olecranon and triceps now being held proximally with a towel-clip, the whole of the lower end of the humerus can be examined and the ulnar nerve retracted with a tape and watched carefully throughout. The fracture can be repositioned and held temporarily with Kirschner wires while the various components are fixed. With a T-fracture, the first step is to insert a transverse screw to close up the vertical component of the fracture. The re-assembled lower fragment can then be attached to the shaft with a small one-third tubular contoured plate applied to each condylar fragment. When these plates lie on the side of the shaft, compression can be applied by drilling the holes for the screws at the upper end of each hole in the plates, so that when the screws are driven home, compression is applied to the fracture complex. With comminuted fractures, additional screws may be needed at various points but it is usually possible to reconstruct the articular surface of both the capitellum and the trochlea so that the degree of post-traumatic arthrosis is minimal. When the operation on the humerus is completed, the olecranon is replaced and a long cancellous screw is inserted in the hole previously drilled down the shaft. A small transverse hole is drilled in the shaft of the ulna distal to the osteotomy site, and a wire passed through this and upwards as a figure-of-8 round the neck of the screw in the olecranon. This wire is twisted up, the ends buried and the screw driven fully home.

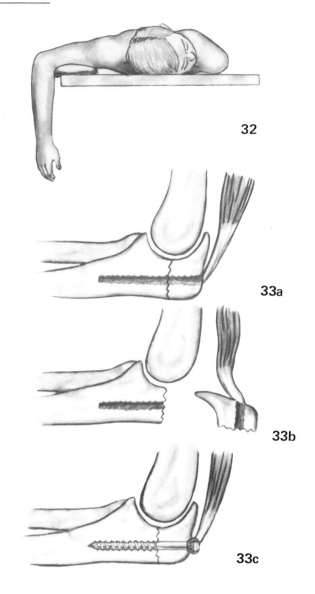

32

33a

33b

33c

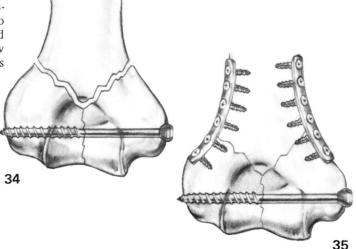

34

35

T-fractures of the knee

Whether these occur in the femur or the tibia, they are well fixed by transverse cancellous screws inserted so as to close snugly the vertical fracture but each fragment may need an additional plate to exert compression axially and thus to stabilize the other parts of these fracture complexes. The special condylar plate has an application both at the lower end of the femur and the upper end of the tibia.

The ankle

Uni-, bi- and tri-malleolar fractures can all be treated by internal fixation, which has the advantage of allowing active movement, as well as making more certain of accurate restoration of the articular surfaces. An especially designed malleolar screw is self-drilling and exerts compression because it is not fully threaded. It can be inserted into the medial malleolus or from the fibula into the tibia in order to close the ankle mortice.

36, 37 & 38

With a comminuted or an oblique fracture causing shortening of the fibula, it is important first to restore the full length of the fibula; this may be done either with one or more small transverse lag screws or by the application of a one-third tubular plate, contoured to fit the outer side of the fibula. The medial malleolus can be satisfactorily fixed by a single malleolar screw, but because the fragment may pivot round this screw, a Kirschner wire should be driven alongside the screw to prevent this. A third posterior tibial fragment can be well fixed by a cancellous screw inserted from the front of the tibia, so that its thread is entirely within the small posterior fragment, and draws it firmly into place.

Suction drains are used after any of these operations.

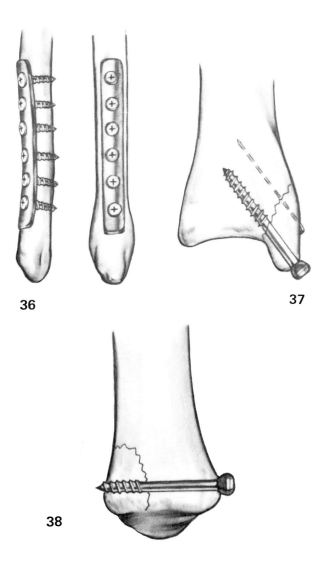

36

37

38

39

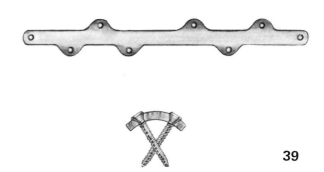

39

Plating without compression

Most of the plates that have been used without any attempt at compression are incapable of fixing fractures rigidly. Rigidity can be achieved without compression by using the specially designed and unusually strong plate of Hicks. As with compression plates, however, this needs to be used with both skill and a clear understanding of its proper application. Its strength makes it difficult to alter its shape and its bulk may make it difficult to close skin over it when the plate is subcutaneous.

With these plates it is customary to use self-tapping screws and a drill the size of the core of the screw. Such screws grip well in strong bone, from which they may be impossible to remove later, but they get only a poor grip in soft spongy bone.

Removal of plates

Whether or not plates are used for compression, it is desirable to remove them eventually, partly because of their liability to corrosion (which is not very high in the case of stainless steel plates) and also because a strong plate bears some of the load, which prevents the normal stresses from falling on the bone deep to the plate. These stresses help the bone to remodel and regain its natural strength. It is, therefore, wise to remove plates from the lower limb after 18—24 months, and from the upper limb between 12 and 15 months in most instances. After the removal of a plate the patient must exercise cautiously for some weeks, while the internal architecture of the bone is restored. It has been found that the functional assessment of the limb improves noticeably after the removal of a plate, but in most cases the final functional result depends on the severity of the fracture.

INTERNAL FIXATION USING WIRES

In addition to cerclage wiring, which has an occasional place for fixing a 'butterfly' fragment to the shaft as mentioned above, the main place for wire fixation is in fractures of the olecranon, fractures of the patella and for fixing back comminuted fractures of the greater trochanter of the femur, and of the medial or lateral malleolus. For these fractures the wire is used as a tension wire to resist distraction forces.

Fractures of the olecranon

40

A simple oblique fracture of the olecranon can be conveniently fixed with one compressing screw inserted from the point of the olecranon, directed obliquely downwards and forwards to gain a grip on the coronoid process but with other fractures of the olecranon, especially when there is some comminution or the fracture is transverse, it is better to use two Kirschner wires and a length of flexible wire as described below.

41a & b

A transverse 2 mm hole is drilled through the ulna distal to the site of the fracture. Two Kirschner wires are then driven downwards through the tip of the olecranon parallel with each other but their proximal ends are left projecting an inch or two. A length of wire is then prepared with a small eye at its mid-point and one end is passed through the drill hole and brought up to go round the end of the Kirschner wires. The small eye in the wire is left on one side and the loose ends are twisted together on the other side. The loose ends and the eye in the wire can be tightened simultaneously, thereby applying an equal stress on each side. The ends are buried and the Kirschner wires are each bent to 180°, cut short and hammered flush with the bone from above.

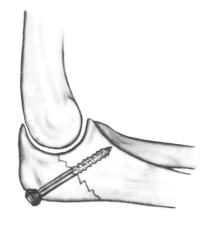

40

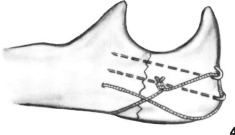

41a

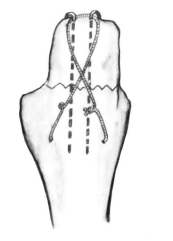

41b

42

Kirschner wires and tension wires can be used in exactly the same manner for awkward fractures of the greater trochanter of the femur, for the medial and lateral malleolus and for the patella.

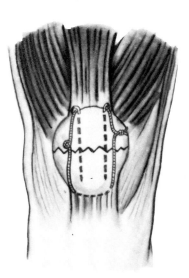

42

Kirschner wires

Kirschner wires may be used for internal fixation of small fragments and especially in phalanges and metacarpals and metatarsals as medullary fixators. It is best to use an open method because it can be difficult to achieve the desired position of the fracture and the wire in any other way. An incision is made over the fractured bone, retracting the extensor tendon, and the wire is then passed through the medullary canal of the distal fragment in a distal direction. When it has emerged through the skin at the appropriate point, it is possible to pass it proximally to its full extent while holding the fracture reduced. Wires may be left buried under the skin or better left bent over or protected with a cork outside the skin over the flexed joint. When the fractures are firm, all the wires are removed and the joints can be exercised.

This method is not very satisfactory with comminuted or oblique fractures and particularly for metacarpals, the plates provided in the A.O. small fragment set give better fixation for irregular fractures and especially those near the joints. For severely smashed hands, it is sometimes helpful to hold some alignment between the metacarpal bones by drilling a Kirschner wire transversely through all the metacarpals; more than one wire may be used in this manner. It may then be possible to institute early activity to keep the metacarpophalangeal joints in action.

Kirschner wires are also useful by themselves for fractures of the epicondyles, condyles or supracondylar region of the lower end of the humerus, especially in childhood. Fractures of the medial or lateral epicondyles in children are safely fixed with temporary Kirschner wires which are left projecting under the skin and removed as soon as stability is obtained. This may be done quite safely without interfering with the growth of the part. In the occasional case of supracondylar fracture for which open reduction is required, it is quite satisfactory to pass a Kirschner wire through each epicondyle in a proximal direction, crossing over each other and obtaining a purchase in the cortex of the metaphysis on each side. These wires may be removed when the fracture is stable.

Cerclage

Loops of wire wrapped round or partly round a bone offer a useful way of holding spiral fragments together, perhaps supplementing a Küntscher nail, or holding in place fragments that for one reason or another cannot be screwed and, temporarily, for assembling comminuted fractures that are to be fixed by other means. Wire loops used definitively in this way should be double and must be applied and remain snugly against bone all the way round; they are dangerous when they are loose, not because they are too tight.

43 a&b

It is important when using cerclage to employ the right thickness of wire, and it is convenient to have spools prepared for use in the theatre marked 'fibula', 'tibia' and 'femur' respectively. Temporary cerclage is of great value when dealing with comminuted fractures, during the application of a plate, or while screwing fragments together: a single loop suffices for this. The most convenient variety for temporary use during an operation is a fairly stout wire with a small eyelet on one end. This is passed round the bone with the help of a tubular wire-passer and the end is then threaded through the eyelet.

A suitable wire-tightener is applied and the wire bent over to hold the bony fragments together. The wire can be left in place while the plate or screws are applied, having just bent it over to hold the wire in a 180° kink. It can be removed before closing the wound but if a plate is applied on top of the wire, it is important to remove the wire before the screws are finally driven home, lest it becomes trapped and cannot be extracted. It is often possible to apply the plate loosely to the bone and then pass the cerclage wire round both the bone and the plate together, holding the fragments up towards it. When the plate has been screwed home and all is secure, it is a simple matter to cut the wire and remove it, together with the wire-twister (Müller, Allgöwer and Willenegger, 1970).

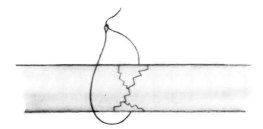

43a

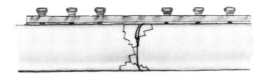

43b

OPEN REDUCTION WITHOUT INTERNAL FIXATION

There are a few occasions when having exposed a fracture it is sufficient to set it in place and close the wound; one such is the overlapped transverse fracture of one or both bones of a child's forearm that has resisted closed manipulation, but even these should be fixed if their shape or a defective hinge makes the fracture unstable in any acceptable position.

EXTERNAL SKELETAL FIXATION

Whenever vessels or nerves are injured and have had to be repaired, it is difficult to hold a fracture by plaster; the soft tissue damage often makes plate or screw fixation impracticable. It is then helpful to have available one or other of the appliances that can give external skeletal fixation. The simplest of these uses two Steinmann pins passed transversely through each of the main fragments of long bones, the ends of the four pins being joined by bars on the medial and lateral sides of the limb. A single pin in each fragment does not prevent movement at the fracture. With a transverse fracture it can be arranged that compression is applied if the lateral bars are provided with thumb screws to push the ends of the Steinmann pins towards each other.

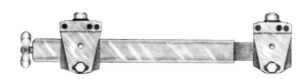

44a

44 a, b & c

The disadvantage of using Steinmann pins is that they may become loose so that pin-track infection is a common complication. This may be avoided by using screws rather than pins and the best apparatus for this purpose is that devised by Wagner; it was originally intended for leg-lengthening operations, but has been found to be just as good for holding a fracture rigidly or for applying compression. This instrument consists of a very strong square-section bar enclosed in a square-section tube, provided with clamps that can be held rigidly at each end by nuts. Screws are driven into the bone, which has been drilled with a 3·6 mm drill. The screws get a very powerful purchase on the bone, penetrating both cortices. Two screws are placed in each main fragment and each pair can be set well apart to allow for dressings and skin grafting procedures or to leave a wound open, if necessary. Each pair of screws is held rigidly by the special clamps to the inside bar and the outside tube of the external fixator. The nuts can be loosened to allow adjustment of the angle of the screws and then tightened to get a very powerful purchase. The fracture is then rigidly stabilized by the outside bar.

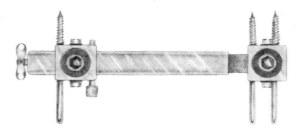

44b

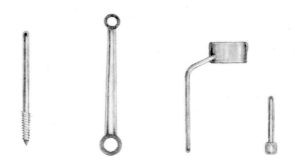

44c

INTERNAL FIXATION IN THE TREATMENT OF NON-UNION

Only the principles are to be dealt with here.

(*1*) Ensure rigid fixation.

(*2*) Do not disturb the fracture except to correct unacceptable deformity.

45

(*3*) Bulging callus may be removed with a chisel for the sake of letting a plate fit snugly, but a plate may be bent to fit offset fragments, which may themselves be trimmed with advantage.

(*4*) Bone grafts should be used to span a gap or a length of dead bone, that is bone that has no callus fixing it.

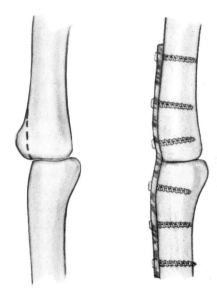

45

INTERNAL FIXATION OF OPEN FRACTURES

This is not the place to argue the case for internal fixation of open fractures, but merely to remind surgeons who choose to do so of the steps that are important in their pursuit of success.

(*1*) Blood sufficient to replace that already lost and that will be lost, particularly when a tourniquet is not used.

(*2*) Thorough cleansing of the skin around the wound.

(*3*) Gentle but thorough exploration of the wound followed by the painstaking removal of all foreign matter, clot and dead or doomed tissue. In the case of bone, completely separate fragments may have to be retained for the sake of accurate restoration of the fracture.

(*4*) Repeated irrigation of the wound with Ringer's solution helps to remove clot and bacteria.

(*5*) What metal is used must be sufficient for its purpose but should be used in such a way as not further to reduce the ability of the wound to heal.

(*6*) It may be advantageous not to close the wound until 3—5 days after fixation.

Removal of metal

Operations for removal of metal implants may be easy or difficult. The indications for removal of metal depend partly on the type of metal that has been used, what function the implants are performing and whether there have been any complications.

When a fracture that has been internally fixed becomes infected, if the fixation remains firm and is firmly holding a fracture that has become infected, it should be left in position; such operations as are required may proceed and irrigation drainage should be employed. When, however, metal implants are loose in the presence of infection, they are certainly harmful and should be removed, after which treatment can be continued with external splintage, external fixation devices or occasionally the re-application of a better and more rigid implant. It is often helpful in addition even at this stage to insert cancellous bone.

Implants should be removed when there is a danger of corrosion, which may happen with all stainless steel plates and screws in the second or third year, especially if they have been damaged during insertion.

Screws used independently for compression in the medial malleolus, for example, may be left because they do not prevent the transmission of stress in an axial direction and, if not in contact with a plate, they will not corrode. The transverse screw applied in a malleolar fracture from the fibula to the tibia should be removed at 8 weeks in order to restore the normal movement at the inferior tibiofibular joint.

There may be difficulties in the removal of plates and these chiefly concern the shape of the plate, the overgrowth of bone, or the use of self-tapping screws. The plate may be difficult to remove if it is of an irregular shape, or if some of the screw holes have not been filled so that bone has grown into them. If a plate has been inserted under the periosteum it is quite common for bone to grow over the ends of the plate and sometimes over its whole surface so that its removal may require the use of an osteotome. There is finally the difficulty of removing a plate which has been inserted with self-tapping screws, when bone has grown into the flutes at their tips so that it is impossible to turn them. When screws cannot be turned and it is imperative to remove the plate, their heads may be cut off with a diamond wheel and the shafts of the screws removed with the help of a trephine.

Medullary nails are probably better removed in all cases and certainly if they cause discomfort, especially by sticking out too far. It should be remembered, however, that progressive expulsion of a nail is a sign that the fracture is still moving.

The patient should be so placed as to render the proximal end of the nail most easily accessible and this end should then be displayed, which makes it much easier to engage the extractor hook firmly. If it should happen that the nail jams while only partly out, it should be cut short with a hacksaw.

References

Allgöwer, M., Perren, S. M. and Matter, P. (1970). 'A new plate for internal fixation – the dynamic compression plate (DCP).' *Injury* **2**, 40
Heim, U. and Pfeiffer, K. M. (1974). *Small Fragment Set Manual*. Berlin: Springer-Verlag New York: Heidelberg
Lowbury, E. J. L. and Lilley, H. A. (1975). 'Gloved hand as applicator of antiseptic to operation sites.' *The Lancet* **II**, 153
Müller, M. E., Allgöwer, M. and Willenegger, H. (1970). *Manual of Internal Fixation*. Berlin: Springer-Verlag New York: Heidelberg

[*The illustrations for this Chapter on General Techniques of Internal Fixation of Fractures were drawn by Mr. G. Lyth.*]

Injuries at the Elbow

P. S. London, M.B.E., F.R.C.S.
Surgeon, Birmingham Accident Hospital

APPROACHES TO THE ELBOW

1

The elbow can be approached from either side, from in front and from behind. The operations described are based upon the traditional bony and muscular landmarks but it must be remembered that the recently injured elbow is usually so swollen, and often deformed as well, that precise identification of the landmarks is at least difficult. It is, therefore, wise to make a generous cut in the skin and direct the deeper levels of the approach along the course of any already existing disruption of the tissues, which is usually first identified by an eruption of blood (*see Illustration 1*).

When there is already a wound adjoining the fracture, if it is practicable to do so, the approach should be made through the wound so as to make use of existing damage and add as little as possible.

A tourniquet should be used.

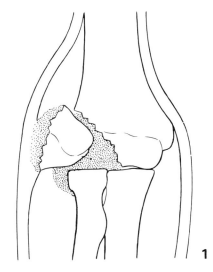

1

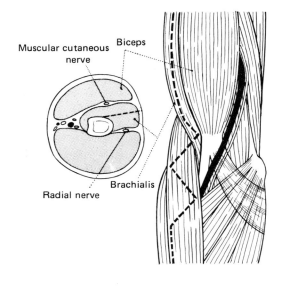

2

ANTERIOR APPROACHES

Henry's

2–5

This has the advantage of being extensile in either direction, but if it is made with a straight cut through the skin this causes the scar to web across the creases and the corrective Z-plasty can be anticipated by making a zig-zag in the first place.

The cut starts above a finger's breadth lateral to the outer edge of the belly of biceps brachii and follows a line that takes it to the medial edge of Henry's 'mobile wad of three' extensor muscles. After dividing the deep fascia the brachialis is split obliquely to the middle of the front of the humerus. Note that a strip of brachialis remains to protect the radial nerve (*see Illustration 2*). As the elbow is approached this cut can split brachialis right down to the coronoid process and in front of the elbow the space between this muscle and the three extensors is opened up. As this is done it is necessary to secure, divide and ligate a leash of branches from the brachial artery, and the veins accompanying them. The capsule of the elbow joint is split vertically and separated and reflected from its attachments sufficiently for the purposes of the operation.

Indications

This approach is most useful for dealing with dislocation of the head of the radius that is not corrected by manipulation, for re-attaching the avulsed tendons of biceps and for getting at high fractures of the shaft of the radius. It would also be useful if the head of the radius and the capitulum needed to be exposed at the same time.

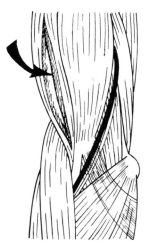

3

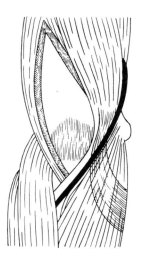

4

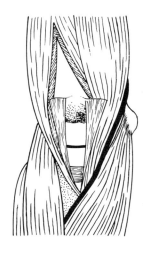

5

6&7

Transverse approach

This may be used when it is necessary to expose the brachial artery and its branches or the median nerve. It is transverse only in front of the elbow, otherwise following the general line of the neurovascular bundle. It must be remembered that this bundle may be stretched over the sharp edge of the humerus and pressed firmly against skin that has had the fat scraped from its deep surface.

The median nerve is damaged in continuity and usually recovers well enough to make any later operations unnecessary. The brachial artery may require no treatment, ligation or resection of a damaged segment and repair of the defect.

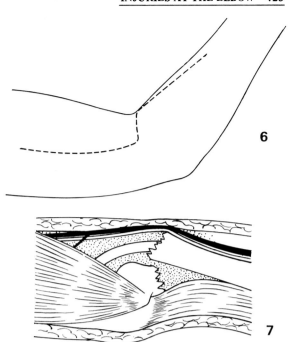

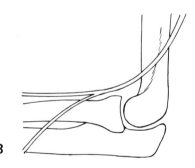

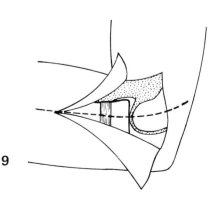

LATERAL APPROACHES

These may be thought of as being major or minor.

8

The minor approach

A straight cut is made from a little above its lateral epicondyle down to the humerus, the joint cavity, the head of the radius and the orbicular ligament, which is not divided. The upper part of the common origin of the extensor muscle is split. This incision carries no risk to the radial nerve above or its posterior interosseous branch below.

Indications

The approach is most useful for removing the head of the radius.

9

The major approach

Access to the elbow is greatly increased if the simple split in the extensor muscle is made into a T by detaching the soft tissues from the humerus in front of and behind the split. This enables loose bodies to be removed from almost any part of the joint, fractures of the lateral condyle, capitulum and some fractures of even the olecranon process to be dealt with. Access is further improved if the head of the radius has to be removed.

MEDIAL APPROACH

A straight cut is made down to the medial epicondyle and of sufficient length for the purpose of the operation.

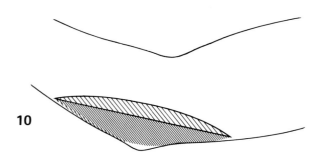

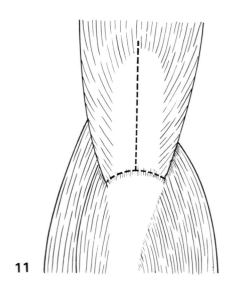

Indications

Extraction and replacement of the medial epicondyle, exploration and transplantation of the ulnar nerve and exploration of the brachial artery and the median nerve.

POSTERIOR APPROACHES

These leave the triceps brachii intact, split it or turn down its tendon or divide the ulna and turn it and the triceps upwards.

10

Simple approach

The cut starts a little above the point of the elbow, curves gently to the outer side and back towards the subcutaneous border of the ulna. The flap is undermined enough for it to be raised from the olecranon process and the upper part of the shaft of the ulna. If the upper end of the radius has also to be exposed the length and curvature of the cut are both made greater.

Indications

Fixation of fractures of the proximal quarter of the ulna with or without removal of the head of the radius.

11

Splitting the triceps brachii

A straight cut down the middle of the back of the arm goes down to bone and as far as is necessary along the two sides of the olecranon process. The two flaps so created are held apart by suitable forceps or by levers placed in front of the humerus. With the extensive exposures the ulnar nerve should be displayed and protected.

Indications

This approach gives adequate exposure for the reconstruction and fixation of even the most complex fractures of the lower part of the humerus, but any upward extension must be made with the radial nerve in mind.

Turning down the tendon of triceps brachii

The approach is not recommended because it does much more damage to the muscle than simply splitting it and it gives no better exposure. In any case, the tendon is not a simple block, but more like a wedge with its largest expanse on the surface and its bulk diminishing towards the olecranon process.

12a&b

Dividing the ulna

The ulna is first drilled so that it can be screwed back afterwards, it is then cleared so that it can be divided into the olecranon notch. While this is being done the articular cartilage of the humerus must be protected by levers, which are inserted after pulling the two bones apart. After being divided, the lower end of the ulna is freed from the soft tissues on either side so that it and the triceps can be turned upwards for as far as is necessary. It gives even more extensive access to the humerus than splitting the triceps but there are few cases when this is necessary.

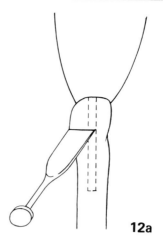

12a

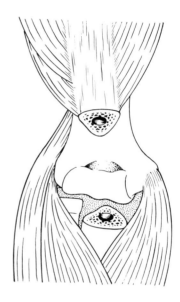

12b

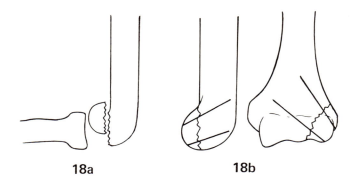

18a

18b

FRACTURES OF LATERAL CONDYLE OF THE HUMERUS

18a-e

IN ADULTS

The fracture is rare as an isolated injury and may be either a shearing off of the anterior third or so of the capitulum or separation of the condyle. In either case the major lateral approach (*see Illustration 9*) should be used, extending the dissection well across the front of the humerus. If the sheared off fragment is completely detached it should be removed because if it is replaced and fixed it may become degenerate and impair the action of the joint. If it is large enough to have a substantial stalk of soft tissue this should be preserved and the fragment fixed accurately in place with one or two Kirschner wires. It is usually easiest to insert these from an anterolateral direction and they should be completely buried in bone. This is best done by first cutting partway through the wires by rotating them slowly in the lightly closed jaws of a wire cutter. The groove should be made where it will be just below the surface of the cartilage; having been driven in that far the wire can be snapped by bending it sharply.

If the whole condyle has been broken off it can be fixed securely in place by means of a single A.O. cancellous screw about 30 mm long inserted above the articular surface and taking care not to have its point sticking out into the olecranon fossa.

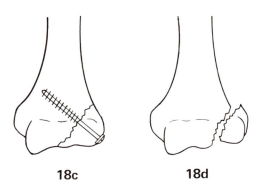

18c

18d

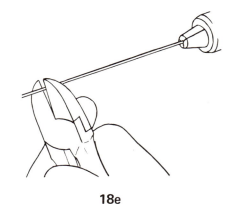

18e

IN CHILDREN

The usual fracture-separation of the lateral condyle's epiphysis nearly always has to be operated on because of the marked displacement and the difficulty of effecting and maintaining a good position by closed methods. The approach should be the same as with adults and the fragment can be fixed adequately usually with one Kirschner wire; there is no objection to having it cross the epiphyseal cartilage but it should be left long enough to be easily removed after about 3 weeks. It is not necessary to use a screw but merely to stitch the soft tissues is not always reliable.

19

It should be mentioned that the operation is often carried out as the primary method of treatment; even at this stage it is wise to have a good view of the inside of the joint because the fragment is a good deal bigger than the ossific nucleus that shows up in the x-ray films and it may include a fair amount of the trochlea. In some cases, however, the initial displacement is only slight but increases so much that after 10—14 days it is unacceptable. By this time a good deal of careful dissection is necessary if the displaced fragment is to be fitted accurately in place. Because of the risk of progressive displacement even the mild fractures should be radiographed two or three times during the first fortnight.

FRACTURES OF MEDIAL CONDYLE OF THE HUMERUS

These are rare and should be treated in the same way as fractures of the lateral condyle, using a medial approach.

FRACTURES OF MEDIAL EPICONDYLE OF THE HUMERUS

These occur in isolation or in association with dislocation of the elbow. They need to be operated on only if there has been damage to the ulnar nerve or if the epicondyle has become trapped in the joint. Otherwise, if the fragment is left alone it tends to be drawn up towards its rightful place as the lesion heals and any remaining deformity is reduced as growth takes place.

If the fragment is operated on it is usually enough to repair the soft tissues; it is in most cases big enough to take a Kirschner wire but not big enough to take a screw without splitting.

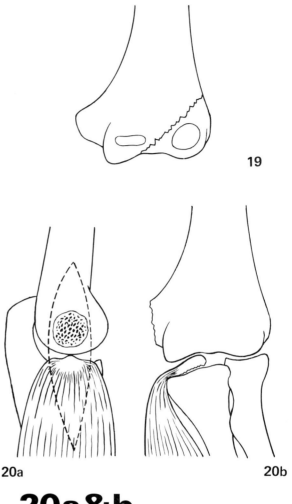

19

20a   20b

20a&b

THE EPICONDYLE TRAPPED IN THE JOINT

It is not always easy to recognize that this has happened; one should look carefully in any case of dislocation of the elbow of a child to see if the medial epicondyle has been pulled off. Knowing that it has been puts the manipulator on his guard. When the elbow has been put back in joint it is usually possible to flex it 30° or 40° beyond a right angle but if only 20° or so is possible it is likely to be because the epicondyle is in the joint and blocking movement. It can often be extracted by gently stimulating the flexor muscles by a faradic current; failing this it should be exposed by the medial approach, extracted from the joint and fixed in place.

COMPLICATED FRACTURES OF CONDYLES OF THE HUMERUS

21a,b&c

These vary from simple Y- and T-shaped fractures to extensive comminution of the lowest quarter to third of the humerus. In elderly patients, if the surgeon lacks experience of such operations it is wisest to treat the fracture by means of a sling and early movements. If operation is undertaken it is most conveniently done within the first few days and it requires a generous posterior approach using the position shown in *Illustration 14*.

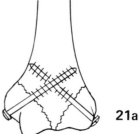

21a

The objective is to have the fragments squeezed tightly together in perfect position, for which A. O. cancellous screws are particularly well suited. Y-fractures are among the easiest to treat in this way. T-fractures can be dealt with by a λ-shaped plate or by a combination of screws and plate such as is shown in *Illustration 21b*. The lowest screw should be inserted first, followed by the lowest one holding the plate, after which the upper and lower elements should be compressed. More complicated fractures may require screws alone (*see Illustration 21c*) or screw and a plate or sometimes Kirschner wires to hold small, key fragments in place. When using multiple fixative devices it is important to ensure that they do not get in each other's way. The main requirements are ingenuity, technical skill and the right surgical equipment.

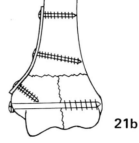

21b

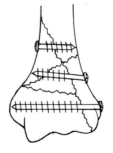

21c

FRACTURES OF HEAD AND NECK OF RADIUS

22 & 23

FRACTURES OF THE HEAD

There is much less readiness to remove the head of the radius than there was some years ago. It should certainly be done when it is obviously blocking movement, which is rare, and when it is combined with a fracture in the proximal quarter of the ulna that needs to be fixed. The size and number of the fragments are not the most important reasons for removing the head.

In the adult, the minor lateral approach (*see Illustration 8*) is used for fracture confined to the head of the radius, which is made conveniently accessible by passing curved levers behind and in front of the neck of the bone, which is divided little by little with an osteotome while the bone is rotated. Any spikes are then removed with nibbling or cutting forceps. This approach may suffice for repairing the orbicular ligament and for removing conveniently placed loose bodies.

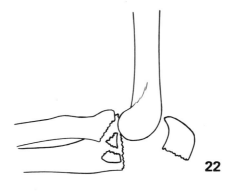

22

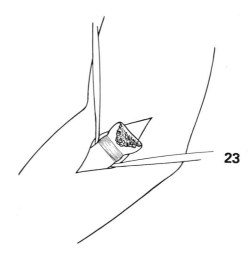

23

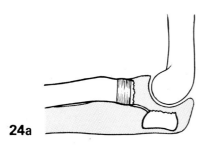

24a

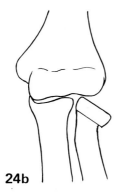

24b

24 a & b

FRACTURES OF THE NECK

These fractures nearly always occur in children and they require operation only if the head has been completely separated or is tilted by more than about 40° on the neck and cannot be pressed back into place from without. For the latter condition the minor lateral approach (*see Illustration 8*) will suffice, but to replace and fix the radius's head will require wider access (*see Illustration 9*).

FRACTURE - DISLOCATIONS OF RADIUS AND ULNA

MONTEGGIA'S INJURIES

25a, b &c

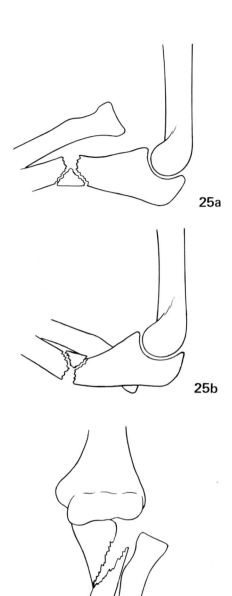

25a

25b

25c

The accepted characteristics of these injuries are dislocation of the head of the radius forwards, backwards or laterad, in each case with fracture of the ulna. It is often possible to obtain a sufficiently good position by manipulation and hold it by plaster of Paris but it is not unusual for the ulna to heal only very slowly and for the elbow and radio-ulnar joints to become very stiff after perhaps months in plaster. For this reason, there is much to be said for operation if a perfect position is not obtained, and after middle age. It is quite often found that once the ulna has been set and fixed in place the head of the radius is back in joint. If this should not be so it should be exposed by means of a lateral incision and any obstruent soft tissue extracted from the joint. The orbicular ligament should be repaired if it does not lie neatly in place.

The ulna is best fixed by a plate applied with compression and there are reasons to believe that doing this after 7 or 10 days (in plaster) reduces the risk of delayed union. If the fracture is very high it may be fixed by means of a screw, hook-plate or Kirschner wires and a figure-of-8 wire loop. In each case a straight or slightly curved incision with a lateral bow is used with the patient placed as shown in *Illustration 4*.

Plating the ulna

The ulna is exposed by stripping periosteum and muscles as one layer. If a flat plate cannot be fitted neatly to the ulna a semitubular one should be used and, as with the dynamic compression plate, it is not necessary to undertake the separate steps of applying compression.

26

The hook plate

This is particularly useful if the proximal fragment is too small to be plated in the usual way or screwed. The hook is embedded first and pulled snugly home at the same time as the fracture.

As with other sorts of plate, one must ensure that the proximal screws do not enter the elbow joint.

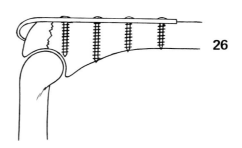

26

27&28

Screwing the ulna

The skin needs to be cut a little way up the back of the arm in order that the tip of the olecranon can be exposed and cleared enough to keep the drill clear of the tendon of triceps. The subcutaneous border of the ulna is drilled 2 or 3 inches from the tip of the olecranon and the spike of Charnley's clamp set in the hole while a claw in the other arm of the clamp is set against the olecranon. The clamp is then closed and held closed by means of the cross-bar and screw. The tip of the olecranon is drilled and fixed with a good strong screw. If A.O. equipment is not used the proximal fragment must be drilled oversize to allow the screw to exert compression. The screw should be long enough to grip cortex where the marrow cavity begins to narrow some 2–4 inches distal to the tip of the olecranon and it must be remembered that the spike in the cortex may encroach too far to let a screw be driven past it.

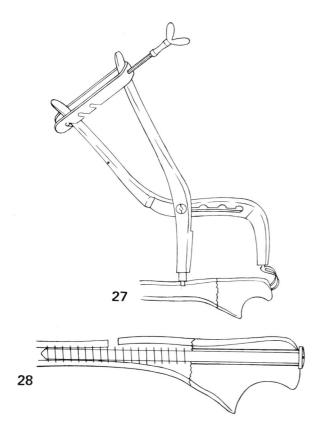

27

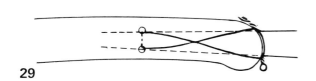

28

29

Wire loop and Kirschner wires

The fracture is exposed and set and held in place as described. A hole is then drilled across the cortex about 2 inches distal to the tip of the olecranon and size 20 stainless steel wire is passed through it. Two stout Kirschner wires are then driven distad well past the fracture on slightly converging courses. The two ends of the wire are passed round them to form a figure-of-8, pulled tight and twisted off, taking care that the twisted ends will not stick out under the skin. The ends of the Kirschner wires are then cut short, turned over and hammered down. This method has a particular advantage with comminuted fractures. Rush and Küntscher nails should not be used because they did not give compression and may not make the fracture immovable.

29

COMPLEX INJURIES

These may comminute all three bones of the elbow and be open fractures as well. There is no set method of dealing with such injuries but the following general rules apply.

(*1*) Ensure prompt healing of the wound, using delayed primary closure in appropriate cases and a skin flap if necessary.

(*2*) Fix the fragments accurately and securely in place by whatever means are appropriate. This requires an adequate exposure (*see Illustrations 10* and *11*), a wide range of equipment, skill, ingenuity and determination.

(*3*) If accurate and secure fixation is not possible it may be best to excise some or all of the bony fragments and treat the operation as a simple arthroplasty, for which the retention and screwing of some fragments is carried out and, as with arthroplasty, the patient is required to start moving the joint as soon as possible.

(*4*) A combination of inadequate internal fixation and external splintage is liable to give a result of a sort that can be made worse only by infection.

Reference

Rowell, P. J. W. (1975). 'Arterial occlusion in juvenile humeral supracondylar fracture.' *Injury* **6**, 254

[*The illustrations for this Chapter on Injuries at the Elbow were drawn by Mr. F. Price.*]

Emergency Operations on the Forearm

P. S. London, M.B.E., F.R.C.S.
Surgeon, Birmingham Accident Hospital

The principal emergency operations on the forearm are for internal fixation of fractures, which is dealt with in the Chapter on 'General Techniques of Internal Fixation of Fractures', pages 400—420, and the exploration and repair of wounds and fasciotomy for incipient ischaemic contracture, which are dealt with below. Exposures are dealt with on pages 393—399.

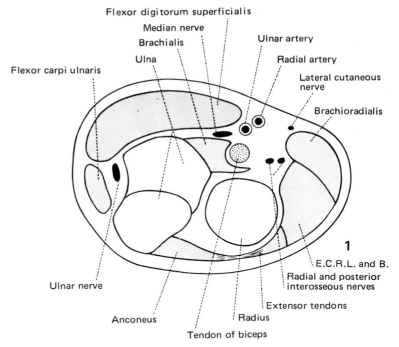

Flexor digitorum superficialis
Median nerve
Brachialis
Ulna
Ulnar artery
Radial artery
Lateral cutaneous nerve
Flexor carpi ulnaris
Brachioradialis
1
E.C.R.L. and B.
Radial and posterior interosseous nerves
Ulnar nerve
Extensor tendons
Anconeus
Radius
Tendon of biceps

EXPLORATION OF DEEP WOUNDS OF FOREARM AND WRIST

1, 2 & 3

One of the more testing experiences for a young surgeon dealing with the victims of accidents is to have to treat a deep wound between the elbow and the hand where there are so many important structures that have to be identified correctly and repaired accurately. Perhaps the most useful guide to such a task is a clear recollection of cross-sectional views of the limb in its uppermost, middle and lowermost thirds.

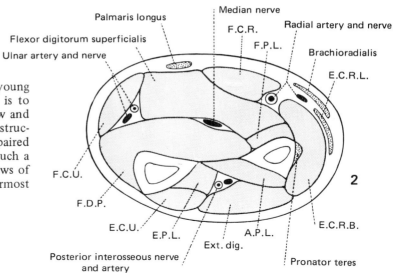

Palmaris longus
Median nerve
F.C.R.
Radial artery and nerve
F.P.L.
Flexor digitorum superficialis
Brachioradialis
Ulnar artery and nerve
E.C.R.L.
F.C.U.
2
F.D.P.
E.C.R.B.
E.C.U.
E.P.L.
A.P.L.
Ext. dig.
Posterior interosseous nerve and artery
Pronator teres

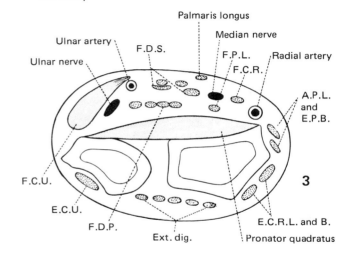

Palmaris longus
Median nerve
Ulnar artery
F.D.S.
F.P.L.
Radial artery
F.C.R.
Ulnar nerve
A.P.L. and E.P.B.
F.C.U.
3
E.C.U.
E.C.R.L. and B.
F.D.P.
Pronator quadratus
Ext. dig.

Preparing for operation

There is often brisk bleeding, for which a firm, bulky dressing is required and this should be left in place until a tourniquet has been applied to the limb. If the wound is large, with many structures cut, the

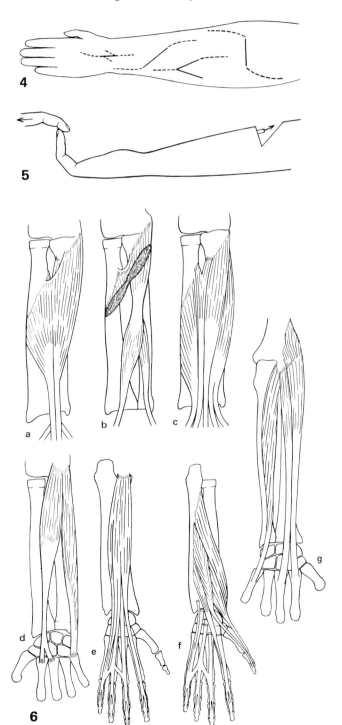

(*a*) Flexor digitorum superficialis — superficial part. (*b*) Flexor digitorum superficialis — deep part. (*c*) Flexor digitorum profundus. (*d*) Flexors of the wrist. (*e*) Extensor digitorum. (*f*) Deep layer of extensor digits. (*g*) Extensors of the wrist.

duration of the operation is likely to make regional and intravenous analgesia inadequate.

The limb should be prepared so as to give room for the wound to be extended several inches in a proximal direction and to allow the hand and fingers to be uncovered so that the actions of the distal stumps of muscles and tendons can be identified.

4

Extension of the wound

The larger the wound, the less need there is to extend it; a transverse wound down to both bones can usually be dealt with without extending it, smaller wounds will need more or less extension in a generally longitudinal direction. V-Shaped wounds usually need to be extended from the apex and perhaps from the deeper of the two limbs. If longitudinal wounds have to be extended into the hand, this should be done with due regard for the creases there. Z-Plasty at the wrist may be desirable but it should not be carried out as a primary procedure unless it can be expected to heal uneventfully. When the wound has to be extended the extension should allow it to be held open with no more than gentle pressure on the tissues.

5

Inspection

When the wound is a tidy one, careful inspection of the cut surfaces combined with gentle retraction of individual masses of tissue and passive movements of the wrist and digits may allow all the divided structures to be identified without any formal dissection. Final distinction between the distal stumps of deep and superficial flexors of the fingers is easily made by applying passive resistance to a fingertip while pulling on a flexor tendon. This illustration shows that it is the superficial tendon that is being tested.

6

When the wound is untidy, identification may be much more difficult, especially if it is necessary to cut away large amounts of damaged muscle with the result that there is no longer any correspondence of shapes and sizes on the two sides of the wound. In these circumstances it is helpful to be reminded of the different shapes of the muscles and the arrangement of their several masses of flesh and tendons.

Aids to identification

The distal cut tissues are usually easier to identify than the proximal, among which one then looks for the corresponding shapes and positions.

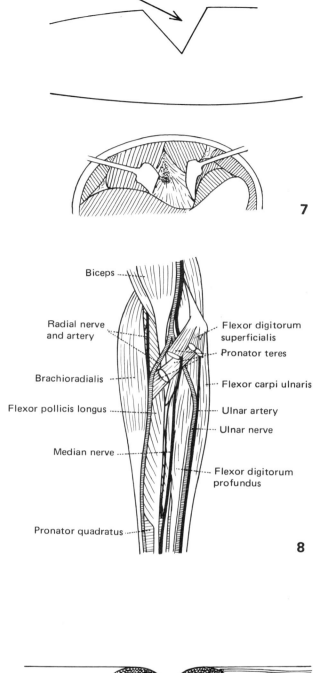

7&8

All movable structures have more or less well defined sheaths, along which they can withdraw. As they do so they leave a small amount of blood in their wake and this may enable one to recognize either the entrance to the tunnel or the side of it. This is particularly true of separate tendons such as those of flexor pollicis longus and flexor carpi radialis and it also applies to nerves, but because nerves cannot retract far it is usually possible to 'milk' the proximal end down and to produce the distal end by flexing the wrist and digits. If these actions are unsuccessful the nerve should be sought by formal exploration proximal and distal to the point of division, to which it is then traced.

7

Biceps

Radial nerve and artery

Brachioradialis

Flexor pollicis longus

Median nerve

Pronator quadratus

Flexor digitorum superficialis

Pronator teres

Flexor carpi ulnaris

Ulnar artery

Ulnar nerve

Flexor digitorum profundus

8

9

It is, regrettably, necessary to point out the ease with which the median nerve has been mistaken for palmaris longus at the level of the wrist. When both structures are present there is not likely to be confusion, but this easily arises when palmaris longus is absent and the nerve is the most superficial structure in front of the wrist. Careful inspection of the cut surface of a nerve shows the characteristic bundles, with the accompanying vessels on its anterior surface, but error is most likely to occur when the possibility of error is not considered and inspection is accordingly cursory.

It must be emphasized that dissection should be carried out only when it is necessary to do so in order to display or secure a structure and it should be avoided as far as possible until all the tissues visible in the cut surfaces have been identified and, if necessary, marked for future reference. Tendons can be prevented from retracting by temporarily transfixing them with needles. The more dissection is carried out the more the fascial and aponeurotic partitions are disturbed, so rendering identification more difficult.

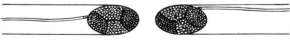

9

10

Examination of the cut surfaces should continue until all the structures at risk have been identified as being either damaged or undamaged. When the wound is of an obliquely penetrating nature it may be necessary to extend it (along the dotted line) in the direction of penetration and to dissect the superficial tissues quite extensively in order to display and identify the deeper damage.

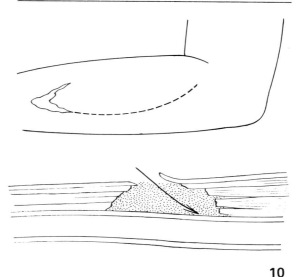

10

PRINCIPLES OF REPAIR

Once all the damaged structures have been identified the process of repair can be planned.

Arteries

If one main artery remains undamaged the other can safely be ligated. Although the hand can certainly survive ligation of both the radial and the ulnar arteries when both have been cut it is wise to repair whichever is the larger or more likely to remain patent for other reasons.

Nerves

Primary repair should be carried out only by a competent surgeon when the nerve has been cleanly divided and will lie in a bed with little scar in it and with every reason to expect prompt healing of the

wound. If these favourable conditions are not present the ends should be tacked neatly together so as to prevent retraction and without one being twisted upon the other.

Muscles and tendons

Flexores carpi radiales, pollicis longus, carpi ulnaris and digitorum profundus should be repaired whenever it is possible to do so. Flexor digitorum superficialis should be repaired if it has been damaged in isolation but there is no need to do so if repairing it is likely to lead to a solid mass of scar that will bind all the muscles together and so interfere with their actions. If the tendons are cut near the wrist the distal ends should be shortened so that they will not become stuck to the wall of the carpal tunnel.

11

Simple double right-angle stitches suffice for both tendons and muscles and should include the sheaths or aponeurotic parts of muscles. Individual structures should be repaired individually and not by mass suture.

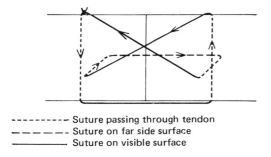

--------- Suture passing through tendon
— — — —- Suture on far side surface
——————— Suture on visible surface

11

DECOMPRESSION OF THE FLEXOR MUSCLES

Ischaemic contracture of the flexor muscles may follow damage to the brachial artery by a supra-condylar fracture of the humerus but this is now less often the cause than crushing or bruising of the forearm, and sometimes quite mild fracture of the radius and ulna.

Diagnosis

The most important features of the condition are pain in the forearm, which is swollen, hard and exquisitely tender and the fact that the patient will not allow the fingers to be extended because this hurts too much. The hand can at the same time be pink with pulses present at the wrist.

12

Treatment

What makes the muscles ischaemic is a rise in pressure within their unyielding envelope of bone, interosseous membrane and deep fascia and the pressure can be reduced by slitting the deep fascia far enough to allow all the swollen muscles to bulge out and change back from a congested to a healthy colour. The skin must also be divided because blind fasciotomy is both difficult and dangerous.

The wound should be covered with a firm, bulky dressing, the limb elevated and movement of the hand and fingers encouraged. In a few days' time it may be possible to sew up the skin, but if it is not the raw surface should be covered with a split-skin graft. The fascia need not be closed.

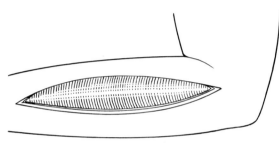

12

Other considerations in treatment

Management of arterial damage at the elbow is dealt with in the Chapters on 'Injuries at the Elbow', pages 421—434 and 'Arterial Suture and Anastomosis', pages 91—97, and the treatment of established contracture in The Hand volume of this series.

[*The illustrations for this Chapter or Emergency Operations on the Forearm were drawn by Mr. F. Price.*]

Fractures of the Wrist

Geoffrey R. Fisk, M.B., B.S., F.R.C.S., F.R.C.S.(Ed.)
Senior Orthopaedic Surgeon, Princess Alexandra Hospital, Harlow
and St. Margaret's Hospital, Epping;
Hunterian Professor, Royal College of Surgeons of England

SMITH'S AND BARTON'S FRACTURES

Smith's fracture, first described in 1847, is sometimes called a reversed Colles' fracture. It occurs within 1 inch (2·5 cm) of the lower articular surface of the radius with forward displacement and anterior tilting of the lower fragment. The inferior radio-ulnar joint is usually not disrupted.

Barton's fracture was described in 1838, and differs from Smith's fracture in being a fracture-dislocation of the wrist in which the carpus is displaced forwards upon fragments broken from the anterior articular surface of the lower end of the radius. Thomas (1957) has described three varieties of volar displacement of the carpus which incorporates these two named fractures.

1a,b&c

(1) An oblique fracture in which the carpus is displaced forwards and proximally upon a triangular fragment of radius.
(2) A comminuted fracture of the radial articular surface which carries the carpus anteriorly.
(3) A forward angulation of the lower part of the radius with or without comminution.

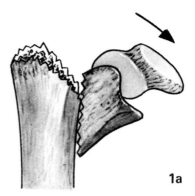

1a

A fourth variety may be added; namely, a volar displacement of the lower radial epiphysis in the immature skeleton.

The injury is said to occur by a fall on the dorsum of the flexed hand but it is more likely to result from a fall backwards onto the outstretched hand with the forearm fully supinated, thus exerting a pronation force upon the lower radius. Others may be sustained in motor cyclists when the handle-bar is thrust against the heel of the palm. A stable fracture may be reduced by traction and manipulation, restoring the alignment of the lower radial articular surface, which is normally tilted forwards by some eleven degrees to the long axis of the radius. Smith's fracture is usually immobilized in some dorsiflexion of the wrist, but Barton's fracture may be displaced even further anteriorly if this position is adopted. Thomas recommends immobilization in full supination in order to maintain the reduction, but this position has the disadvantage that pronation of the forearm may never be fully regained.

Ellis's buttress plate is an excellent and safe method of restoring and retaining the unstable anterior lip of the radial articular surface, but it does not prevent collapse of the fracture towards the radial side. The operation is carried out under tourniquet and the lower end of the radius and the carpus are exposed through an anterior approach. A vertical incision is made down the centre of the forearm; this forms the proximal part of the anterior approach to the carpal tunnel and the volar aspect of the wrist joint. Flexor carpi radialis is retracted laterally and flexores profundus and sublimis and the median nerve retracted medially. Pronator quadratus is divided over the lower end of the radius and the fracture is identified and reduced.

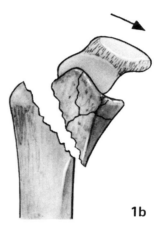

1b

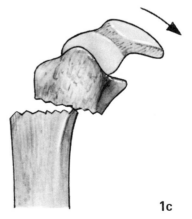

1c

2 & 3, a & b

The fracture is found much more proximally than the x-ray appearance suggests. It is reduced under direct vision, the buttress plate is placed across the distal fragment and held by two screws through the radial shaft. A T-shaped plate may be used if the distal fragment is sufficiently large to take one or more screws.

Woodyard (1969) suggests that the Ellis plate is most effective in those comminuted fractures which enter the wrist joint.

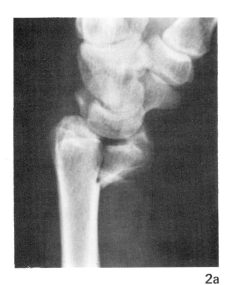

2a

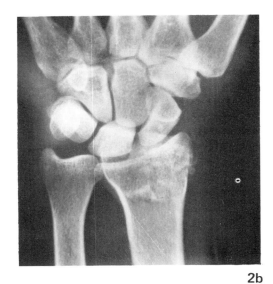

2b

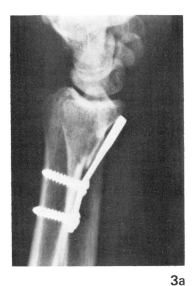

3a

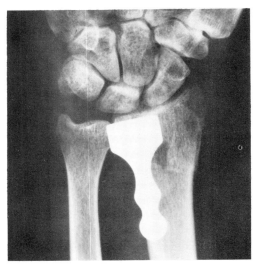

3b

COLLES' FRACTURE

This common injury was first described in 1814. It is caused by a fall on the outstretched hand with the forearm pronated so that it is essentially a dorsi-flexion-supination injury. The fracture occurs within 1 inch (2·5 cm) of the lower articular surface, producing four deformities: (*1*) the lower fragment is displaced backwards; (*2*) the articular surface tilts backwards; (*3*) it is driven upwards; and (*4*) it is tilted towards the radial side.

4a&b

The fracture is usually accompanied by avulsion of the tip of the ulnar styloid carrying the ulnar collateral ligament. Reduction is achieved by manipulation under local or general anaesthesia, each deformity being reduced in turn, with immobilization of the wrist in some palmar and ulnar flexion. Most cases do not require immobilization of the elbow, but if reduction can be achieved only in pronation the elbow must be included. In many cases the reduction cannot be maintained and the fracture collapses and unites with some shortening and radial angulation. This is not incompatible with a good functional result but it is inevitably associated with disruption of the inferior radio-ulnar joint. The ulnar head may be displaced backwards, giving rise to one variety of Madelung's deformity. Sarmiento (1975) has suggested that the tension exerted by brachioradialis on the lower fragment is the cause of displacement. He recommends splintage of the wrist in ulnar and volar flexion, the forearm fully supinated with the elbow flexed.

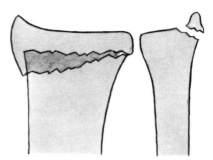

4a

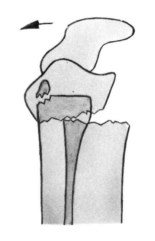

4b

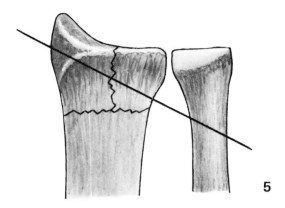

5

5&6

Many attempts have been made to stabilize the comminuted Colles' fracture by internal fixation, such as impaling the lower end of the radius to the ulnar shaft by one or more obliquely placed Kirschner wires as recommended by DePalma. Alternatively, a fine Steinmann pin may be passed through one or more metacarpals and another through the proximal ulna. The fracture is reduced, traction is applied and the pins are incorporated in a plaster cast (Green, 1975). Mal-union of Colles' fracture is common but is rarely worth surgical correction, since the functional result is often acceptable to the patient and the surgeon. Late surgical correction is often surprisingly difficult to achieve. The radius is divided through a laterally placed incision about 1 inch (2·5 cm) proximal to its articular surface. Deformity is reduced by using the osteotome as a lever. This leaves a wedge defect which may be filled either by a graft cut from the iliac crest or using the medial aspect of the ulnar head (Jackson Burrows' operation).

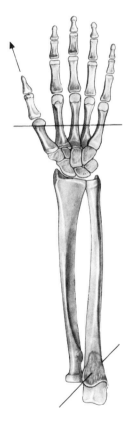

6

7

Malunion is associated with dislocation of the inferior radio-ulnar joint resulting in a prominent and painful ulnar head and loss of rotation of the forearm.

Darrach's operation consists of excising the head of the ulna. It is important that an excessive amount of the ulna should not be removed since this will lead to dorsal dislocation of the ulnar shaft with pain and crepitus. Displacement can be minimized by suturing flexor and extensor carpi ulnaris together over the cut end of the ulna.

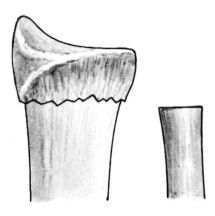

7

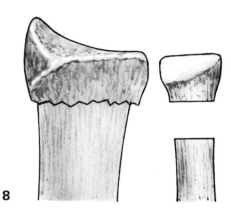

8

8

A preferable operation in many cases is that attributed to *Baldwin*, which consists of excising the neck of the ulna so that the head drops back into its correct relationship with the radius. This not only restores the normal appearance of the wrist with preservation of its contour, but also allows rotation to take place at the pseudarthrosis established at the neck of the ulna. It is wise to suture the periosteum over the exposed ends of the bone to prevent union of the osteotomy.

9

Lauenstein's operation comprises excision of the neck of the ulna with fusion of the ulnar head to the lower end of the radius by a transversely placed transfixion screw. This additional procedure is not usually necessary unless there is persistent painful dislocation of the ulnar head.

Injury to the dorsal aspect of the radius may result in rupture of the extensor pollicis longus tendon as it passes round Lister's tubercle. Inability to extend the thumb usually occurs spontaneously some 3–6 weeks after wrist injury. It is usually not possible to repair the tendon directly since it has undergone attrition and necrosis, but transfer of extensor indicis proprius to the distal end of the extensor pollicis longus results in restoration of normal function.

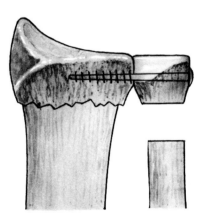

9

FRACTURED RADIAL STYLOID

This uncommon traction injury usually unites with simple plaster immobilization. Occasionally periosteum and soft tissue is turned in between the fracture surfaces, preventing accurate apposition and easy union. In these circumstances the fracture may be fixed by crossed Kirschner wires or a screw.

FRACTURED CARPAL SCAPHOID

Fracture of the scaphoid is a common injury. It is often undiagnosed — either because the patient does not seek treatment, or x-ray examination carried out soon after the injury fails to reveal the fracture. In those cases in which physical signs and symptoms suggest this injury, it is important that the wrist be immobilized in a well-fitting plaster cast for 3 weeks and then examined again in four planes by x-rays. Eighty or ninety per cent of these fractures will unite by immobilization for 6–8 weeks in some 30° of dorsiflexion and radial deviation. If the wrist is symptom-free at the end of this period in spite of the x-ray appearances normal use of the hand should be advised (London, 1961). As such a high proportion of uncomplicated fractures of the scaphoid will unite with conservative care there is no justification for routine internal fixation.

In the author's view the key to the prognosis in this fracture depends upon the associated ligamentous injury involving the mid-carpal joint (Fisk, 1970). Carpal instability can be diagnosed from two criteria: the first is increased anteroposterior mobility at the wrist joint, and the second the zig-zag or 'concertina' deformity seen in the lateral x-ray view. The indications for surgical intervention may be summarized as follows.

Early

(*1*) If the fracture is undisplaced and the carpus stable plaster fixation for 6–8 weeks is carried out then treatment is abandoned.

(*2*) In the event of the fracture's not uniting and remaining painful, screw fixation by open or closed methods is performed.

(*3*) If the fracture is displaced or the carpus unstable, primary screw fixation and plaster immobilization is carried out.

(*4*) If the fracture is associated with other carpal fractures or dislocations, they are reduced, primary screw fixation is carried out and the wrist is immobilized in plaster.

(*5*) With avascular necrosis of the proximal fragment screw fixation is preferred to prolonged plaster immobilization.

Late

(*1*) In unsuspected old fracture with recent injury the sprain should be treated by plaster fixation for a few weeks.

(*2*) In an ununited fracture without stability or resorption but persisting symptoms, peg grafting is performed as described by Murray (1946) or iliac chip grafting as described first by Matti (1937) and later by Russe (1960).

(*3*) An ununited fracture with instability and resorption and angulation of the scaphoid fragments is best treated by wedge grafting and plaster immobilization.

(*4*) Resorbed or mal-united fractured carpal scaphoid with scaphoradial osteo-arthritis, excision of radial styloid only is carried out.

(*5*) Periscaphoid osteo-arthritis: (*a*) excision of proximal row of carpal bones to give a mobile weak wrist or (*b*) periscaphoid arthrodesis to preserve some wrist movement, or preferably (*c*) panarthrodesis of the carpus from the radius to the base of the third metacarpal.

Screw fixation

This is best performed using a lag screw as designed by McLaughlin (1954) or Maudsley (1972) by closed or open methods.

Closed methods

X-ray control is essential. A 0·5 inch incision is made over the lateral aspect of the carpus centred over the tuberosity of the scaphoid. This can be identified by flexing the hand to the ulnar side with a little dorsi-flexion, which will bring the tuberosity of the scaphoid from under the trapezium. Armstrong (1945) has shown that the long axis of the scaphoid is vertical if the forearm is supinated to 60° and the elbow flexed to 45°, and the hand may be placed on a special rest for this purpose.

10 & 11a & b

A guide wire is inserted and the position and length checked by x-ray films in two planes or under the image intensifier. A calibrated, cannulated crown drill is then slipped over the guide wire so that it penetrates the bone right up to the scapholunate joint. The drill is removed leaving the wire in place. A cannulated lag screw of appropriate length is then passed over the wire which is then removed. The screw must grip the proximal fragment and the head lie flush with the tuberosity or its compression effect will not be exerted.

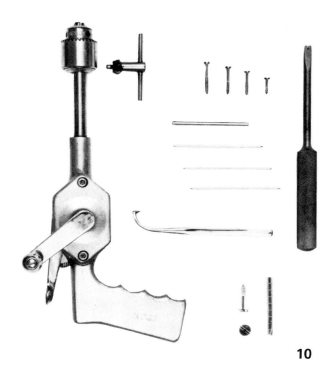

10

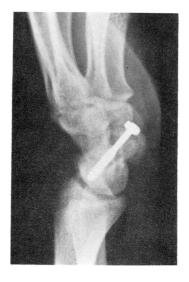

11a

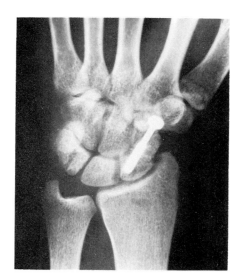

11b

12, 13 & 14

Open method

A bayonet incision is made along the radial aspect of the lower end of the radius and the wrist joint. The dorsal branch of the radial nerve is identified and retracted, since its damage produces painful neuromas and unpleasant paraesthesia out of all proportion to the size of the nerve. The radial styloid is stripped of its periosteum, the extensor pollicis longus tendon is retracted backwards and the abductor and extensor tendons forwards. The radial collateral ligament carrying the radial artery is detached from the tip of the styloid process. The bone is now divided about 0·5 inches (1 cm) proximally to the tip, the osteotome being directed distally at 45° to the long axis. When the radial styloid process is removed the articular surface of the scaphoid is exposed and the fracture located. The tuberosity of the scaphoid is identified. Care must be taken to preserve the vessels entering the distal fragment. Screwing is then performed as above but it is now much easier to direct the wire down the long axis of the scaphoid. The radial styloid process need not be replaced provided that the periosteum and the radial collateral ligament are carefully sutured back into position.

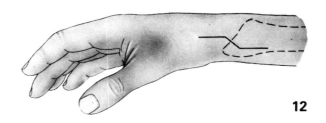

12

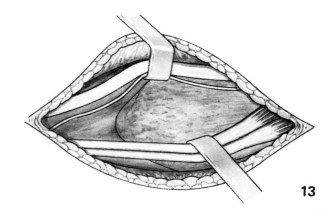

13

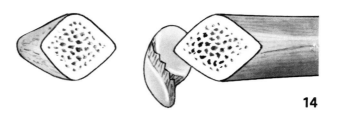

14

Bone peg grafting

The same procedure is followed as outlined above, but a cortical bone graft removed from the olecranon, the tibia or iliac crest is passed down the prepared drill hole and gently tapped home; a rather larger calibre of drill is required.

The Matti-Russe operation

The ununited scaphoid is approached from the front by a vertical incision just to the lateral side of the tendon of flexor carpi radialis, this is retracted to the ulnar side and the radial artery protected. The capsule of the wrist joint is incised and the fracture identified.

It is curetted until normal bone is observed. A bone graft is taken from the opposite iliac crest about 0·5 inches long, shaped as a peg and tapped gently into the prepared gutter in the line of the long axis of the scaphoid. Bone chips are taken from the same site and pressed gently around the bone peg filling the cavity. The wound is closed in layers and immobilized in a plaster cast for 3 or 4 months.

Wedge grafting of the ununited fractured scaphoid (Author's operation)

In the presence of carpal instability the proximal fragment tilts backwards with the lunate and the distal fragment forwards with the capitate. This opens up the fracture at the dorsal aspect and is one cause for the fracture not uniting. Resorption of the anterior margins of the fracture takes place so that the scaphoid collapses in length and becomes 'hump-backed', the distal and proximal poles pointing forwards.

15, 16 & 17a & b

The radial styloid process is removed through the incision outlined above, but the excised bone is carefully preserved. The fracture is identified and is cleared of fibrous tissue. If the concertina deformity is corrected by traction and anterior displacement of the carpus, the defect in the scaphoid is disclosed as wedge-shaped based anterolaterally. The fractured surfaces are curetted, but if they are excessively sclerosed multiple fine drill holes are made into both fragments. The carpus is then manually re-aligned by an assistant and a wedge of appropriate size and shape is cut from the radial styloid process, fitted into the defect and tapped home with a bone punch. When the traction is released the resilience of the soft tissue holds the graft firmly in position and it is not necessary to transfix it by wire or screw. Any protruding corners of the bone wedge are trimmed and the wound is closed in layers and immobilized in a plaster cast for 2—3 months.

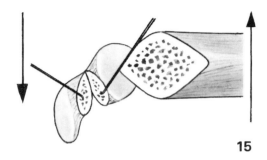

15

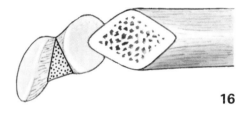

16

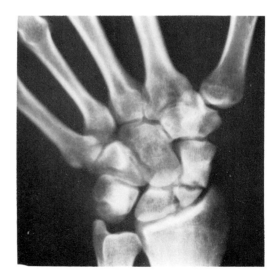

17a

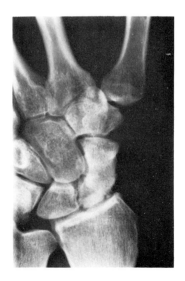

17b

Excision of the radial styloid process

This is performed when there is a local scaphoradial arthritis. The operation has already been outlined above. It is important not to carry out this operation where there is a pseudarthrosis of the scaphoid because there is a danger that the distal pole will prolapse on to the cut surface of the radius.

Arthrodesis of the wrist

Many operations have been described in an attempt to immobilize the scaphoid while preserving some carpal movement, such as scaphoradial, scapholunate and scapholunocapitate fusions; panarthrodesis of the wrist, however, provides such excellent function that it makes partial fusions hardly worthwhile. The wrist may be fused through a dorsal incision running from the base of the third metacarpal to the lower radius. The tendon of extensor pollicis longus is detached from its tunnel around Lister's tubercle and displaced proximally. The articular cartilage from the carpal bones is removed as far as possible. A gutter is cut with a twin saw from the third metacarpal to the radius, the wrist being held in a little dorsiflexion and ulnar deviation. The extremities of this gutter are undercut into the radius and medullary cavity of the metacarpal. A curved graft is now cut from the iliac crest by the same twin saw, each end trimmed on the flat by about 0·5 inches to half its thickness. The wrist is flexed, the graft is slipped into the gutter and into the cavity of the bone at either end and when the wrist is dorsiflexed the graft is held firmly in place. The extensor pollicis longus tendon is rerouted through a sling constructed from local fascia, the skin closed and the hand immobilized in plaster for 2–3 months.

References

Armstrong, J. R. (1945). *Bone-grafting and the Treatment of Fractures*. Edinburgh: Livingstone
Barton, J. R. (1938). *Medical Examiner* **1**, 365
Colles, A. (1814). *Edinburgh Medical and Surgical Journal*.
Ellis, J. (1965). *J. Bone & Jt Surg.* **47B**, 724
Fisk, G. R. (1970). *Ann. R. Coll. Surg. Engl.* **46**, 63
Gonçalves, D. (1974). *J. Bone & Jt Surg.* **56B**, 462
Green, D. P. (1975). *J. Bone & Jt Surg.* **57A**, 304
London, P. S. (1961). *J. Bone & Jt Surg.* **43B**, 237
McLaughlin, H. L. (1954). *J. Bone & Jt Surg.* **36A**, 765
Matti, H. (1937). *Zentbl Chir.* **64**, 2353
Maudsley, R. H. and Chen, S. C. (1972). *J. Bone & Jt Surg.* **54B**, 432
Murray, G. (1946). *J. Bone & Jt Surg.* **28A**, 749
Russe, O. (1960). *J. Bone & Jt Surg.* **42A**, 759
Sarmiento, A., Pratt, G. W., Berry, N. C. and Sinclair, W. F. (1975). *J. Bone & Jt. Surg.* **57A**, 311
Smith, R. W. (1847). *A Treatise on Fractures in the Vicinity of Joints*. Dublin: Hodges & Smith
Thomas, F. B. (1957) *J. Bone & Jt Surg.* **39B**, 463
Woodyard, J. E. (1969) *J. Bone & Jt Surg.* **51B**, 324

[The illustrations for this Chapter on Fractures of the Wrist were drawn by Mr. F. Price.]

The Acute Injured Hand

Adrian E. Flatt, M.D., M.Chir., F.R.C.S.
Professor of Orthopaedics, University of Iowa Hospitals, Iowa City;
formerly First Assistant, Orthopaedic and Accident Department, The London Hospital

PRE - OPERATIVE

General principles

The fate of an injured hand is determined by its primary operative care, and a comprehensive plan of treatment must be found, taking into account the patient's age and occupation. This should yield a final result in one operation in all but the most extensive injuries.

In major injuries in which normal function cannot be preserved a choice will often have to be made between the two basic functions of pinching or gripping. Pinching requires an opposable thumb and a pillar against which it can act; this should preferably be a mobile digit towards the radial border of the hand. Gripping is a stronger action than pinching and is dependent on the breadth of the palm and mobility at the metacarpophalangeal joints. Every effort must be made to preserve the length of the thumb and its mobility at the carpometacarpal joint.

The general principles applicable to care of hand injuries do not differ from those of general traumatic surgery, but since the hand has little excess tissue there must be the minimum sacrifice of tissues during toilet.

It is important to avoid infection and fibrosis since scar tissue will prevent functional recovery. Immediate and complete skin cover is, therefore, of paramount importance. It is permissible to sacrifice tissues of doubtful viability which might delay healing and cause fibrosis if their removal does not compromise basic hand function.

Special equipment

Plastic and ophthalmic surgical instruments are needed. In particular, forceps which have many small teeth are much less traumatic than the larger rat-tooth type. A power drill capable of carrying 6-inch (15 cm) lengths of Kirschner wires is of great use. Any monofilament fine suture material, including wire, is suitable for skin closure; 8/0 or 10/0 monofilament material should be used for nerve suture.

Pre-operative preparation

Shaving, irrigation and gross trimming precede more careful cleaning with a mild detergent. It is often better to do this with a pneumatic tourniquet in place and inflated. Minor injuries can frequently have most of their toilet performed by the patient himself. The flexor aspect of the forearm is usually used as the donor site for split-skin grafts and should also be given a thorough pre-operative cleansing.

In cases in which grafts are to be taken from the forearm it should be prepared, the graft taken and the donor area sealed with an occlusive dressing before the wounded area is cleansed.

Chemotherapy

Antibiotics are no substitute for proper surgical toilet. When indicated, adequate cover with a broad-spectrum antibiotic can be obtained by timing an injection to reach maximum blood level at about the time the tourniquet is released. By this means, the clot that forms in the wound is heavily loaded with the drug employed.

Anaesthesia

General anaesthesia is acceptable but axillary block intravenous lignocaine or local nerve block is of particular use in the treatment of ambulant patients. Metacarpal nerve block is preferable to digital nerve block since the finger is not distended. Adrenaline must never be included with any anaesthetic agent injected into the hand.

PROCEDURE

1

Subungual haematoma

Crush injuries of the distal phalanx frequently produce a haematoma beneath the nail which is extremely painful because of the pressure built up within the closed space. Immediate relief can be obtained by trephining the nail. This can be done by drilling a hole with the point of a fine-bladed scalpel. An equally satisfactory method is to open out a paper clip, heat the end of this in a match or cigarette lighter and then press on the centre of the nail with the hot end. It will immediately penetrate the nail, the haematoma will well out and cool the hot end of the paper clip. No pain is felt by the patient and immediate relief is obtained by the decompression of the haematoma. A small occlusive dressing should be placed over the nail hole for a matter of a few hours and the patient encouraged to keep the finger dry for a few days.

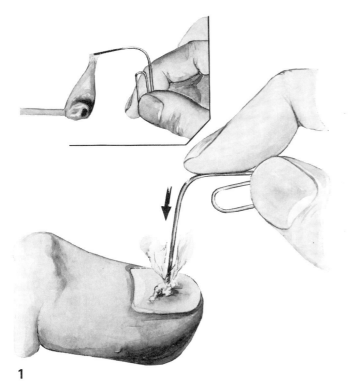

1

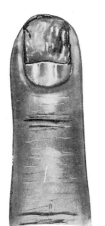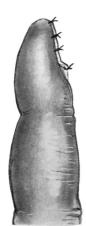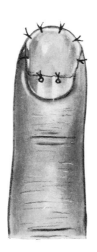

2

2

Nail bed injuries

Slicing wounds which remove part of the nail bed but leave the nail root intact are best treated by immediate covering with a thin split-skin graft. The graft should be sewn into place and holes can be drilled through the nail remnant to secure adequate fixation. When a portion of the finger tip has also been lost the graft should be cut thicker at one end to allow this portion to be used to cover the lost tip.

As the nail grows the graft will be incorporated into the nail bed until normal structure is regained.

3

Partial amputation

If one of the vascular bundles has been left intact the distal portion of the finger should be sutured back, even if the injury has severed the bone. The hand should be kept elevated and the finger cooled as much as possible by applying only the minimum of dressings.

When flexor or extensor tendons, or both, have also been damaged amputation of the finger can be considered. The decision must take into account the state of the rest of the hand and the patient's occupation, but in general it is best to preserve the finger as a primary measure. When only pulp has been lost the tactile skin may be replaced by a thenar flap (*see* pages 486 and 492).

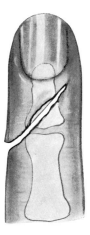

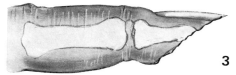

3

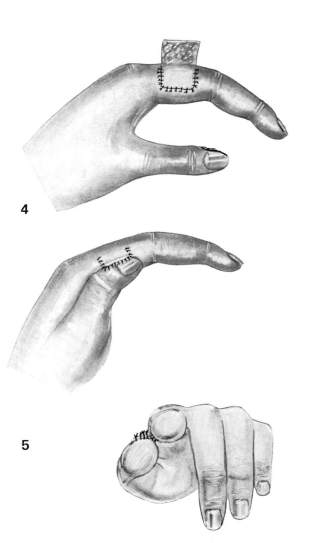

4

5

Index to thumb flap

4

Donor site

Pulp lost from a finger tip is best treated by a thenar flap but similar losses from the thumb cannot be treated in this way. A flap can be raised from the area of the base of the little finger, but a much more satisfactory donor area is the radial side of the index finger. (Some prefer to use the dorsum of the middle phalanx of the long finger as a donor site.)

5

Attachment of flap

After the edges of the thumb wound have been trimmed, a flap is designed to the width of the lesion and based on the dorsum of the finger. Fat should be included in the flap but care must be taken not to damage the digital bundle. The edge of the flap should not encroach on the palmar surface of the index finger.

A split-skin graft is sewn into the donor area before the flap is attached to the thumb defect. The thumb should be placed on the grafted area (being separated by tulle gras and a few layers of gauze) and the flap sewn in as far as possible so that little gap exists between the thumb and the index finger.

The flaps can be safely detached in 14 days.

Phalangeal recession

6

Preservation of distal phalanx

Preservation of the distal phalanx with its highly specialized tactile sense can be accomplished in wounds which leave both soft tissue and bony gaps proximal to the nail bed. If a viable soft tissue bridge containing a functioning artery and nerve (or reparable nerve) has been left, it will be sufficient to nourish an unwounded finger tip and recession of the phalanges will give good results.

The operation should not be attempted unless an adequate nerve supply can be ensured and unless there is sufficient bone to give greater finger length than would be obtained by amputation.

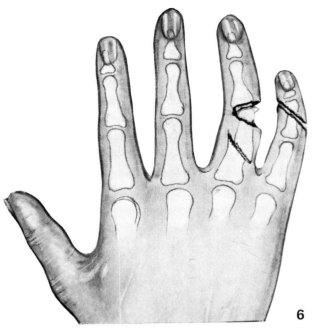

6

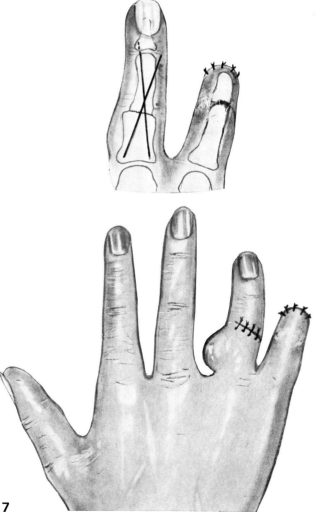

7

7

Method

After sparing excision of the skin wound any frankly loose spicules of bone must be removed. Formal trimming of bone-ends sacrifices too much length and the irregular bone-ends should be impacted together. Fixation is obtained either by Kirschner wires or by suturing of soft tissues such as periosteum and joint capsule with stainless steel wire.

Severed tendons should be trimmed and approximated even though tenolysis may be required later. Any obvious 'bleeders' must be ligated, and after trimming back to normal tissue the cut ends of the digital nerves must be joined end-to-end with interrupted 8/0 silk sutures. The shortening of the finger will have left excess tissue on the side of the intact skin bridge. This must be allowed to bulge in a smooth arc, otherwise vessel kinking and thrombosis may occur.

Any excess flexor tendon length will be taken up by muscle retraction fairly early and the skin bulge will subside in 3—4 months.

Complete finger amputation

8

Distal phalanx

The immediate treatment of complete digital amputation is to obtain skin cover with preservation of the maximum length of the finger.

In injuries of the distal phalanx the turning up of a palmar flap is the most suitable treatment. The bone will have to be nibbled back until the flap can be sutured without undue tension.

When the head of a phalanx is exposed it is better to remove the articular cartilage and allow the pulp of the flap to gain firm attachment to the bone.

Exposed nerves should be cut cleanly across as they lie in the wound; there is no advantage in pulling them distally before trimming.

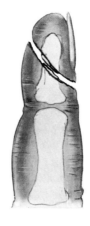
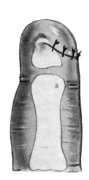

8

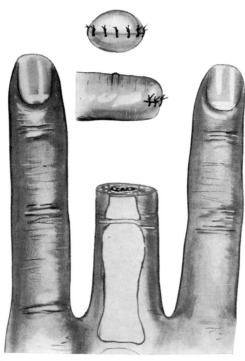

9

9

Middle or proximal phalanx

In amputations through the middle or proximal phalanges the use of a dorsal or lateral flap may be dictated by the type of injury.

The fish-mouth or equal-flap amputation is a useful procedure and is indicated in clean-cut amputations. The flexor and extensor tendons must not be sutured together over the bone-ends or the balance of movement in the hand will be impaired.

If an amputation will leave less than one-half of a middle phalanx it may be best to consider re-amputation to the proximal joint as a primary measure. The flexion power of such short stumps is often limited and they are liable to protrude during fist-making and gripping.

Multiple amputations

10

Utilization of severely injured finger as skin flap

A finger which has had its flank severely injured can often be utilized to supply skin to adjacent areas of loss. By this means, local skin with the appropriate nerve supply can be used to fill defects which would otherwise have to be treated by less satisfactory methods, such as grafting, or the application of a flap from a distance.

In the injury shown the long finger has lost the neurovascular bundle on its ulnar side, the proximal phalanx is fractured, the distal phalanx partially amputated and the flexor tendons damaged. Both the ring and little fingers have been traumatically amputated near their base.

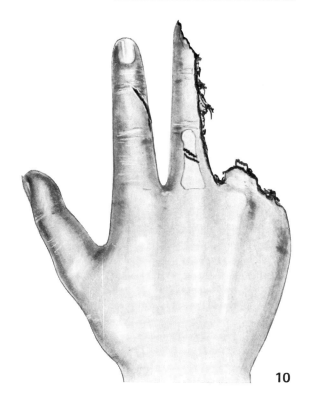

10

11

Method

When a damaged finger is to be filletted great care must be taken not to jeopardize the blood supply of the skin which will be used as a flap. Frequently, dorsal veins draining the finger can be traced over the metacarpophalangeal joint. These veins must be preserved as they often carry a major part of the venous return. The phalanges must be removed together with the flexor and extensor tendons, which should be pulled distally before being cut cleanly off and allowed to retract proximally.

Cartilage should be removed from the heads of the metacarpals over which the flap is to be sutured but the bones should not be shortened. The digital nerves of the amputated fingers should be cut back so that their ends lie deep in the palm, and the digital vessels should be ligated with fine catgut.

All the fat should be retained in the finger flap, which should be sutured into place with no tension. If any excess skin is present in the width of the flap, dorsal rather than palmar skin should be removed, but care must be taken not to infringe the length/breadth ratio of the flap. There should be no tension on the flap and good eversion of the suture line must be obtained.

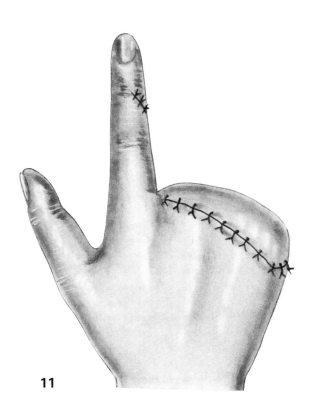

11

12

Phalangeal fractures

Fractures of the proximal phalanx can be immobilized satisfactorily by pinning, and in open fractures it is the method of choice if the finger is likely to survive. The wire is usually best introduced through the head of the phalanx in its more dorsal part and to one side of the mid-line. It is passed down to, but not through, the base of the phalanx and is cut off beneath the skin over the proximal interphalangeal joint. This method allows some movement to the finger, and although it is often advisable to supplement the fixation with some external splint this should be removable to allow daily supervised motion.

Middle phalangeal fractures can be treated in a similar fashion although size sometimes makes the procedure technically more difficult.

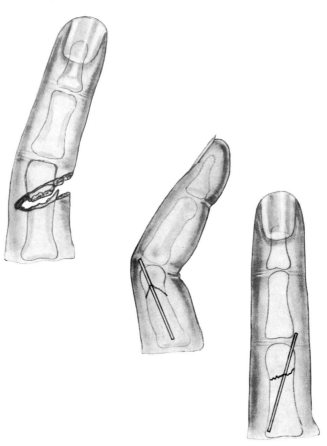

12

Metacarpal shaft fractures

13

Kirschner wire fixation

Transverse fractures of the metacarpal shafts are frequently unstable, particularly on either border of the hand, and if transfixed by Kirschner wires no plaster of Paris is needed and active movements can be carried out throughout treatment.

Open fractures can be successfully treated by this method and even comminuted fractures can be held reduced by the careful insertion of more than one wire.

Frank sepsis should be considered a contra-indication to the use of wire fixation, but fresh contaminated compound wounds are no contra-indication to the method if proper surgical toilet is carried out.

When the fracture is in the region of the neck of the bone a transverse wire passed into the adjacent metacarpal will give the necessary antirotation stabilization.

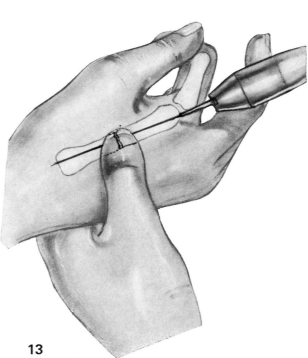

13

14

Method

Kirschner wires between sizes 1·0 and 1·5 mm in thickness are suitable. The wires can be placed by using a hand chuck or a standard drill, but a power drill is the easiest means of introduction. With the finger held well flexed at the metacarpophalangeal joint the wire can be introduced through the head of the metacarpal while the fracture is held reduced by the thumb and fingers of the other hand. It is usually not necessary to pass the wire into the carpus but this can be done if it gives better fixation.

When fixation is satisfactory the wrist-joint is firmly flexed and the wire passed through the skin on the dorsum of the wrist. It is then withdrawn until there is free metacarpophalangeal movement, and is cut off so that it lies beneath the skin.

Before the wire is allowed to exit, the skin over the wrist should be pulled to one side so that the puncture wound does not lie directly over the protruding wire end.

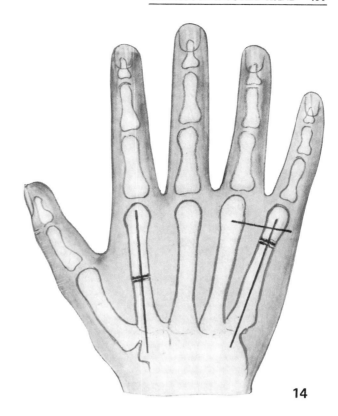

14

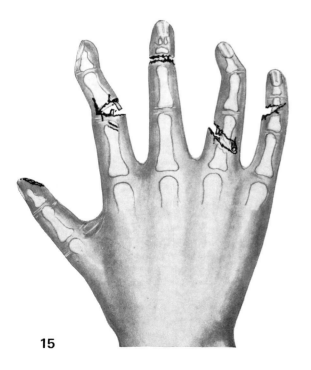

15

Multiple open fractures

15

Preservation of finger length

There is the greatest variation in these injuries and they can be associated with any combination of skin loss, neurovascular bundle injury and tendon damage. The principle of primary treatment is to preserve as much length as possible, and potential stiffness of interphalangeal joints is no contra-indication to salvage if the metacarpophalangeal joint is intact.

Cross-finger flaps and filletting of irreparably damaged fingers may be needed to supply skin to fingers whose length would otherwise have to be sacrificed.

A typical case with multiple open fractures illustrates well the principles of treatment.

16

Method

Since both the index and ring fingers have damage to their pair of digital bundles and to the tendons, they cannot be saved. The index finger was treated by turning up a palmar flap and the ring finger by removing the base of the proximal phalanx before completing the amputation.

The long finger tip wound was closed by a fish-mouth type of amputation to preserve as much length as possible. The area of skin loss on the thumb was repaired by sewing in a full thickness skin graft cut from the amputated tip of the long finger.

The little finger has damage to the digital bundles on the radial side and some laceration of the extensor tendon, but the probable stiffness of the distal interphalangeal joint is acceptable in view of the length saved; the fracture should, therefore, be pinned with a Kirschner wire and the skin wound sutured.

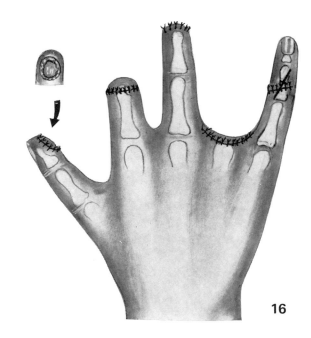

16

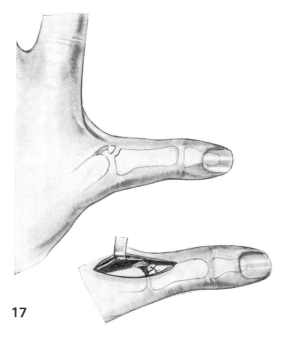

17

17

'Sprained thumb'

Lateral strain of the metacarpophalangeal ligament of the thumb can produce complete rupture or avulsion of a bone chip from the base of the proximal phalanx. This is a serious injury and, if on the ulnar side of the joint, can be crippling since the integrity of the pinch mechanism is destroyed.

Operative repair is essential and can be carried out through a dorsal incision centred over the joint.

Because of the risk of painful neuromata, great care must be taken to preserve and retract any branches of the radial nerve in the area. The repair or replacement of the bone chip can be accomplished with either fine catgut sutures or stainless steel wire using the pull-out technique. The tie-over button will be placed on the radial side of the thumb and the pull-out wire will exit on the ulnar side of the meta-carpophalangeal joint. This wire should be left in place between 2 and 3 weeks before it is removed.

Postoperatively, the thumb should be immobilized in plaster in semiflexion for 3 weeks, but the inter-phalangeal joint can be left free.

18

Dislocated thumb

Manipulative reduction of a dorsal dislocation of the thumb metacarpophalangeal joint frequently fails. Open reduction is then essential. An approach on the dorsolateral side of the joint shows that the metacarpal neck is tightly gripped by the capsule of the joint which has been split in a vertical direction by the forward-thrusting metacarpal head. Occasionally, the flexor pollicis longus tendon or the sesamoid of the flexor pollicis brevis is interposed between the joint surfaces.

By gradually increasing the length of the vertical split with repeated attempts at reduction, the dislocation can be corrected without too much further damage to the joint capsule. Occasionally it may be necessary to cut transversely across the line of capsular attachment to obtain sufficient relaxation.

No attempt should be made to repair the rent in the joint capsule and the thumb should be rested in a plaster splint in semiflexion for 3 weeks with the interphalangeal joint left free.

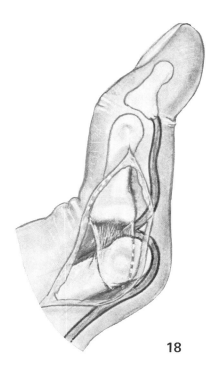

18

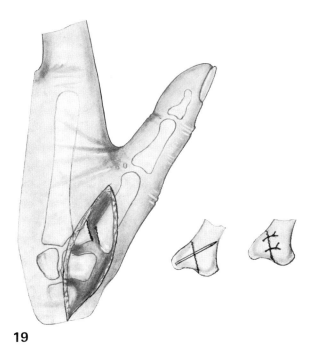

19

19

Fracture-dislocation of the thumb

In Bennett's fracture of the thumb the palmar articular process constitutes the small triangular fragment which remains in place while the main metacarpal shaft dislocates proximally or proximolaterally. Reduction is best obtained by placing the metacarpal shaft in opposition.

While closed treatment by traction on the thumb combined with a well moulded plaster can give satisfactory results, radiography may show that the reduction is not satisfactory. The joint is too important to the hand for indifferent results to be acceptable and there should be no hesitation in performing open reduction of the injury if closed methods fail.

The decision to operate must be taken early, before the traumatic inflammatory reaction has made the operation technically difficult. Exposure of the joint is easy through an incision on the radial side. The fracture can usually be held reduced by sutures of catgut or fine wire through the adjacent soft tissues, but it is often necessary to obtain firm reduction by pinning the fragments together with a Kirschner wire. The reduction site will have to be protected by distal traction on the thumb for several weeks or by transfixing the first and second metacarpal shafts with a Kirschner wire.

Degloving injuries

These injuries are difficult to treat and frequently lead to unsatisfactory results.

20

Fingers

Avulsion of the skin cylinder of the ring or little fingers occur after a ring has caught on some protruding hook. The skin usually takes with it both digital neurovascular bundles and leaves the flexor and extensor tendons exposed but unharmed. Full flexion and extension of the digit is possible.

Palm

Catching the palm on protruding objects can lead to varying degress of avulsion of the palmar skin. The plane of cleavage is usually between the subcutaneous tissues and the palmar fascia. These injuries raise flaps which frequently appear to have adequate arterial supply and may even have vessels spurting from the edges, but their venous return will have been almost completely cut off.

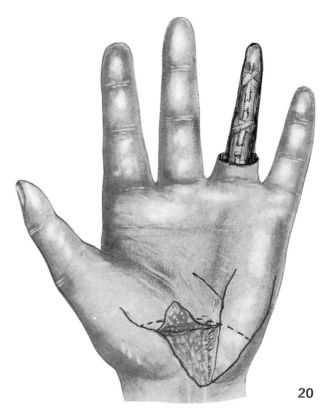

20

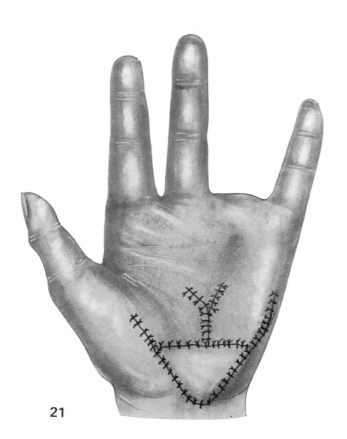

21

21

Method

Because of the excellent movement of the finger it is tempting either to replace the skin if available or to place the raw digit under an abdominal flap. Experience shows that the results of either procedure are so poor that primary amputations is by far the best treatment. The most successful treatment for fingers in which, for occupational reasons, attempts at salvage must be made is to wind strips of split-skin graft about 2·5 cm in width around the finger in a spiral fashion. These must be sutured in place. At best, the result will be a partially stiff insensitive finger.

In the case of palmar injury the inevitable venous congestion in these flaps will lead to necrosis of a variable amount of the tips. The narrow peninsular type will have a considerable loss. The best primary treatment is to suture all these flaps back into place. Immediately the area of loss is defined, it should be excised and the granulation beneath will form a good base for a thick split-skin graft.

Injuries of dorsum

22

Restoration of skin loss by rotation flap

Anything but a trivial injury of the dorsum of the hand must involve the extensor tendons and frequently also involves the metacarpal shafts and the metacarpophalangeal joints.

The dorsum is the only area of the hand in which it is possible to restore skin loss by a rotation flap. The amount of loss that can be compensated for is small and the flap should be planned on a generous scale to overcome the tension produced when a fist is made. Open injuries involving skin loss, tendons and metacarpal shafts can all be treated at the one operation.

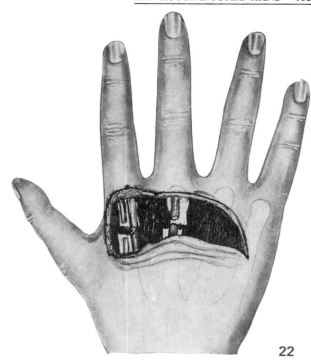

22

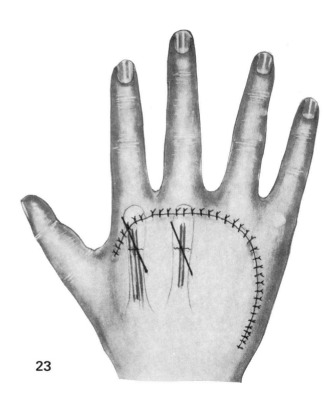

23

23

Method

In the injury illustrated the flap is based proximally and can, therefore, be sutured back without any fear as to the efficiency of its venous return. The skin loss over the first metacarpal area can be corrected by extending the line of the wound along the ulnar side of the hand and rotating the skin in a radial direction.

The transverse fractures of the metacarpal shafts are each immobilized by transfixion with a single Kirschner wire. The end of the wire is left protruding through the side of the head of the metacarpal so that it can be withdrawn through a small nick in the skin.

The cut extensor tendons should be repaired by buried stainless steel sutures.

The hand should be immobilized in the position of function.

24

Major injury yielding 'pincer'

In this illustrative case there is: (*1*) a soft tissue wound of the thenar eminence; (*2*) destruction of both neurovascular bundles of the index finger; (*3*) a small flap raised on an otherwise intact long finger; (*4*) gross destruction of the distal part of the ring finger with a wound on the palmar surface of its proximal phalanx; and (*5*) an open fracture of the head of the fifth metacarpal with destruction of the flexor tendons and the neurovascular bundle on the ulnar side of the finger.

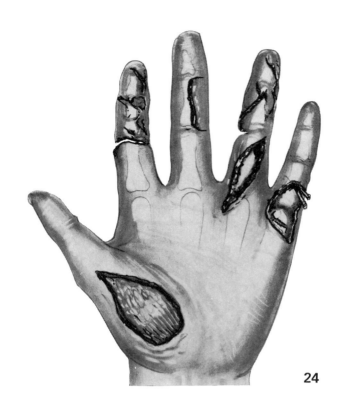

24

25

Analysis of injuries

(*1*) The thenar wound can be closed without tension by slightly increasing its length.

(*2*) The index can be preserved at a level just proximal to the proximal interphalangeal joint.

(*3*) The small flap on the long finger can be sewn back into place.

(*4*) The multiple injuries of the ring finger distal to the proximal interphalangeal joint combined with the severance of both flexor tendons over the proximal phalanx mean that no more than the proximal phalanx of the finger can be preserved.

(*5*) The little finger injuries are such that it is beyond salvage.

The object is, therefore, to produce a pincer hand by suturing the palmar wounds on the thenar eminence, the long and the ring fingers. The index length is preserved by a fish-mouth amputation and that of the ring finger by turning up a palmar flap. The fifth metacarpal is trimmed off obliquely through the fracture site and a dorsal flap brought down to the palmar wound.

The result is a pincer hand in which lateral pinch is possible between the side of the index and the thumb and tip pinch between the long finger and thumb.

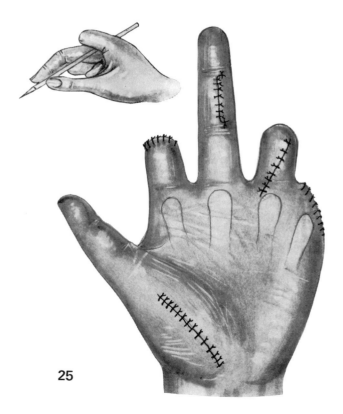

25

26

Major injury yielding 'vice'·

The injuries in this illustrative case are: (*1*) small wound of tip of thumb; (*2*) virtual destruction of the index finger; (*3*) destruction of both digital bundles and an open fracture of the long finger proximal phalanx; (*4*) an open fracture of the ring finger with tendon damage and destruction of the terminal phalanx; and (*5*) a crush fracture of the tip of the little finger.

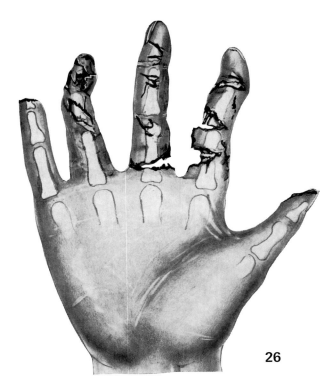

26

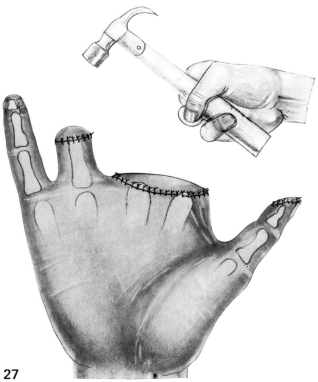

27

27

Analysis of injuries

(*1*) The thumb can be repaired by simple suture.

(*2*) Both the index and long fingers are beyond recall and will have to be amputated at the metacarpophalangeal joint level.

(*3*) The ring finger can be saved at the proximal interphalangeal joint level.

(*4*) The little finger will lose very little length by trimming the tip.

The object is, therefore, to produce a power grip hand by completing the amputation of the index and long fingers, saving length of the ring finger by turning down a dorsal flap, and the length of the little finger by turning up a palmar flap.

The result is a power grip hand in which breadth of the palm has been preserved and in which there is length and mobility on the ulnar side together with a normal thumb.

Splinting of hand

28

Mason and Allen universal splint

After the majority of procedures on the hand, it is necessary to apply some form of temporary rest by splinting.

Malleable aluminium strips 1·25 cm in width make excellent splints for holding individual digits in flexion, but in many cases it is better to put the hand at rest. While this can be achieved adequately by a properly moulded plaster of Paris slab, a splint has been specifically designed for the purpose.

The universal splint of Mason and Allen is moulded from aluminium and is so designed that it can be used for either hand, and for a great variety of conditions including fractures. It is of particular value in the first-aid and early treatment of hand injuries since it gives support to the whole palmar side of the hand and the forearm. It allows compression dressings to be applied without the risk of pressure on bony prominences.

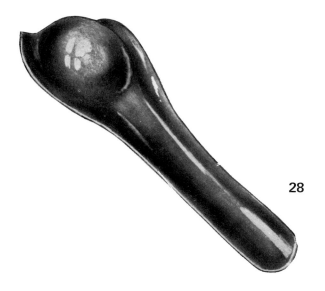

28

29

Application

The splint can be used for the treatment of soft tissue injuries associated with fractures which have or have not been immobilized with internal fixation. It is not radio-opaque and it will often be found that fractures can be held in a satisfactory reduction position when the hand is bandaged to the splint.

It may be used for virtually any type of hand injury except those in which parts of the hand require temporary immobilization in more extreme positions following the repair of tendons or nerves. It is particularly valuable in the early care of crush injuries in which the hand needs firm support in the position of function. It is not suitable for the care of already swollen hands since the oedema will hold the hand away from the splint and fractures will rapidly angulate.

Great care must be taken to maintain the exact position of the splint in relation to the wrist. Should the splint be allowed to slip proximally, angulations will be produced at the fractures, which would be crippling should the bones unite. Frequent inspections and x-ray films must be made during the first few days of treatment on this splint.

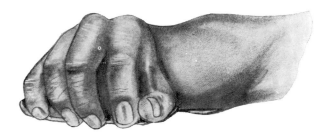

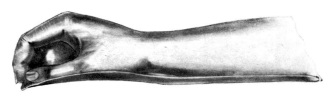

29

SPECIAL POSTOPERATIVE CARE AND COMPLICATIONS

Swelling

Postoperative swelling is inevitable but its severity is directly dependent upon the trauma inflicted both before and during the operation. It is best controlled by elevation of the limb and compression dressings. The pressure should be supplied by a thick fluffed-out gauze dressing which can be held in place by either crêpe or cotton bandages. The fingers must be separated by several thicknesses of gauze to prevent maceration and pressure between adjacent bony points.

Crush injuries are particularly prone to swelling and healthy looking areas of skin may die in the early postoperative days.

Particular attention must be paid to the intrinsic muscles in crush injuries of the palmar area. These muscles are sheathed in strong deep fascia and intolerable internal pressure can rapidly build up. Pain, paralysis and increasing pain on passive stretching of these muscles are diagnostic of recoverable ischaemic contracture. Surgical decompression through multiple dorsal incisions is then essential. If the surgeon is doubtful prophylactic surgical decompression is advisable.

First dressing

This should always be applied at least by the fifth postoperative day and should be changed right down to the tulle gras layer. The position of the hand should be maintained so as not to disturb any tendon or nerve repair that may have been carried out.

Later postoperative care

Movements

Return of hand function should be supervised under the active care of an occupational or physical therapist trained in the care of these particular conditions, and special attention must be paid to the shoulder and elbow on the injured side. To keep the arm in a sling without actively exercising these joints will induce stiffness and may on occasions lead to the crippling shoulder—hand syndrome.

While uninjured portions of the hand must be exercised from the start of treatment, motion in freshly injured areas will promote exudate which will later organize into fibrous tissue. Splinting should, therefore, be retained for the injured parts until they are sufficiently repaired to withstand movement. Simple wounds can be moved from about the tenth day, but if tendons or nerves have been repaired then splinting should be maintained for about 3 weeks. When motor nerves have been sutured the appropriate splintage for the paralysed muscles must be retained until recovery is well advanced.

Tendon and nerve repairs should be protected from involuntary damage by 2—3 weeks of night splinting after movement has been resumed.

Children

Compressive dressings are not sufficient to immobilize small fingers and it may be necessary to secure the fingers to the splint by stainless steel sutures passed through the tips of the nails.

A light plaster of Paris protective cover to the dressings made into an above-the-elbow plaster is the best form of immobilization.

Children are not inhibited by stiff joints or 'compensationitis' and very rarely is any formal physiotherapy needed.

References

Bunnell, Sterling (1951). 'The early treatment of hand injuries.' *J. Bone Jt Surg.* **33A**, 807
Entin, M. A. (1964). 'Crushing and avulsion injuries of the hand.' *Surg. Clins N.Am.* **44**, 1009
Evans, E. M. (1954). 'The injured hand.' In *Progress in Clinical Surgery*. London: Churchill
Flatt, A. E. (1972). *The Care of Minor Hand Injuries*, 3rd ed. St. Louis: Mosby
James, J. I. P. (1962). 'Fractures of the proximal and middle phalanges of the finger.' *Acta orthop. scand.* **32**, 401
Riordan, D. C. (1954). 'Primary treatment of soft tissue injuries of the hand.' *J. La St. med. Soc.* **106**, 300
Swanson, A. B. (1970). 'Fractures involving the digits of the hand.' *Orthop. Clins N. Am.* **1**, 261

[The illustrations for this Chapter on The Acute Injured Hand were drawn by Mr. G. Lyth.]

Operative Treatment of Fractures of the Hand

D. A. Campbell Reid, M.B., B.S.(Lond.), F.R.C.S.
Consultant Plastic Surgeon, Sheffield Royal Hospital,
Sheffield Royal Infirmary, Sheffield Children's Hospital,
Hallamshire Hospital, Chesterfield Royal Hospital;
Honorary Clinical Lecturer, University of Sheffield

PRE-OPERATIVE

General principles

The majority of phalangeal and metacarpal fractures may be satisfactorily treated by the generally accepted means of external splintage. There is a good case, however, in a number of instances for some form of internal fixation. This involves accurate apposition at the fracture site, which frequently necessitates surgical exposure, followed by complete internal fixation. Cumbersome external splintage is dispensed with, allowing early movement of uninvolved joints and digits.

Indications

Internal fixation is indicated for open injuries with multiple fractures or when fractures are associated with gross displacement. Establishment of skeletal stability by internal fixation of the fractures enables one to proceed with the soft tissue repair, which may involve skin replacement or tendon suture.

Closed transverse fractures of the phalanges with marked deformity, particularly when manipulation has failed to reduce the displacement or when early redisplacement has occurred, are also best treated by internal fixation. Transverse fractures near joints are, owing to muscle action on one fragment, particularly difficult to control by simple splintage. Examples of this type of fracture may be seen in the necks of the proximal and middle phalanges and at the base of the distal phalanx.

Occasionally, transverse fractures are seen at a later stage when established non-union is present. These fractures, when occurring in the proximal and middle phalanges, may cause considerable disability, and operative treatment is indicated.

For fractures of the metacarpals with gross overlap and when manipulative methods fail, internal fixation is recommended. Fractures at the proximal end of the first metacarpal may sometimes be difficult to control adequately by external splintage, in which case it is better held internally. Oblique fractures of the phalanges or metacarpals associated with rotational deformity or wide displacement are difficult to control by external splintage, and internal fixation is better treatment.

Intra-articular fractures of the phalanges or metacarpal heads are another indication for internal fixation, provided that comminution does not preclude it. Malunion of fractures may occur due to failure of primary treatment and corrective treatment may be required subsequently to overcome the deformity by an appropriate osteotomy followed by internal fixation at the site.

Anaesthesia

Ring block anaesthesia is useful for treating fractures of the middle and distal phalanges. A bloodless field is achieved by securing a soft rubber tube around the base of the finger.

Other cases will require the application of a pneumatic tourniquet to the exsanguinated extremity to ensure a bloodless field. This will necessitate a general anaesthetic, a brachial plexus block, axillary block or the production of analgesia by intravenous injection. This latter technique is very suitable for these cases. A dilute solution of lignocaine is injected after the tourniquet has been applied and complete analgesia of the hand and arm is obtained. It avoids the complications of brachial plexus block, especially pneumothorax. The latter may also be avoided, however, by an axillary block.

Special equipment

Kirschner wires of varying lengths and pointed at either end must always be available. An easily controlled Kirschner wire introducer is essential, a power-operated one being the most efficient. With such an instrument it is easier to place a wire with precision, particularly when passing it obliquely through cortical bone, than is the case with a hand operated introducer. Other instruments may be attached to the power-driven handpiece, e.g. drills, reciprocating saws for cutting bone grafts and performing osteotomies and burrs for fashioning grafts. These mechanical aids enable one to undertake precision work with minimum of effort and considerable saving of time. Other equipment includes a watchmaker's anvil on which to support the hand when working on the bone and on which to fashion a bone graft. Graduated reamers are needed to prepare the intramedullary cavity when inserting a peg-type bone graft. Small bone-holding forceps and small periosteal elevator/bone spikes are also invaluable.

THE OPERATIONS

KIRSCHNER WIRE FIXATION FOR MULTIPLE METACARPAL FRACTURES

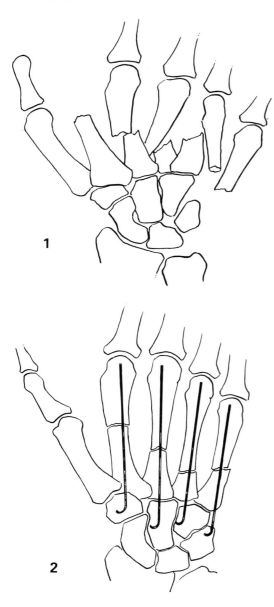

1

Kirschner wires are widely used at the time of injury to control multiple or grossly displaced fractures of metacarpals or phalanges. Grossly displaced fractures will almost certainly be open injuries. The one illustrated is a tracing of the x-ray appearance in such a case.

2

The fractures are reduced in turn and Kirschner wires passed across them. This is most easily done by passing the wire in a retrograde fashion through the distal metacarpal segment and out through the metacarpophalangeal joint. The wire is then driven back into the proximal segment and out through the dorsal aspect over the carpus where it is withdrawn so far as to ensure that the distal end lies within the metacarpal. The proximal end of the wire may be bent over in open injuries or alternatively, cut flush with the skin and allowed to retract beneath the surface.

KIRSCHNER WIRE FIXATION FOR FRACTURE OF DISTAL PHALANX

3

Transverse fracture

Transverse fractures through the proximal end of the distal phalanx result in this characteristic deformity. The forward tilting of the basal fragment is caused by the strong pull of the flexor digitorum profundus tendon which is inserted into the base of the distal phalanx.

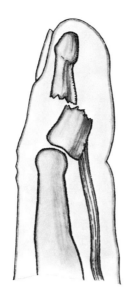

3

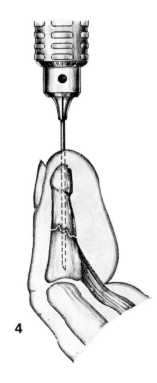

4

4

Insertion of wire

For closed injuries, the fracture is first reduced by manipulation. This involves flexing the distal interphalangeal joint to relax the flexor digitorum profundus tendon. The distal fragment may now be aligned satisfactorily. The Kirschner wire is inserted through the terminal pulp close beneath the finger nail and driven down the centre of the distal phalanx until it engages the basal fragment. A resistance is felt when the point of the wire impinges on the joint surface.

5

Completion of wiring

The distal phalanx is extended and the wire driven onwards into the head of the middle phalanx for a distance of about 1 cm. The wire is then cut off flush and left buried beneath the surface.

Open injuries

In open injuries the wire may be passed under direct vision. In these circumstances it may be easier to pass the wire in a retrograde direction through the distal fragment first and partially withdraw it through the pulp before driving it back through the proximal fragment from the other end. This technique on a metacarpal fracture is illustrated on page 473.

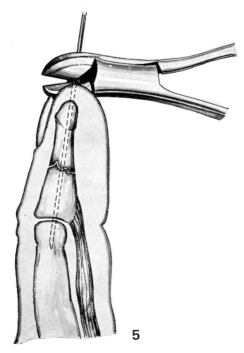

5

KIRSCHNER WIRE FIXATION FOR FRACTURE OF MIDDLE PHALANX

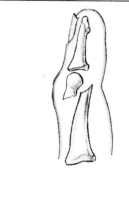

6

Displaced fracture of middle phalanx

Fractures through the neck of the middle phalanx tend to be unstable. The head of the phalanx displaces dorsally and angulates. Redisplacement may follow closed reduction and Kirschner wire fixation is then indicated.

Exposure of fracture and insertion of Kirschner wire

A longitudinal incision is made in the mid-lateral line of the finger 3 cm long, starting just beyond the distal crease and extending proximally over the distal interphalangeal joint. The neck of the phalanx is exposed by raising the periosteum just proximal to the distal joint. The fracture site is exposed and the fracture reduced by manipulating the fragments into opposition. A Kirschner wire is driven obliquely through the neck of the phalanx into the main fragment and cut flush with the surface. The skin incision is closed.

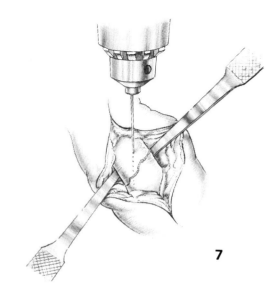

7

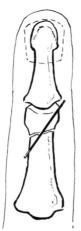

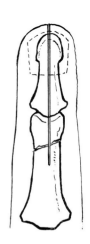

8   9

Kirschner wire fixation

The advantage of this method is that the distal interphalangeal joint is not immobilized. The wire is removed 3 weeks later.

Alternative method of fixation

The Kirschner wire may be passed through the terminal pulp of the finger, driven across the distal interphalangeal joint and then on to secure the fracture.

15

Insertion of wire

The incision is deepened down to the fracture site, which is exposed, and the fracture surfaces are cleared in the usual way. A Kirschner wire is passed in a retrograde direction along the medullary cavity of the first metacarpal. The thumb is held acutely flexed at the metacarpophalangeal joint and the wire emerges through the joint and the skin overlying it.

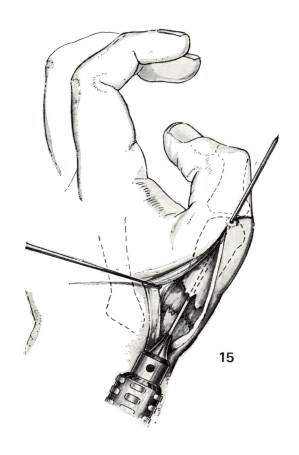

15

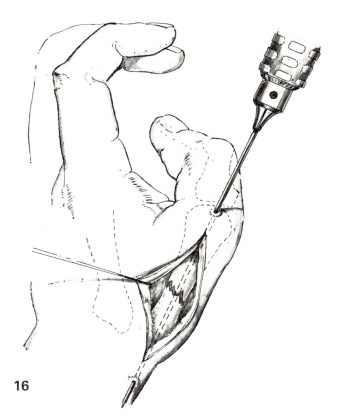

16

Positioning of wire at fracture site

16

Distal end

The introducer is transferred to the distal end of the wire which is further withdrawn until its proximal end lies at the fracture site. The fracture is manipulated into alignment and the Kirschner wire is driven proximally into the base of the metacarpal and onwards through the carpus. The thumb is held with the metacarpal flexed at the carpometacarpal joint during this stage of the procedure, and with the wrist in full ulnar deviation the wire is driven proximally until it emerges through the skin overlying the carpus.

17

Proximal end

The introducer is again switched to the proximal end of the wire which is then withdrawn backwards through the metacarpophalangeal joint until the distal end of the wire lies just within the head of the metacarpal. The proximal end is cut flush with the skin and left buried. This technique may be used with other metacarpal fractures particularly multiple ones in open injuries as shown in *Illustrations 1* and *2*. The same applies to phalangeal fractures.

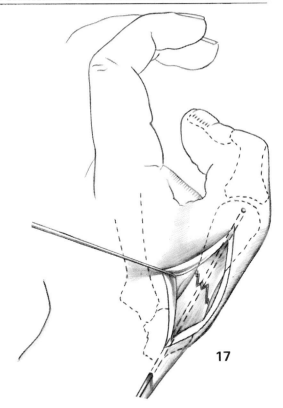

17

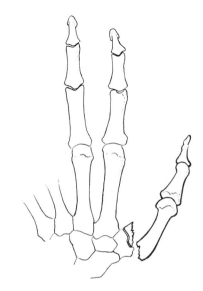

18a

18a & b & 19

Bennett's fracture

A Bennett's fracture may be similarly held by a Kirschner wire. If the detached fragment is of sufficient size a small screw provides an excellent means of fixation (*see* below).

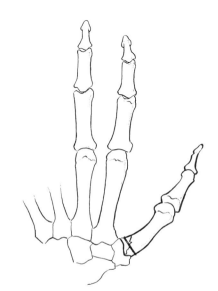

18b

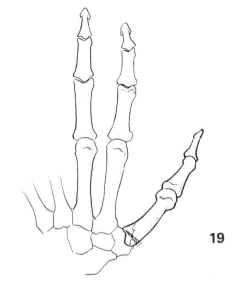

19

FIXATION OF FRACTURE BY A SINGLE SCREW

20

Oblique fracture of fifth metacarpal

The oblique type of fracture of a metacarpal with gross displacement or rotational deformity is readily reduced and held by means of a single screw.

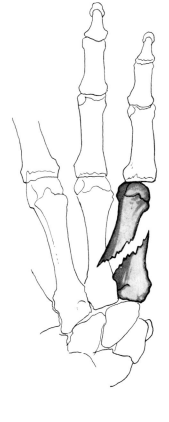

20

21

The incision

A longitudinal incision is made in the line of the fifth metacarpal on the dorsum of the hand.

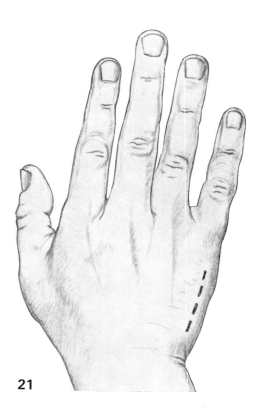

21

22

Mobilization of fracture fragments

The extensor digiti minimi tendon is exposed and the incision deepened through the deep fascia on the ulnar side. The tendon is then retracted radially and the fracture site exposed. The periosteum is stripped for a short distance along the fragments enabling each to be mobilized. The fracture surfaces are cleared of blood clot and soft tissues and manipulated into opposition. Accurate reduction having been achieved, it is maintained by means of a small clamp whilst the bone is drilled in such a way as to take a satisfactory bite of both fragments.

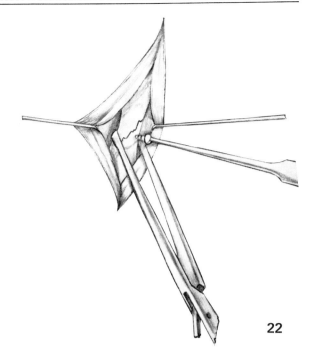

22

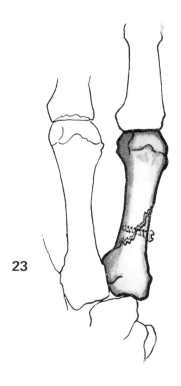

23

23

Insertion of screw

A screw is then placed and driven across the fracture. The wound is closed in layers. The screw may be left in place permanently.

BONE PLATE FOR PHALANGEAL FRACTURE

24

The incision

An incision is made in the mid-lateral line of the finger over the fractured phalanx.

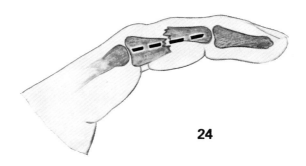

24

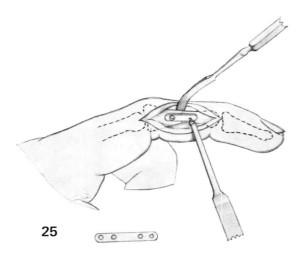

25

25

Fixation by Vitallium plate

The incision is deepened to the periosteum and the fracture site exposed. The periosteum on either side of the fracture is stripped, the haematoma removed and the bone ends reduced where they may be held by small bone spikes. A small Vitallium plate is then held in position and secured by two or four screws.

INTRAMEDULLARY BONE GRAFT FOR NON-UNION OF A METACARPAL FRACTURE

The graft is most conveniently taken from the sub-cutaneous surface of the ulna just below the olecranon. A length of bone 5 cm × 0·5 cm is cut with a power-driven oscillating saw.

26

The incision

The site of the old fracture is exposed by a longitudinal incision over the second metacarpal and on the radial side of the extensor tendons to the index finger. The incision is deepened directly to the periosteum and it may be necessary to divide the proximal part of the extensor hood. The fracture site is exposed.

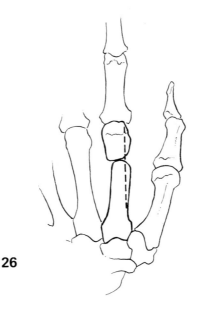

26

27

Preparation of bone for the graft

The sclerosed bone is removed from the ends of both fragments. The bone proximal to the fracture is now mobilized and prepared for reception of the graft. Whilst the bone is held in a pair of small bone-holding forceps, the medullary cavity is enlarged by reamers of graduated sizes. It is important to extend this process well down the shaft of the bone. The distal end is then similarly prepared.

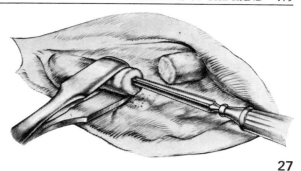

27

28

Preparation of bone graft

The bone graft is fashioned into a peg of circular cross-section and of a diameter which will just fit securely into the prepared cavity of the metacarpal. To achieve this, the graft is held in a special clamp and fashioned to size over a watchmaker's anvil, using a power-driven burr. The diameter of the graft may be checked at intervals using a drill gauge until it approximates to the size of the largest reamer used in preparing the medullary cavity.

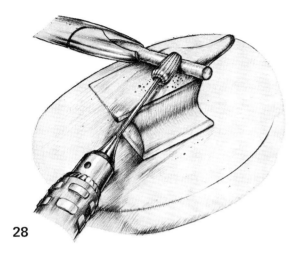

28

29

Insertion of graft

At this stage, the graft is driven into the cavity prepared in the proximal bone fragment and as far proximally as it will go. It is most important to ensure this before shortening the graft distally. The graft will now be projecting from the proximal fragment for anything from 1·25 to 2·5 cm. It should be shortened to about 1·25 cm. The distal fragment is levered over the projecting peg which should then slip into the cavity prepared in the distal bone fragment.

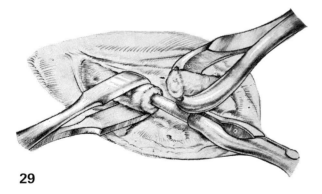

29

30

Completion of operation

Finally an impacting force is applied over the head of the metacarpal with the metacarpophalangeal joint flexed to 90°. The gap should close and the bone ends at this stage should be in contact. If they fail to do this it may mean that the graft is too long and will have to be adjusted.

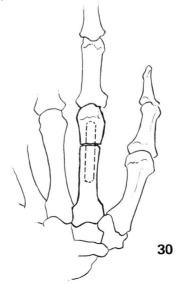

30

WEDGE OSTEOTOMY FOR ANGULATION DEFORMITY DUE TO MALUNITED FRACTURE (CONDYLE OF PROXIMAL PHALANX)

31

The deformity

The ulnar deviation deformity of the right ring finger may result from malunion following a condylar fracture of the head of the proximal phalanx.

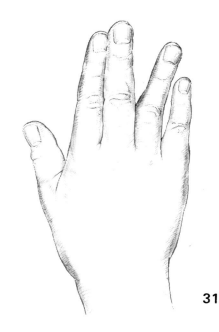

31

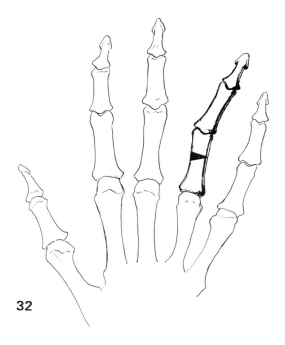

32

32

Plan for correction

A wedge osteotomy is planned. A wedge, open on the radial side, is marked out in the proximal phalanx of the ring finger.

33

The incision

A longitudinal incision about 3 cm long is made in the mid-lateral line on the radial aspect of the proximal phalanx of the finger. The intrinsic insertion is retracted dorsally and the incision deepened to the periosteum, which is raised. Periosteal elevator/bone spikes act as retractors to expose the bone.

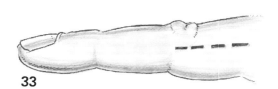

33

34

Marking the wedge

The wedge of bone to be removed is marked out with Bonney's blue. The amount of bone removed must be consistent with the degree of angulation to be corrected.

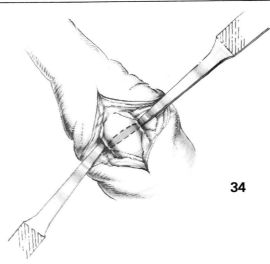

34

35

Removing the wedge

The bone wedge is removed by the use of an oscillating saw. The cut should not divide the cortex on the ulnar side. The small bone bridge left in this way is then greenstick-fractured and the wedge closed on the radial side.

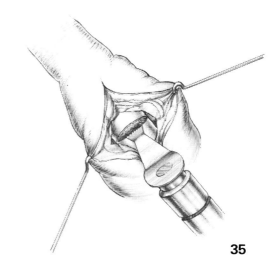

35

36 & 37

Kirschner wire fixation

The osteotomy site is now secured by two Kirschner wires introduced by a powered appliance and cut flush with the bone.

The wound is sutured and the hand bandaged over a wire-wool pad. No additional fixation is required. The fingers are mobilized at 10 days.

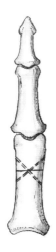

37

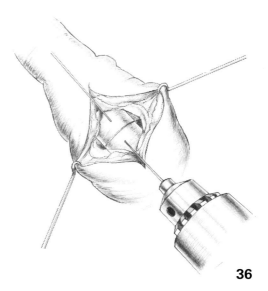

36

ROTATION OSTEOTOMY FOR ROTATIONAL DEFORMITY IN METACARPAL

38a & b

This deformity was due to malunion of a spiral fracture of the fourth right metacarpal. Note that the finger nail shows clearly that the ring finger is rotated towards the ulnar side so that on making a fist this finger over-rides the little finger.

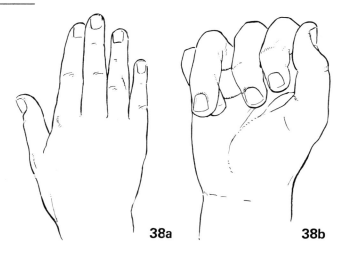

38a   38b

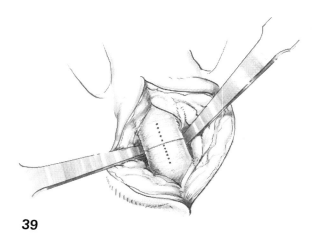

39

39

An incision is made in the line of the fourth metacarpal on the dorsum of the hand. The extensor is retracted to one side and the periosteum raised. A longitudinal mark is made at the site of the proposed osteotomy and stained with Bonney's blue. The bone is then divided transversely through this line using an oscillating saw.

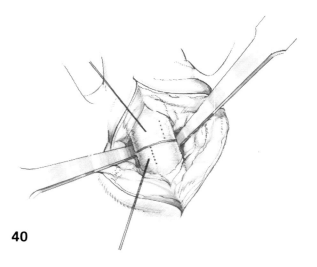

40

40

The bone is then rotated at the osteotomy site. The degree of rotation must be estimated and is related to the degree of deformity. The longitudinal guide marks now assist one in effecting the rotation. The site is secured by two Kirschner wires passed obliquely.

41

The pre- and postoperative appearances of the oste-otomy site. The x-ray film taken initially shows the degree of ulnar rotation of the metacarpal head. Postoperatively the normal projection of the meta-carpal head has been restored by the osteotomy.

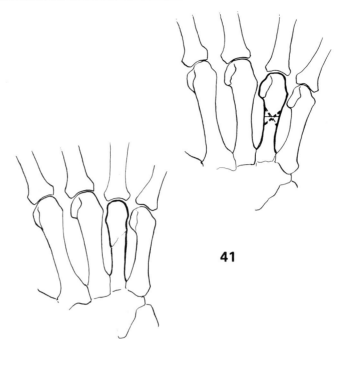

41

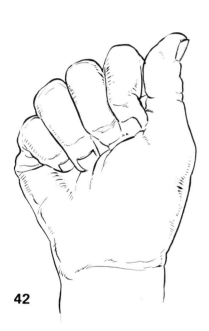

42

42

The wound is sutured and the hand bandaged over a wire-wool pad. Movements begin at 10 days. On making a fist the ring finger now flexes normally into the palm.

POSTOPERATIVE CARE

In the case of a fracture of the distal or middle phalanx held by a Kirschner wire, a simple occlusive dressing or protective wash leather finger stall is all that is required. No additional fixation is necessary. Movement of the proximal interphalangeal joint is encouraged from the start.

For more extensive injuries or when open reduction has been employed, the following routine is followed. The hand is bandaged in a functional position by incorporating a pad of sterile household steel-wool in the palm. Suitably sized bundles of steel-wool enclosed in a layer or two of gauze and sterilized by autoclaving are kept available. Apart from supporting the hand in the optimal position, this spongy mesh prevents maceration of the skin. The hand is elevated for 48 hr to control oedema, during which time the patient is encouraged to move the fingers by squeezing the enclosed pad. The dressing may be dispensed with at a week and replaced by a simple occlusive one for the wound. At this stage more active movement of all uninvolved joints is encouraged.

Open injuries receive a course of penicillin to cover the early postoperative period.

Kirschner wires are removed at 3—4 weeks, depending on the nature of the injury and subject to the radiological appearance of the fractures. When these wires have crossed joint surfaces further mobilization is required. Joint surfaces do not appear to be damaged by the wires and movement is soon regained. Buried wires are extracted through small incisions directly over their ends after infiltrating with local anaesthetic or by using a ring block. In certain cases it may be necessary to apply a tourniquet to the arm, in which instance an appropriate anaesthetic is given. Once the point of the wire has been located it is grasped by a pair of extracting forceps and withdrawn by a combination of traction and rotation.

Management following corrective osteotomy for malunited fracture follows similar lines. Buried Kirschner wires, provided they are well away from joints, may be left *in situ* and removed only should they cause discomfort.

References

Holmes, C. McK. (1963). 'Intravenous regional analgesia. A useful method of producing analgesia of the limbs.' *Lancet* 1, 245
Hoyle, J. R. (1964). 'Tourniquet for intravenous regional analgesia.' *Anaesthesia* 19, 294
Milford, L. (1971). 'Hand Surgery.' In *Campbell's Operative Orthopaedics.* London: Kimpton
Pulvertaft, R. G. (1966). 'Injuries of the phalanges and metacarpal bones and joints.' In *Clinical Surgery—The Hand*, p.80. London: Butterworths
Reid, D. A. C. (1956). 'Experience of a hand surgery service.' *Br. J. plast. Surg.* 9, 11
Reid, D. A. C. (1974). 'Corrective osteotomy in the hand.' *The Hand* 6, 50
Vom Saal, F. H. (1953). 'Intramedullary fixation in fractures of the hand and fingers.' *J. Bone Jt Surg.* 35A, 5

[*The illustrations for this Chapter on Operative Treatment of Fractures of the Hand were drawn by Mr. A. S. Foster.*]

Skin Replacement and Scar Correction in the Hand

P. J. Whitfield, F.R.C.S.
Consultant Plastic Surgeon, Plastic Surgery and
Burns Centre, Queen Mary's Hospital, Roehampton

PRE - OPERATIVE

Skin loss on the hand is usually caused by injury but may be the result of operation for malignant disease and occasionally as a sequel to infection. Replacement is of paramount importance and failure to undertake this adequately will lead to fibrosis, stiffness and incapacity of the hand. Furthermore, any reconstructive operation will be prejudiced by such stiffness.

Skin cover is obtained by the use of free grafts or flaps.

Free grafts

The survival of free grafts depends on the blood supply of the bed on which they are placed. It is futile to place free grafts on bare bone, bare tendon and cartilage. In these situations skin flaps are required.

Free grafts take well provided that haemostasis is ensured with immobilization of the graft. Failure to achieve haemostasis will lead to haematoma, and the graft fails to take. It also serves as a nutrient medium for bacteria and any resulting infection will certainly destroy the graft.

Free grafts used on the hand will be of either split-skin (Thiersch) or full-thickness (Wolfe).

Split-skin grafts take more rapidly than Wolfe grafts because they are rapidly vascularized and have a high resistance to infection.

Wolfe grafts have better durability, tactile gnosis and appearance than split-skin grafts and in addition there is less likelihood of contraction.

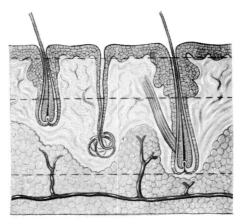

Split skin grafts

Full thickness grafts

485

Flaps

Flaps are much to be preferred to free grafts in some instances because they provide soft tissue padding and they possess a certain blood supply if they are planned correctly.

They are necessary where bone, tendon or cartilage is exposed or infection and sloughing of these structures will occur.

Local flaps should be used wherever possible as they convey better tactile sensibility. This is not always possible and in these cases or when the back of the hand is concerned, skin from a distant site may have to be used.

Whether local or distant, the success of a flap is dependent on careful planning and the use of sensible proportions in the vascular base or pedicle.

Flaps should always have an adequate layer of fat. If too bulky they may be thinned later.

Flaps usually leave a secondary defect, which is closed with a split-skin graft and tie-over packs. Occasionally, primary closure is possible but it should be avoided if it may kink the base of the flap.

It is extremely important that distant flaps be planned with consideration of the scarring produced by the secondary defect. It is not justifiable to make elegant flaps from cosmetically unacceptable sites when less conspicuous sites can be selected.

SPLIT-SKIN GRAFTS

Indications

As emergency cover following any injury where skin loss does not expose cortical bone, cartilage or bare tendon.

As a definitive cover where skin loss results from a full-thickness burn or removal of a skin tumour. In the release of contractures.

Anaesthesia

When the area of skin lost is small, local analgesia or regional block may be used. However, general anaesthesia is preferred for large grafts.

FULL-THICKNESS GRAFTS

Indications

Small defects of the palm or flexor aspects of the fingers where better durability and tactile gnosis is required than that provided by split-skin grafts.

Anaesthesia

Local or regional analgesia is used but general anaesthesia is preferable for nervous or excitable patients.

TOE PULP GRAFTS

Indications

These are used only in children when only the pulp of the finger has been lost. The defect in the toe is closed by suture of a small split-skin graft.

Anaesthesia

General anaesthesia is preferred.

LOCAL FLAPS

The thenar flap

Indications

This type of repair is applicable to traumatic amputations of any of the fingers through the distal phalanx, especially when the end of the bone has been exposed or cleanly cut off at right angles to the length.

The flap should result in a nicely rounded end of the finger with good sensibility. It obviates the necessity for shortening the phalanx in order to bury the exposed end of the bone.

The texture of palmar skin is similar to that of the finger tip and gives better recovery of tactile sensibility than would result if more distant skin were employed. This method is unsuitable for elderly patients, when stiffness may follow the period of immobilization, and in every case before commencing the operation the surgeon should make sure that the finger tip can reach the palm with ease.

Anaesthesia

General anaesthesia is preferred for children. In adults digital block can be employed with local infiltration of the donor site.

The palmar flap

Indications

These are much the same as with the thenar flap but a palmar flap is used principally when there is skin lost from the distal part of the thumb. It may have the disadvantage, however, of leaving a tender scar.

Anaesthesia

Local or general.

The cross-finger flap

Indications

This method is indicated when skin lost from the flexor surface of the finger or thumb is of such thickness that repair by a free split-skin or Wolfe graft is likely to result in marked deformity or loss of tactile appreciation.

It is particularly suitable for oblique, slicing injuries of the ends of the digits.

Anaesthesia

General anaesthesia or digital block is satisfactory.

Transposition flaps

Indications

These are few and usually occur with defects on the volar aspect of the middle phalanx or on the dorsum. They are hazardous in elderly patients and when there is crushed or burnt skin in the intended flap or its base.

Anaesthesia

General anaesthesia is used.

Volar advancement flap (Moberg)

Indications

This flap is used to replace a small insensitive scarred area at the tip of a thumb, where the loss of feeling is important. A strip of skin up to 15 mm wide can be moved by such a manoeuvre.

Anaesthesia

General anaesthesia is preferred.

DISTANT FLAPS

The abdominal skin flap

Indications

This operation replaces scarring on the back of the hand by an abdominal skin flap. It is suitable for cases of severe scarring of the dorsum involving the extensor tendons and causing a 'frozen' hand. It is also suitable for trauma to the dorsum and occasionally for localized burns.

While the flap to be described is a large one, smaller abdominal flaps may be used for finger defects.

In women a small flap may be raised from the inframammary fold, where the secondary defect is largely concealed.

Anaesthesia

General anaesthesia is necessary for the first stage of the operation; for the subsequent part, general or local infiltration is all that is required.

The groin flap (McGregor)

Indications

This flap is based on the superficial circumflex iliac vessels and is used to cover the dorsal or palmar surface of the hand. It can be used in acute degloving injuries of the hand as well as for elective reconstruction.

Anaesthesia

General anaesthesia is preferred.

The pectoral flap

Indication

This is of particular use in degloving injuries affecting the thumb but it is contra-indicated in women because the secondary scarring is unsightly. The abdomen may be used for this purpose but the flap tends to be bulkier and requires thinning.

Anaesthesia

General anaesthesia is preferred.

The cross-arm bridge flap

Indications

This operation is designed to effect a full-thickness skin repair on the volar aspect of a finger by means of a flap from the opposite forearm. Repair by this method is indicated in the following circumstances. (*1*) Flexion contracture on the volar aspect of any finger involving the flexor tendon or digital nerves and vessels. (*2*) Severe skin shortage between the distal interphalangeal joint and the base of the finger. (*3*) To supply suitable skin cover where the flexor tendon sheath has been destroyed in addition to the skin and subcutaneous tissues and a free tendon graft will be required later. This condition is commonly seen in electrical burns.

Anaesthesia

A general anaesthetic is suitable; alternatively brachial block may be used for the affected arm, with local infiltration of the donor area of skin on the opposite forearm.

The Z-plasty operation

Indications

The principle

Many linear scar defects in the hand are correctable by Z-plasty.

It has two effects: (*1*) it lengthens the scar by a ratio of $1 \cdot 7 : 1$ when the angles of the Z are $60°$; (*2*) it breaks up the scar line so that any contracture only opens the limbs of the Z.

Z-plasty is indicated for linear scars on the hand which (*a*) run across skin, (*b*) by their linear contracture reduce the range of movement, (*c*) are confined to skin and subcutaneous fat, or (*d*) are surrounded by healthy skin.

Anaesthesia

General or local infiltration anaesthesia is required.

The neurovascular island flap

Indications

(*1*) Where there is sensory loss on the contiguous sides of the index finger and thumb.

(*2*) When a skin flap has been used to reconstruct the thumb the restoration of sensibility promotes the function of the whole hand.

Anaesthesia

General anaesthesia is preferred.

THE OPERATIONS

THE SPLIT-SKIN GRAFT

1

Cutting the graft

The graft is taken freehand from the back of the thigh, using a board to steady the skin and a skin graft knife lubricated with liquid paraffin. A small graft may be taken from the forearm in men and from the buttock in women.

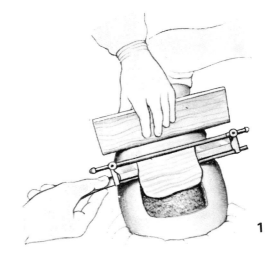

2

Severance of graft

The graft is cut off with scissors. The donor site is dressed with tulle gras and gauze dressings re-inforced with wool.

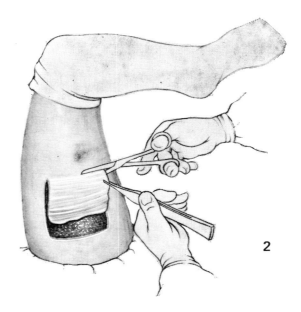

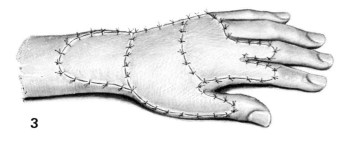

3

Application of graft

The graft bed is prepared and the graft sutured into position as shown. It is secured with tie-over sutures tied over wet wool or flavine wool.

THE FULL-THICKNESS OR WOLFE GRAFT

4

The donor area

The best site is the medial side of the arm just above the epicondyle, where the skin is slack and scarring is inconspicuous and will not cause contracture.

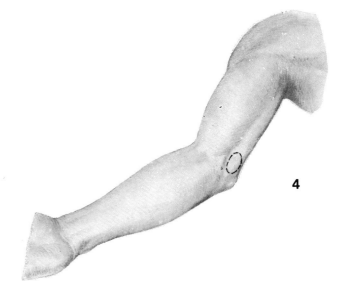

4

5

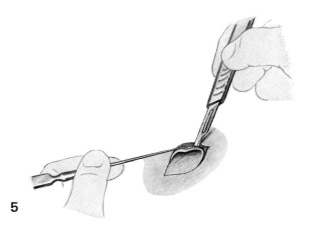

5

Removing the graft

The size and shape of the graft is marked out before the skin is incised and the graft lifted with a hook and dissected free. The resulting defect can then be closed by sutures.

6

Thinning the graft

The graft is supported on the surgeon's index finger while the fat is cut off with curved scissors.

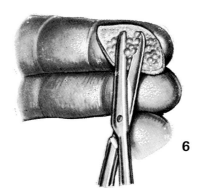

6

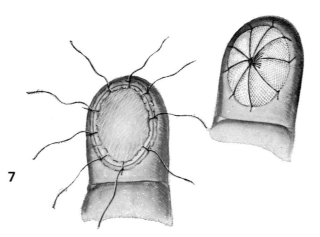

7

7

Suturing the graft

The graft is sutured in position and held with tie-over packs.

THE TOE PULP GRAFT

8

Estimation of pulp loss

A pattern of area of skin lost is made, using a piece of jaconet.

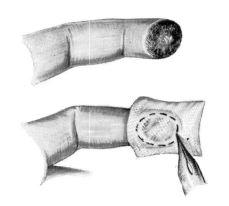

8

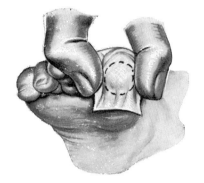

9

9

Removal and transference of donor pulp

Before removing the toe pulp, the toe pulp is marked as shown. The graft is sutured in position on the finger tip and split-skin graft is applied to the toe.

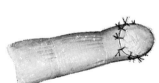

THE THENAR FLAP

First operation

10

Estimation of defect

The defect is cleaned and the skin trimmed so that the free edge of the dermis is clearly defined. The finger is flexed until the tip meets the palm, where it leaves a circular blood stain corresponding to the defect.

The incision

Using the blood stain on the thenar area as a guide. a jaconet pattern is cut to correspond with the flap of skin required. The two corners of the base of the pattern are stitched temporarily to the skin. The

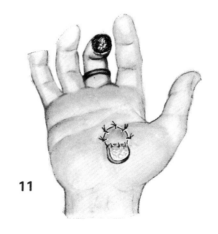

10

pattern hinged on the stitches is placed in contact with the finger tip to check length and alignment. After this test the pattern is laid back on the thenar skin, and the flap to be raised is marked out with Bonney's blue.

11

Raising the flap

The skin flap is raised in the subcutaneous fat layer. A small split-skin graft from the inner aspect of the arm is placed over the thenar defect and tied in place with a wool pack.

11

12 & 13

Attachment of flap

The thenar skin flap is sutured to the finger tip, fixation being obtained by a strip of zinc oxide strapping, another piece round the wrist fixing the two ends securely. It is advisable to place a small pad of wool or orthopaedic felt between the strapping and the dorsum of the proximal interphalangeal joint to prevent a pressure sore.

Second operation

Two weeks later the flap is divided under local analgesia, trimmed and stitched neatly in place.

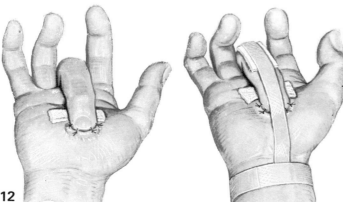

12

13

THE PALMAR FLAP

14

Raising the flap

The raising of the flap is undertaken after marking of the area with a jaconet pattern.

Closure of secondary defect

A split-skin graft is sutured to the bed from which the flap was raised before the flap is attached to its new site.

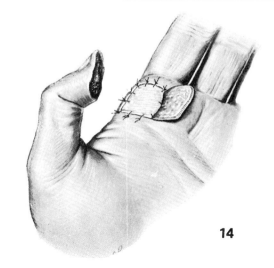

14

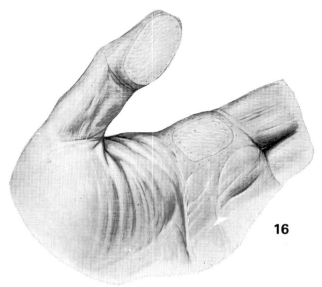

15

15

Attachment to thumb

This is undertaken with interrupted fine silk sutures, and there must be no tension in the flap.

16

Inset of flap

This is undertaken at 3 weeks, the base being divided and trimmed in the usual way.

16

THE CROSS-FINGER FLAP

First operation

17

Estimation of defect and raising of flap

A jaconet pattern is cut out and stitched at its base to the donor finger. By bringing its surface in contact with the defect on the recipient finger and then laying it back on the donor finger, the exact extent of the flap required is estimated. The outline of the pattern is marked out on the donor finger with Bonney's blue. The flap is then raised, dissecting in the subcutaneous fat. This dissection should never be taken beyond the mid-lateral line lest a tender lateral scar result.

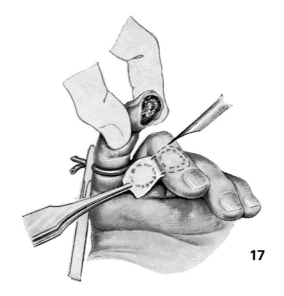

17

18

Flap suture

The flap is sutured with fine silk or nylon to the margins of the defect, which have been undermined slightly to permit accurate apposition.

The donor area is covered with a sheet of split skin carefully sutured to its margins. Several of the stitches are left 'long' and tied over a small pack of wool laid on the graft (omitted from the illustration for clarity).

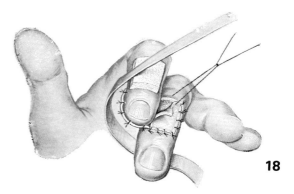

18

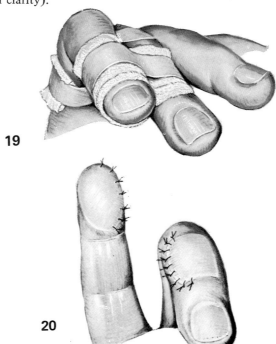

19

20

19

Immobilization technique

After dressing, the two fingers are strapped together with strips of adhesive strapping suitably padded across the dorsum of each finger.

Second operation

20

Separation of flap

The flap can be divided at the end of 2 weeks with local analgesia. As an out-patient operation the two free edges are seen set in to their respective fingers.

THE TRANSPOSITION FLAP

21

Principle

The unsatisfactory area is excised and an incision made as shown. (Note that the flap is broader and much longer than the area it is to replace.) The flap is undermined and used to cover the defect. The secondary defect is closed with a split-skin graft. The buckling at the base of the flap gradually disappears.

21

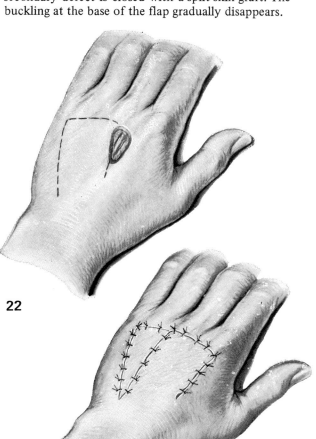

22

23

22&23

On dorsal defects of the hand

Illustration 22 shows removal of the lesion and planning of flap.
Illustration 23 shows the flap inset and split-skin graft on the defect.

24&25

On proximal phalanx of finger

Illustration 24 shows removal of the lesion and planning of flap.
Illustration 25 shows the flap inset and split-skin graft on the defect.

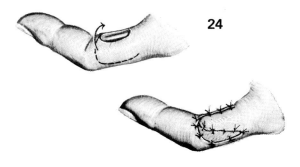

24

25

VOLAR ADVANCEMENT FLAP (MOBERG)

26

Incisions are made in the mid-lateral line on each side and the ventral skin is elevated with the neurovascular bundles. The scarred area is excised.

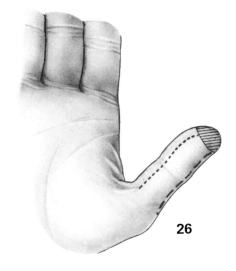

26

27

The flap is advanced distally to close the tip defect.

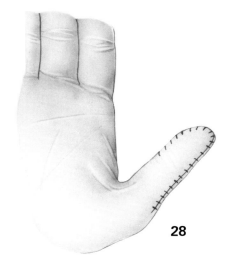

27

28

The flap is sutured into its new bed and the arm is elevated and the thumb left exposed with the digit in flexion.

28

THE ABDOMINAL FLAP

First stage

29

Scar excision

A tourniquet is applied to the arm and thorough dissection of all scar tissue is carried out in a bloodless field. The tourniquet is then removed and bleeding stopped.

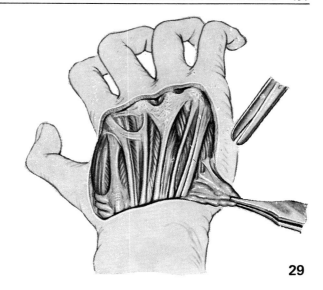

29

30

Planning of skin flap

A jaconet pattern is cut to the shape of the defect. It is laid upon the hand, making sure that there is ample length to reach the furthest point without tension. Two stitches through the skin fix the base of the pattern at the points where the attachment of the flap is to lie.

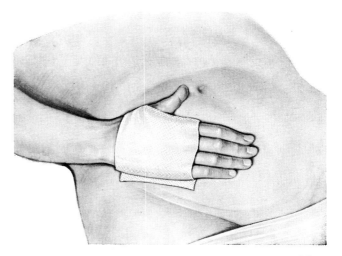

30

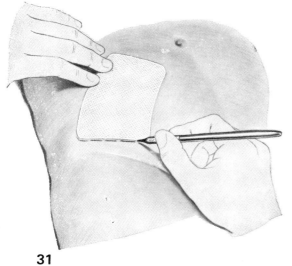

31

31

Marking of skin flap

The hand has been withdrawn and the pattern smoothed out to rest on the abdomen. The flap is then marked out on the skin with Bonney's blue.

32

Covering the secondary defect

The skin flap is incised and elevated, dissecting the subcutaneous fat to an even thickness. The defect on the abdomen is covered with a sheet of split-skin taken from the thigh and stitched in round the margins. A few sutures are left long to be tied over a pack of wool.

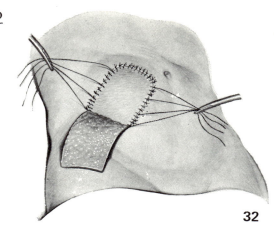

32

33

Suture of the flap

The pack of wool is tied in position and the flap of skin carefully sutured into the defect on the back of the hand.

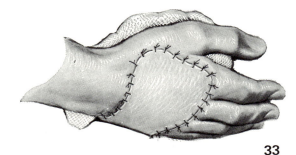

33

34

Fixation of the arm

The arm is fixed by strips of extension Elastoplast padded where pressure might occur. It is of the utmost importance that the fixation be secure while the patient is recovering from the anaesthetic.

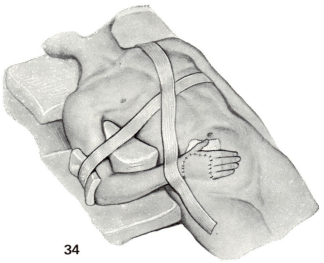

34

35

Second stage

Provided that the flap has taken well on the hand the second stage can be carried out 3 weeks after the first. It consists of dividing the base of the flap, trimming and setting it into the ulnar border of the hand, and closing the small remaining defect on the abdomen.

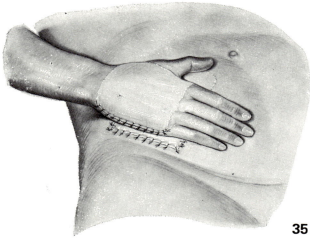

35

THE GROIN FLAP (McGREGOR)

First stage

36

The site is chosen on the groin so that the hand lies in comfortable proximity to it.

The inguinal ligament and the femoral artery are marked to establish reference points before marking out the necessary size of flap.

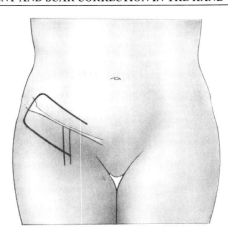

36

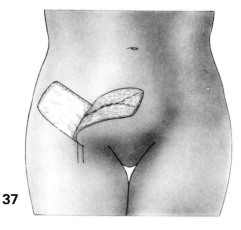

37

37

The flap is raised down to fascia and is based on the superficial circumflex iliac vessels, to the level of the sartorius muscle (to avoid damage to the feeder vessels).

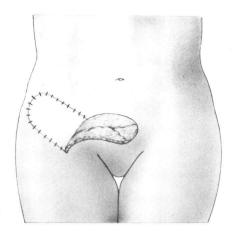

38

38

The bed of the flap is closed with a split-skin graft (occasionally direct closure is possible).

39

The flap is inset into the hand defect.

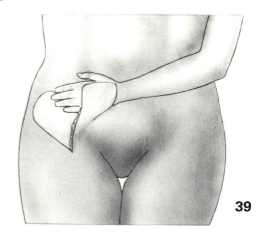

39

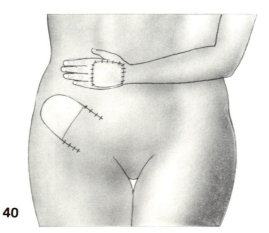

40

Second stage

40

The flap is divided at 3 weeks but not inset. Dressings are applied.

Third stage

41

The flap is trimmed and inset into the hand after further week.

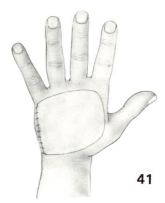

41

THE PECTORAL FLAP

42

Planning of flap

The patient is positioned on the table in a comfortable position and the flap is marked on the chest wall in a suitable position for attachment to the thumb.

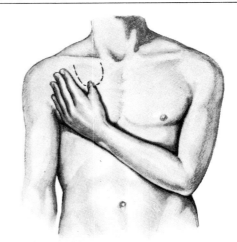

42

43

Raising the flap

The flap is raised and thinned evenly but leaving a modest amount of fat.

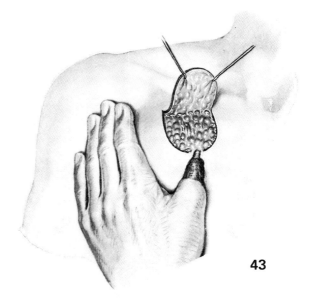

43

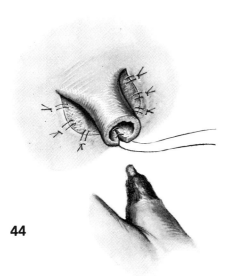

44

44

Refining the flap

The flap is 'tubed' and a split-skin graft used to cover the secondary defect.

45

Attachment of tube

The tube is attached to the thumb carefully and the arm is strapped to the side with a pad in the axilla.

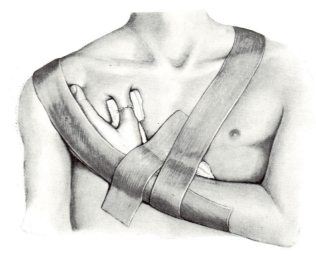

45

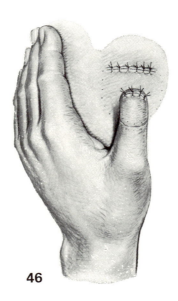

46

46

Division of the flap

The flap is divided at 3 weeks and inset.

THE NEUROVASCULAR ISLAND FLAP

47

Estimation of defect

The defect in the thumb is marked on the pulp of the ulnar side of the ring finger.

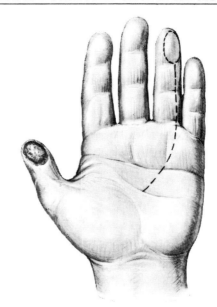

47

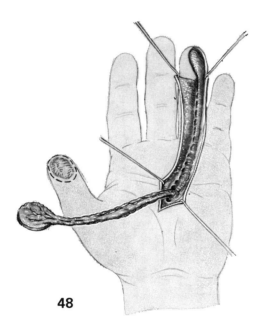

48

48

Dissection of island flap

The donor area is dissected free with its intact neurovascular bundle, which has to be separated into the palm.

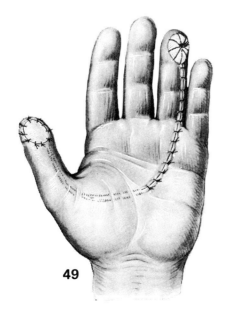

49

49

Inset of island flap

Via a tunnel made from the palm to the thumb tip the hemipulp attached to its bundle is passed to its future site.

The secondary defect in the ring finger is closed with a split-skin graft sutured with tie-over packs.

THE CROSS-ARM BRIDGE FLAP

Position of patient

The primary dissection of the finger is carried out with the patient supine and the hand resting on an arm board by the side of the table. The skin of both arms is prepared and each is towelled separately to the elbow. The rest of the body is covered with a sterile sheet up to the axillae. The arm on the side of the lesion is exsanguinated with an Esmarch bandage and pneumatic cuff tourniquet inflated to 240 mm.

50

Pre-operative appearance

The type of deformity for which the procedure is most suitable is illustrated.

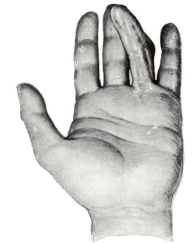

50

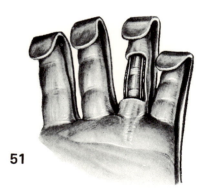

51

51

Scar excision

A lead hand splint keeps the fingers extended while removal of all scar tissue limiting extension is carried out, but preserving digital vessels and nerves. The flexor tendon sheath may in some cases have to be removed, leaving only enough of the pulleys to prevent 'bowstringing' of the tendons.

52

Planning the flap

After completing the dissection the skin edges should be quite loose when the finger is fully extended and should lie along the mid-lateral lines of the finger. An oblong defect remains to be covered.

The tourniquet is then removed and bleeding stopped. The forearms are crossed in front of the chest and the dissected finger laid along the postero-medial aspect of the donor arm. The outline of the recipient finger is drawn on the arm and a flap of suitable width and length marked out.

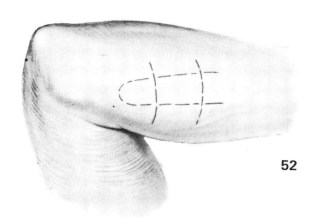

52

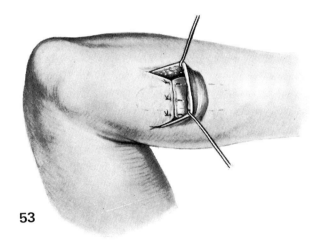

53

53

Preparation of skin bridge

The bridge is incised, undermined and raised. The skin defect beneath the bridge is closed by undermining and approximation. Alternatively a split-skin graft can be applied and stitched to the margins.

The recipient finger will come to lie between the split-skin graft and the skin flap.

54

Attachment of flap

The finger is passed beneath the bridge of skin and the wrist is bandaged to the donor forearm. To secure the finger in correct alignment a single stitch of strong nylon has been passed through the free edge of the finger nail and the adjacent forearm skin. The bridge flap should completely cover the exposed defect on the finger and only a few marginal sutures are required to unite the opposed edges.

Bands of Elastoplast suitably padded hold the arms together, leaving the good hand free so that the patient can feed himself.

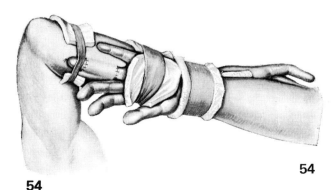

54

54

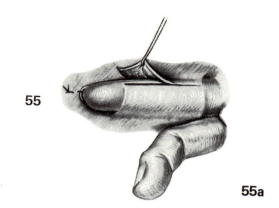

55

55a

55 & 56

Later procedures

Ten days later the anterior attachment of the bridge is divided with local analgesia, leaving sufficient skin to inset the edge on the mid-lateral line of the finger without tension. Another 10 days later the posterior attachment of the bridge is divided and inset in the same way as at the previous operation.

On the donor forearm the two ends of the flap are trimmed and inset.

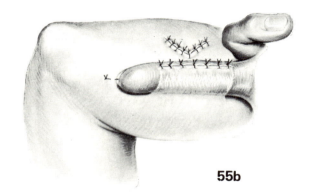

55b

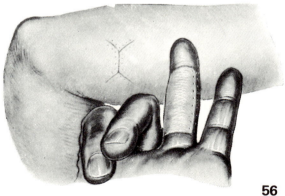

56

THE Z-PLASTY

57

The incisions

The area of scar to be excised has been marked with Bonney's blue and two triangular skin flaps outlined. The angle of apex of the flaps should not be less than 45° and preferably more. They must be carefully planned to be of equal size and in such a direction that when transposed their adjacent sides will lie in a normal skin line, in this case the middle palmar crease.

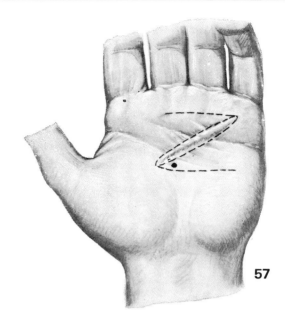

57

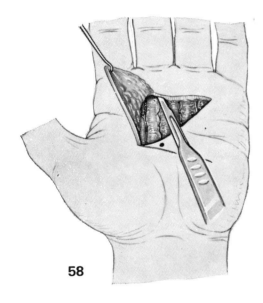

58

58

Excision of scar

The scar is excised and the two flaps dissected up in the subcutaneous layer. Hooks rather than forceps should be used for holding up the skin and the undermining should be carried beyond the base of each flap.

59

Transposition of flaps

The flaps are transposed and sutured into their new position without tension. A light-pressure dressing is applied over the whole palm.

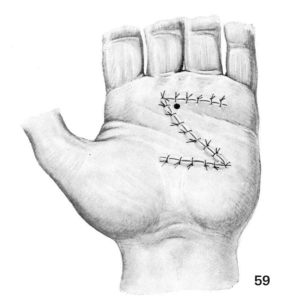

59

POSTOPERATIVE CARE

All free grafts must be kept elevated at shoulder level for 72 hr. Thereafter the hand must be kept in a sling for 2 weeks.

All flaps must be inspected regularly so that changes in position do not kink the base nor put tension on the suture line. They should be 'rolled' gently and regularly to obviate collection of haematomas.

The split-skin graft

This may be inspected and dressed at 6—7 days and then re-dressed. When healing has occurred gentle grease massage is commenced.

The Wolfe graft

This is best left for 10 days before dressing and inspection. A firm dressing is re-applied for a further 10 days and grease massage started.

The toe pulp graft

Sutures are removed at 10 days.

The thenar flap

The patient is kept under observation as an out-patient and encouraged to use the rest of the hand as much as possible. The sutures and wool pack are removed on the tenth day, but the strapping fixation must be retained until the flap is divided, after which the repaired finger should be protected by a finger-stall from rough usage for a further 3 weeks.

The cross-finger flap

The patient can be discharged the day after the first operation to attend as an out-patient and is encouraged to use the rest of his hand.

Should the implantation of the flap on the recipient finger have failed to 'take over' at least two thirds of the defect, it is advisable to allow a longer interval between the two operations.

The transposition flap

The split-skin graft is re-dressed at 6 days and the flap sutures removed after 8 days.

Volar advancement flap

The hand is kept elevated for 10 days. The sutures are removed after 8 days.

When first used the digit should be protected by a finger-stall until the tip becomes 'weathered'.

Groin flap

Gentle finger movements may be allowed when the flap is attached and they can be graduated during the 3 weeks before detachment of the flap.

When the flap is detached movements may be continued but reduced for 5 days after it has been finally set in place.

The hand should be kept elevated after detachment of the flap and remain so for 10 days after formal insetting. Then, with exercises, the limb may be allowed gradually lower positions.

The abdominal and pectoral skin flaps

Ten days after the first operation the sutures in the flap are taken out and the pack over the graft is removed.

The cross-arm bridge flap

When the finger is soundly healed exercises and wax baths are used to restore function.

The neurovascular flap

The split-skin graft is inspected at 6 days and the sutures are moved from the thumb at 8 days.

The Z-plasty

The hand should be elevated in a sling until the sutures have been removed, which should be after 10 days. Gentle active movements can then be commenced but full extension of the previously restricted digit should not be attempted until the scar is soundly healed.

References

Clarkson, P. W. and Pelly, A. (1962). *General and Plastic Surgery of the Hand*. Oxford: Blackwell
Gillies, H. D. and Millard, D. R. (1957). *The Princuples and Art of Plastic Surgery*. London: Butterworths
McGregor, I. A. (1968). *Fundamental Techniques of Plastic Surgery*, 4th ed. Edinburgh: Livingstone
McGregor, I. A. and Jackson, I. T. (1972). *Br. J. plast. Surg.* **25**, 3
Moberg, E. (1964). *J. Bone Jt Surg.* **46A**, 817
Rank, B. K., Wakefield, A. R. and Hueston, J. T. (1968). *Surgery of Repair as Applied to Hand Injuries*, 3rd Edition. Edinburgh: Livingstone

[*The illustrations for this Chapter on Skin Replacement and Scar Correction in the Hand were drawn by Mr. R. N. Lane and Mr. F. Price.*]

Amputations

H. Graham Stack, F.R.C.S.
Consultant Orthopaedic Surgeon, Harold Wood Hospital, Essex,
Consultant in Hand Surgery, Regional Centre for Plastic Surgery,
St. Andrew's Hospital, Billericay, Essex

PRE-OPERATIVE

General preparation

Amputation of any part of the hand should be approached as a full surgical procedure. The patient has to live with his stump for the remainder of his life. It is not an operation to be approached lightly in a casualty department.

The aim is a smooth, pain-free, non-tender, mobile stump, covered with soft mobile skin, with normal sensibility.

In cases where injury has caused severe mutilation, a plan for the best possible restoration of function should be formulated. It may be advisable to retain parts of the hand, of no value in themselves, to aid the task of later reconstruction.

General anaesthesia and a pneumatic tourniquet are required. Fine instruments are used, scaled to the size of the structures to be handled. It is particularly important to use fine suture material on fine needles: 5/0 or 6/0 silk or nylon is recommended.

Painful stumps

Excessive length of bone relative to a shortage of skin can cause a painful stump, as can a fragment of nail bed remaining, or an epidermoid cyst in the scar.

The most common cause of a painful stump is the presence of a neuroma attached or too close to the skin. The regenerating nerve fibres may even be involved in the scar.

In the past, re-amputation achieved a bad reputation because the nerve or the neuroma became involved again at the new level. Long continued discomfort may lead to ineradicable pain, but true causalgia is a rare complication.

A painful stump therefore should at least once be treated by exploration with removal of the neuroma, and shortening of the nerve. This operation must be done with the greatest possible care by an experienced surgeon.

Levels

Length should be preserved as far as possible, particularly in the mutilated hand. This applies especially to the thumb, where length is all-important for opposition function even if one or more joints are stiff.

In each segment of the fingers, as much length of bone as possible should usually be preserved since small fragments tend to be painful and flexed but it is a mistake to leave a stump with a stiff joint that makes it stick out awkwardly beyond the other digits.

The best levels in practice are: (1) not more proximal than the middle of the distal phalanx; (2) as near the neck of the middle and proximal phalanges as possible; (3) through the metacarpophalangeal joint if the palm is to be preserved intact; (4) through the proximal third of the metacarpal shaft if the remaining fingers are to be approximated.

If all the fingers are to be removed, as much of the metacarpus should be saved as possible, to provide an opposition post for the thumb.

The undamaged thumb alone is of immense value because it carries the tactile sensibility that a prosthesis does not possess.

Incisions

Incisions must be planned in accordance with the principle that they should not cross flexure lines at right angles, and should be sinuous rather than linear. Where the latter is unavoidable, breaking the scar with Z-plasties may be necessary.

Vessels

Haemorrhage may result from a partially divided vessel, particularly from the branching veins on the dorsum of the hand. Care must be taken that all vessels are cleanly cut across. Holding a vessel in a haemostat for a few minutes is often enough to prevent further bleeding. Lavish ligation of many vessels leaves much foreign tissue behind, so minimal ligation is advised.

The main vessels on the volar side may require ligation. Release of the tourniquet before the final suturing of the skin will reveal the necessity for ligation.

THE OPERATION

1

Flaps

Flaps often have to be designed for each case, due to the loss of tissue by trauma. They may have to be of equal length, with a terminal scar. Preferably, the volar flaps should be a little longer, making the scar slightly dorsal. 'Dog-ears' must be avoided by excision and by tailoring the flaps to fit carefully.

There is a tendency for flaps to shrink even before suture; this tendency should be allowed for in the design of flaps, as it is essential that the final stump must be covered by free mobile skin.

The flaps must not be under tension, or a shiny painful stump will result.

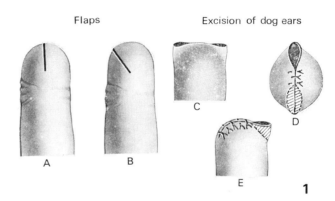

Flaps   Excision of dog ears

A   B   C   D   E

1

2

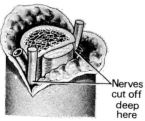
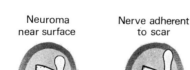

Neuroma near surface   Nerve adherent to scar

Nerves cut off deep here

POOR RESULTS

2

Nerves

The treatment of the nerves is all important. The individual digital nerves should be carefully sought, separated and explored proximally. The nerves should all be shortened considerably to ensure that the inevitable neuromata will not be subject to pressure on gripping, and to ensure that the fibres growing out from the end of the nerve cannot infiltrate or become adherent to the scar. The nerves should be cut across cleanly with a sharp knife or razor blade, to ensure the minimum of damage. The end should be buried under muscle or fat if possible. The extremely tender 'electric finger' is due to nerve involvement in scar.

3

Tendons

Fixation of a tendon to the stump or deep in the hand can cause considerable interference with function, both of the stump or the uninjured fingers. The tendons must not be sutured to each other across a stump, but should be excised well back into the stump or the hand.

Tenderness in the palm can also be caused by a retracted tendon or tendon sequestrum.

Due to the common origin of the tendons of the flexor digitorum profundus to the middle, ring and little fingers, adhesion of a cut tendon may seriously interfere with the function of the tendons in an adjoining finger. This has been described by Verdan (1966) as the 'syndrome of the Quadriga'. In these cases the long flexor tendons of the damaged fingers should be excised well up in the palm, through the proximal palmar, or even the thenar crease.

It used to be stated that the short stump of a finger consisting of the proximal phalanx only was useless, as there were no muscles attached to it, preventing it being moved. This is not the case. There are enough attachments of intrinsic muscles to the stump to move it satisfactorily, and the stump maintains the integrity of the hand as a whole, particularly in preventing the fingers falling together, when the damaged finger is the middle or ring finger.

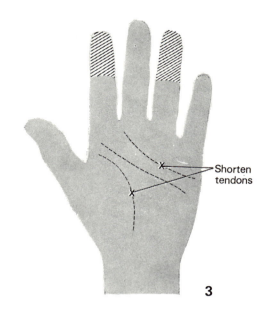

Shorten tendons

3

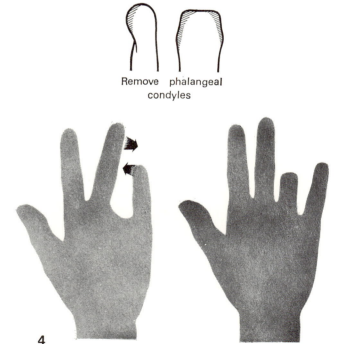

Remove phalangeal condyles

4

4

Bone

Bone stumps should not be left so long that they cause tension in the overlying skin. Bone should be carefully cut, to avoid splintering which may be followed by sequestration. The shaft of the bone should not be cut across in one bite.

The protuberance of the condyles of the phalanges, both anteriorly and laterally must be removed, in order to prevent bulky stumps.

Very short phalangeal stumps tend to flex, and amputation is better performed through the more proximal joint.

Proximal phalanges should be preserved if possible, as this stump prevents the fingers deviating.

5 & 6

Transverse sections

These two diagrams, taken from fetal cross sections, are to illustrate the size and position of the bones, and also the position in which to search for the digital vessels and nerves. *Illustration 5* shows the transverse section through the middle phalanx. *Illustration 6* shows the transverse section through the proximal interphalangeal joint.

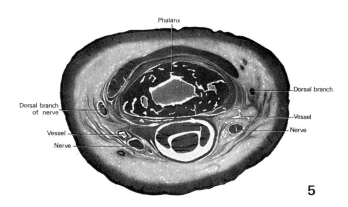

5

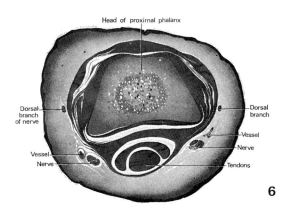

6

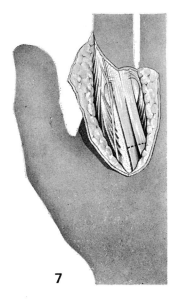

7

AMPUTATION THROUGH THE METACARPO-PHALANGEAL JOINT, PRESERVING THE HEAD OF THE METACARPAL

7

The incision

Make an asymmetrical dorsal racket incision. The lateral flap should be larger and extend nearly halfway down the shaft of the phalanx. This has to reach the web of the adjoining finger after suture, without tension. The two limbs of the incision at the web should meet at an angle to prevent a 'dog-ear'.

8

Exposure

Deepen dorsally until the extensor tendons are exposed. Divide the extensor tendon and turn it distally. Separate the expansion round the base of the proximal phalanx. Divide the collateral ligaments of the metacarpophalangeal joint. On the volar side divide the flexor tendons as far proximally as possible. Divide the volar plate. Cut through the remaining soft tissues, ligating the vessels and shortening the digital nerves, and remove the finger.

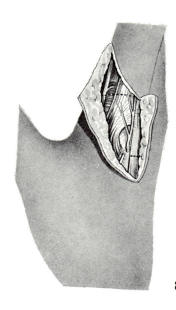

8

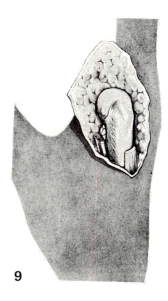

9

9

Reduction of bulk of scar

Trim away the ligamentous tissue round the metacarpal head, the volar plate, the collateral ligaments and the fibrous flexor tendon sheath, in order to reduce the bulk of the scar.

10

Closure

Arrange the skin flap to give good cover of the metacarpal head, trimming if necessary.

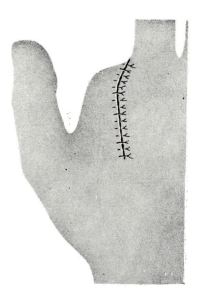

10

COSMETIC AMPUTATION THROUGH THE META-CARPAL SHAFT

11

The incision

The same skin incision is used, but the proximal limb is extended more proximally. Preserve sub-cutaneous tissue with the flaps.

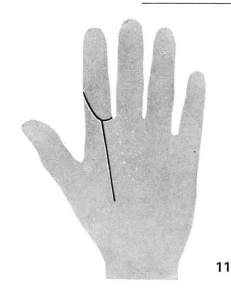

11

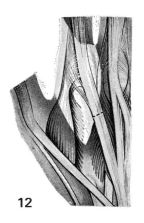

12

12

Exposure

Separate the extensor expansion with the attachment of the intrinsics.

13

Division of tendons, vessels and nerves

Divide the extensor tendon and turn distally. Separate the interossei from the shaft of the metacarpal. Deepen the volar incision and divide the vessels and nerves. It is simpler to divide straight through to the flexor tendons and then attend to the vessels and nerves definitively when the amputated finger is out of the way.

The amputation

Cut the metacarpal across, at about the junction of the proximal and middle thirds. Bevel both dorsally and radially. Turn the volar flap medially; ligate and shorten the vessels, and shorten the nerves. Remove the fibrous flexor tendon sheath, and shorten the flexor tendons as deep as possible in the palm.

The lumbrical muscle will also be removed at the same time.

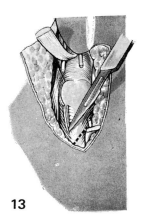

13

14

Closure

Proximally

Suture the sheath of the first and second dorsal interosseous muscles together, if possible, to give soft tissue cover to the end of the bone.

Distally

Suture the attachment of the first dorsal interosseous to the extensor expansion of the middle finger, in order to restore its function in pinch grip.

Release the tourniquet and ensure haemostasis.

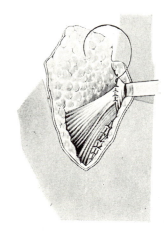

14

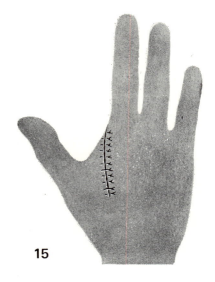

15

15

Skin closure

Suture the skin, allowing enough skin to cover the stump without tension.

FINGER TRANSFER

16

The incision

Use a dorsal racket incision, surrounding the base of the finger to be amputated, and extend it upwards over the metacarpal of this finger, to approach the base of the finger to be transferred.

Cut the extensor tendon, and expose the metacarpal of the finger which is to be transferred, by separating the interosseous muscles from it.

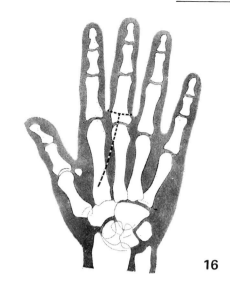

16

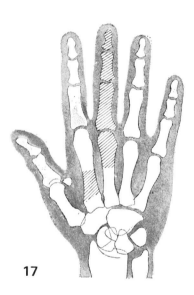

17

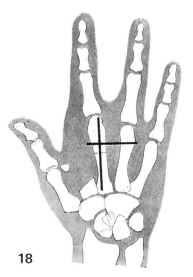

18

17

Amputation of finger

Divide this metacarpal through at about the middle of the shaft.

Deepen the volar incision to the front of the finger to be amputated, dividing the vessels and nerves and tendons.

The finger to be amputated can now be removed. Carefully approach the metacarpal of the finger to be transferred in the same way, and divide it at the same level. Remove the proximal part of the shaft of this metacarpal by cutting it obliquely near its base.

The volar plate—transverse ligament of the palm system—can now be visualized, and needs to be shortened by suture or removal of a portion.

The intrinsic muscle on the same side of the removed finger as the transferred finger becomes functionless and is in the way of the transfer and should be removed. The muscle on the other side of the removed finger can be used to reinforce the muscle on the transferred finger.

18

Stabilization

The transferred finger is fixed to the base of the metacarpal of the amputated finger with Kirschner wires. Transverse wires piercing the metacarpals of adjoining fingers may be used to stabilize the finger.

THE KUTLER REPAIR

19

Suitable in selected cases of transverse amputation of the distal segment, in order to cover the stump with normal digital skin with normal sensibility.

The skin is cleansed and dead tissue is removed. The edges of the divided bone are rounded off to provide support to the flaps without interfering with the blood supply.

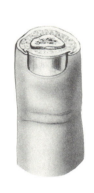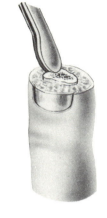

19

20

A triangular flap is designed on each side of the finger, each with the apex directed proximally, in line with the lateral line of the finger. The sides should be approximately 6–7 mm in length, and the base should be a little less.

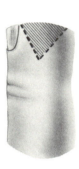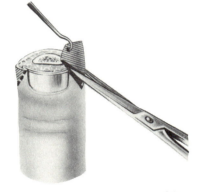

20

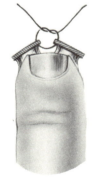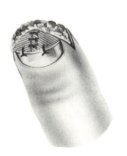

21

21

The incisions are deepened to the pulp, care being taken not to damage the neurovascular supply approaching from the pulp of the finger. Just enough tissue is freed to allow the flaps to be approximated over the end of the bone.

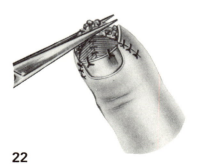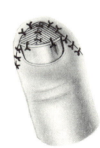

22

22

The bases of the flaps are approximated over the end of the bone and are sutured carefully with the very fine needles and suture material to avoid any loss of viability.

The two flaps will lie just anterior to the nail bed, and the volar flap of skin will be sutured to the two approximated flaps.

THE TRIANGULAR VOLAR FLAP

23

An alternative method to cover exposed bone is useful for transverse but not for volar oblique amputations (Atasoy *et al.*, 1970). The remaining part of the phalanx may need shortening.

24

A triangular flap is fashioned on the volar surface of the finger with the base on the cut surface. The width should be at least equal to the width of the amputated nail matrix.

The distally based flap is developed by cutting through the full thickness of the skin only, and carefully preserving the nerves and blood vessels to the flap. The subcutaneous fibrofatty tissue should be separated from the underlying periosteum and tendon sheath to mobilize the flap, which is then advanced to reach the cut edge of the nail.

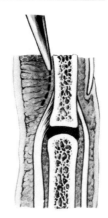
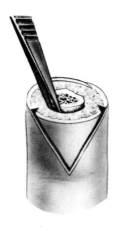

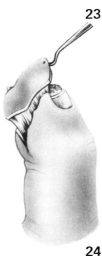
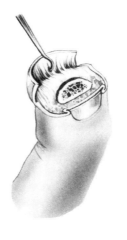

23

24

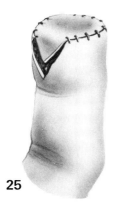
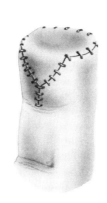

25

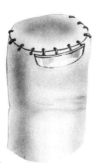
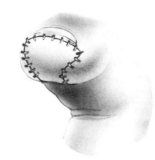

26

25

After suturing with 6/0 fine sutures of the V-incision on the volar surface is closed to convert it into a Y.

A small skin graft may be necessary in addition, to fill small uncovered areas.

26

This method gives a good contour and padding to the tip of the finger and there is normal sensation of the finger tip.

Stiffness is minimal because immobilization is unnecessary.

References

Atasoy, E., Ioakimidis, E., Kasdan, M. L., Kutz, J. E. and Kleinert, H. E. (1970). 'Reconstruction of the amputated finger tip with a triangular volar flap.' *J. Bone Jt Surg.* **52A**, 921

Fisher, R. H. (1967). 'The Kutler method of repair of finger-tip amputations.' *J. Bone Jt Surg.* **49A**, 317

Kutler, W. (1947). 'A new method for finger tip amputation.' *J. Am. med. Ass.* **133**, 29

Verdan, C. E. (1966). In *Hand Surgery*, Edited by J. E. Flynn, p.225. Baltimore: Williams and Wilkins

[*The illustrations for this Chapter on Amputations were drawn by Mrs. C. Clarke.*]

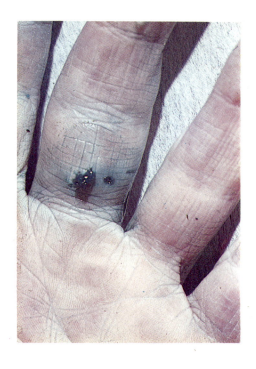

Illustration 1 from page 522

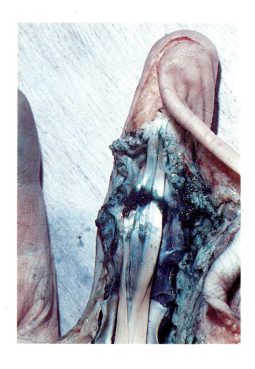

Illustration 3 from page 523

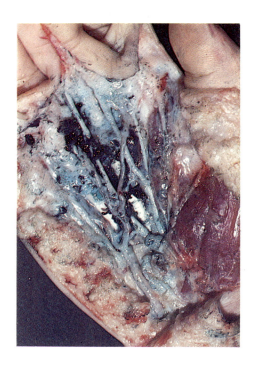

Illustration 11 from page 526

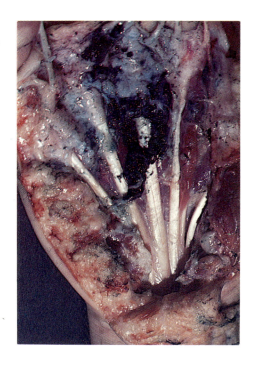

Illustration 12 from page 526

Tendon Injuries in the Hand

R. Guy Pulvertaft, C.B.E., Hon.M.D., M.Chir., F.R.C.S.
Emeritus Orthopaedic Surgeon, Derbyshire Royal Infirmary;
Honorary Civil Consultant, Royal Air Force

INTRODUCTION

General

The problems set by tendon divisions in the hand are complex and their treatment varies with the site of injury. There are certain observations which have a general application. A tendon heals readily when held in apposition and the union is sufficiently strong at 3–4 weeks to withstand slight strain. Damaged tendons have a marked tendency to become adherent to the surrounding tissues, limiting their gliding movement. A gentle and precise technique is essential and this implies the use of the finest instruments and a suture material which does not provoke a tissue reaction. A bloodless field, using a tourniquet, is necessary. The tourniquet is removed at the completion of the operation and complete haemostasis obtained before the wound is closed.

EXTENSOR TENDONS

Distal interphalangeal joint (Mallet deformity)

Rupture or division of the extensor attachment to the distal phalanx is best treated by splintage in extension for 6–8 weeks, or for longer if the treatment has been delayed. The splint needs to be tolerable to the patient and effectively maintained. Several patterns of splint have been described; the one illustrated

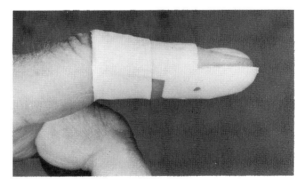

(devised independently by Parker and by Stack) is suitable, and is used in preference to plaster and to internal fixation.

Operative treatment is reserved for those cases in which conservative treatment has failed or are seen late. The choice lies between arthrodesis of the distal joint or repair of the tendon. Tendon repair is effective only when the passive joint range is complete or nearly complete. Operative treatment is also advisable when a considerable fragment of bone has been avulsed with the tendon or when there is a subluxation.

Proximal interphalangeal joint (Boutonnière deformity)

The extensor tendon divides over the proximal phalanx into a central band which is attached to the base of the middle phalanx, and into two lateral bands which bypass the proximal interphalangeal joint and join to be inserted into the base of the distal phalanx. Division of the central band allows the proximal joint to flex and the distal joint is drawn into hyperextension. The lateral bands migrate forwards and act as flexors of the proximal joint. Secondary ligamentous contractures lead to a fixed deformity of both joints.

When a rupture or division of the central band is seen within 5 or 6 weeks after injury, a good result can usually be obtained by splintage in extension for a period of 4–6 weeks, followed by protective mobilization in a dynamic splint. A suitable static type is the Bunnell splint which is fitted as illustrated

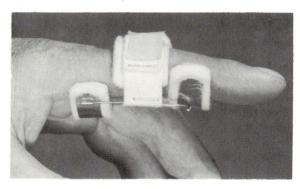

to permit flexion of the distal joint. The Capener dynamic splint is recommended for the mobilization phase. It may also be used to correct a moderate flexion contracture.

Operative treatment is reserved for those cases which fail to respond to conservative measures and for those that are manifestly unlikely to do so.

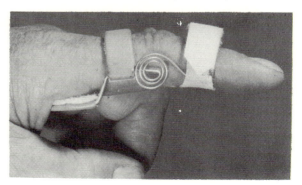

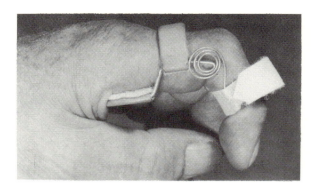

Hand and wrist

Tendon retraction after division over the metacarpophalangeal joint is usually slight and an early case may be treated successfully by splintage in extension. If there is any doubt, and always in later cases, surgical repair is advisable. Tendons divided in the central and proximal parts of the hand and over the wrist joint always require repair. In late cases it may not be possible to obtain apposition of the tendon ends and a tendon graft or a tendon transfer may be needed.

FLEXOR TENDONS

Flexor digitorum profundus in the finger

When the profundus tendon alone is divided beyond the superficialis attachment, good results can be obtained by immediate suture. Delayed suture is possible if the vincula are intact and retraction has been prevented.

If retraction and shortening of the muscle has occurred or if the tendon has been severed proximal to the superficialis attachment, consideration should be given to the replacement of profundus by a free graft. A thin tendon, preferably plantaris, is used and reaches from the proximal palm to the distal phalanx. The undamaged superficialis tendon is not disturbed. This operation is justified for someone whose occupation demands finger tip action and for children. The purpose is to achieve perfection and, as the possibility of disturbing superficialis function exists, the operation should only be undertaken when the indications are clear and the surgeon is experienced in tendon grafting.

The alternative procedure is fixation in suitable flexion of the distal joint by arthrodesis or tenodesis.

Flexor digitorum profundus and superficialis in the finger

During recent years there has been a movement towards the wider use of primary suture of flexor tendons divided within the digital theca, the technique of which is described in the next chapter. It must be stressed that the results are likely to be disappointing unless the facilities and the technique are of the highest order; failure will foul the ground for subsequent tendon grafting. Primary suture is not recommended unless the surgeon has studied the subject fully and has had adequate training in the exacting technique. When these conditions are not satisfied, it is wiser to do no more than clean and suture the wound and leave the case for tendon grafting later. The tendons are replaced by a graft when the digit has recovered from the initial trauma and all reaction has resolved; this may take 4–6 months. Apart from the inconvenience to the patient, there is no inherent harm in the delay for excellent results can be achieved even after the lapse of years, provided the digit is in good overall condition. It is useless to expect tendon grafting to succeed in the presence of severe scarring, contracture or complete sensory loss. If these conditions prevail, consideration should be given to the two-stage operation for tendon reconstruction described in The Hand volume of this series.

Flexor pollicis longus

Division of flexor pollicis longus in the distal part of the thumb should be treated by immediate suture. In the region between the metacarpophalangeal joint and the wrist the tendon is in close relationship to the sensory nerves of the thumb and the motor branch to the thenar muscles. These structures are at risk during a tendon repair and, if injured, lead to a worse disability than the lack of distal joint flexion. If the surgeon is inexperienced, it is better to perform skin suture only with a view to tendon grafting later.

In general, function can be restored in all late cases by tendon grafting. Occasionally it is possible to perform a late secondary suture in the distal part of the thumb; when this is not feasible it is more satisfactory, in the author's experience, to use a graft rather than elongate the tendon above the wrist.

Palm

Suture of the superficialis and profundus tendons divided at the same level in the palm is apt to be followed by cross-union which limits the flexion action to superficialis. Meticulous suture of sharp cut tendons will avoid this complication, but when the tendon ends are ragged it is advisable to cut back superficialis and restrict the repair to profundus. Secondary suture may be practicable if the proximal end is held by the lumbricalis muscle, but in late cases end-to-end contact may not be obtainable and the gap should be closed with a free graft taken from superficialis.

Wrist

Tendons divided at the wrist level retract severely and their muscles shorten and prevent apposition, even in a fairly recent case, which necessitates the use of multiple bridge grafts for reconstruction. It is imperative, therefore, to perform immediate suture of tendons in this region if the wound conditions permit. End-to-end suture of all the tendons is performed, using the more rapidly applied double right-angle stitch rather than the criss-cross stitch.

Anaesthesia

General anaesthesia is used unless there is some special indication for plexus or local nerve block anaesthesia.

OPERATIONS FOR INDIVIDUAL TENDON INJURIES

Tendon junctions

Suture material

Stainless steel wire causes no tissue reaction and has proved a most satisfactory suture material. Care must be taken to avoid kinking; a reef knot is tied and the wire may be cut off flush with the knot leaving no protruding ends. Monofilament wire (British wire gauge 40) can be obtained swaged to 2·5 cm bayonet-ended malleable needles which were specifically developed for tendon surgery. Synthetic fibres (4/0) are also widely used.

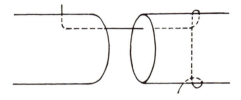

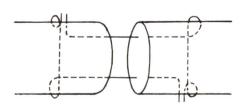

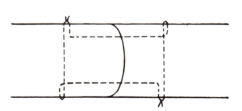

2

1

Bunnell criss-cross stitch

The Bunnell criss-cross stitch is the usual choice for joining two tendons of equal cross-section. A single wire with needles at both ends is used and there is only one knot required.

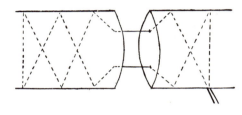

1

2

Kessler grasping stitch

This stitch has the advantage of requiring fewer penetrations of the tendon and it is claimed that it has less tendency to compress the tendon ends and embarrass the blood supply.

3

Bunnell double right-angle stitch

This stitch can be inserted more rapidly than the criss-cross method and is a convenient and adequate technique to use when many tendons are divided at the wrist level.

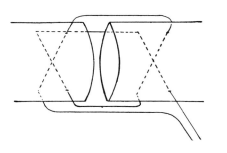

3

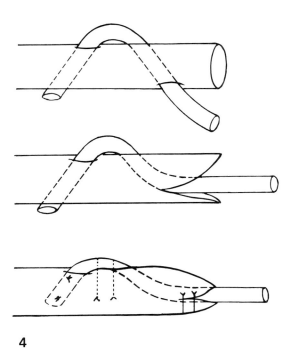

4

4

Interlacing method

The interlace and fish-mouth technique is recommended when a slender tendon needs to be joined to a larger tendon and is suitable for the proximal attachment of a graft. It combines the neatness of an end-to-end junction with the strength of an interlacing suture.

5

Bunnell withdrawal stitch

The Bunnell withdrawal stitch is a neat method of attaching the distal end of the tendon and it may also be used for the attachment of a tendon graft. The wire passes on either side of the phalanx to emerge through the finger end where it is tied over a dental wool roll. The tendon end is snugged into the angle between the bone and the profundus insertion. The accurate passage of the wire can be facilitated by the use of hollow needles, through which the wire is passed (*see Illustration 7* and accompanying text).

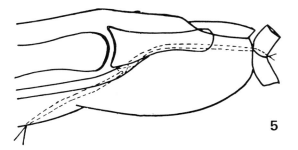

5

6

Alternative method of graft attachment

A disadvantage of the Bunnell stitch for a graft is that the length of the graft cannot be estimated accurately until the wires have been passed through the finger pulp and held while the tension is being tested. An alternative method was devised to overcome this difficulty. The graft, which needs to be slender, is drawn through the stub of the profundus tendon and through the finger pulp by a Reverdin needle. A small cross-action haemostat grips the graft to permit the tension to be tested by moving the wrist and fingers. When the length of the graft has been judged to be correct, the graft is stitched to the profundus remnant. The finger is then flexed and the graft withdrawn a little from the finger and cut short.

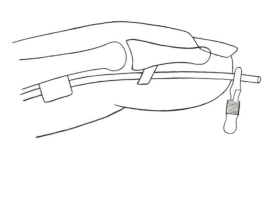

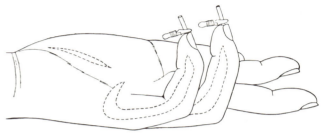

6

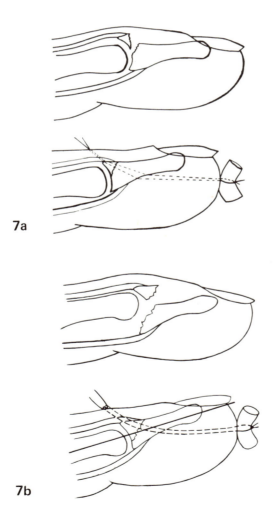

7a

7b

7a&b

Re-attachment of extensor tendon and bone fragment

The withdrawal stitch is a convenient way of re-attaching the extensor tendon when it has avulsed a fragment of bone. The wire passes through drill holes in the phalanx and is tied in the manner already described. Hollow needles may be passed in the retrograde direction through the pulp and the drill holes to receive the wire. Small fragments of avulsed bone may be ignored and this injury is adequately treated by splintage alone.

The fracture subluxation of the distal joint caused by a direct blow upon the finger tip (cricket or baseball injury) is not, strictly speaking, a tendon injury. An accurate lateral x-ray will reveal the joint displacement which requires reduction and fixation as described. It is advisable to secure the position with a Kirschner wire passed across the joint.

SECONDARY REPAIR OF MALLET DEFORMITY

8

The incision

The incision is angled. The transverse arm is placed midway between the distal interphalangeal joint and the nail root. The longitudinal arm follows the mid-lateral line to midway between the interphalangeal joints.

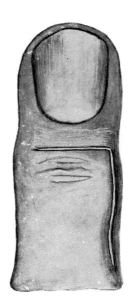

8

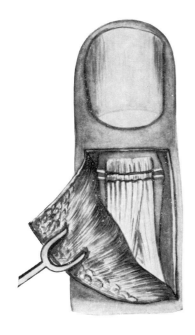

9

9

Exposure of extensor tendon

The flap is raised exposing the extensor tendon. The two lateral bands are seen joining to form the single tendon which is inserted into the dorsal surface of the base of the distal phalanx. Here is seen the original division or rupture which has united by scar tissue producing lengthening of the tendon.

10

Removal of scar tissue and adhesions

The scar tissue is removed and the adhesions between the proximal part of the tendon and the periosteum are severed. The excision must be strictly limited to scar tissue or it will be found impossible to close the gap between the tendon ends. A Bunnell stitch is inserted into the proximal end.

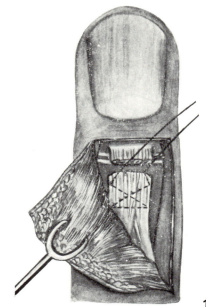

10

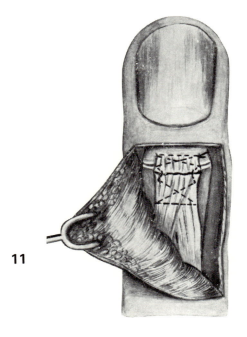

11

11

Apposition of tendon ends

The wire is passed into the distal part of the tendon and the tendon ends snugged together by drawing upon the wire which is then tied and the ends cut short. A few tidying stitches of very fine wire are used if the junction appears ragged. Vilain (1962) has reported good results from division and plication of the posterior surface of the scar, leaving the anterior surface intact.

SECONDARY REPAIR OF BOUTONNIERE DEFORMITY

12

The incision

A curved incision is used which passes forwards almost as far as the mid-lateral line of the joint. The transverse crease lines over the dorsal surface of the joint are avoided.

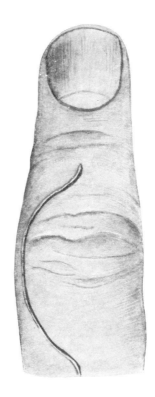

12

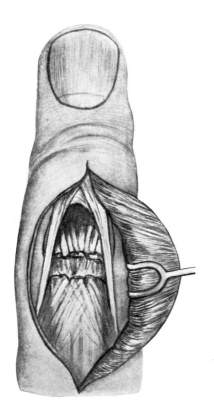

13

13

Exposure of extensor tendon

The skin and subcutaneous tissue are turned back revealing the extensor tendon. Here is seen the central band divided and the gap has become filled with scar tissue. The two lateral bands are passing by the side of the joint to become one tendon over the middle phalanx.

14

Removal of scar tissue

The scar tissue is removed and the joint is seen. At this stage it is advisable to separate the central band completely from the lateral components.

The central band is usually found to be adherent to the neck of the proximal phalanx. These adhesions must be freed so that the tendon moves easily when drawn in the distal direction.

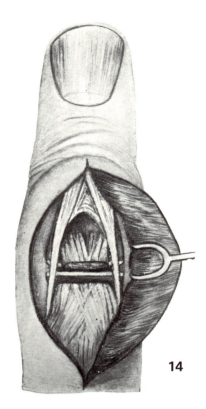

14

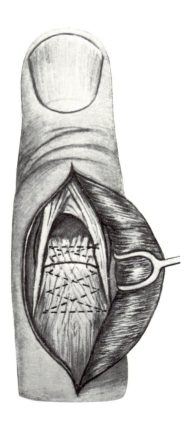

15

15

Suture of central band to distal remnant

The central band is sutured to the distal remnant with a Bunnell stitch. The lateral bands, which may need to be released when they are displaced volarwards, are held in contact with the sides of the central band with a few fine catgut stitches (not illustrated). The final tension should allow the finger to lie in the correct position relative to the other fingers.

In a neglected case, it may not be possible to reconstitute the normal anatomy. Matev (1964) corrects the deformity by transposing one of the lateral bands to the base of the proximal phalanx and lengthens the other band to overcome the hyperextension of the distal phalanx. Littler and Eaton (1967) centralize the lateral bands over the proximal joint, relying on the oblique retinacular ligament of Landsmeer and the lumbrical muscle to extend the distal joint. These operations are described in The Hand volume of this series.

REPAIR OF TENDONS ON THE BACK OF THE HAND

16

The incision

A curved longitudinal incision is made so that the scar does not overlie the tendon junction, and the dorsal veins are avoided.

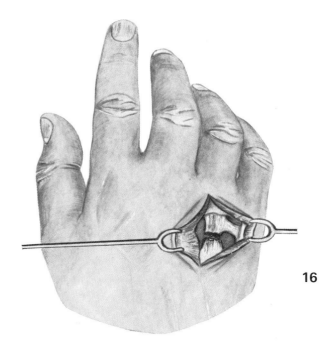

16

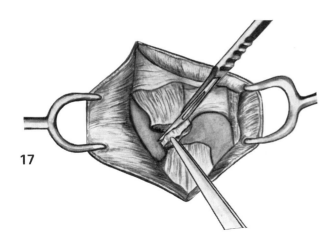

17

17

Preparation of the tendon ends

A thin shaving of the damaged tendon ends is removed so that even and freshly cut tendon fibres will meet. This ensures a neat union with the minimum of scar tissue.

18

Suture of the tendon

The Bunnell stitch is used and the tendon ends drawn together. Here is shown the stage before final tightening and knotting of the wire.

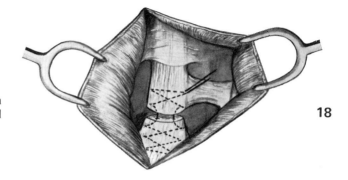

18

FLEXOR TENDON DIVISIONS SHOWING SUITABLE METHOD OF REPAIR

19

A. Primary suture should be performed if wound conditions are satisfactory; otherwise suture the skin and perform secondary suture or a tendon graft later.
B. Primary suture or secondary graft depending upon the circumstances.
C. Primary suture should be performed if wound conditions are satisfactory; otherwise suture the skin and perform secondary suture or bridge graft later.
D. Primary suture is highly desirable. Delay necessitates bridge grafting (*see* page 544).

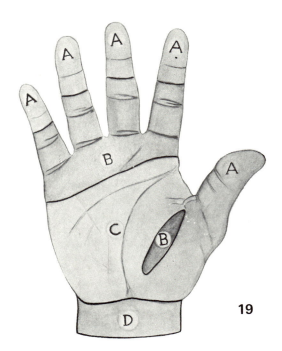

19

TENDON GRAFT OPERATION

The graft source

Palmaris longus, plantaris and extensor digitorum longus are suitable. Flexor digitorum superficialis is ideal for a short bridge graft but is less suitable to use as a full length graft. Palmaris muscle occasionally extends down the tendon too far to leave sufficient length of pure tendon. It is exposed through a short transverse incision above the wrist and a similar incision in the mid-forearm and drawn out. Plantaris is sufficiently long to serve as two grafts and is of appropriate size; occasionally it is very thin and should not be used. Its presence cannot be determined until the first incision is made on the medial border of the tendo Achillis. A second incision is made in the mid-calf, three finger breadths behind the medial border of the tibia. The gastrocnemius muscle is retracted and the plantaris is seen on its deep surface; it is divided in the distal wound and drawn out of the proximal wound. Although a tendon stripper is commonly used, it has been found more satisfactory to remove these tendons in the manner described. A toe extensor tendon is best removed through a full exposure and is of ample length if divided above the extensor retinaculum. A leash of four tendons may be taken if required, but it must be remembered that the fifth toe does not possess a short extensor muscle and will drop into flexion if its sole extensor tendon is removed.

20

The incisions

In the case of the index finger, the incision is made in the exact mid-axial line from the nail root to the thenar crease, which it then follows to the proximal part of the palm. A similar incision is used for the little finger, but the palmar incision follows the distal crease for about 3 cm and then is continued into the proximal palm parallel to the thenar crease. For the middle and ring fingers, separate palmar incisions are made in the appropriate crease lines; these may be joined to the finger incision if it is found necessary to expose the base of the finger.

The thumb requires three separate incisions: mid-axial in the thumb, the thenar crease and above the wrist just medial to the tendon of flexor carpi radialis.

The Bruner zig-zag incision is commonly used for the finger and gives an excellent exposure. The mid-axial approach is more suitable for the operative technique to be described.

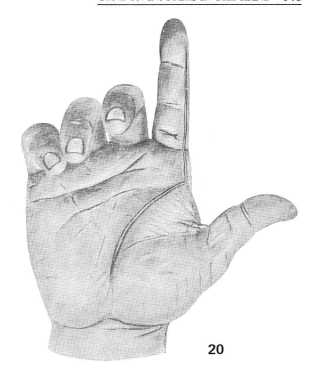

20

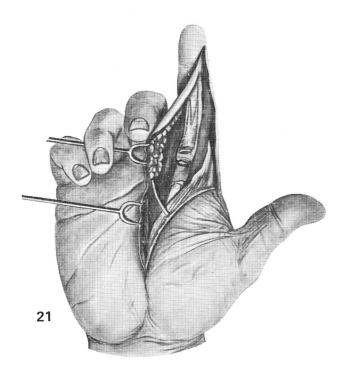

21

21

Exposure of the digital theca

The incision is deepened, passing posterior to the digital vessels and the digital nerve which are carried forwards in the flap. Care must be taken not to injure these structures which are shown crossing the operative field. The dorsal branch of the digital nerve arises just beyond the base of the proximal phalanx (not illustrated). It is not always possible to preserve this small nerve, but it should be looked for and retained if it does not unduly embarrass the exposure. This sensory branch assumes particular significance when the digital nerve has been injured more distally.

The digital theca containing the tendons is fully exposed. The lumbrical muscle is seen on the radial side of the finger.

22

Selective excision of the digital theca and insertion of the graft

The theca is cut away leaving three bands to serve as pulleys. These are situated in front of the metacarpo-phalangeal joint, and the mid-parts of the proximal and middle phalanges. The two proximal pulleys are essential to prevent bowstringing and should be reconstructed if adequate pulleys cannot be fashioned from a damaged and fibrosed theca. The profundus tendon and the proximal part of the superficialis tendon are completely removed. The distal part of the superficialis tendon is not removed if it is firmly adherent and its excision would leave raw tissue along the course of the graft. The graft is inserted and its proximal end attached to the profundus or the superficialis tendon, whichever is found to possess the better amplitude of movement. The fish-mouth technique (*see Illustration 4)* is used. When the graft is attached to profundus, the junction is covered by the lumbricalis muscle provided this muscle is not fibrosed and will cause a lumbrical plus syndrome. The superficialis of the little finger is a weak muscle and is not suitable to use as a motor. It is helpful to hold the proximal part of the motor tendon by a trans-fixation needle during this stage of the operation.

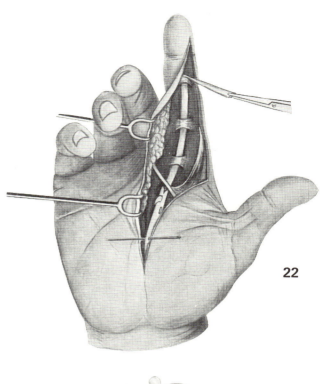

22

23

Distal attachment of the graft

The graft is attached to the stub of the profundus tendon by the technique described (*see Illustration 6*), or by the Bunnell method (*see Illustration 5*).

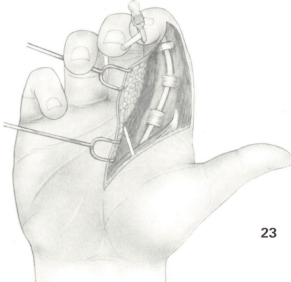

23

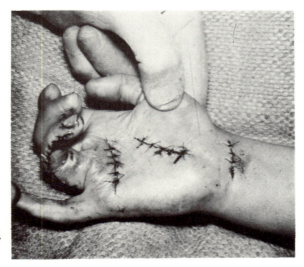

24

(Reproduced from 'Hand Surgery', Figure 13, page 305 by kind permission of J. E. Flynn and Williams and Wilkins Co.)

24

Tension of the graft

The tension must be carefully adjusted until the finger lies in a slightly more flexed position than would appear correct in relation to the other fingers. This patient has had tendon grafts for the middle and ring fingers.

25

Completion of the operation

The hand is covered with a moist dressing and held well elevated, combined with tilting of the table, and the tourniquet is removed from the arm. This position is maintained for 8—10 min and it is not unusual to find that bleeding has ceased by the end of this time. Any persistent haemorrhage is controlled by bipolar coagulation or ligation. Perfect haemostasis is essential and the wound is washed clear of blood before it is closed.

The wound is dressed with tulle gras. A little fluffed dry gauze is placed between the fingers and the palm is filled with steel wool, over which the fingers are bandaged in moderate flexion with the wrist in the position of rest. Firm, but not compressive, crêpe bandaging is used reinforced by adhesive strapping. A plaster cast reaching to above the elbow is used in children. The limb is kept elevated for 48 hr.

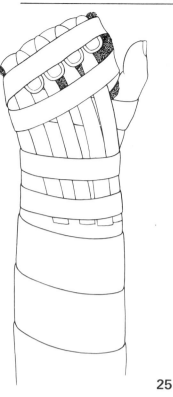

25

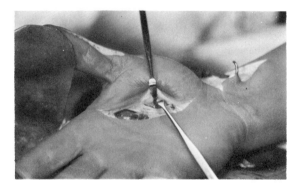

26a

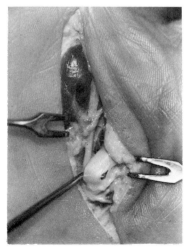

26b

26a & b

Tendon graft for flexor pollicis longus

The three incision are: mid-axial in the thumb reaching from the base of the nail to just proximal to the metacarpophalangeal joint; almost the full length of the thenar crease and above the wrist medial to the flexor carpi radialis tendon. Through the thenar crease incision, the palmar aponeurosis is incised to expose the first lumbrical muscle, the digital nerve to the radial side of the index finger, both digital nerves to the thumb and the flexor pollicis longus tendon lying between these two nerves.

(Reproduced from Am. J. Surg. Volume 109, Figure 18, page 350 by kind permission of Dunn-Donnelly Publishing Co.)

TENDON DIVISIONS IN THE PALM

27

Suture

The incision is determined by the position of the existing wound or scar, bearing in mind that a wide exposure is needed to repair nerves in addition to the tendons and that the tendon is likely to be divided at a more distal level than the wound would suggest. In a secondary repair one can expect to find considerable scar tissue which demands a painstaking dissection. The superficialis and profundus tendons are both sutured when conditions are suitable, but if there is a risk of cross union it is wiser to cut back superficialis and suture only the profundus tendon as illustrated. Tendons severed in the distal part of the palm are considered to be in region B (*see Illustration 19*) and treated accordingly.

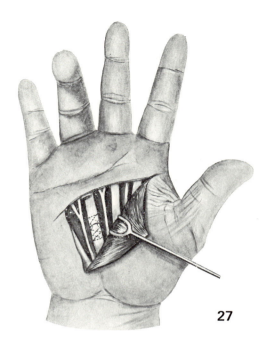

27

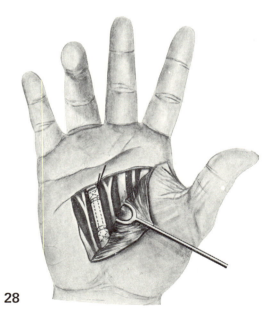

28

28

Bridge graft

In cases where there has been a delay of some months it may be difficult or impossible to bring the tendon ends into apposition. An effective repair may be performed by using a short superficialis graft to bridge the gap in the profundus tendon. The suture passes through the graft in the manner shown; in this illustration the wire has not yet been drawn tight and knotted.

TENDON DIVISIONS AT THE WRIST

29

The first step in dealing with a major injury of this kind is to enlarge the wound in distal and proximal directions and identify the structures. Respect should be paid to the angles of the flaps and in this illustration the angles are made too sharply.

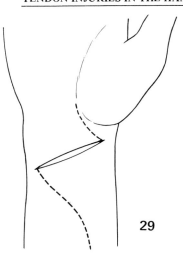

29

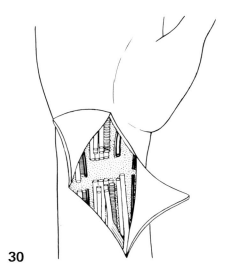

30

30

There are twelve tendons, (palmaris longus not shown), two main nerves and two main arteries on the flexor aspect of the wrist and two tendons—abductor pollicis longus and extensor pollicis brevis on the radial aspect. All may be divided and it is not surprising that confusion arises when searching for the corresponding ends. Once the anatomy is clearly seen, the surgeon can proceed in confidence with the repair work which may take several hours to complete.

Although many hands have survived the loss of both main arteries, this cannot be taken for granted, particularly in older persons, and in any case problems associated with vascular insufficiency may arise later. At least one of the arteries should be anastomosed. All tendons, with the possible exception of palmaris longus, should be sutured when they are divided proximal to the carpal tunnel. It is probably wiser to ignore the superficialis tendons when they are divided within the tunnel.

Opinion differs about the wisdom of primary or secondary suture of nerves divided under these circumstances; if a formal suture is not performed the nerves should be held together to prevent shortening and to preserve the orientation.

In a later reconstructive operation it is not possible to bring the tendon ends together without excessive positioning of the joints. Continuity can be restored to the essential tendons by the interposition of bridge grafts taken from superficialis when the conditions are favourable. The alternative procedure is tendon transference.

POSTOPERATIVE CARE

At the stage—some 3—5 weeks after tendon suture—when it is customary to permit movements, there is a special risk of the tendon junction giving way. This is due to two factors: the union is immature and, in addition, adhesions limit the free gliding of the tendon which in a normal hand allows the strain to be taken up gradually.

For these reasons it is unwise to allow complete freedom immediately the primary splintage is removed. Some form of protective splintage is advisable such as a check rein strap or elastic, or a spring device.

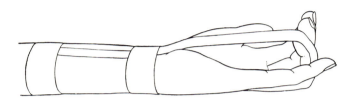

Movements return slowly and the patient requires constant encouragement. He should be kept under personal supervision until the final state is reached which may not be for 6—9 months after operation.

Occasionally, the operation of tenolysis is indicated for cases in which the active range fails to attain the passive range of motion.

EXTENSOR TENDONS

Mallet deformity

The finger is splinted with the distal interphalangeal joint extended and the proximal interphalangeal joint slightly flexed for 5 weeks followed by 3 weeks' spring splintage (long Capener splint).

Boutonnière deformity

The finger is splinted with the proximal interphalangeal joint extended for 4 weeks followed by 3 weeks' spring splintage (short Capener splint). The distal joint may be left free.

Back of the hand

The forearm, wrist and fingers are splinted with the wrist in the position of rest and the metacarpophalangeal and the interphalangeal joints in slight flexion for 4 weeks. The fully extended position of the fingers is unnecessary and can lead to joint stiffness. During the following 2 weeks, flexion of the fingers is limited by a pad of steel wire bandaged into the palm against which the fingers can squeeze.

FLEXOR TENDONS

Fingers, palm and wrist

The wrist is held by a firm supportive bandage in a position of rest and the digits in moderate flexion for 3 weeks. After the removal of splintage, digit extension is limited for a further week (2 weeks in children, for whom a plaster cast is used in the first stage) by the use of an elastic check rein strap. This strap allows flexion exercises to be practised but prevents excessive extension.

PHYSIOTHERAPY

Supervised active exercises are useful, particularly in young children, but the patient's own intelligent co-operation is the most important factor in the after-care. As tendon union becomes stronger more active work in the Occupational Therapy department is given.

References

Bruner, J. M. (1967). 'The zig-zag volar digital incision for flexor tendon surgery.' *Proc. Br. Club Surg. Hand,* May, p. 33

Bunnell, S. (1970). *Surgery of the Hand.* 5th Edition. Edited by J. H. Boyes. Philadelphia: Lippincott

Fetrow, K. O. (1967). 'Tenolysis in the hand and wrist.' *J. Bone Jt Surg.* **49A,** 667

Flynn, J. E. (1975). *Hand Surgery,* 2nd Edition. Baltimore: Williams and Wilkins

Kessler, I. (1973). 'The grasping technique for tendon repair.' *The Hand* **5,** 253

Littler, J. W. and Eaton, R. G. (1967). 'Re-distribution of forces in the correction of the Boutonnière deformity.' *J. Bone Jt Surg.* **49A,** 1267

Matev, I. (1964). 'Transposition of lateral slips of the aponeurosis in treatment of long-standing Boutonnière deformity of the fingers.' *Br. J. plast. Surg.* **17,** 281

Pulvertaft, R. G. (1948). 'Repair of tendon injuries in the hand.' *Ann. R. Coll. Surg. Engl.* **3,** 3

Pulvertaft, R. G. (1956). 'Tendon grafts for flexor tendon injuries in the fingers and thumb.' *J. Bone Jt Surg.* **38B,** 175

Pulvertaft, R. G. (1960). 'The treatment of profundus division by free tendon graft.' *J. Bone Jt Surg.* **42A,** 1363

Pulvertaft, R. G. 'Flexor tendon grafting after long delay.' In *The Hand,* Edited by R. Tubiana. Philadelphia: W. B. Saunders (awaiting publication)

Rank, B. K., Wakefield, A. R. and Hueston, J. T. (1973). *Surgery of Repair as Applied to Hand Injuries.* 4th Edition. Edinburgh: Churchill-Livingstone

Reid, D. A. C. (1966). 'Tendon injuries.' In *Clinical Surgery,* Vol. 7, Edited by Charles Rob, Rodney Smith and R. G. Pulvertaft. London: Butterworths

Souter, W. A. (1967). 'The Boutonnière deformity.' *J. Bone Jt Surg.* **49B,** 710

Symposium on Tendon Surgery in the Hand. Philadelphia 1974. Published 1975. St. Louis: Mosby

Verdan, C. E. (1972). 'Half a century of flexor-tendon surgery.' *J. Bone Jt Surg.* **54A,** 472

Vilain, R. (1962). 'Repair of the extensor of the finger at its distal extremity.' *Proc. Br. Club Surg. Hand,* May, p. 19 (These Proceedings are now (1975) published entitled *The Second Hand Club,* Edited by H. G. Stack and H. Bolton. London: The British Society for Surgery of the Hand.)

[*The illustrations for this Chapter on Tendon Injuries in the Hand were drawn by Dr. K. Velis and by Mr. F. Price. The Parker–Stack Splint was supplied by Pryor and Howard Ltd., Willow Lane, Mitcham, Surrey; the Bunnell Splint by Zimmer Orthopaedic Ltd., Bridgend, Wales and the Capener Splint by the Devonian Orthopaedic Association, Wonford Road, Exeter.*]

Primary Tendon Repair within the Digital Theca

H. Bolton, Ch.M., F.R.C.S.
Consultant Orthopaedic and Accident Surgeon to
the Stockport Group of Hospitals

INTRODUCTION

1

The area of operation to be considered is the shaded area in *Illustration 1*; it will be noted that, in the case of the fingers, it includes the area between the distal palmar skin crease and the proximal interphalangeal joint; in the thumb, it includes the areas within the thenar muscles and as far as the insertion of the flexor longus pollicis tendon. In the author's view it should also include the area within the carpal tunnel, where conditions similar to those in the digital theca exist.

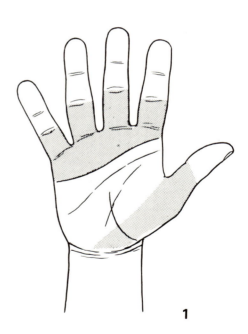

1

PRE-OPERATIVE

General

Whether or not the operation should be attempted has remained a point of controversy amongst Hand Surgeons for many years and it has been customary to teach that when tendons have been cut within the area shown in *Illustration 1,* the wound should be cleaned and sutured, leaving the tendons for repair by secondary suture or by grafting, when the original wound has healed without infection and when an experienced Hand Surgeon would be available. This advice was the result of the poor outcome of many attempts at primary repair, performed usually under difficult circumstances when the primary wound was sustained. With improvements in surgical techniques there can now be no doubt that primary repair of the tendon may be the correct treatment in some cases, but it must be stressed that strict criteria must be adhered to if good results are to follow.

Main requirements

(*1*) The type of wound causing the tendon division is important in deciding which cases are suitable for surgical repair and only clean wounds caused by knife or glass are usually suitable.

(*2*) There should have been no pre-operative interference with the wound by blind exploration at the initial examination in conditions of doubtful sterility with instruments which may not be sterile; blind groping with Spencer-Wells forceps to stop bleeding is particularly harmful. Most bleeding in the hand can be stopped by firm pressure and elevation of the limb.

(*3*) Operation should be considered only when it can be performed within the first 3 or 4 hr of injury. Alternatively, it may be done as a secondary procedure if the original wound has been cleaned and closed within the time limits suggested above and has healed without infection.

(*4*) The patient should be fully protected by a booster dose of tetanus toxoid injection and by antibiotics.

(*5*) An experienced surgeon, versed in the exacting techniques of hand surgery, should be available to perform the operation, which has to be done in proper surroundings with correct instruments and, of course, using a bloodless field afforded by an inflatable tourniquet.

(*6*) Operation should usually be done under general anaesthesia, but brachial block has been shown in many centres to be equally effective and it may be possible in these circumstances to perform an operation on a patient who is unsuitable for the administration of a general anaesthetic.

(*7*) The patient's after-treatment, the use of suitable splintage and of other splints and measures to restore movement should be under the personal control of the surgeon performing the operation.

AREA OF OPERATION

To the areas shaded in *Illustration 1* should be added the carpal tunnel, where the conditions are similar to those in the digital theca of the fingers, that is a fibro-osseous tunnel which is largely occupied by unyielding tendons.

Tendon suture

Formerly tendon repair was carried out using 4/0 white silk mounted on atraumatic curved needles. The peripheral tendon repair was performed with 5/0 black silk on atraumatic needles. Recently, because of observations on the slight reaction which can occur around silk sutures, a trial has been made of the use of multifilament stainless steel wire and two sizes are in current use, a thicker seven strand 0·08 mm wire to perform the apposing mattress suture and a finer three filament strand of 0·05 mm for the peripheral interrupted sutures.

Repair in children

When repairing the tendons in a child's hand, who is of such an age as to make co-operation in the postoperative treatment difficult, it may be advisable to leave this needle in place to prevent inadvertent traction at the suture line and remove it when the sutures are removed at the end of 3 weeks. It is almost always necessary to give the child a short anaesthetic for that to be achieved. When the tendon ends are delivered into the wound, it is often noted that in the type of wound where tendon repair is to be performed, the tendon ends are cleanly cut and do not need further trimming. Reliance must be placed on careful wound cleansing and the use of antibiotics to prevent infection.

Repair of one or both tendons

When both the superficialis and profundus tendons are divided in the finger it is usually preferable to repair only the profundus tendon, for if the superficialis is also repaired and the two repairs lie at the same level, adhesions may develop, thus impairing the finger movements subsequently. In a small number of patients, usually children, good results have followed where both tendons have been repaired. The advice to repair both tendons in children and some other selected cases, has been given by some authors notably Verdan (1972) and Kleinert (1975).

2

The technique is illustrated. It will be noted that a simple mattress suture properly inserted gives adequate and secure fixation and is preferable to the use of a Bunnell type of suture, which of necessity damages the tendon over a longer area than does the mattress suture and is, therefore, more likely to cause adhesions of the tendon to surrounding structures. When delivered into the wound the proximal tendon is best held in place by perforating it well proximal to the suture line by a fine straight skin suturing needle which is removed at the conclusion of the repair.

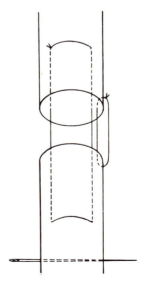

2

3

In adults when the profundus tendon only is repaired the superficialis should be removed as described. One of the slips of insertion should be removed as near as possible to its point of attachment to the middle phalanx. The other slip is cut transversely about 1·2 cm from its insertion; the slip thus created is rerouted to lie outside the fibrous tendon sheath and is sutured to the para-osseous tissues of the proximal phalanx with the proximal inter-phalangeal joint in slight flexion. This is to prevent the troublesome hyperextension of the proximal interphalangeal joint which sometimes develops when the superficialis is removed completely. The fibrous tendon sheath should be removed for a distance of approximately 0·6 cm on either side of the suture line in the tendon to prevent the tendon becoming adherent to it during the healing process. Similarly, the flexor retinaculum should not be sutured at the completion of a primary tendon repair in the carpal tunnel.

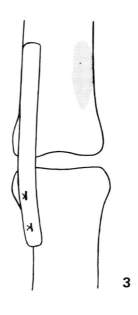

3

4

Extension of incision or wound

Should access to the finger or thumb be inadequate, the wound can be extended in a bayonet or V or W fashion (illustrated) as recommended by Bruner. Occasionally, a small accessory incision is necessary in the palm at the base of the affected finger or fingers to recover the proximal ends of divided tendons.

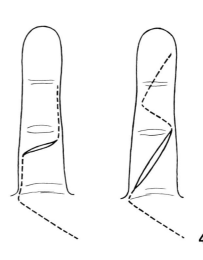

4

Skin closure and dressing

It is essential that the skin is carefully closed at the completion of the tendon repair and this can be very difficult as the finger will lie in a flexed position. Non-absorbable sutures of fine monofilament nylon mounted on a small curved needle should be used. The dressing immediately next to the wound should be of gauze moistened with saline, which prevents the dressing sticking when the blood which oozes from the wound on the release of the tourniquet comes in contact with that dressing. This dressing is further held in place by a copious mass of fluffed gauze carefully applied with the fingers in semiflexion and the

thumb in the position of palmar abduction. Immobilization is secured by the application of a dorsal, padded, aluminium splint which is fastened to the skin of the forearm by adhesive strapping and the compression dressing complete with cotton crêpe bandages incorporating the splint within it. A plaster of Paris dorsal slab is an acceptable alternative. Splintage of the wrist in easy flexion should be the aim. The dressing and splintage is retained for a total of 3 weeks. In the last week of this period of immobilization gentle movements of the affected finger or thumb are permissible. Postoperative elevation of the limb for a period of 48 hr is usual and subsequently the patient should carry the affected limb in a sling to prevent swelling of the hand.

After-treatment

The sutures are removed when the dressing is taken off at the end of 3 weeks. Fine nylon causes no tissue reaction and can safely be left for this period or longer. The patient then recovers movement by frequent warm soapy water washing, olive oil massage and active exercises, if necessary under the supervision of a physiotherapist who is knowledgeable in this type of work. If the affected finger shows any tendency to remain in a flexed position, a spring extensor splint can be applied to assist in mobilizing the affected digit. The 'armchair' or clothes pin splint is the one usually employed.

TENOLYSIS

It has been found necessary in some cases, when active recovery ceases, to advise the patient to undergo tenolysis. This is an extensive operation which involves opening the whole area of tendon damage, dividing the adhesions which may be limiting the excursion of the repaired tendon and closing the wound. Instillations of cortisone into that wound should never be practised as this increases the chance of tendon rupture after the operation. Tendon rupture may occur even when cortisone is not used, for it is essential, after the performance of tenolysis, to make the patient begin active exercises within hours of the operation, otherwise adhesions will re-form and the value of the operation will be lost. The patient should usually be warned that there is a danger of tendon rupture following this procedure. Tendon rupture may necessitate further surgical treatment and the use of either a free tendon graft or a Silastic rod if the bed of the tendon is very scarred.

OTHER METHODS

It is important to mention the work of certain surgeons who have for some years been advocating primary tendon repair in suitable cases. Verdan uses stainless steel pins to transfix the repaired tendons proximally for 3 weeks postoperatively, thus immobilizing the site of tendon suture with more certainty. Richards advocates careful repair of the tendons and their sheath. He has taken this view as a result of microscopic studies of healing tendons and believes tendons can heal from within. This is contrary to the widely accepted views of Potenza, who showed that healing was by invasion from the surrounding synovial tissues. Kleinert uses magnification to achieve a more accurate repair, using fine synthetic sutures of 6/0 or 7/0 size to produce a smooth junction. He has also introduced a postoperative method of immobilization using a dorsal plaster splint and rubber band traction from the finger nail to the front of the forearm. During the period of splintage the patient is encouraged to perform guarded extension exercises against the resistance of the rubber band, which otherwise holds the finger flexed and protects the site of repair. Kleinert's improved results have led to further trials of this method by other surgeons. As previously mentioned both Verdan and Kleinert advocate repair of both flexor tendons in children and certain cases in adults, believing that the tendon's circulation through the vincula is more certainly restored by so doing, and, in their hands this gives improved results.

References

Bolton, H. (1960). The Second Hand Club (London). *Br. Soc. Surg. Hand* **54**

Boyes, J. H. (1970). *Bunnell's Surgery of the Hand*, 5th Edition. Philadelphia: Lippincott

Kleinert, H. L. and Stormo, A. (1973). 'Primary repair of flexor tendons.' *Orthop. Clins N. Am.* **4**, 865

Kleinert, H. L. (1975). *Symposium on Tendon Surgery in the Hand*, p. 91. American Academy of Orthopaedic Surgeons. Philadelphia: C. V. Mosby

Koch, S. L. (1952). Personal communication

Mason, M. L. and Allen, H. S. (1951). Personal communication.

Potenza, A. D. (1970). 'Flexor tendon injuries.' *Orthop. Clins N. Am.* **1**, 355

Rank, B. K., Wakefield, A. R. and Hueston, J. T. (1973). *Surgery of Repair as Applied to Hand Injuries*, p. 149. Edinburgh: Churchill Livingstone

Richards, H. J. (1975). 'Hunterian Lecture.' *Ann. R. Coll. Surg. Engl.*, (In press)

Verdan, C. E. (1961). 'Tendon suture in no-man's land.' The Second Hand Club. p. 104 *Br. Soc. Surg. Hand*

Verdan, C. E. (1972). 'Half a century of flexor-tendon surgery.' *J. Bone Jt Surg.* **54A**, 472

[The illustrations for this Chapter on Primary Tendon Repair within the Digital Theca were drawn by Mr. F. Price.]

Repair of the Ulnar Collateral Ligament of the Thumb with and without Chip Fractures

Bertil Stener, M.D.
Professor of Orthopaedic Surgery, Sahlgren Hospital, Göteborg

PRE - OPERATIVE

Clinical examination

When the thumb has sustained a violent hyperabduction the main purpose of the clinical examination is to determine whether or not the stability of the metacarpophalangeal joint has been impaired. Sometimes it is necessary to eliminate the stabilizing function of the adductor pollicis muscle by anaesthesia. When testing stability comparison should always be made with the uninjured joint because the normal range of movement varies from person to person. To ensure that instability is not overlooked the test should be made with the joint in flexion (*see Illustration 1*). In extension, the ulnar collateral ligament is relaxed, and consequently normal lateral stability found in extension does not preclude complete rupture of the ligament.

1

Radiographic examination

Radiographic examination is always indicated because various types of skeletal injury frequently occur in association with rupture of the ligament. A fragment can be *avulsed* from the base of the phalanx or, less frequently, from the metacarpal head, and a fragment can be *sheared off* from either the ulnar part of the base of the phalanx or the volar part of the radial condyle of the metacarpal head, or from both, when these skeletal parts come into violent contact during radiovolar displacement of the phalanx after the ligament has ruptured. A complete radiographic examination includes a true lateral view of the joint. The more easily obtained oblique lateral view, in which the ulnar condyle makes up the volar contour of the metacarpal head, may fail to demonstrate a shearing fracture of the radial condyle.

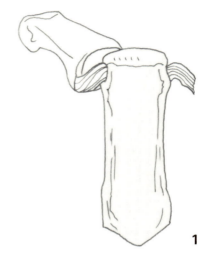

1

Indication for operation

When the metacarpophalangeal joint is found to be unstable following violent hyperabduction of the thumb, surgical treatment is indicated because the ulnar collateral ligament, having ruptured at its distal end (the usual site), often becomes folded back so that it sticks out beyond the proximal edge of the adductor aponeurosis (*see Illustration 4*), this structure thus being interposed between the ligament and its place of insertion on the phalanx (*see Illustration 6*). Operation should be undertaken, and the sooner the better because the formation of granulation tissue quickly obscures the pathological anatomy.

THE OPERATIONS

2 - 9

A curved incision is made over the ulnar side of the joint. During the following dissection care must be taken not to injure the thumb's ulnar cutaneous branch from the radial nerve. It is advisable to start the dissection by isolating the adductor aponeurosis. It will then usually be clear whether the torn end of the ligament has been displaced outside the aponeurosis (*see Illustration 4*), or not (*see Illustration 5*).

The next step—assuming the rupture is not proximal is to sever the adductor aponeurosis at right angles to the line of its fibres (*see Illustrations 6* and *7*). This will disclose the location of the rupture and the ligament, if it has been displaced, can be returned to its proper position. Even if the ligament has not been folded back it may have become retracted so that there is a considerable gap at the site of the rupture (*see Illustration 7*). Naturally, direct suture is employed if the rupture is situated some way from the bone. However, this method can also be used when the ligament has ruptured just where it attaches to the phalanx. The ligament is fastened with a few sutures to the tendon of the adductor pollicis (*see Illustration 8*), the role of the sutures being to hold the ligament close to the phalanx while the injury heals. After suture of the ligament, the adductor aponeurosis should be reconstructed carefully.

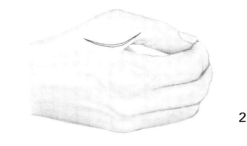

2

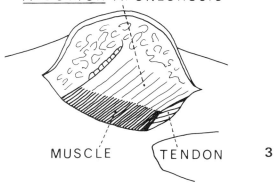

ADDUCTOR APONEUROSIS

MUSCLE   TENDON   3

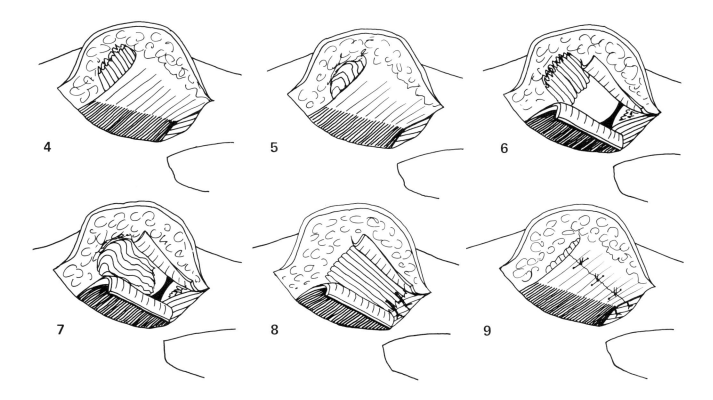

4

5

6

7

8

9

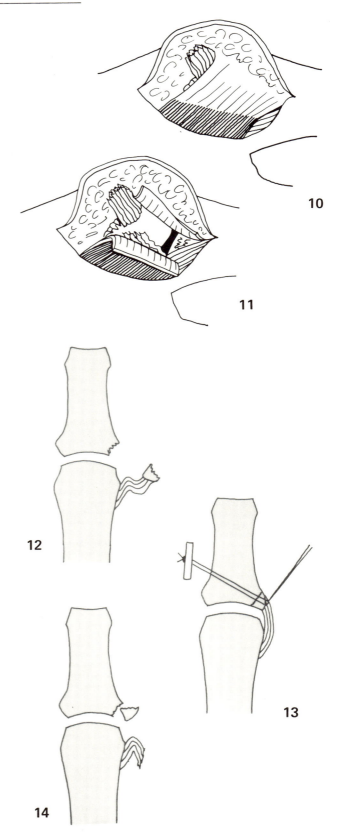

10

11

10 & 11

Sometimes the ulnar collateral ligament proper has been ruptured near its distal attachment whereas the accessory collateral ligament has been ruptured near its proximal attachment. It is important to recognize this because otherwise the mistake could be made to suture the proper and accessory ligaments to each other with insufficient stability as a result.

After suture of the skin, a plaster cast enclosing the thumb, the hand as far as the proximal transverse skin crease, and the forearm should be applied, special care being taken to ensure that the plaster is moulded with a dorsal groove between the first and second metacarpals to prevent ulnar deviation of the first metacarpal by the first dorsal interosseous muscle. Otherwise this muscle may achieve, albeit indirectly, abduction at the metacarpophalangeal joint, because the thumb is prevented by the plaster cast from moving with the metacarpal bone. The plaster is removed after 5–6 weeks.

Management of chip fractures associated with rupture of the ligament

If the ligament has avulsed a small fragment of bone, which does not interfere with the joint surface, the fragment can be either removed or placed in its proper position, whereupon the ruptured ligament is repaired in the same manner as in cases without skeletal lesion.

12

13

14

12, 13 & 14

If the fragment is larger and involves the joint surface it and the ligament can be fastened to the phalanx, using the pull-out wire technique. The same technique can be employed if a large fragment, instead of being avulsed by the ligament, has been sheared off from the base of the phalanx during radiovolar displacement of the phalanx after the ligament has ruptured.

Small, sheared-off fragments that are loose should be removed. Fragments of bone sheared off from the volar part of the radial condyle of the metacarpal head, usually displaced in a radioproximal direction, do not as a rule call for any treatment. If such a fragment is loose and is readily accessible through the joint space from the ulnar side it is probably best to remove it before repairing the ligament.

The plaster fixation should be the same and kept for an equal period of time irrespective of whether or not the rupture of the ligament is associated with a skeletal lesion.

[The illustrations for this Chapter on Repair of the Ulnar Collateral Ligament of the Thumb with and without Chip Fractures were drawn by the Author.]

The Neurovascular Flap

D. A. Campbell Reid, M.B., B.S.(Lond.), F.R.C.S.
Consultant Plastic Surgeon, Sheffield Royal Hospital,
Sheffield Royal Infirmary, Sheffield Children's Hospital,
Hallamshire Hospital, Chesterfield Royal Hospital;
Honorary Clinical Lecturer, University of Sheffield

PRE - OPERATIVE

There are few occasions for the use of neurovascular flaps in the immediate treatment of the injured hand but for those few occasions the method is of particular value when carried out by a suitably experienced surgeon.

General principles

The operation of transferring a flap of skin with its intact nerve supply from one part of the hand to an adjacent part or a more remote part means that it is possible to restore the all-important sensation, termed tactile gnosis, to an area where this is essential to efficient function, the only other available method being by pollicisation. There are many cases, however, where the latter procedure would not be justifiable. In addition to providing gnostic sensation the transfer also enhances the blood supply to the part, which is of particular value when it is undertaken for a tubed pedicle reconstruction.

The neurovascular flap is usually taken as an island of skin isolated entirely on its neurovascular bundle. The most suitable donor site is the ulnar aspect of the ring or middle finger but this may depend on special circumstances in individual cases. Generally speaking, it is more important to preserve the radial tactile aspects of the fingers for pinch grip between them and the thumb. The length of the flap may also be varied, but usually an adequate length will be provided by taking the flap from the distal two segments. An island of skin may be advanced on its two neurovascular bundles in terminal amputations or to replace scarring. This would apply particularly to thumb defects.

The Kutler-type flap repair for distal pulp defects consists, in fact, of two small island flaps mobilized on pulp pedicles containing neurovascular tissue.

Local sensory flaps may also be used as rotation or transposition flaps to transfer sensation from a relatively unimportant area, e.g. the back of a finger to a more important adjoining area such as the tactile surface of the finger or to cover an amputation stump.

Filletted finger flaps are based on the same principles and are of value in covering defects, where the palmar aspect of a badly mangled finger is spared with its intact neurovascular bundles.

An innervated cross-finger flap may also be employed occasionally to restore pulp with nerve supply to a damaged thumb. Radial nerve fibres on the back of the index finger are dissected out and incorporated in such a flap.

Indications

The neurovascular pedicle flap is indicated in the following instances.

(1) Loss of nerve function. This may be the result of irreparable digital nerve injury in the thumb. It may also follow a median nerve injury where adequate recovery has failed to occur after nerve suture or where repair has not been possible. In such a case it will be necessary to re-innervate the tactile surface of thumb or index finger, preferably the former.

Loss of sensation on the radial side of the index finger pulp due to division of the digital nerve in the distal crease may be quite disabling. Provided the digital nerve to the ulnar side of the finger is intact an island flap from this side of the pulp may be transferred. Failing this, an island flap from the middle finger may be used.

(2) Loss of thumb pulp due to trauma or infection. Terminal loss may be restored by a local neurovascular flap. Total loss will usually necessitate transfer of an island from a finger. Alternatively, it may be possible to use an innervated cross-finger flap from the back of the index finger.

(3) Degloving injuries of the thumb treated initially by tube pedicle cover.

(4) Certain mutilating injuries of the hand.

(5) Thumb lengthening by tube pedicle and bone graft following loss of the thumb at the metacarpophalangeal joint level. The alternatives here are lengthening by the Gillies method, or pollicisation where a partially amputated finger is available.

(6) Autograft of the amputated thumb.

THE OPERATIONS

LOCAL NEUROVASCULAR FLAP FOR DISTAL THUMB DEFECT

1

The incisions

The flap is outlined by longitudinal incisions extending from the defect in a proximal direction and at either edge of the pulp as far as the proximal interphalangeal joint where they are joined by a transverse incision. The longitudinal incisions are also extended onto the proximal segment of the thumb to provide access to the neurovascular bundles.

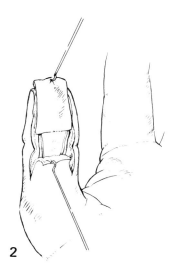

2

Mobilizing the flap

The longitudinal incisions are made and the neurovascular bundles isolated over the proximal phalanx. These are carefully mobilized and the transverse incision made through the skin over the interphalangeal joint of the thumb. Care is taken to protect the neurovascular bundles as they enter the flap. The distal edge of the flap is now mobilized and dissected at a level deep to the bundles. The flap is thus completely freed and advanced distally.

3

Suture of flap and repair of secondary defect

The distal edge of the flap is lightly sutured over the end of the thumb and the advanced edges similarly sutured. It is important to avoid any tension on the flap. The secondary defect is closed by applying a full-thickness free graft which is sutured in place, some of the sutures being left long. These are then tied over a small pad of cotton wool wrung out in saline. Excessive pressure on the underlying neurovascular bundles must be avoided. The island flap must be left partly exposed so that its circulation may be periodically checked.

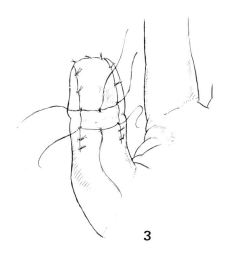

NEUROVASCULAR FLAP TRANSPOSED FROM ULNAR TO RADIAL SIDE OF INDEX FINGER PULP

4

The incisions

An island flap is marked out on the ulnar half of the terminal pulp of the index finger. This extends from the mid-line to the mid-lateral line on the ulnar border and from the tip of the finger distally to the terminal crease proximally.

A zig-zag incision extends from the flap, proximally in the finger to the distal part of the palm. The skin over the radial side of the pulp is similarly marked out.

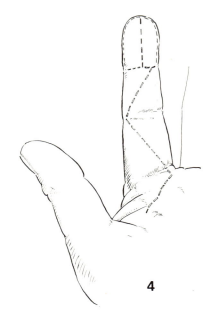

4

5

Mobilization of flap and neurovascular bundle

The incision is made in the finger and the triangular flaps reflected to expose the neurovascular bundle on the ulnar side of the finger. This is followed distally into the pulp flap at the end of the finger, which is now raised. Distally the dissection is carried deeply to ensure avoiding damage to the neurovascular bundle. A corresponding defect is now created on the radial side of the pulp by excising the skin. This may be used as a free full-thickness graft to repair the secondary defect.

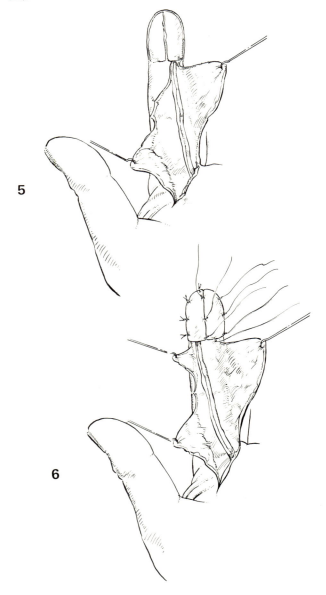

5

6

6

Transfer of island flap and repair of secondary defect

The island flap which has now been completely mobilized on its neurovascular pedicle is transferred to fill the defect on the radial side of the pulp. It is lightly sutured in position. The secondary defect is covered with a full-thickness free graft. The skin removed from the radial side may be utilized for this purpose and it is secured by the tie-over dressing technique. The zig-zag incision is then closed by sutures.

INNERVATED CROSS-FINGER FLAP FOR THUMB DEFECT

7

The incisions

The defect to be replaced is marked out on the palmar aspect of the thumb. A pattern of this is made in material, e.g. rubber dam. This is then applied to the dorsal aspect of the proximal segment of the index finger where a flap of similar dimensions is marked out with its base sited at the mid-lateral line of the finger. A longitudinal incision is extended proximally on the dorsal aspect of the thumb/index web from the base of the flap at its proximal extremity. This is in the line of the fibres of the radial nerve.

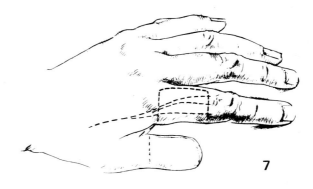

7

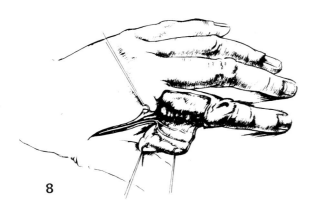

8

8

Raising the flap and exposing the radial nerve

The flap is turned off the back of the index finger at the level of the paratenon overlying the extensor tendon. The radial nerve fibres are then exposed over the thumb/index web, mobilized and traced into the flap.

9

Transfer of cross-finger flap and radial nerve fibres to thumb

The defect is prepared on the palmar aspect of the thumb by excising the appropriate skin or scarring. A longitudinal incision is then made from the defect on the thumb along its dorso-ulnar aspect to link up with the other longitudinal incision at the proximal part of the thumb/index web. The radial nerve fibres are then transferred to the thumb defect in continuity with the cross-finger flap which is now sutured into the defect on the palmar aspect of the thumb. The longitudinal incisions are sutured and the secondary defect on the index finger covered with a split skin graft.

The cross-finger flap is divided and inset 2 weeks later.

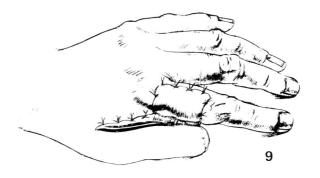

9

TRANSFER OF HETERODIGITAL ISLAND FLAP TO THUMB

10

The incisions

The flap is outlined on the ulnar aspect of the donor finger, in this case the middle finger. It comes to the mid-line on the volar aspect and extends proximally to the level of the proximal interphalangeal joint. The line is broken over the distal interphalangeal joint to overcome the risk of a contracted scar. The posterior edge of the flap extends beyond the mid-lateral line on to the dorsal aspect of the finger. The incision continues from the proximal end of the flap in the mid-lateral line to the base of the finger. From here it extends in an S-shaped manner towards the proximal part of the palm using the skin creases as far as possible. The recipient area is outlined on the tactile surface of the thumb. This should cover the ulnar aspect of the palmar surface of the thumb and extend over the tip where possible. At the base of the thumb the incision is continued for a short distance on to the thenar region.

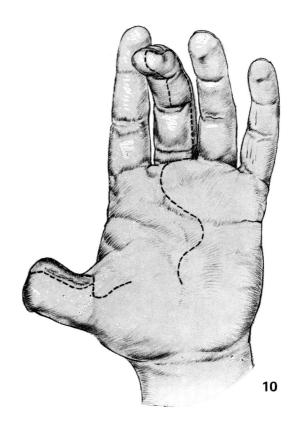

10

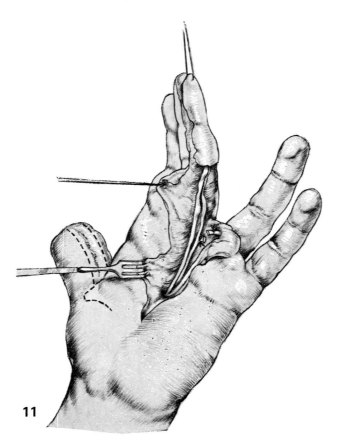

11

11

Dissection of neurovascular pedicle

The dissection commences in the palm after reflecting the skin flaps. The neurovascular bundle to the middle-ring finger cleft is exposed. The digital artery to the radial side of the ring finger is clamped, divided and ligated whilst the nerves to the adjacent sides of the cleft are separated from one another into the palm. This is readily achieved by blunt dissection. The digital artery and nerve to the ulnar side of the middle finger have now been isolated as far as the base of the finger. They are then dissected distally to the island flap. Next, the dissection is switched to the distal end of the finger when the island flap is dissected free in a proximal direction taking the pulp with the overlying skin. Once the dissection has reached the proximal extremity of the flap, the latter will have been isolated on its neurovascular pedicle to the level of the mid-palm. During the dissection of the pedicle, branches of the digital artery are carefully ligated.

12

Transfer of island flap

The recipient site is prepared on the thumb. Where there has been a tubed pedicle reconstruction the original seam is opened up. In any event, the aim should be to place the flap towards the ulnar aspect of the tactile surface. The incision at the base of the thumb extends on to the thenar region. The bridge between this and the main palmar incision is undermined with scissors at a level immediately subjacent to the palmar aponeurosis. The island flap is now gently pulled through, taking care not to kink its pedicle. There should also be some slack on the pedicle to prevent any risk of tension and congestion of the flap which is the main hazard to its viability.

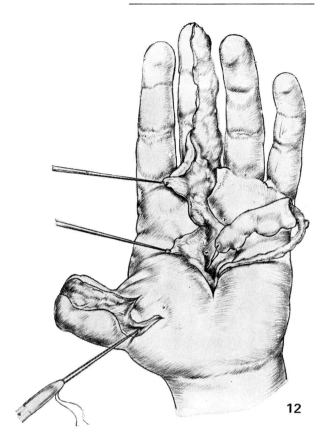

12

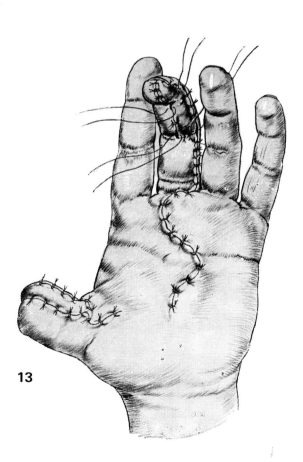

13

13

Closure of defects

Having transferred the island flap, the tourniquet is released and the hand elevated until bleeding is controlled. The secondary defect on the finger is covered with a full-thickness free skin graft sutured into place. Some of the sutures are left long and tied over a dressing to prevent haematoma. The remaining finger incision is sutured, as are the palmar incisions. The island flap is sutured loosely into the thumb defect.

14

Autograft of amputated thumb, degloving injuries and bone graft lengthening procedures

Sometimes in amputation of the thumb, the avulsed part is preserved intact and is brought in with the patient. It may be used as an autograft as follows. The nail is avulsed and the skin dissected off the amputated part. This is then re-attached to the thumb stump by means of a Kirschner wire driven across. The severed tendons are sutured if possible. The condition now resembles that of a degloving injury or a bone graft lengthening procedure, and the subsequent management is the same.

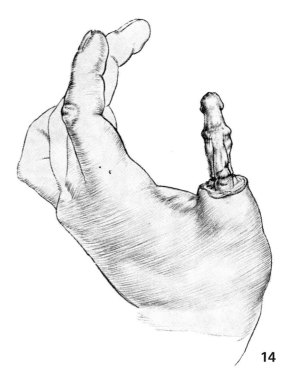

14

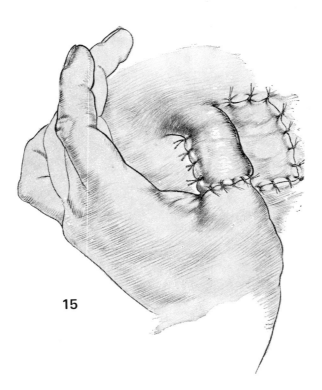

15

15

Skin cover

Skin cover for the thumb autograft, degloving or bone graft is provided by means of a tubed pedicle raised on the chest wall. This is obtained by raising a flap 7·5 cm × 7·5 cm, the base of which is staggered in such a way that when it is tubed the seam will lie along the ulnar aspect of the thumb. The thumb is now inserted into the tube which is then stitched circumferentially around the thumb base. The secondary defect is covered with a split-skin graft.

An excellent alternative is the use of a groin flap which has the additional advantage of providing access for the taking of a bone graft, when this is required, through the same incision.

Transfer of island flap

The chest end of the tube is divided at 3 weeks, the seam excised and the island flap brought through as previously described.

POSTOPERATIVE CARE

The hand is dressed with a layer or two of gauze and orthopaedic wool and is then bandaged over a pad of steel wool in the palm. This serves to keep the hand in a functional position and exerts a mild, uniform pressure. The distal part of the neurovascular flap is left exposed for observation. The hand is kept elevated for 24—48 hr. The flap may appear a little congested initially but this soon wears off. Undue congestion at an early stage should be treated by firm periodic pressure on the flap with a gauze pad in order to express the congested blood. This is rarely necessary provided the flap has been sutured loosely and there is no tension on the pedicle. The patient is encouraged to squeeze the enclosed pad periodically from an early stage. The dressing is left for a week when the donor site is inspected. The dressing is then renewed and the stitches are removed at 2 weeks. Free use of the hand is then encouraged. In his rehabilitation, the patient should start using his hand and particularly the thumb as soon as it is soundly healed. The sensation in the island flap will be referred to the donor finger. As the patient becomes used to the new state of affairs and learns to think of the flap as belonging to the thumb he will use it with increasing efficiency. Eventually, he may come to think of the flap as being an integral part of his thumb, although this involves a certain voluntary discipline on his part.

Once the flap has been established for 6—12 months it is frequently possible to increase its overall size by excising excess tissue and advancing the neurovascular flap. This particularly applies when it has been used in association with a tubed pedicle reconstruction.

References

Adamson, J. E., Horton, C. E. and Crawford, H. H. (1967). 'Sensory rehabilitation of the injured thumb.' *Plastic reconstr. Surg.* **40**, 53
Hueston, J. (1966). 'Local flap repair of finger tip injuries.' *Plastic reconstr. Surg.* **37**, 349
Joshi, B. B. (1970). 'One stage repair for distal amputation of the thumb.' *Plastic reconstr. Surg.* **45**, 613
Joshi, B. B. (1974). 'A local dorso-lateral island flap for restoration of sensation after avulsion injury of finger tip pulp.' *Plastic reconstr. Surg.* **54**, 175
Littler, J. W. (1956). 'Neurovascular pedicle reconstructive surgery of the hand.' *J. Bone Jt Surg.* **38A**, 917
Littler, J. W. (1961). 'Neurovascular skin island flap transfer in reconstructive hand surgery.' *Transactions of the International Society of Plastic Surgeons,* 1959, Edinburgh: Livingstone
Moberg, E. (1955). 'Discussion of paper on The Place of Nerve Grafting in Orthopaedic Surgery—Donal Brooks.' *J. Bone Jt Surg.* **37A**, 305
Moberg, E. (1958). 'Objective method for determining the functional value of sensibility in the hand.' *J. Bone Jt Surg.* **40B**, 305
O'Brien, B. (1968). 'Neurovascular island pedicle flaps for terminal amputations and digital scars.' *Br. J. plast. Surg.* **21**, 259
Reid, D. A. C. (1966). 'The neurovascular island flap in thumb reconstruction.' *Br. J. plast. Surg.* **19**, 234
Tubiana, R. and Duparc, J. (1961). 'Restoration of sensibility in the hand by neurovascular skin island transfer.' *J. Bone Jt Surg.* **43B**, 474
Wilson, J. S. P. and Braithwaite, F. (1964). 'The autografting of an amputated thumb.' *Transactions of the International Society of Plastic Surgeons,* 1963, Amsterdam: Excerpta Medica Foundation

[*The illustrations for this Chapter on The Neurovascular Flap were drawn by Mr. A. S. Foster.*]

Microsurgical Techniques

John R. Cobbett, F.R.C.S.
Plastic Surgeon, Queen Victoria Hospital, East Grinstead

Microsurgical techniques are time-consuming and have to be learned by practice. Their use is indicated where it can be shown that a procedure is more likely to produce a favourable result where such techniques have been used.

It is possible to repair a digital artery of 1 mm external diameter using an ophthalmic loupe alone but it is extremely difficult, and workers in digital replantation surgery using an operating microscope and proper microsurgical equipment have found their overall success rate to be far greater than that of workers using loupe alone.

Millesi has demonstrated the great value of microsurgical precision in the suture of nerves and nerve grafts.

The added operative time for the patient and training time for the surgeon are therefore well justified in nerve and blood vessel work in the hand.

INSTRUMENTATION

The microscope

Ideally this should have several 'heads' so that two or three surgeons or assistants may have binocular vision and therefore truly assist rather than observe. A light source co-axial with the visual optical system is ideal and genuinely shadowless. Zoom magnification ranging from X3 to about X20 is ideal. Foot control of focus and zoom mechanisms helps to keep the operators hands where they are needed.

All these things are available—at a price. At the other end of the scale a simple X6 or X8 binocular table-mounted microscope is still a very valuable tool.

Surgical instruments

1

These are all designed so that they may be used with the operator's hand resting on its ulnar border and small finger, largely eliminating tremor.

Straight and angled spring scissors, a long Barraquer or O'Brien needle-holder and both straight and curved needle point jewellers forceps are the basic equipment, and equipment is best kept as basic as possible. The spring on all the instruments should be weak, as the necessity for firm pressure in gripping the instrument—pencilwise—will increase the degree of tremor and the rate of onset of fatigue. The needle-holder should have no lock as the action of this causes unwanted movement at the point of the instrument. Vascular clamps for microsurgery come with and without an approximation apparatus and in various shapes and sizes. An appropriately weakened Scoville Lewis neurosurgical aneurysm clip makes a good all-purpose clamp but here again individual surgeons will find their own favourites.

Suture material

10/0 Nylon mounted on curved taper point needles of from 3 to 6 mm in length is readily available from several manufacturers. The surgeon will choose whichever needle he finds suits him best. Finer suture material is not required for clinical work.

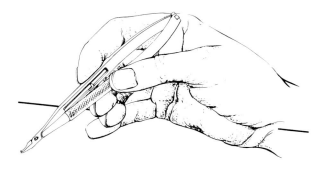

1

It cannot be over-emphasized before approaching a clinical case that microsurgery requires practice. This is best undertaken in the animal laboratory where blood vessel or nerve repair may be tried. Even working on a small vessel taken off the surface of a sheep's brain bought at the local butcher's shop will give valuable experience in using the microscope and fine instruments.

THE REPAIR OF A SMALL BLOOD VESSEL

Clamps are applied to the divided vessel and the ends of the vessel washed clear of blood and clot with a solution of heparin, 1000 units in 100 ml of Ringer's solution. As far as possible no instrument should touch the inner endothelial surface of the vessel, as even slight intimal damage can produce local thrombosis. Thus the vessel ends are washed by a jet of fluid, rather than by inserting a cannula into the lumen.

Next excise loose adventitia by pulling a cuff of it down over the vessel end, and cutting it off with scissors.

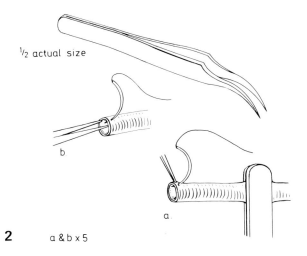

½ actual size

b

a

2   a & b × 5

2

The next step is the most difficult—the first suture. Hold the end of the vessel by a pinch of muscle only—not the full thickness of the vessel wall—and pass the needle from without inwards close to the point of the forceps. If this proves impossible, it is permitted, only as a last resort, to place the tips of the forceps within the lumen and use these as counterpressure for the first suture. Passing this suture from within out on the second vessel end is a far simpler procedure. Tie the knot, and leave one suture end long as a stay. The second suture should be placed on the same aspect of the vessel, about one-third of the circumference around. It too should have one long end.

3

Traction on these two stay sutures will now present the opposing vessel walls between them for the insertion of more interrupted sutures. These should be placed rather less than twice the thickness of the vessel wall from the cut edge, and in the case of an artery spaced about 0·3 mm apart. Once sufficient sutures have been placed between the two stays appropriate manipulation of stay sutures and clamps will rotate the vessel to show the unrepaired two-thirds of the circumference. The unequal placing of the stay sutures lets the posterior vessel edges fall back out of the needle's way after preparing the anterior suture line, thus lessening the chance of sewing the front of the vessel to the back.

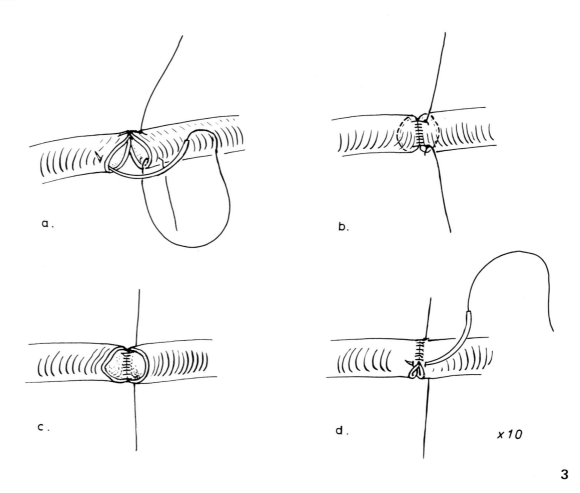

a.

b.

c.

d.   x 10

3

Once all sutures have been inserted the long ends of the stays are cut, and the clamps removed. Firm digital pressure, gradually lessened over 60 sec, will control local oozing between sutures. Rarely an extra stitch will be required to complete a watertight seal.

Once the clamps have been released it is inadvisable to re-apply them unless the stagnant blood in the anastomotic area is rapidly washed out, as under these circumstances local thrombosis is likely.

The repair of a small vein is accomplished in the same manner, but fewer sutures are required.

[*The illustrations for this Chapter on Microsurgical Techniques were drawn by Miss J. Graham.*]

Digital Replantation

John R. Cobbett, F.R.C.S.
Plastic Surgeon, Queen Victoria Hospital, East Grinstead

INTRODUCTION

The replantation of a totally amputated digit by microvascular techniques was first successfully performed by S. Tamai in Nara, Japan in 1965. Since then many hundreds of successful replant cases have been reported.

PRE-OPERATIVE

1

Indications for attempting digital replantation

Provided the patient is fit for the prolonged surgery required:

(*1*) *Thumb amputation* through the proximal phalanx or more proximally

(*2*) *Multiple digital amputations* and

(*3*) Any amputation through the proximal phalanx in a child, are all absolute indications for attempting replantation.

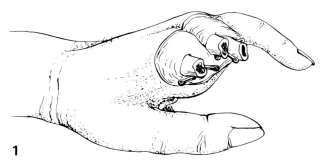

1

A single finger amputation

This situation requires considerable consultation between patient and surgeon. Surgical treatment may well be prolonged, and a somewhat stiff partially anaesthetic aching digit the only result after months of treatment. If, however, this digit happens to be the left ring finger of an unmarried girl even this is well worth having. The patient's work, social status and special wishes must all be balanced against the chances of success and the morbidity entailed.

Contra-indications

The success rate in the replantation of digits that have been avulsed or have been severely crushed is so poor as to render these injuries unacceptable for attempted replantation except in the most unusual circumstances.

Anaesthesia

General anaesthesia is the rule for replantation procedures, which may last from 2 to more than 8 hr, depending on the number of digits to be replanted, and the amount of reconstruction performed on each one. Brachial plexus block has been used by some workers.

2

Cooling

As soon after the injury as possible the amputated part should be placed on (but not in) ice; freezing should be avoided. At room temperature irreversible changes start in nerve and muscle after about 5 hr. With cooling to 4°C survival has been reported after replantation at over 24 hr.

If the amputation is incomplete and a skin bridge remains it should be left intact as it may contain a valuable vein, rendering venous anastomosis unnecessary.

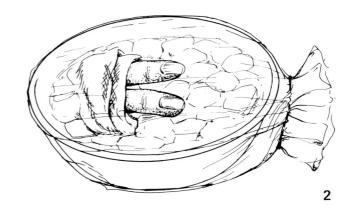

2

THE OPERATION

Preparation

If two surgical teams are available the hand and the amputated digit can be explored simultaneously. Otherwise the digit should be explored first to ascertain its suitability for replantation, before anaesthetizing the patient.

Perfusion of the amputated digit with heparin or any other substance is not recommended. A recent experimental series in animals showed that perfusion of any sort reduced the replantation success rate (Harashina and Buncke, 1975).

3

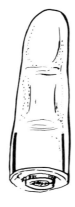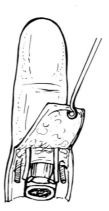

3

In a clean cut guillotine amputation, or one with minimal local crushing, the digital arteries will not be difficult to find, but direct longitudinal incisions over the digital bundles are advised. Once found, it is essential that all damaged artery be excised. Anastomosis of a crushed artery will inevitably result in failure. In the avulsion type of injury the artery is frequently divided at a completely different level from the skin, and a long 'tail' of vessel may be hanging from one or other stump. Such a 'tail' must have been extremely severely stretched, and is unsuitable for repair. Considerable difficulty may be encountered in locating the opposite end of the vessel and this, together with the very long vascular defect gives such injuries their deservedly unpopular reputation. One or more dorsal veins should also be found at this stage, but should this prove difficult they may be left until after the arterial repair, when back bleeding will make them obvious.

4

It is usual to explore the proximal side of the amputation under a tourniquet, releasing this when all vital structures have been found, and appropriate vascular clamps put on the main vessels. A few workers prefer not to use any vessel clamps, but to perform their microsurgical vessel repair under the tourniquet alone.

Longitudinal incisions over the digital bundles will also be helpful on the proximal side of the amputation. Here again it is essential to excise all damaged blood vessel. It should be emphasized at this point that proposed digital replantation does not excuse the surgeon from performing a full and proper surgical debridement of both proximal and distal wounds. All non-viable tissue, barring that which will be revascularized in the replantation must be excised. Replantation surgery is difficult enough without the added complications of postoperative wound infection or skin slough.

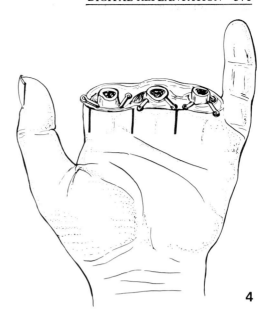

4

5

Bony fixation

Bone shortening achieves two objects—it removes potentially contaminated bony surfaces and also allows easier approximation of divided soft tissues. This is particularly important in the case of the blood vessels, which may be too short for a tension-free anastomosis after their debridement. Over-enthusiastic bone shortening to achieve direct vascular repair is to be discouraged—it is better to use a reversed vein graft to fill the vascular defects.

Bony fixation as a first stage is essential to achieve a stable platform for later work. Longitudinal Kirschner wires may be used for this, at a price of some later joint stiffness. It is better, if bone length allows, to drill two transverse holes through the bone ends and use a 'square' twisted wire.

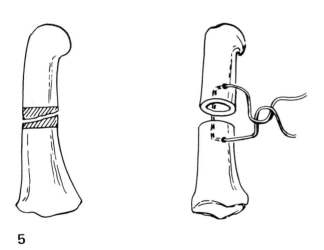

5

6

Extent of primary suture

Following bony fixation further procedures depend on the amount of primary surgery anticipated. Secondary surgery—particularly on the digital nerves —will involve a difficult dissection of the digital bundle in scar tissue, with a very real danger of arterial damage and possible loss of the digit. The surgeon should consider how he would manage the nerve and tendon injuries if no vascular problem existed. Nevertheless, considering the difficulties of secondary surgery, when in doubt, he may well opt for primary nerve repair under less than ideal conditions.

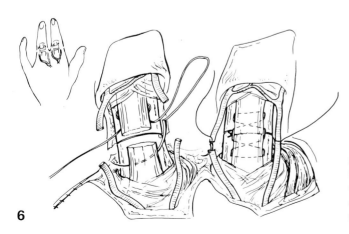

6

7, 8 & 9

If conditions are favourable those workers with experience will repair bone, extensor tendon, dorsal vein, or veins, dorsal skin, digital arteries, nerves, one or both flexor tendons, and flexor skin in that order.

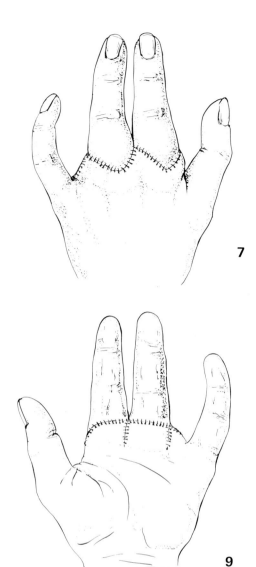

7

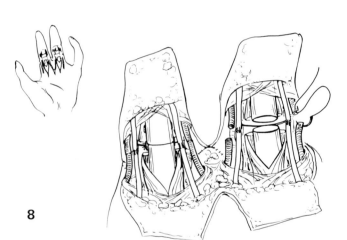

8

9

At the other end of the scale the novice replant surgeon may well be content to achieve bony fixation, repair one digital artery only and then suture the skin loosely, letting the digital veins bleed into bulky dressings. This bleeding will cease after about 48 hr, and approximately 1 litre of blood will be lost in this time. Several digits have been successfully replanted by this technique (Snyder, Stevenson and Browne, 1972).

Blood vessel repair

The technique of microsurgical repair of blood vessels is described in the Chapter on 'Microsurgical Techniques', pages 566—568.

One arterial repair is adequate—if time permits the repair of both arteries gives an added sense of security. Longitudinal tension in the vessel repair may be avoided by using a reversed vein graft. The superficial veins on the flexor aspect of the forearm are of a suitable calibre and easily accessible.

The more veins repaired the more physiological is the postoperative situation. Multiple vein repair seems to have little effect on the degree of most postoperative oedema. If only one vein is repaired the velocity of the blood flow therein is greatly increased and this probably lessens the chance of anastomotic thrombosis. One vein repair per digit is the author's practice.

Failure of satisfactory blood flow into the digit immediately following the arterial repair is common, in spite of an apparently patent anastomosis. Local warmth, papaverine to the proximal vessel, time and the rapid infusion of 50 ml of low molecular weight dextran (LMWD) solution will usually restore a colour return to the digit under these circumstances. Failing this, vascular clamps should be re-applied and the adequacy of the proximal input checked by removing some sutures from the anastomosis and briefly releasing the proximal clamp. Failure of flow under these circumstances is usually due to proximal vascular damage, and the hand should be explored more proximally with this in mind.

POSTOPERATIVE CARE AND COMPLICATIONS

The hand should be elevated just above heart level. Analgesics and appropriate prophylactic antibiotics are administered as required.

Frequent (at least half-hourly) observations of the replanted digit are vital. Colour, colour return, warmth and the tissue tension in the pulp should all be assessed. Some degree of postoperative oedema is inevitable, but a tense pulp with an over-rapid colour return—usually to light purple—indicates a venous block. A pale lavender digit with lost pulp tension has an arterial block. In either case the treatment is prompt return to the operating theatre and re-exploration.

Prophylaxis of arterial spasm

Chlorpromazine 25 mg twice daily is given orally, and oral alcohol intake encouraged. Most patients benefit from a stellate ganglion block before recovering from anaesthesia, and this may be repeated if arterial spasm appears to be a problem.

Prophylaxis of anastomotic thrombosis

Low molecular weight dextran in intravenous infusion is given as a dosage of 500 ml twice daily for the first few days. Aspirin has definite antithrombotic properties and in the absence of a contra-indication most workers use 600 mg 4-hourly.

Heparin is not required where a technically satisfactory anastomosis exists, and may result in haematoma formation. Where there is doubt about the quality of the anastomosis, heparin may be used— appropriately controlled—but it is advisable to delay its use for 24 hr after the completion of surgery. The coumarol derivatives do not appear to have been used in replantation work, and their ability to prevent thrombosis at a suture line in a vessel is in doubt. It should be emphasized once more that the key to success is a technically adequate vessel anastomosis, which can only be gained by previous practice in microsurgical techniques.

References

Harashina, T. and Bucke, H. J. (1975). *Plastic reconstr. Surg.* **56**, 542
Komatsu, S. and Tamai, S. (1968). *Plastic reconstr. Surg.* **42**, 374
Snyder, C. C., Stevenson, R. M. and Browne, E. Z. (1972). *Plastic reconstr. Surg.* **50**, 553

[*The illustrations for this Chapter on Digital Replantation were drawn by Miss J. Graham.*]

Replacement and Fixation of Posterior Lip of Acetabulum
(following Posterior Fracture-Dislocation)

E. Letournel, M.D.
Professor of Orthopaedic Surgery and Traumatology,
Centre Medico-Chirurgical de la Porte de Choisy, Paris

PRE-OPERATIVE

Indications

The replacement and fixation of a fracture of the posterior lip of the acetabulum is advisable because the restoration of the articular crescent restores the stability of the joint and allows a natural distribution of intra-articular pressure, thereby preventing post-traumatic osteo-arthrosis.

Furthermore the surgical correction allows one to clear the joint of any small fragments which are not visible with x-rays and can give troubles later on. It enables the surgeon to recognize the fractures in which the external part of the posterior wall is separated into one or more fragments, whereas the inner part is impacted into the underlying cancellous bone and has to be dislodged and replaced in contact with the femoral head. Good fixation allows early walking without weight-bearing and avoids all kinds of postoperative immobilization.

The only contra-indication is small fragments that are too small to be screwed.

Time of operation

The dislocation has to be reduced as soon as possible after injury. Usually the head is stable, but the fragments remain displaced. Rest in bed with slight external rotation of the limb avoids recurrent dislocation; traction is not necessary.

If the hip cannot be reduced (because, for example, of a big intra-articular fragment) or is unstable after reduction because of the extent of the fracture, operation should be carried out as an emergency.

Provided that the reduced head remains in the joint, replacement of the posterior fragment can be easily performed during the first 6 or 8 days after injury, so there is plenty of time in which to prepare the patient.

Anaesthesia

General anaesthesia is necessary and blood should be available.

1

Position of patient

The patient is placed prone on an orthopaedic table.

To relax the sciatic nerve and avoid damaging it during the posterior approach, the knee should be flexed about 45° and a transcondylar Steinmann pin allows traction on the limb.

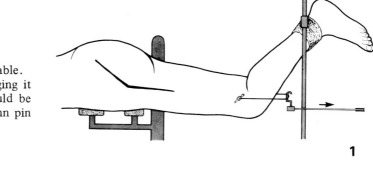

1

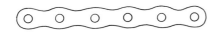

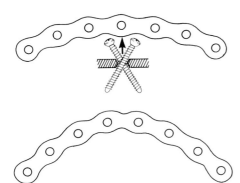

2

2

The device

Screws are used; plates may also be necessary.

The plates do not need to be very thick and wide and they must be capable of being shaped to lie perfectly on the reconstructed posterior wall. Vitallium Sherman's plates are satisfactory because they can be easily shaped in all directions. There are also curved Vitallium Letournel acetabular plates with 6, 8 or 10 holes and two curvatures.

To give them the desired shape one can use special benders or, more commonly, two big forceps grasping the plate at the right places. It is essential to shape the plate to follow perfectly the contours of the posterior column where it must lie; it is easy to make it too much or too little curved and so to spoil the position of the fragment(s) when the screws are driven home.

3

Special tools

It is helpful to have an instrument to push fragments into place and it should be protected by a shield 4 mm from its end.

A special retractor may be inserted in either sciatic notch; it takes a good hold because of its distal hook, and it presents a convex surface to the nerve, but it must be kept closely against the bone (sciatic spine upwards, ischial tuberosity downwards) in order to avoid compression of the nerve by one or other side of its hook.

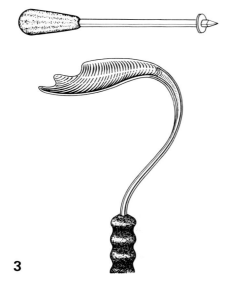

3

THE OPERATION

4a&b

Kocher-Langenbeck approach

The skin incision has two limbs centred on the superior part of the greater trochanter; the upper runs two-thirds of the way towards the posterior-superior iliac spine and the lower passes down the lateral aspect of the thigh.

The gluteus maximus and the fascia lata are split in the line of the incision. The gluteus maximus is split only as far as the first important vascular pedicle.

The tendon piriformis is divided, lifted up and attached by a stitch to the internal lip of the incision. Lifting the muscle exposes the sciatic nerve and gives access to the greater sciatic notch and to the neuro-vascular pedicle of the gluteal muscles.

The obturator internus and the gemelli are also divided through their terminal tendons, secured with a stitch and freed carefully from the bone. The under-lying synovial bursa is opened and gives access to the lesser sciatic notch, into which the special retractor can be inserted and where it will remain separated from the nerve by the obturator tendon. The whole of both sciatic notches must be reached and exposed.

The upper pole of the ischial tuberosity has to be cleared of muscular insertions but it is not always necessary to divide the quadratus femoris.

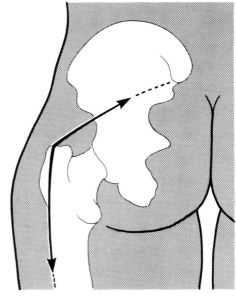

4a

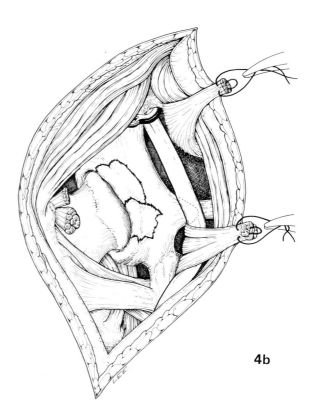

4b

5a&b

Posterior wall fracture

The posterior wall fracture can then be displayed. It varies from case to case. The most typical is separate fragments with a part of the articular surface and a part of the retro-acetabular surface; these fragments may or may not remain attached to the capsule and other soft parts. Fragments are often embedded in the underlying cancellous bone and must be carefully looked for. Sometimes there are isolated fragments of the articular or of the posterior cortical surface. Both the extent of the posterior wall avulsion and the number of fragments vary greatly from one case to another. The displaced fragments and the tear of the capsule allow access to the joint. Although it is difficult to avoid some stripping of the soft tissues from these fragments, such dissection should be kept to a minimum.

Clearing the joint

The joint must be cleared of any fragments that are in the acetabular fossa and one must not forget to remove the fragment that is sometimes attached to the ligamentum teres, which generally remains attached to the head.

With the aid of traction one gains an excellent view of the joint and should easily recognize both free and impacted fragments.

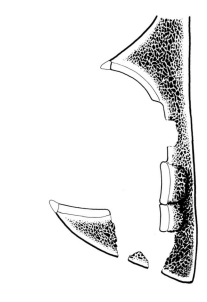

5a

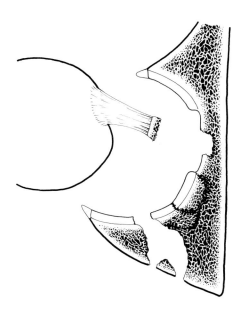

5b

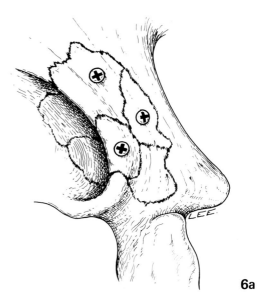

6a

6a&b

The reduction

When traction is released the head takes its place under the roof and the anterior part of the articular crescent, but one must ensure that the contact is perfect. The fragments are then replaced. First, any impacted fragments are gently mobilized with a chisel or a lever, trying to keep their cancellous part intact and they are set in place upon the head of the femur. The posterior fragments are then replaced. It is easy when there is only one fragment, it is more difficult when there are several pieces, which have to be put in their right places as carefully and perfectly as the pieces of jigsaw puzzle. This takes time and may require many trials and errors. When there is a combination of separated and impacted fragments there may be found to be a gap after they have been re-assembled as best one can; if this is likely to impair the stability of the reconstruction it should be filled with cancellous bone from the ilium or from the greater trochanter of the femur.

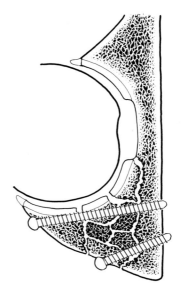

6b

7a,b&c

Fixation

In the case of small fragments two or three isolated screws may suffice; this is most likely to be so when the fragments bear a small portion of articular surface. A single big fragment may be fixed by several screws inserted in different directions. These screws are inserted into the posterior aspect of the fragment and are directed to the quadrilateral surface of the iliac bone where they obtain a good hold. One must always take care to avoid the joint and the head and it is wise to test the movement of the head in its socket so as to be sure that there is no grating. A finger passed through the great sciatic notch tests the length of the screws.

In most cases plates are needed as well as screws. Two or three screws are used to hold the fragments in place. Then a plate has to be fitted to the posterior column, from the upper pole of the ischial tuberosity to the posterior part of the wing or above the roof of the acetabulum, depending on the size and the exact site of the posterior fracture(s). The plate follows the long axis of the articular fragments. Whether straight or curved, the lower end of the plate is given a sharp bend to follow the contour of the 'infra-acetabular groove'. The rest of the plate is shaped to follow exactly the contours of the posterior column so as to be in perfect contact with the bone. The gluteal muscles' pedicle is very carefully freed from the bone if it is necessary to insert the plate under it. The plate is then screwed down, taking care not to enter the joint. The lowest screw is inserted into the ischial tuberosity, where it finds a very strong hold and may be 40 or 45 mm long. The screws over the roof may be 30–40 mm and those into the posterior part of the wing, 25–35 mm. The intermediate screws, like the separate ones, take hold of the quadrilateral surface. If possible, one should insert two screws beyond each extremity of the fracture site.

One must always test the freedom of the joint after plating.

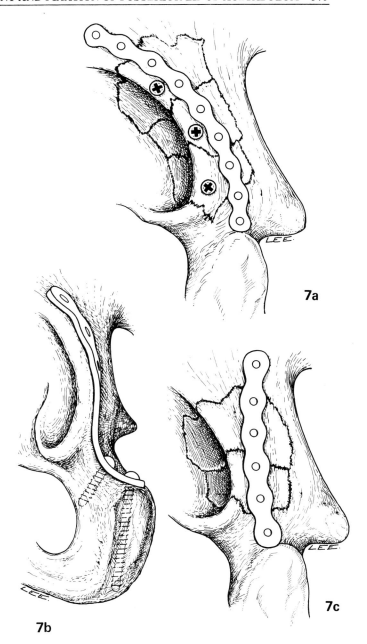

7a

7b

7c

Closure

Piriformis and obturator internus are re-attached to their tendons and sewn together side to side in order to provide a muscular pad between the sciatic nerve and the plate.

One or two suction drains are required.
Gluteus maximus is sutured and the skin closed.
The transcondylar traction pin is removed.

POSTOPERATIVE CARE

No plaster, splint or traction is required, only bed rest.
The patient is allowed to move his limb.
Passive exercises begin on the second or third day.
Suction drains are removed after 5 or 6 days.
Walking without weight-bearing is allowed on the eighth to the tenth day.
Full weight-bearing is allowed after 75 days.

[*The illustrations for this Chapter on Replacement and Fixation of Posterior Lip of Acetabulum (following Posterior Fracture-Dislocation) were drawn by Mrs. G. Lee.*]

Fractures at the Upper End of the Femur

P. S. London, M.B.E., F.R.C.S.
Surgeon, Birmingham Accident Hospital

FRACTURE OF NECK OF FEMUR

Choice of treatment

The surgeon has to decide whether to remove the head or to retain it and if he is going to retain it he has to decide which method of fixing it to use.

1-4

The head should be retained in children and in adults with Garden's Stage 1 and Stage 2 fractures. Some surgeon's retain the head also after Stage 3 and Stage 4 fractures, others replace it. The distinction between Stages 3 and 4 is based upon the direction of the trabeculae in the head of the femur; they are disposed abnormally in Stage 3 and normally in Stage 4 and the implication is that with Stage 3 the fragments are still connected by soft tissues whereas with Stage 4 they are not. This means that there is a better possibility of achieving and maintaining a good position with Stage 3 than with Stage 4 fractures.

Unfavourable features that favour removing rather than keeping the head are:

(1) a large posterior fragment;

(2) displaced fractures that are more than a few days old and have as a result become mutually adapted in deformity;

(3) pathological fractures;

(4) fractures in the old and frail, for whom one reliable and fairly quick operation is desirable.

Patients from mental hospitals are liable to have their hips dislocated after prostheses have been inserted and are usually better dealt with by a conservative operation.

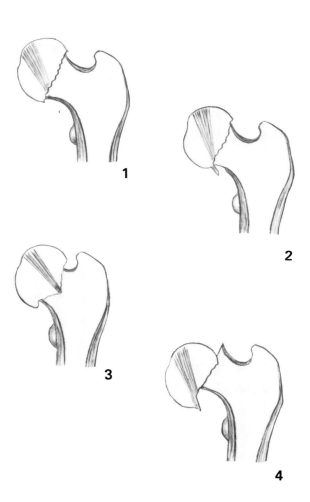

FIXATIVE OPERATIONS

Anaesthesia

Local anaesthesia can be used for inserting multiple pins but general anaesthesia requires much less tolerance on the part of the patient and can much reduce the length of the operation.

5 & 6

Manipulation

The patient should be fully relaxed, when it is sufficient to turn the abducted limbs inwards as far as they will comfortably go before fixing them to an orthopaedic table. Traction is not necessary.

Alternatively, the operation can be performed on an ordinary operating table with the knees bent over the sides and the feet supported on stools so that the legs are vertical. This rotates the thigh far enough medially.

If manipulation fails to achieve an acceptable position the surgeon has to choose between open reduction of the fracture (*see* page 591) and removing the head of the femur.

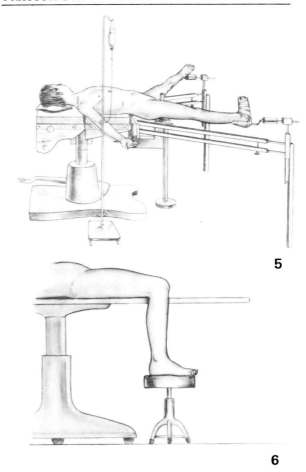

5

6

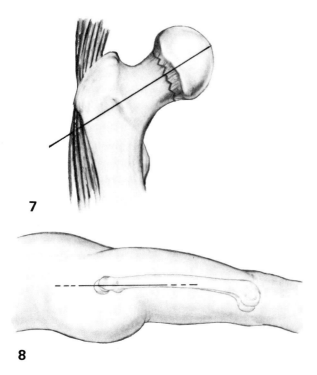

7

8

7 & 8

Exposure

The point of entry of pins or nails is usually an inch or so below the ridge that separates vastus lateralis from the gluteus medius. It is chosen so that when a nail is used it will lie as near as possible to the long axis of the neck; when multiple pins are used it does not matter very much whether they are parallel or not; length is perhaps more important than direction.

The incision

This should start at the tip of the great trochanter in thin patients and 2 or 3 inches higher in fat ones and it should extend downwards on the lateral face of the thigh for the same distance below the point of entry to the bone. If a nail-plate is used, the downward extension may have to be 6 or more inches long.

9

If the incision is made a little behind (posterior to) the mid-line of the femur as seen from the side, the lower edge of the wound needs little retraction and it enables the surgeon to keep behind tensor fasciae latae, which can bleed briskly. If vastus lateralis is split in the line of its fibres by blunt dissection it does not usually bleed much whereas an approach by cutting along the posterolateral septum followed by turning vastus lateralis forwards from the femur is liable to make the perforating arteries bleed.

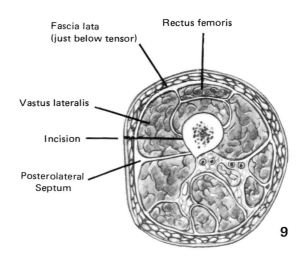

Fascia lata
(just below tensor)

Rectus femoris

Vastus lateralis

Incision

Posterolateral
Septum

9

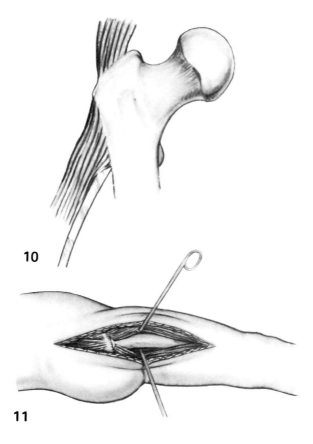

10

11

10 & 11

The lateral surface of the bone is cleared with a periosteal elevator pushed upwards into the angle between muscle and bone. The ridge should be clearly seen, to which end it is often necessary to make a small cut through the aponeurotic origin and at right angles to the length of the femur.

Having been cleared, the bone is kept exposed by bone levers. Once these are in place there is often little bleeding from the muscle but there are sometimes spurting vessels in the other layers and these should be dealt with as they are encountered.

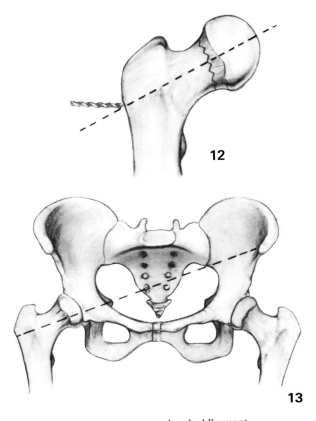

12

12, 13 & 14

Inserting the guide wire

If image-intensified radiography is available the wire is driven in under the guidance of the eye. Otherwise its passage can be guided in several ways but may require more than one attempt.

   If the cortex is thin the guide wire can be driven straight through it, otherwise it is easier first to make a hole with a drill that is slightly larger than the guide wire and directed in the intended line of the guide wire. The necessarily oblique direction should not be adopted until a start has been made with the drill perpendicular to the bone. Some surgeons direct the wire at the anterior, superior spine of the opposite ilium, others aim for the shadows of clips put over the head of the femur before applying the towels. The femoral artery crosses the head of the femur between its middle and medial thirds and the inguinal ligament forms a tangent to the head.

   If the neck of the femur is parallel to the floor the guide wire is directed horizontally, but if not, due allowance must be made for this deviation.

13

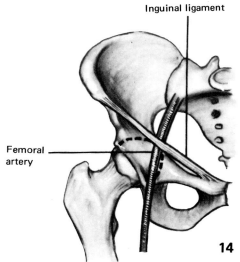

Inguinal ligament

Femoral artery

14

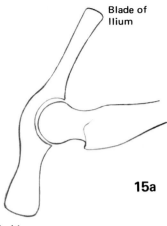

15a

A warning

15a & b

If x-ray films are used it is necessary to be sure that the lateral view is the right way up and that in a fat person the head can be made out. The unwary may fail to recognize that when both are not visible in the lateral view the blade of the ilium may be mistaken for the ischium, with the result that the film may be read upside down.

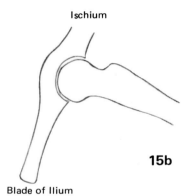

15b

16a & b

In the lateral view, the guide wire should be as nearly as possible in the long axis of the neck but if, as is not unusual, the head and the neck are not perfectly aligned, it is desirable that the wire should be so placed that as much as possible of it shall lie within the head while yet leaving room for the nail to lie within the cortical walls of the neck.

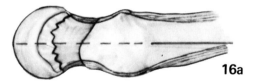

16a

In general, a well-placed guide wire can be inserted quite easily by hand; if it enters the bone through a comfortably sized hole in the cortex the surgeon can recognize the characteristic crunching of passage through cancellous bone. Any obstruction to the onward movement requires radiographic explanation and once the wire has been inserted the surgeon must ensure that a nail can be driven over it. Some surgeons prefer to insert two or even three wires before calling for x-rays and if one is not sure whether the first is in a good position a second should be inserted.

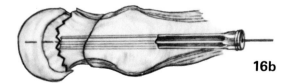

16b

Multiple pins

17a & b

These are favoured for children's fractures because the force required to drive a nail into the tough, young bone can cause considerable harm. They may also be used for fractures with little displacement in case a nail should enter the head slightly off centre and tilt it, and bend the guide wire at the same time.

18

A confident surgeon or image intensification makes a guide wire unnecessary, three or four pins being driven in under direct vision so that their tips reach the subchondral bone of the head. Those with the outer part threaded are secured by running nuts up to the bone and holding them by twists of wire. The unwanted lengths are then cut off. If unthreaded pins are used they are less likely to slide out if they are not parallel to each other.

Nails

These are driven in over a guide wire and the process is made easier if the cortex of the femur is first broached.

19

Simple, three-flanged nails are not recommended because even with Pidcock's cross-pin they can slide out of the head of the femur and a nail plate is preferable. If the nail is passed through a comfortably large hole that has been drilled through the cortex it is much less likely to cause a subtrochanteric fracture than the heavy blows that are required to drive a broaching tool through what may be thick cortex. Surgeons who favour a steep nail should bear this in mind.

Such a hole can be made with a cannulated drill passed over a suitably placed guide wire, or Hudson's brace can be used to breach the femur, after which a guide wire is passed through the hole, which can, if necessary, be enlarged with nibbling forceps.

20

Of the nail plates, McLaughlin's is the easiest to use because the angle between the nail and the plate can be adjusted to suit the individual case. After putting a guide wire in an acceptable position the further steps are as follows.

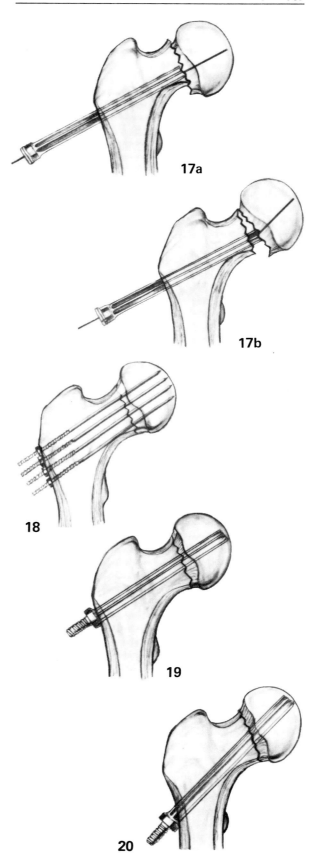

17a

17b

18

19

20

21-26

(*1*) Measure the length of wire that is in the femur. Both guide wires and rulers are 7 inches (18 cm) long.

(*a*) Add a little if the tip of the guide wire is more than ¼ inch short of the cortex as seen on the film.

(*b*) Subtract a little if the fracture is slightly widened and therefore likely to settle and shorten.

(*c*) Allow ¼ inch for the nail that occupies the space between the plate and the outer surface of the femur.

(*2*) Screw the chosen nail to the handle and pass it over the wire so that the bevelled tip will fit the curvature of the subchondral bone of the head.

(*3*) Drive the nail in. If it passes in to its full length without heavy blows x-ray films need not be exposed until it has been driven home. If, however, it becomes difficult to drive the nail in the surgeon must use x-rays (preferably with intensified images) to find out why.

The usual causes of difficulty are:

(*a*) The nail is excentric and has come up against cortex in one or other view.

(*b*) The nail has tilted the head and bent the wire. If this happens the nail and then the wire must be withdrawn and a new wire inserted higher up in an attempt to correct the tilt; if it does so, it should then be driven into the pelvis so as to fix the head and used either for a new nail, perhaps of a different length, or as a guide for a new guide wire.

(*4*) Fit the hole in the top end of the plate over the threaded outer end of the nail.

(*5*) Apply the locking washer.

(*6*) Apply the locking nut. This should be made finger tight.

(*7*) Place the plate snugly against the shaft of the femur.

(*8*) Screw it in place. For fractures of the neck of the femur a plate with only one hole will suffice.

(*9*) Tighten the nut fully.

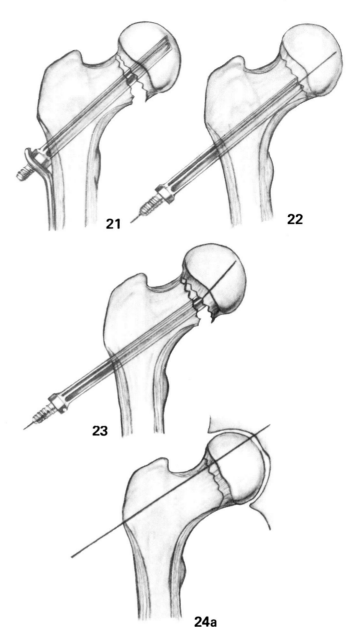

21   22

23   24a

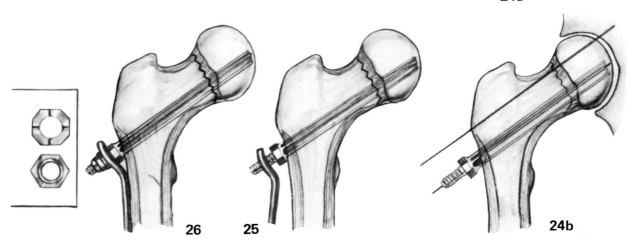

26   25   24b

27, 28 & 29

Fixed angle nail-plates

Capener-Neufeld and Jewett's nail plates are less bulky on the outer side of a thin person's thigh than are McLaughlin's but they are in some ways more difficult to use and require a different technique for their insertion.

(*1*) Exposure of the femur is as has already been described.

(*2*) Choose the point of entry of the nail by first laying a nail plate with the appropriate angle (120°, 130°, 135° for Capener-Neufeld's and 130° and 150° for Jewett's) on the x-ray film in the position that it is intended to occupy and note how far below the ridge this is. Allow for about 20 per cent magnification when marking this place on the bone.

(*3*) Broach the femur as described.

(*4*) Insert a guide wire through the centre of a large hole, using a guide of the chosen angle.

(*5*) Determine its position with the aid of x-rays, and insert other wires if necessary. If having done this the acceptable wire is too close to the hole to enable the nail to pass over it the hole may be suitably enlarged with the aid of nibblers.

(*6*) Choose the length of nail as already described.

Although an experienced surgeon may be able to remove an ill-placed guide wire and insert a nail plate having corrected its position in his mind's eye this is not recommended because without a guide wire to steady the head a nail is likely to displace it.

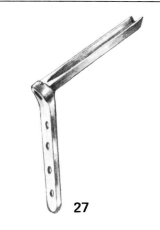

27

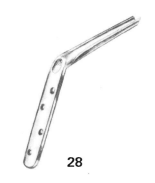

28

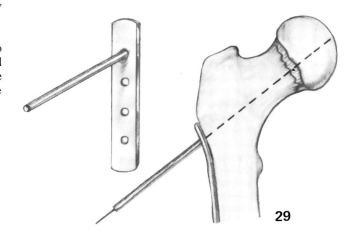

29

Other methods of fixation

There are so many methods in use that it is impracticable to mention them all. Most surgeons settle down to perfect their use of one or two methods and the author has described those that he uses but the use of crossed screws has much theoretical argument in its favour.

30 & 31

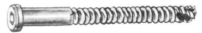

30

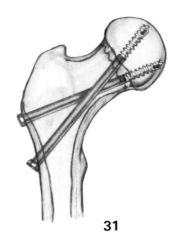

31

Garden's screws (Garden, 1964)

These are cannulated and passed over guide wires after breaching the cortex with a cannulated drill. The screws should lie in contact and one should lie in the line of the weight-bearing trabeculae. The screw's head has a socket by means of which it is screwed into place.

The method is attractive in that it gives secure fixation; the presence of a second guide wire or screw prevents the head from being twisted as the screw is inserted and the smooth shafts of the screws allow them to help to draw the head snugly down onto the neck, but it requires considerable technical skill.

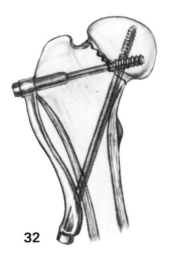

32

32

Triangle pinning (Smyth *et al*., 1964, 1974)

Two screws are used with a metal bar between them. The method is as effective as any that is carried out by its deviser, but it requires considerable skill and it does leave a large prominence.

DISPLACED PROXIMAL EPIPHYSIS OF FEMUR

33

Manipulation

The safest way of doing this is by using traction and a rotation bandage in bed before the operation. With a history of a recent, acute slip this may be completely successful in correcting the deformity. Manipulation with general anaesthesia can also be used both successfully and safely but must be carried out very gently as described for fracture of the neck of the femur.

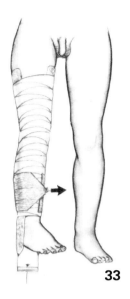

33

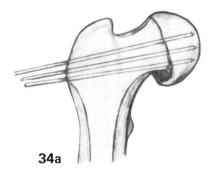

34a

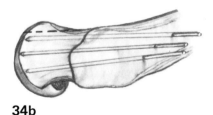

34b

34a & b

Accepting deformity

If the displacement of the head of the femur does not exceed about one third of its diameter there need be no hesitation in accepting it. Greater displacement than this can also be accepted and the deformity later corrected by removing the prominent forward bow of the neck of the femur.

35a & b

Correcting deformity

Dunn (1964) has described a corrective osteotomy but it needs to be done with great care to preserve the lateral epiphyseal arteries and few surgeons have matched Dunn's results or been prepared to recommend the operation.

The essence of the operation is a good exposure that allows the surgeon to see clearly what he is doing and what he must protect.

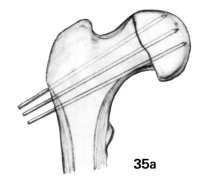

35a

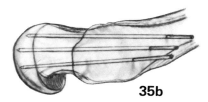

35b

36

The approach

Gibson's is satisfactory, the incision running up the side of the thigh and at the tip of the greater trochanter bending slightly to reach the iliac crest 2 — 3 inches in front of its posterior superior spine. Gluteus maximus and tensor fasciae latae are separated and the latter retracted forwards after splitting the fascia lata in its grain.

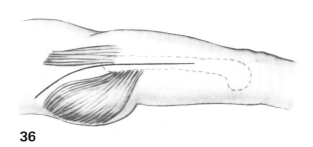

36

37 & 38

The greater trochanter is cut off and turned upwards to expose the capsule of the hip, which is then cut first longitudinally and then round its attachment to the acetabulum. The synovial membrane is then divided in the long axis of the neck and round only the front of the acetabulum, so as not to jeopardize the blood supply of the head of the femur. The head has then to be carefully eased off the neck so that the posterior spur on the neck can be removed and the neck shortened without endangering the blood vessels. Trimming the neck enables the head to be replaced without stretching its blood supply.

Fixation

Multiple pins should be used; three will suffice but four are preferable.

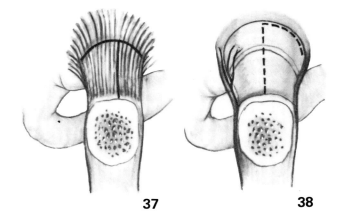

37　　　　　　**38**

OPEN CORRECTION OF DEFORMITY AFTER FRACTURE OF THE NECK OF THE FEMUR

This can be used when manipulation of a Stage 3 or 4 fracture fails to put it in an acceptable position and the surgeon does not want to put in a prosthesis.

39

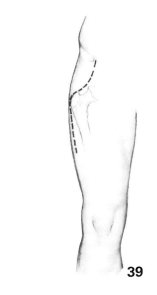

39

The usual approach is through an angled incision from the anterior superior spine to the tip of the great trochanter and then down the outer side of the thigh as already described. The hip is approached between tensor fasciae latae and sartorius and then rectus femoris and psoas major are retracted medially (displacing the femoral vessels) while looking out for the troublesome ascending branch of the lateral circumflex femoral artery. It is helpful in some cases to detach rectus femoris from the pelvis.

40

The capsule is then opened in the line of the neck with a cross-cut at the edge of the acetabulum. The corners should be held apart by Kocher's forceps or by stitches, not by bone levers, which may damage any remaining arteries to the head of the femur. It may then be quite easy to correct the position of the head on the neck of the femur with the aid of lateral rotation and adduction of the thigh by adjusting the table and of distraction of the fracture by means of a bone clamp or hook inserted through the vertical, lateral part of the incision. The position of the head should be adjusted gently and carefully, for which purpose an awl or periosteal elevator can be useful in that it gets a grip and does little or no damage. A bone lever or a hook may have to be inserted into the fracture but the surgeon must take care not to risk disrupting the lateral epiphyseal vessels.

These actions may be easy and successful but the surgeon may be handicapped by the fact that the correct fit of neck and head is not recognizable so that radiographic confirmation should be carried out. Once an acceptable position has been achieved the fracture is fixed as has been described.

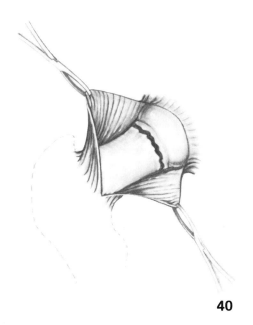

40

Closure

The wound is closed in three layers around one or two suction drains.

Dressing

Although a ready-made adhesive dressing may suffice for covering the wound, with restless, old patients it may be wise to protect it with a bandage.

REPLACING HEAD OF FEMUR

Choice of approach

The posterior approach is the easier because it gives better access but it is a bigger exposure, the incision is more likely to be contaminated by urine and faeces and there is an appreciable risk of dislocation of the hip.

The anterior approach allows earlier and more comfortable walking and it is less likely to be con-taminated or followed by dislocation but it is not such a comfortable approach as the posterior.

Choice of prosthesis

Moore's prosthesis requires more bone to be removed and consequently requires more effort for its insertion but it does not require cement. Thompson's prosthesis is easier to use; cement is often used, but not by Dr. Thompson himself.

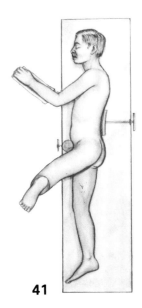

41

41

THE POSTERIOR APPROACH

The patient lies on the uninjured side and close enough to the 'front' of the table for the injured, upper thigh to be carried right down over the edge of the table. The trunk must be firmly secured without obstructing the upper thigh.

Suction and diathermy should be available and the towels secured so that little more than the field of operation is exposed in spite of the wide range of movement to which the injured limb is subjected.

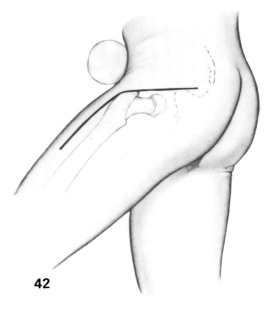

42

The incision

42

This runs for 4 – 6 inches along the side of the thigh and at the top of the great trochanter it bends sharply across the buttock and is taken 4 – 6 inches towards the posterior, inferior spine of the ilium. Fascia lata and gluteus maximus are split in their grains, using a knife and then scissors for the former and blunt dissection for the latter. This enables a group of vessels near the inner end of the split to be identified and dealt with rather than divided and perhaps lost.

43

The tough, aponeurotic angle of the flap so formed is drawn medially to expose the gluteus medius, piriformis and the 'short rotator' group of muscles (quadratus femoris and the gemelli), which are more or less hidden by connective tissue that is easily swept aside with gauze. The sciatic nerve is easily found, and must be identified, in the medial part of the wound.

The rotator group and piriformis and an inch or so of gluteus medius are cut with diathermy so as to leave enough on the femur for the muscles to be repaired. One should not cut below the rotator group, where the medial circumflex femoral artery comes into the field and can cause troublesome bleeding. This and the next step are facilitated if an assistant flexes, adducts and medially rotates the limb at the hip joint so as to tauten the structures behind it.

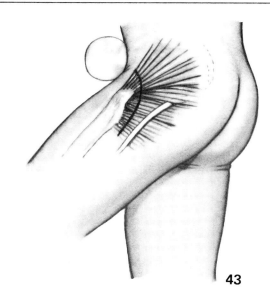

43

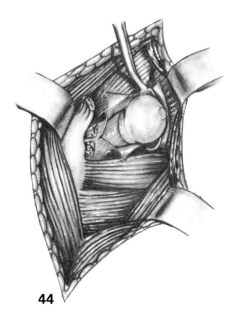

44

44

The capsule is cut cross-wise and in the line of the neck the cut is taken as far as the edge of the acetabulum. With the further aid of the assistant, who must be warned of the fragility of the femur, the fracture line is then opened up widely so as to allow room for the head of the femur to be removed. This can be done conveniently with the aid of a curved gouge that is slipped between it and its socket. The sharpness of this tool usually makes it easy to divide the ligamentum teres. The size of the head is measured; there is no harm in using a prosthesis that is *very* slightly larger than the head of the femur but when the size cannot be matched exactly it is wiser to use a smaller rather than a larger implant.

45

The stump of neck should be cut square, remembering that because there is often a fragment of bone broken from the posterior cortical layer of the neck much more bone needs to be removed from the front than from the back. Notwithstanding careful retraction it is not usually possible to cut the neck neatly, even with Gigli's saw, but the irregularity left by trimming with nibbling forceps is acceptable. It is also important to remove enough neck, especially when little or no cortical loss has occurred. If Moore's prosthesis is to be used it is helpful to cut away at this stage part of the superior cortex of the neck so that the shoulder of the prosthesis can rest snugly in the great trochanter. This is easier than removing the bone with a rasp.

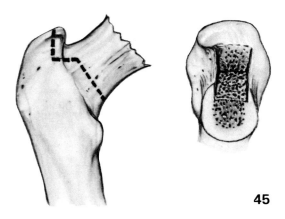

45

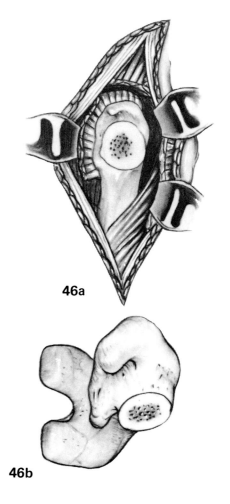

46a

46b

Preparing the socket

According to the texture of the bone this may be hard work or very easy. The assistant must place the thigh in as much flexion and medial rotation as possible so that the broken surface of the neck is clearly accessible; otherwise the rasp fouls the soft tissues. It is sometimes helpful to draw the femur away from the pelvis by means of a large bone hook.

46a & b

The surgeon must now ensure that he has the position of the shaft of the femur clearly in his mind's eye lest he inadvertently drive the tip of the rasp out through the lateral cortex of the shaft, which requires less force than might be supposed and is particularly likely if a nail or nail plate has already made a hole in the cortex.

47

False passages are less likely when the rasp can be used without hammering and this is often the case when using that for Thompson's prosthesis. There need be no misgiving about using a hammer with Moore's rasp if it can be seen that its passage is being blocked by the medial and lateral sides of the neck but the rasp should be withdrawn after three or four blows so that it acts as a rasp and not as a wedge that will split the femur. As mentioned, one should now remove lateral rather than medial bone.

48a & b

It is also important to concentrate on removing bone on the deeper (anterior) side of the neck rather than, as is easier, from the posterior side.

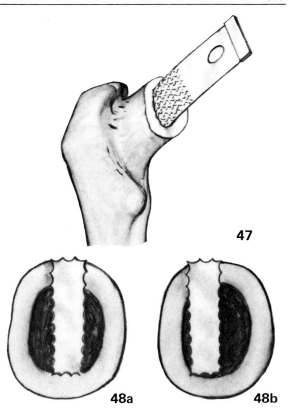

47

48a   48b

When the rasp can be driven fully home in the femur the chosen prosthesis should be tried for size. It should be a tight enough fit to require a few firm blows with a hammer but not so tight as to split the calcar when it is driven home.

If cement is to be used it should not be mixed until the surgeon is satisfied with the socket, and the anaesthetist should be told of what is to be done. It is wise to pass a plastic catheter well down the socket before inserting the cement, which is most easily done by means of a special 'gun'. Otherwise the fingers provide as good a way as any of ramming down suitably narrow rolls of doughy cement. Because it gives out heat, surplus cement must not be placed even temporarily on the patient's skin.

The venting tube must be removed before the prosthesis is driven home.

Replacing the hip

This is done mainly by the surgeon, who pushes the ball back into the socket with a tool that fits the curvature of the ball; the assistant's task is to assist by causing the limb to follow the path required by the replacement of the joint. If he tries to guide it back he may break the femur. With the upper thigh resting on the lower the wound is ready to be closed.

Closure

Two suction drains should be used if there has been more than slight bleeding. Although it is not necessary to close the capsule this should be done when possible, followed by respectively rotator group of muslces, gluteus maximus, tensor fasciae latae and, finally, the skin.

Dressing

If the wound is dry enough for an adhesive strip dressing to be used it is wise to protect this with a bandage.

Postoperative care

Because of the risk of dislocation of the hip it is necessary to prevent flexion, adduction and medial rotation at this joint.

On the way back to the ward the limb must not be allowed to assume this position.

In bed it is sufficient to suspend the limb in two slings and to maintain abduction by skin traction but special care needs to be taken when it is necessary to roll the patient onto the sound side, because this may allow the limb to adopt a dangerous position.

When sitting in a chair it is wise to keep the patient's knees apart with a pillow.

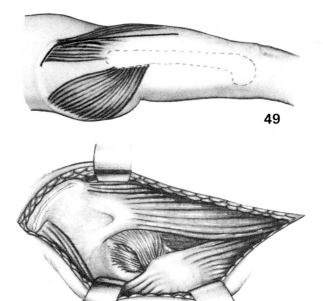

THE ANTERIOR APPROACH

49 & 50

Smith-Petersen's approach is used, cutting along the iliac crest and then down the front of the thigh for 4–5 inches. Tensor fasciae latae and gluteus medius are stripped from the ilium and the front of the hip is exposed between the tensor laterally and sartorius and rectus femoris medially. The lateral cutaneous nerve of the thigh passes over sartorius an inch or so below the anterior superior iliac spine and should be preserved. The ascending branch of the lateral circumflex femoral artery should be identified and ligated a couple of inches below the joint.

51

The capsule should then be cut along the upper edge of the neck and from its attachment to the anterior intertrochanteric ridge. The neck may be cut across at this stage, or after opening up the fracture and removing the head. The line of division should be fairly close to the lesser trochanter.

For presenting the neck of the femur it is necessary to be able to lower the thigh past the edge of the table as well as rotating it laterally. The socket is made and the prosthesis inserted as has already been described.

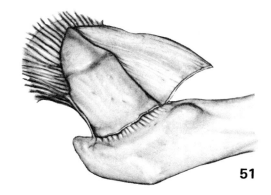

Closure

Capsule, muscles and skin are each closed. Suction drainage is necessary and an adhesive dressing should be protected by a bandage.

Activity

There is less need for caution than after the posterior approach.

FRACTURES OF TROCHANTERIC REGION OF FEMUR

There are four main patterns of fracture that can be treated along similar lines by means of nail-plates. The approach to these fractures and the insertion of the implant have already been described for fractures of the neck of the femur (*see* page 582) but there are important differences with different patterns of fracture. In this section only the special steps required for a given fracture will be described.

Manipulation

This is as for fractures of the neck of the femur with the exception that if the fracture is comminuted the limb should be rotated only far enough to make the patella face directly up at the ceiling. Full medial rotation can easily be effected at the fracture, which compounds the deformity.

FRACTURES OF THE BASE OF THE NECK OF THE FEMUR

52 & 53

These fractures are liable to sag into a varus position and if such deformity is corrected before the nail-plate is put in it may recur and either bend the nail or the plate or cause the nail to erupt through the head and neck. The fracture sags until the under-surface of the neck of the femur gains the support of the calcar femorale, and this gives a clue to treatment.

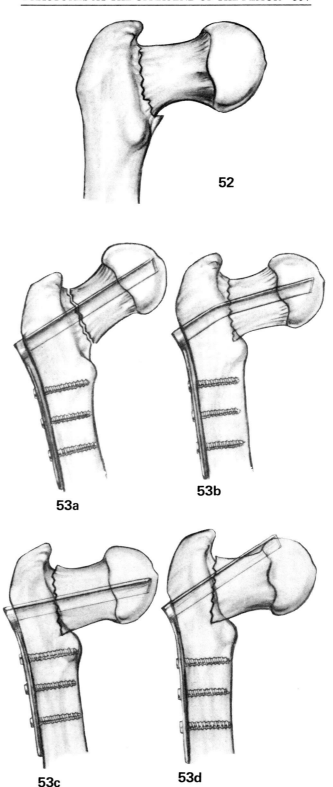

52

53a

53b

53c

53d

54 & 55

(1) Accept the varus deformity in which the fracture comes to rest and fix the fracture in deformity, which is acceptable in most cases, but not for the younger or more active person that usually sustains this sort of fracture.

(2) If varus deformity is unacceptable, first nail the fracture in a good position, then carry out osteotomy and fix this in 20 — 30° of abduction. McLaughlin's nail and plate has obvious advantages for this operation.

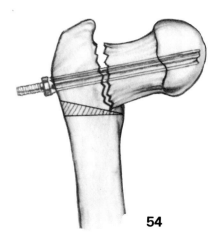

54

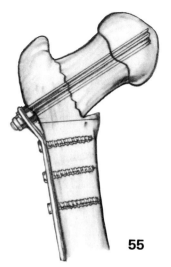

55

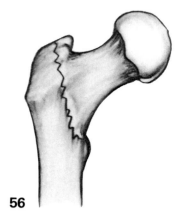

56

56

SIMPLE PERTROCHANTERIC FRACTURES

These are the easiest to deal with; a good position can be both attained and maintained with a nail-plate.

COMMINUTED FRACTURES

57a & b

The fracture is usually both per- and intertrochanteric and unless the fragments are few and not much separated they cannot be kept accurately in place by any sort of internal fixation. As with the fractures of the base of the neck, deformity is limited only when the main proximal fragment is supported by the main distal fragment(s). The safest policy is to accept this deformity at the outset, recognizing that it is almost certain to occur in the end, metal or no.

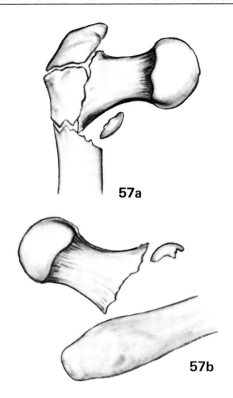

57a

57b

Manipulation

This usually has to be carried out with the fracture exposed. It is therefore advisable to make the incision longer than usual, especially at its proximal end, and so to allow the proximal fragment to be brought into view.

The incision

Because the fragments of bone may be quite widely separated the incision cannot be planned as accurately as with simpler fractures and the surgeon will have to accept a good deal of bleeding and he will have to allow for the fact that the main fragment of shaft drops (posteriorly) from the main proximal fragment.

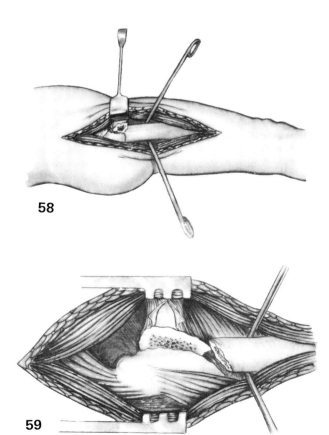

58

59

58 & 59

Large levers such as Lane's should be used to open up the incision and it may be necessary to use an angled retractor such as Morris's or a large self-retaining retractor to discover the proximal fragment. If the fracture has passed through the basal attachment of the capsule of the hip joint it may be necessary to split and detach this for half an inch or so to allow the cortex to be seen.

The lowest part of this fragment is often tilted upwards (i.e. flexed) by some fibres of the psoas or pectineus muscles and it may have to be pressed downwards to bring it into line with the rest of the femur. It may be possible to re-assemble the fragments more or less correctly and then insert a nail-plate but this is not likely to result in more than temporary improvement and the attempt is not worth making.

Making the best of a bad job

60-63

The following steps are recommended.

(*1*) Insert one or more guide wires into the proximal fragment, ignoring the others.

(*2*) When a guide wire is suitably placed, drive a nail in over it. Because the proximal fragment is fairly easily moveable it is best to use McLaughlin's nail. Jewett's nail-plate can be used but the presence of the plate can be inconvenient. Capener-Neufeld's nail-plate is not recommended because the V-section cannot be relied upon to follow the guide wire.

It should be noted that the nail may need to be 2 – 3 inches rather than 3 – 4 inches long.

(*3*) The shaft should now be lifted up and placed partly below the proximal fragment so as to provide support for it. This is most conveniently done with the aid of a large pair of bone clamps, such as Hey Groves's.

(*4*) The plate is attached to the nail and screwed to the shaft of the femur. There is no advantage in using a very long plate: the weakness is where nail and plate join or at the top screw hole in the plate.

There is no need to try to secure or replace the lesser or greater trochanters when these have been broken off but if more or less of the greater trochanter remains attached to the shaft there need be no hesitation in cutting it off; in some cases it can be drilled so that the hole in it can then be slipped over the nail that has already been driven up the neck. Alternatively, it may be possible to set the main fragments in place, then make the hole and insert first a guide wire and then the nail through it.

It will be recognized that this is not an easy operation; it will be least difficult for a surgeon that has taken the opportunity of studying these fractures in the post-mortem or dissecting room. If his experience of them is based on the usual x-ray films and what can be seen through an ordinary incision, any attempt to fix a comminuted fracture of this sort is likely to be bloody, perplexing, prolonged, frustrating and unsuccessful.

The essential requirements are to nail the proximal fragment securely; to have the two fragments fixed securely together with the shaft providing as much *supporting* contact as possible for the main proximal fragment. Other fragments can be ignored.

It is also fair to admit that fingers may have to be used a good deal more than most surgeons would consider reasonable in other circumstances. In these conditions the surgeon will be well advised to protect his rubber gloves by wearing cotton gloves over them.

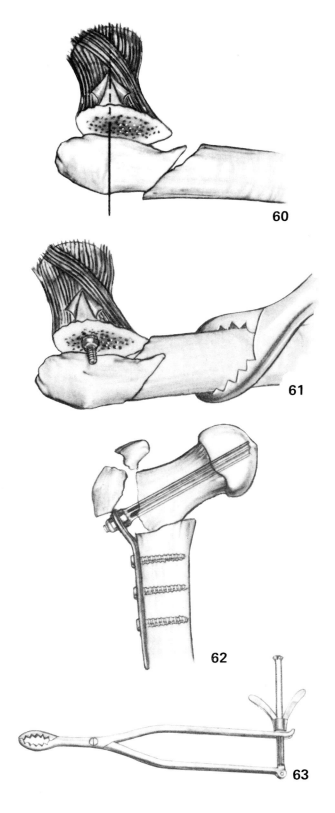

60

61

62

63

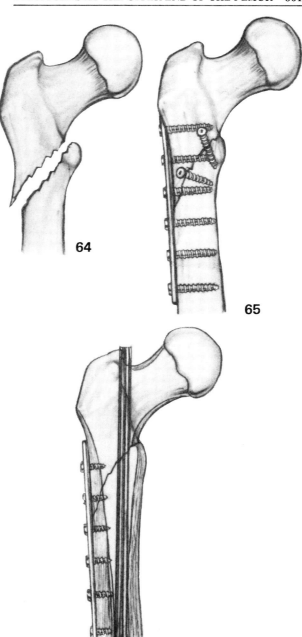

64, 65 & 66

OBLIQUE ADDUCTED FRACTURES

These are often impossible to control with a nail-plate because the forces acting at the fracture can easily bend, break or avulse the implant.

There are three main methods of treatment.

(*1*) Accept the deformity and refrain from operating. This is recommended only for patients with rarefied bones and with little need for activity.

(*2*) Screw the fragments together and apply a protection plate.

(*3*) Insert a Küntscher nail and supplement it with a plate and short screws. This is most successful when the density of the bone and the bore of the marrow allow the screws and the nail to grip well.

Closure and drainage

Two suction drains are required before closing the wound in three layers.

GENERAL POLICY AFTER OPERATIONS ON FRACTURES NEAR HIP

(*1*) The patient is often most comfortable if the limb is suspended in two slings and steadied by skin traction using 5 lb (2 kg) weight.

(*2*) The patient should be urged and assisted to move the hip within 24 hr of operation. When she does this and is otherwise co-operative the traction may be removed. After inserting a prosthesis from the back, however, it may be advisable to retain the traction, between periods of exercise, for a week or 10 days.

(*3*) When the patient can raise the limb unaided from the bed she may get out of bed.

(*4*) Walking is permitted as soon as the patient can be induced and assisted to do it. Two stalwart supporters may be used at first but should be able to give way to a walking frame within a few days. There is no place for crutches in the attempt to get the old, frail, tottery, fearful and confused patient back onto her feet. The comminuted fractures can be treated in this way but walking may not be resumed for a few weeks rather than a few days.

References

Dunn, D. (1964). 'The treatment of adolescent slipping of the upper femoral epiphysis.' *J. Bone Jt Surg.* **46B**, 621
Garden, R. S. (1964). 'Stability and union in subcapital fractures of the femur.' *J. Bone Jt Surg.* **56B**, 630
Smyth, E. H. J., Ellis, J. S., Manifold, M. C. and Dewey, P. L. (1964). *J. Bone Jt Surg.* **46B**, 664
Smyth, E. H. J. and Shah, V. M. (1974). *Injury* **5**, 197

[*The illustrations for this Chapter on Fractures at the Upper End of the Femur were drawn by Mr. G. Lyth.*]

Closed Intramedullary Nailing of the Femur and Tibia

David M. Chaplin, M.B., F.R.C.S.
Department of Orthopaedics, University of Washington School of Medicine

and

Sigvard T. Hansen, M.D.
Department of Orthopaedics, Harborview Medical Center, Seattle

THE FEMUR
PRE - OPERATIVE

Indications

Closed intramedullary nailing of the femur can be used for many fractures of the femur, including transverse, oblique, butterfly, comminuted or segmental fractures. The rigid fixation produced allows healing of the bone at normal length and rotation whilst preserving motion in the hip and knee joints and allows the patient to walk early.

The technique can also be used to fix or even to prevent pathological fractures.

Utilizing special equipment, with this method it is possible to divide the bone from within the medullary cavity in order to correct rotational or other malunion, and it is also possible to remove a segment of bone from the shaft of the femur if it is too long.

Contra-indications

Children with open epiphyses generally heal their fractures quickly and do not require intramedullary fixation.

To achieve fixation in the upper part of the femur it is necessary to have 1 inch (2·5 cm) of intact cortex below the lesser trochanter. A fracture extending above this level is unsuitable for this technique. Similarly, long oblique fractures extending well into the lowest third of the femur are more difficult to hold adequately with an intramedullary nail.

Previous sepsis in or around the femur may rule out any operation on the bone.

Timing of operation

The operation is carried out 5–7 days after the fracture has occurred, by which time the paO_2 has risen to about 80 mmHg and the risk of fat embolism is thought to be less. During this interval the femur is kept out to length by skeletal traction. In the case of fracture through a malignant tumour nailing should be preceded by radiotherapy.

603

1&2

Selection of nail

A '1 metre' film is taken before operation. This film is exposed with the tube 1 metre above the film to ensure standard magnification (about 10 per cent) of the size of the femur. The size of the femur is measured from the film with a special device which allows selection of both the correct diameter and length of the nail from the magnified film. The nail should reach from just outside the greater trochanter to the distal epiphyseal scar of the femur.

A lateral film of the normal femur shows the amount of anteroposterior bowing present and how much the nail should be bent before it is inserted.

If the medullary canal is extremely wide, as in severe osteoporosis, nails need to be interlocked to provide the necessary thickness of nail.

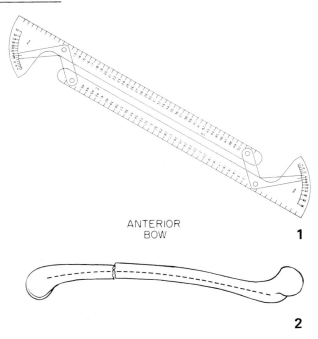

ANTERIOR
BOW   **1**

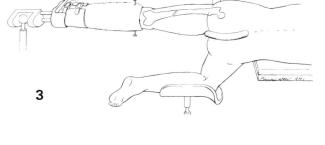

2

3

Preparation and position of patient

Under general anaesthesia, the patient is placed on his side on the table, taking care that the distal part of the leg is in correct rotation when compared to the upper part of the leg and pelvis. The area around the greater trochanter is prepared and draped, the remainder of the leg and, in particular, the fracture being out of the drapes and available for manipulation by an unscrubbed assistant. With a distal fracture, traction on the distal fragment by way of a femoral pin is preferable to traction through the existing tibial pin because it enables one to avoid angulating the distal fragment.

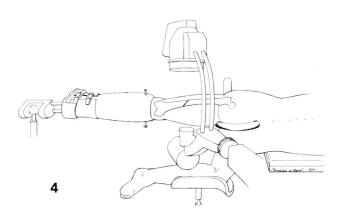

3

4

Special equipment

An image intensifying x-ray machine is necessary with its television screen visible to both the operator and the manipulator. The use of a C-arm makes it possible to get both anteroposterior and lateral views quite easily. A high torque, 300 rev/min driving unit is necessary to drive the long, flexible reamers. The reamers should be available in 0·5 mm increments from 8–20 mm. The 8 mm reamer is end-cutting, and the remainder are side-cutting. Sharp-tipped guide-wires and a bulb-tipped guide are required. A large bone-holding clamp should be available for segmental fractures.

4

THE OPERATION

Trial reduction

The manipulating surgeon makes sure that he can correct displacement at the fracture and also see what he is doing on the television screen. Too much or too little traction can cause difficulty.

5

Incision

A 3 inch (7·5 cm) longitudinal incision is made above the greater trochanter. The deep fascia and gluteus medius are split in line with their fibres, and the greater trochanter is palpated with the index finger.

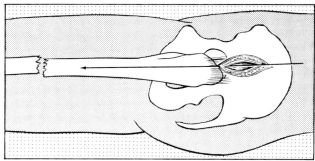

5

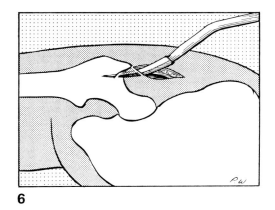

6

6

Entrance site

X-rays will indicate the appropriate position to enter the femur. Usually this is just inside the greater trochanter in the mid-portion of the neck. A sharp awl makes the initial hole, and its position can be confirmed with the image intensifier. When the position is confirmed the hole is enlarged.

7

Correction of deformity

The sharp guide is introduced through the hole in the upper part of the femur and passed down the shaft. The fracture site is displayed on the television screen and the second operator (with lead gloves) manipulates the fracture so that the guide can be passed into the distal fragment. The guide's tip is passed distally and lodged in the cancellous bone in the femoral condyles. Once the sharp guide has been passed the bulb-tipped reamer guide is passed down parallel to the sharp guide-pin, which is then removed. The bulb-tipped reamer guide is used for reaming in case the flexible reamer should break, in which case the broken fragment can be easily extracted.

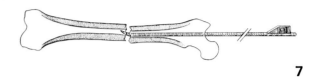

7

8

Reaming

Reaming is commenced with the end-cutting 8 mm reamer. Side-cutting reamers are then introduced at 1 mm increments until the reamer is engaged firmly in both fragments. From this point reaming goes on with 0·5 mm increments to the desired bore. It is usual to over-ream the central portion of the shaft by 1 mm. In order to avoid eccentric reaming it is important to watch with the image intensifier both the manipulation of the fracture and the passage of the reamer by the fracture.

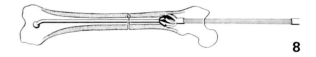

8

9

Insertion of the nail

The bulb-tipped guide is replaced by the sharp-tipped guide and the selected nail is passed over it, through the wound, into the upper part of the femur and hammered down the shaft. The nail is watched with the image intensifier as it crosses the fracture and is driven until it reaches the distal epiphyseal scar. Because the patient is on his side it is important to support the distal fragment by hand so as to avoid nailing the fracture in valgus. If the correct length of nail has been selected, the upper end of the nail should lie about 1 cm outside the greater trochanter. This makes the slot accessible for removal later.

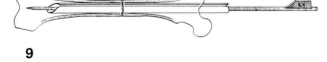

9

Closure

Only the skin is closed, using interrupted sutures.

SPECIAL CIRCUMSTANCES

10

Overlapping fragments

If the fragments are not kept out to length before the operation it may be necessary to use Küntscher's distractor to overcome shortening. The distractor can be applied before the operation and kept on during it.

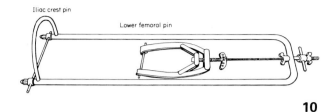

10

Severe osteoporosis

When the largest nail is too small to fit the marrow cavity firmly two smaller nails can be interlocked.

11

Segmental fractures

It is essential that reaming the intermediate fragment(s) be done with 0·5 mm increments, using sharp reamers moved slowly and carefully. External manipulation is not as successful with these fractures as when there is a single fracture. It is often helpful to ream the proximal fragment to 12 or 13 mm and then use a curved, sharp and rigid guide to bring an intermediate fragment accurately in line with the proximal fragment. When the proximal segment is long, it should be finally reamed to a bore 1 mm larger than the nail.

Occasionally, in order to avoid the central fragment's turning with the reamers it is necessary to make an incision over an intermediate fragment and hold it with the bone holder whilst it is being reamed.

11

12

Pathological fractures

It is possible to obtain a sample of tissue from the fracture or tumour by long biopsy forceps introduced before the reamers.

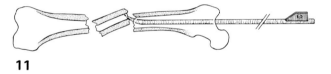

12

13

Oblique fractures and shear-pieces (often referred to as a 'butterfly' fragment)

Usually these fragments fall back into place during the standard procedure, but if this does not occur, one can make a small incision over the fracture and introduce a Parham band to close the fragment around the nail. With distal fractures it is extremely important to support the knee to avoid putting the nail into the distal fragment eccentrically and so producing valgus deformity.

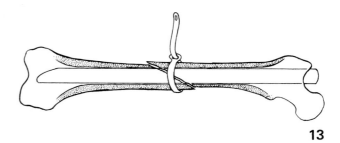

13

14

Proximal fractures

With a proximal fracture the proximal fragment tends to be excessively flexed, which makes it important to remember to approach the greater trochanter from rather further back in order to avoid eccentric reaming. If it is difficult to correct the deformity one can use a 10 mm nail as a handle to control the proximal fragment. The sharp-tipped guide is then passed across the fracture, the small nail is removed and reaming continues as before.

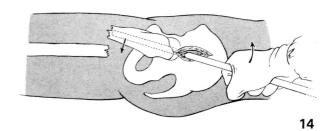

14

POSTOPERATIVE CARE

A well-fixed fracture needs no external support.

The pin through the tibial tubercle is removed at the end of the operation. The leg is elevated on pillows, and the patient starts contracting his quadriceps as soon as possible; he is allowed to get up on crutches as soon as he has quadriceps control, which is usually in 2 or 3 days. Weight-bearing is allowed immediately if the fragments have been fixed in a stable arrangement. Exercise for the knee is encouraged, and movements are usually fully restored at 3 weeks. The progress of healing of the fracture is recorded by x-ray films exposed 1 month, 3 months and 1 year after injury.

Provided that the fracture has united, the nail is removed at 1 year so that the femur can resume its normal function unaided and replace bone lost by reaming.

Complications

It is important not to have the proximal and distal fragments twisted on each other.

Occasionally, with an unstable fracture one of the fragments rotates on the nail and if this is thought possible it should be controlled by splintage, traction or restriction of weight-bearing. Alternatively, a plate can be used, with screws that engage only one cortex.

Delayed union is less frequent than with open nailing, perhaps due to autogenous bone graft produced by the reaming procedure.

Occasionally the nail backs out and produces an uncomfortable bursa at the upper end underneath the gluteus medius and minimus muscles. If the fracture has healed it is sufficient to remove the nail, otherwise it should be replaced by a slightly larger one.

THE TIBIA
PRE - OPERATIVE

Indications

Most fractures of the tibia are successfully treated by external splintage. However, when the initial displacement is severe or the fracture has an unstable pattern internal fixation not only maintains the normal shape of the bone but also protects the soft tissues and allows them to heal rapidly. Similar reasoning underlies the use of nailing in the severe open fracture, which can fairly be looked on as a severe injury of soft tissues that is complicated by loss of their natural bony support. Early movement of the local joints is possible after nailing and this is particularly advantageous to the subtalar joint. Nailing is particularly useful when the state of the skin precludes operation along the shaft.

In cases of delayed or established non-union, closed medullary nailing is an excellent procedure whenever the medullary canal is well aligned; if it is not, a small operation may suffice to align it. Closed nailing is especially useful when there is badly scarred, adherent or grafted skin which rules out an external approach to the fracture. Even residual ulcers or superficial infections may be bypassed by medullary nails.

Contra-indications

The tibia is normally straight, has a wide medullary canal and can accommodate a nail strong enough to support the body's weight, but because of the size of the medullary canal, medullary nails cannot prevent rotation or overlap in the case of fractures of the top or bottom quarters of the tibia. The tibia is brittle when nailed immediately after fracture and this may lead to increased comminution. The tibia is not well covered by soft tissues on the anteromedial surface, so that any interference with the intramedullary blood supply by a nail may be more serious than with the femur.

Tibial nailing is not recommended except for: (1) open fractures in the middle third with marked instability and soft tissue damage but with a stable bony pattern; (2) closed or open segmental fractures, which are not easily aligned by other means; (3) patients requiring wide decompression for a compartmental syndrome associated with tibial fracture. We favour nailing for fractures of the shaft of the tibia associated with intra-articular ankle fractures in order that the ankle may be exercised early, and also when there is a fracture of the femur in the same limb but we accept that this is a matter of preference and not necessity.

Special equipment

The equipment needed is similar to that for nailing the femur and includes a complete set of reamers from 8 to 20 mm with 0·5 mm increments. One of the small reamers should be end-cutting. Reamer guides, awls, nail driving guides, and an image intensifier must be available.

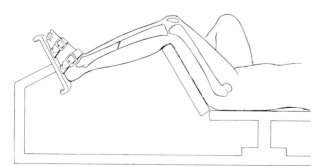

15

15

Preparation and position of patient

The nail length is calculated from a standard 1 metre film (1 metre from tube to film), which magnifies the tibia about 5 per cent. The nail should extend from the upper part of the tibial tubercle to the distal epiphyseal scar. The patient is placed on a table which allows access for the image intensifier with the knee flexed by 70°. The foot is draped out of the field of operation.

THE OPERATION

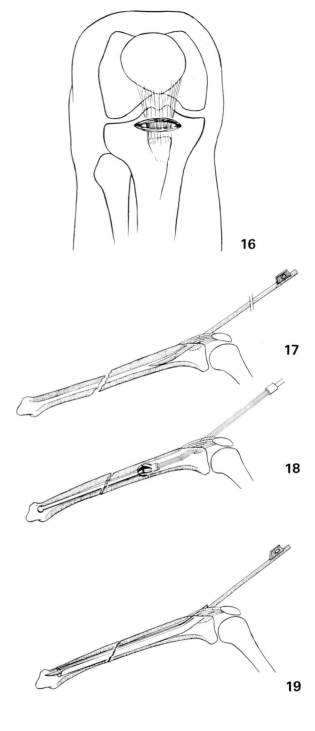

16

16

The incision

A straight transverse incision 3 cm long is made over the mid-portion of the patellar tendon, and deepened to expose this tendon. A longitudinal incision is made through the tendon and fat pad to expose the cancellous bone just proximal to the tibial tubercle.

17

18

17 & 18

Broaching and aligning the tibia

A hole is made into the tibial shaft with the awl. A reamer guide is inserted and guided through the proximal end into the canal of the distal fragment. A gentle bend near the tip and external manipulation are useful aids to this procedure. The image intensifier is used as needed both to accomplish the adjustment of the fragments and to make sure that the bulb-tipped reamer guide is properly positioned throughout the length of the medullary canal.

19

19

Reaming

Reaming is commenced with the 8 mm end-cutting reamer and continued with the side-cutting reamers until good fixation of both fragments is judged to be achievable. As the reamer must be used slightly bent, great care must be observed to avoid eccentric reaming.

Insertion of the nail

The tibial nail has a slight posterior bow at both the proximal and distal ends. The nail is inserted with the longitudinal slot facing backwards and the extraction slot in front. As the nail is driven in, the patellar tendon and overlying skin must be carefully retracted. The size of nail used is generally 11–13 mm in females and 12–15 mm in males. The position of the nail at the distal end is confirmed with the aid of the image intensifier.

Closure

The wound is closed with interrupted sutures for the skin.

SPECIAL CIRCUMSTANCES

Delayed or non-union

In cases of delayed or non-union, insertion of the guide may be difficult because the central canal may be closed by callus or fibrous tissue. In this case, a 6, 7 or 8 mm hand reamer may be used to broach this tissue. Alternatively, a slightly bent, sharp and rigid guidewire of about 4–5 mm diameter may be driven across this area with the image intensifier's aid. When the canal has been re-established, the sharp guide is withdrawn and the slightly bent bulb-tipped reamer guide inserted through this same area.

On some occasions, a small operation is necessary to divide the bone and align the medullary canal. While the fracture is open one or both ends may be drilled as necessary to re-open the medullary canal. The fragments are then aligned and reaming and nailing are carried out as already described.

POSTOPERATIVE CARE

With fresh fractures, a light, well-moulded, short-leg walking cast is recommended for at least 1 month. This is to give support to soft tissues and possibly help with rotation and provide some added immobilization. Partial weight-bearing with crutches is usually recommended.

In delayed cases, the nail produces sound internal fixation by virtue of the larger nail with extra reaming, so that a postoperative cast is rarely needed. Two to five days of elevation may be needed to reduce swelling of the soft tissues. Early weight-bearing is possible and encouraged.

Removing the nail

The nail may be removed after solid union at 18–24 months, but it is not usually recommended unless the patient has discomfort. Discomfort is usually at the patellar tendon and is due to a slightly long nail or some backing out of the nail.

[*The illustrations for this Chapter on Closed Intramedullary Nailing of the Femur and Tibia were drawn by Miss Phyllis Wood.*]

Surgical Technique
for Acute Knee Injury

Don H. O'Donoghue, M.D.
Professor of Surgery, O'Donoghue Orthopaedic Clinic,
Pasteur Medical Building, Oklahoma

INTRODUCTION

It is perhaps not necessary to emphasize that the surgeon who operates on the knee must be prepared to diagnose and treat whatever lesion may be found.

Before undertaking a discussion concerning the proper surgical approaches to treat certain injuries of the knee, it is advisable to discuss the principles of the selection of certain procedures.

When planning to operate on the knee one must bear in mind that all too often the diagnosis is found to be different from what was expected or, even more frequently, that additional lesions may be found that need treatment. In the course of 'simple meniscectomy' it is quite common to discover a torn anterior cruciate ligament. If the surgical approach is one of the 'special meniscus approaches', such as, a curved, more or less transverse incision with the convexity distal or a straight translateral incision, the surgeon may be hard pressed to enlarge this incision in order to get proper access to the lesion. Whenever it is possible, the approach chosen should permit exploration and treatment of whatever condition may be found.

The approaches may be classified according to regions as follows: (*1*) anteromedial: (*2*) posteromedial; (*3*) anterolateral; (*4*) posterolateral; (*5*) posterior, and; (*6*) anterior (transverse).

ANTEROMEDIAL APPROACH

1

The anteromedial approach is a good example of a general utility approach. The full incision extends from 2 cm above the patella medially, continues along the border of the patella, then parallel to the patellar tendon to the tibial tuberosity, at which level it curves posteriorly at about 45° to terminate at about the level of the posterior margin of the tibia.

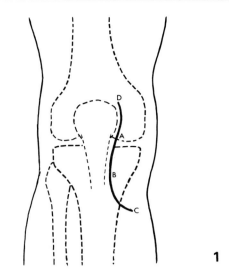

2

The incision is made with the patient supine and his leg hanging over the end of the table with the knee flexed (A–B) 90°. If the anterior cruciate ligament is torn in its fibres or is torn from the tibia, it may be repaired through this incision alone. If on the other hand, the anterior cruciate has been torn from the femur a second incision will be necessary to expose the lateral femoral epicondylar ridge in order to drill holes into the intercondylar notch to re-attach the ligament. This incision is described in more detail on page 616. If the posterior cruciate has been torn from the femur, it can be readily repaired to the lateral side of the medial femoral condyle in the notch through drill holes made through the medial condyle, which is exposed by a slight upward extension of the original incision (A–D) to permit anterior retraction of the vastus medialis in order to make the drill holes for repair of the ligament. See page 617 for a more detailed description. If the patella is found to be damaged and needs treatment, the incision can be extended proximally and so permit tilting of the patella to expose its articular surface. This is described in detail on page 624. If the medial collateral ligament or the pes anserinus needs to be explored, the incision can be extended downward (B – C) and the skin and subcutaneous flap turned back to expose the upper medial aspect of the tibia.

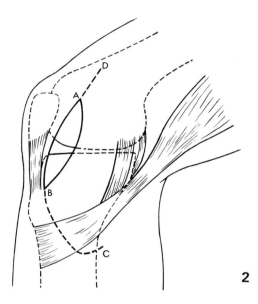

Repair of medial collateral ligament, medial posterior capsule, anterior and posterior cruciate ligament

If there is instability of the medial collateral ligament, the medial posterior capsule, and probably the anterior cruciate ligament, the skin incision is made as in *Illustration 2* (D – C). The skin flap turned back includes all the subcutaneous tissue because this confines the damage to the vessels and nerves to the front of the flap rather than the back. It also helps to preserve the circulation of the skin flap itself. This exposes the fascia of the leg, not the medial collateral ligament. The fascia is a completely distinct structure extending down as a continuation of the fascia of the thigh and to some extent the medial retinaculum. It passes over the pes anserinus whereas the long fibres of the medial collateral ligament pass under the pes anserinus. If it is not known exactly where the tear is, a cut is made just through the fascia along the top of the pes anserinus (*see Illustration 2*). This incision will be relatively far down the leg in front. It will run posteriorly and proximally until it crosses the postero-medial corner of the knee about 2 cm below the top of the tibia. From here it rises up to 1 cm below the level of the knee joint itself. It follows to the top of the pes.

3 & 4

Only the fascia is divided along the top of the pes anserinus, coming down on the long fibres of the medial collateral ligament underneath (shown here torn above the pes). Do not deliberately reflect the fascia of the proximal end off the long fibres as shown but often they are freely separate. Note that the pes is reflected downward. The fascia, and ultimately the proximal end of the ligament, will be reflected upward and backward. In reflecting this fascial flap, great care is taken not to damage the *long fibres of the medial collateral ligament*. These may be found to be pulled out from under the pes, having been torn from the bony attachment to the tibia, or the ligament may be torn near its middle. If the fibres are torn from the bony attachment they can readily be picked up and the whole flap reflected proximally without separating the long fibres of the medial collateral ligament from the fascia. As the incision continues posteriorly along the top edge of the pes it inclines up toward the knee and the flap is reflected backward and proximally. This flap includes the long fibres of the ligament and the fascia. Note that the length of the flap decreases as the incision proceeds posteriorly. At about the level of the mid-point of the medial joint line the incision is about 2 cm below the joint line. Here the incision transects the short capsular fibres of the medial ligament. Further posteriorly the incision is only 1 cm below the joint line where it divides the tibial attachment of the posterior capsule. As the knee joint is approached, the *short capsular fibres* are identified, and the flap is reflected proximally so as not to cause undue damage to these short capsular fibres. It can be determined at this point where the capsular fibres are torn. They may be torn off the femur, off the tibia, or at the line of the joint. If torn off the tibia, they are included in the reflecting ligament and fascial flap. If torn off the femur, the ligament and fascial flap with the superficial fibres is reflected higher in order to expose the femoral condyle and the detachment of the capsular fibres.

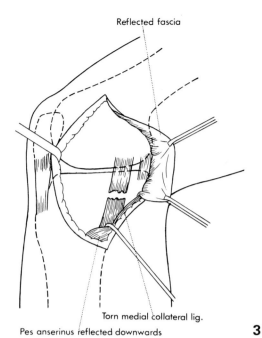

Reflected fascia

Torn medial collateral lig.

Pes anserinus reflected downwards

3

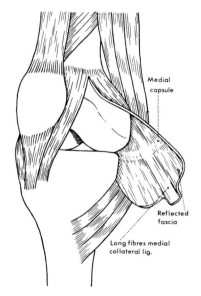

Medial capsule

Reflected fascia

Long fibres medial collateral lig.

4

5, 6 & 7

At this point the *posterior capsule* is inspected. It may be found to be torn in its fibres with a direct transverse tear or it may be found to be avulsed from the tibia. It very seldom is pulled off the femoral attachment. Reflecting the flap gives access to the posterior part of the knee. If the posterior capsule has come off the tibia, drill holes are made from front to back in order to place mattress sutures from front to back through the top of the tibia to pass through the posterior capsule and back through the tibia through the second hole with the aid of a ligature carrier. The star indicates the posterior capsule torn off the tibia. The ligature carrier (*b*) carrying the loop of suture has been passed from front to back through hole (*cc*). The lateral limb of the mattress suture (*a*) has already been passed through the tibia in the first hole and through the capsule. It has been picked up in the loop in the ligature carrier to be pulled through the front. At the same time the first limb of the second mattress suture is pulled forward through this second hole. Usually four holes are used so that three or four mattress sutures are placed in the posterior capsule. If there is a direct tear in the substance of the ligament it can be repaired by direct suture, placing the knots outside the joint.

As a rule the anterior synovial part of the medial capsule of the knee will not have been torn so it will be necessary to divide this below the medial meniscus if the fibres have come off the tibia and above the meniscus if the fibres are off the femur. The *medial meniscus* is examined and is usually removed because it has nearly always been torn; furthermore, it is easier to overlap and tighten up the medial collateral ligament if the medial meniscus is removed. Medial meniscectomy is described in more detail on page 619.

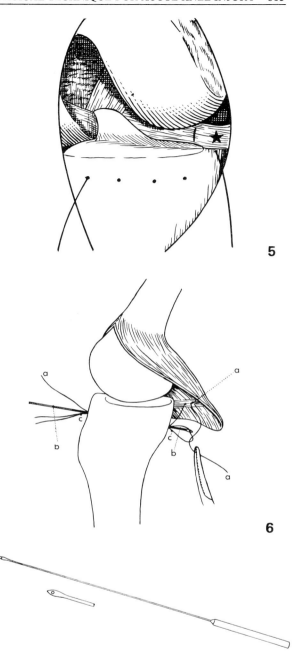

5

6

7

8a & b & 9

If the *anterior cruciate ligament* is found to have been torn, this is usually at or near its attachment. In this case it should be re-attached using drill holes that are made from the medial side of the lateral condyle of the femur, as far back into the notch as it is possible to get, to emerge on the lateral epicondylar ridge and a separate incision. It is preferable to use a smooth pin rather than a drill and to protect it with a sleeve. Mattress stitches are passed through the cruciate ligament and used to pull it up against the femoral attachment by passing them through the drill holes and tying them on the outside of the femur. If the ligament has been torn off the tibia, similar drill holes can be made from the front of the tibia into the area of attachment on the non-articular portion of the tibia in front. Note that there are two separate mattress sutures, one about 1 cm back into the ligament, while the anterior one is at the anterior edge of the tear. The function of the deeper, posterior mattress suture is to flatten out the end of the ligament against the denuded top of the tibia so that there will be good contact of ligament to raw bone. The same manoeuvre can be used if there is a fragment of bone torn up with the ligament and will serve to hold the bone fragment snugly in the vascular bed of the tibia. The mattress stitch should take a wide bite so as not to bunch the ligament where it meets the femur. If the ligament is torn in its substance, it can be repaired by direct suture in the mass of the ligament.

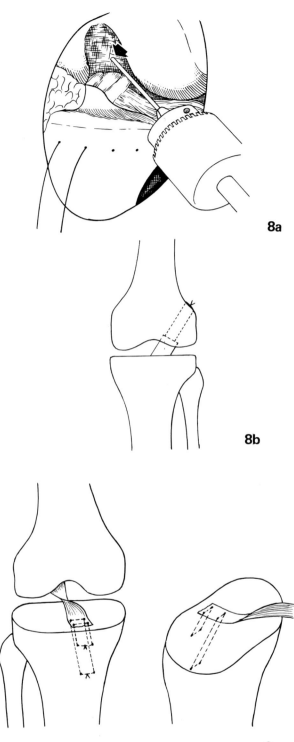

8a

8b

9

10

The posterior cruciate ligament is usually torn off the femur and it is readily repaired through the same incision. The medial epicondylar ridge is readily exposed at the top of the anteromedial incision (*see Illustration 1, A–D*). The vastus medialis is retracted forward and the bone exposed. Drill holes can be made from this ridge into the front of the notch where the posterior cruciate ligament is attached. This femoral attachment is at the extreme anterior edge of the notch just adjacent to the articular cartilage and has a wide attachment so it is important to have the drill holes well separated. They are made parallel about 2 cm apart with the exit points at the very front edge of the lateral side of the medial condyle. It is important to avoid bunching the ligament's end with the mattress suture.

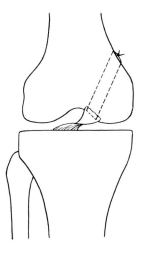

10

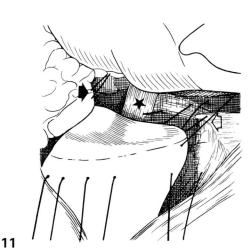

11

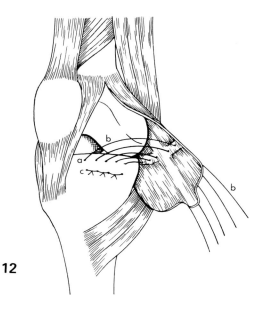

12

11 & 12

After these sutures have been placed but not tied, repair is continued on the medial side of the joint. The three mattress sutures have now been completed going through the posterior capsule in the back of the tibia. The posterior cruciate ligament torn off the tibia (star) is also included in the mattress suture. The right arrow indicates the torn edge of the posterior capsule at the posteromedial corner. Note sutures through the anterior cruciate ligament (left arrow) to be passed up into the medial side of the lateral condyle posteriorly through drill holes made as indicated in *Illustration 8b*.

If the medial capsular ligament is torn partly from the femur and partly from the tibia and there is soft tissue available, it can be repaired by direct suture. If it has been pulled from either the femur or the tibia it may be fastened either to soft tissue by mattress sutures or through drill holes along the rim of the bone if there is not enough soft tissue to permit firm suture. Superficial drills holes (*a*) are made just through the cortex of the tibia and spaced about 1 cm apart. The sutures are passed (*b*) through the holes using a 1 cm curved needle. This drawing shows separate drill holes (*c*) for the posterior capsule with the sutures already tied. In practice, we actually use the same drill holes. That is, the first and most lateral of the medial capsular sutures goes through the same drill hole as the posterior capsular sutures, but are passed through it superficially in a transverse direction with a curved needle. Additional holes are made so that there is a series of holes around the top of the tibia, six or eight in number. If it is not necessary to make the antero-posterior drill holes for the posterior capsule, the drill holes would appear as shown at (*a*).

13

Having placed all these sutures the leg is placed with the knee bent about 30° and the sutures are tied. The long fibres in the fascial flap are then repaired. The proximal one-third of the pes anserinus is then detached from the tibia and reflected downward, permitting the fascia to be sutured to the residual ligamentous stump lying beneath the pes anserinus. The fascia and ligament are brought together so that this fascia, which originally went over the pes anserinus, now goes under it. The pes anserinus is then drawn up over this flap and sewn to it. The skin is closed with suction drainage.

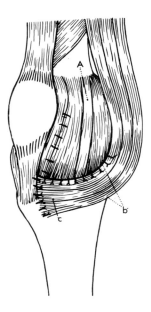

13

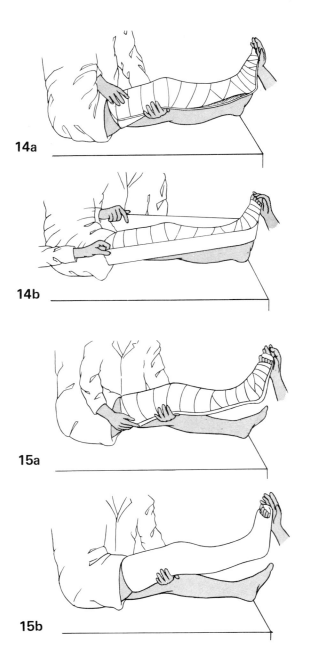

14a

14b

15a

15b

14 & 15

The limb is then placed in a heavy posterior plaster splint running from the gluteal fold to the tip of the toes and a lateral stirrup splint running from the perineum, around the foot, and up to the trochanter. (Note that the extremity is supported constantly by the foot and the thigh permitting the tibia to drop backward and relax the anterior cruciate ligament.) After this has set a single layer of sheet wadding is wrapped from 6 inches above to 6 inches below the knee and covered with a single roll of 6 inch plaster. This is firmly wrapped with gauze. Suction drainage is continued for as long as it is effective, up to 72 hr. At the end of 2 weeks the splint is removed and a solid cast applied. (Note that the extremity is supported by the thigh and the foot to permit the tibia to drop backward to relax the anterior cruciate ligament. The posterior slab is applied with the foot in slight eversion, the ankle neutral and the knee bent 20°. To balance the pelvis the patient should have a shoe with a heel of equal height on the good leg.) The patient wears the walking plaster for another 6 weeks, to a total of 8 weeks' immobilization.

Medial approach for the medial epicondylar ridge

If the repair has been on the lateral side and the medial side is not open, for repair of the *posterior cruciate ligament to the femur*, a second incision will be needed, extending along the medial epicondylar ridge with care to reflect the vastus medialis forward without damage to the muscle. This exposes the bone for drilling into the notch. The technique of placing the sutures has been described on page 617.

Medial meniscectomy

The incision is made (*see Illustration 1*, A–B) with the knee at 90° over the end of the table, which should be

at the height which allows the surgeon to grip the patient's foot between his knees. After the synovial layer has been divided, the leg is lifted into complete extension and the undersurface of the patella carefully examined by palpation and inspection. If it is necessary to carry out some further procedure on the patella the incision should be extended upward (*see Illustration 1*) to D. This should be done now rather than to work through this small incision and make it larger later. If the back of the patella is firm and smooth and if inspection reveals that the cruciate ligaments are normal, if there is no osteochondral damage to the femoral condyles or other lesion, one may proceed with the meniscectomy.

16

If there is no visible tear in the meniscus, use a cartilage feeler which is designed to drop into a gap at the periphery of the meniscus but is blunt so that it cannot be pushed through the capsule. Pass the feeler along the periphery of the meniscus. False catching may occur if the point drops into the posterior fold in this flexed position so extend the knee completely; the fold is eliminated so that if the feeler catches this indicates a posterior peripheral tear.

17 & 18

Sometimes the anterior horn is ecchymotic; sometimes it is overgrown with synovium. Sometimes there are fissures with fibrillation along the medial margin. All these things are indicative of a posterior tear. If there is a tear of the medial meniscus, the anterior end of the meniscus is detached from the non-articular portion of the upper tibia, grasped with a strong-toothed clamp and pulled gently forward. At the same time a tenaculum is attached to the medial retinaculum just above the level of the meniscus. Forward pull on this will expose the sulcus between the meniscus and the capsule. The retraction must be forwards rather than medially, which folds it over and closes up the space, whereas pulling it straight forwards opens it up like a 'Y'.

Using a sharp, strong scalpel, dissection is then carried out just at the periphery of the meniscus so that the front part of the meniscus is freed. At this point the posterior tear can be better defined. Care should be taken with any further sharp dissection not to cut into the ligament, which can easily be damaged.

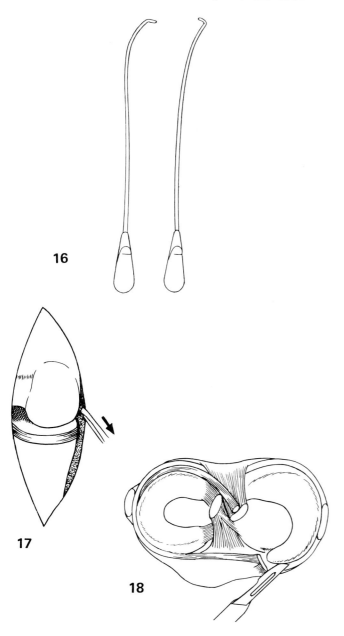

16

17

18

19 & 20

The author then prefers to use the Smillie's meniscotome. (Note that the curvature of the meniscotome should correspond with that of the tibia's margin when the longer tip is resting on the head of the tibia.) This is passed around at a 30° angle above and below, dissecting out the coronary ligament. Pulling forward will pull the meniscus into the notch when there is a defect posteriorly. If it does not, the meniscus can be pulled forward and laterally enough to let the meniscus lie between the femur and tibia, thus holding them apart. It is possible then to pass the Smillie knife between the two bones and dissect the posterior capsule. The author does not believe in using a curved meniscotome and forcibly pushing it back around the back because it has been shown that this can cause severe damage to the articular cartilage. When the meniscus has been pulled through the notch careful dissection, again with the meniscotome, will permit the bony attachment to be divided and the meniscus removed. Meniscectomy is not easy and careful technique is required, *not an attempt to drag it out by its roots*. It must be dissected free with the minimum damage to the other structures. The difficulty for the beginner, who has previously only watched the operation is to appreciate the importance of feel. The knee is thoroughly washed out with sterile saline. Any pannus growing over the femoral condyle is coagulated. The wound is closed in layers with fine stitches for the synovial and subcutaneous layers and stronger material for the capsule and skin.

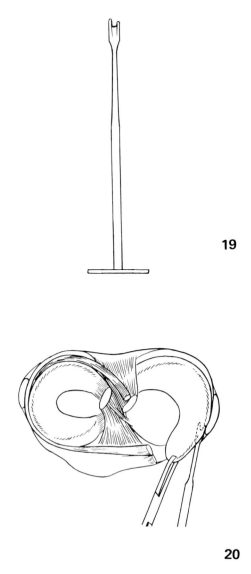

19

20

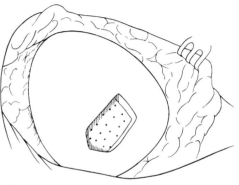

21

21

If the back of the patella feels soft or irregular the incision should be extended proximally (*see Illustration 1*, A–D), the knee can be extended so that the patella can be tilted over. With a discrete shaving brush type of lesion which has good cartilage around it, the author prefers to cut around the softened cartilage leaving vertical margins, curette the softened cartilage down to subchondral bone, then drill this bed with a small Kirschner wire. If it is more diffuse and more superficial, the cartilage should be shaved, using a small scapel to make it as smooth as possible.

22

If the lesion is more severe and confined to one or other *facet of the patella*, that part may be removed. Up to one-third of the patella can be removed without any symptoms apparently referable to this, provided that the remaining patella has normal cartilage. Careful suture of the medial retinaculum to the patella allows postoperative management like that after meniscectomy.

Tears of the cruciate ligaments may also be present and can be repaired at the same time but if the medial collateral ligament is intact and the posterior cruciate ligament has been torn from the tibia, the patient should be turned over and a repair done through the posterior approach, as described on page 632.

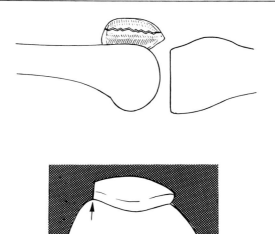

22

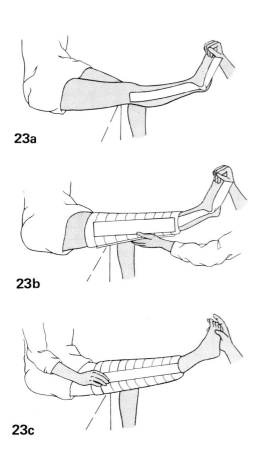

23a

23b

23c

23a, b & c

In the after-care of medial meniscectomy, the leg should be immobilized in the cotton cast, which gives relative stability to the knee but still permits a few degrees of motion. The application is as follows: with the leg extended and supported by the foot, 3 inch adhesive plaster strips are applied to either side of the leg from just below the knee to well beyond the foot. The leg, from upper mid-thigh to the lower part of the leg, is wrapped with five to six rolls of 6 inch sheet wadding. Three 22 inch light, curved wooden strips (yucca boards) are centred at the knee, one on either side and one behind. A gauze bandage is wrapped firmly over this dressing, moulding the boards to the leg. The tape strips are now pulled up over the boards and fastened with gauze. This prevents the dressing from slipping down when standing. The foot is then wrapped with an elastic bandage to prevent its swelling because of pressure above. The author uses this same type of dressing after chrondroplasty or facetectomy of the patella. If any ligament has been repaired, then long leg stirrup splints are indicated.

For immediate postoperative care, the patient can stand the same day if he wants to and is up on crutches with full weight-bearing the first postoperative day. He is given a series of printed exercises (tabulated below) which he should be accomplishing within 2 or 3 days. He is kept in the hospital for about 4 days after operation and in the splint for 2 weeks, after which time the splint is removed, usually without further support. Rehabilitation is continued but if there is synovitis with effusion no loaded flexion exercise is permitted until the swelling subsides.

Rehabilitative Exercises to the Lower Extremity

Each of the following exercises should be done deliberately and to a particular count. In each instance, raise the leg slowly to the count of 3, hold to the count of 3, lower to the count of 3, and rest. Repeat this series 10 times. Rest. Repeat this through three series of 10 times each, 30 times total. The exercise should be repeated two or three times a day, depending upon your tolerance. Whenever you are able to complete this series of 30, add weight and start a new series, gradually adding weight as your strength improves. Build this weight up to 25 pounds (10 kg) if possible. Chart your daily progress and record it. Continue this until the involved thigh is (a) as large as the normal side, (b) as strong as the normal side and (c) normal motion is reached.

The following exercises should be done as indicated above, starting while the leg is still in the cast.

(1) Lying on the back, raise the leg up with the knee straight and not flexing.

(2) Lie on the unaffected side. Raise the leg up with the knee straight.

(3) Lie face down. Raise the leg up with the knee straight.

(N.B. In each instance, increase weight as indicated above, after removal of fixation).

(4) Sitting with the leg hanging and the knee at a right angle, go through the series of exercises with spring resistance or weight. If there is ligamentous damage, a spring or system of pulleys and weight is preferred to hanging the weight on the foot.

(5) Lie face down with weight on the foot, flex the leg to vertical through the same series.

Exercises 1, 2 and 3 should be begun immediately postoperatively, or even started pre-operatively. Exercises 4 and 5 should be done after removal of the cast and should not be done if there is synovitis with effusion.

24

Aspiration may be indicated. In order to aspirate the knee, the knee should be extended and the skin carefully prepared for aseptic puncture. The preferred place to insert the needle is just at the superior edge of the patella and parallel to its posterior surface. This allows the needle to be slipped into the suprapatellar pouch free of any obstructive synovium. Following preparation of the skin, the skin is infiltrated with 1 per cent lignocaine, using a 25-gauge needle. The needle is then pushed in until it encounters the synovium; this is carefully infiltrated with local anaesthetic through an area of about 1 cm in diameter. By careful use of the local anaesthetic the aspiration can be made largely without discomfort. If the knee is likely to be full of blood a 15-gauge needle should be used; for normal synovial liquid a 16-gauge needle is preferable. Careful compression of the suprapatellar pouch and of the knee will permit almost complete evacuation of the effusion.

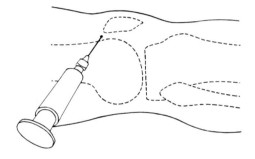

24

Osteochondral fracture

Osteochondral fracture is a frequent injury of the knee. The fracture may be of the patella either following a fall onto it or during dislocation or subluxation of bone over the femoral condyle or by avulsion of the medial edge of the dislocating patella. Alternatively, the fragment can be knocked off the lateral femoral condyle by a dislocating patella. The antero-medial incision gives access to the patella. A fresh osteochondral fragment that can be replaced and fits well can be held in place with Kirschner wires drilled through far enough to be removed later from the outer side of the bone. Ragged and comminuted pieces should be scraped out, the bed carefully curetted down to fresh bone, and then drilled with a small Kirschner wire. If the fragment is avulsed from the patella, it should be removed and the retinaculum carefully re-attached to the patella. In many of these cases of dislocation, there is too much tightness on the lateral side. By elevating or everting the patella and reaching across to the opposite side one can divide the decussating fibres that extend from the iliotibial band up to the patella and beyond some of the vastus lateralis. This release helps to prevent subsequent dislocation. In the case of acute dislocation of the patella there is commonly a complete avulsion of the retinaculum, with or without bone. This should be very carefully and thoroughly repaired after removing any bony fragment and, if the lateral side is tight it should be released. In any of these cases of extensive injury when there has been bleeding with a vascular flap, use of suction drainage for 48–72 hr is often of value in keeping down the postoperative haemorrhage and pain.

Osteochondritis dissecans is usually the result of injury. Unless the fragment is relatively fresh and unless it can be accurately replaced, it is better removed. If, as may happen, the posterior cruciate ligament is attached to it, the ligament can be attached to the defect through the anteromedial incision.

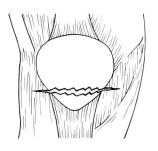

25a

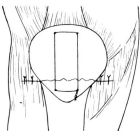

25b

25a, b & c

Avulsion of the distal pole of the patella can be treated either by replacing the fragment or, possibly better, by removing the fragment and sewing the tendon to the patella through drill holes. *Avulsion of the quadriceps tendon* from the top of the patella can be managed through this anteromedial incision with the appropriate extension proximally. In fact, there are more possibilities for the management of injuries through the anteromedial incision than through any of the other incisions.

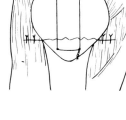

25c

PARAPATELLAR APPROACH

26

For *patellectomy*, the medial parapatellar incision permits comprehensive exploration of the knee. The incision extends through the retinaculum along the medial edge of the patella. The skin flap is reflected and the quadriceps tendon and patellar tendon are then carefully dissected from the patella and the lateral retinaculum is incised beside the patella.

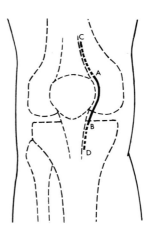

26

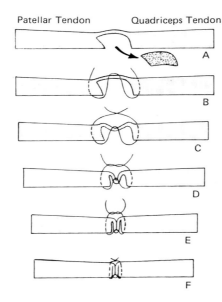

27

27

After the patella has been removed, the edges of the tendons are smoothed and the frayed strips of the two tendon ends are excised leaving the flap intact. When the extensor apparatus remains in continuity in front of the patella the connecting tissue is pulled down into the gap between the quadriceps and patellar tendon. This gives some thickening here to fill the space left by removing the patella.

28

If the patella and the tendinous tissue in front of it are removed, vertical mattress stitches should still be used and will shorten the extensor apparatus.

At this point one should be able to flex the knee to 90° if the tourniquet was applied at 90° flexion. This method shortens the quadriceps somewhat but it maintains full active extension without the extensor lag so frequently seen after patellectomy. One may sacrifice 15° of flexion in order to prevent a 15° extensor lag but flexion has not been difficult to regain.

The treatment of *fractured patella* has been controversial for almost a century. It varies from accurate replacement and firm internal fixation to total or partial patellectomy. The merits of these will not be discussed in detail but if the author cannot leave at least two-thirds of the patella with normal cartilage he prefers to take out the whole patella straightaway rather than later. The medial parapatellar incision is preferred for reasons mentioned previously. If at least two-thirds of the patella seems to be normal, one may dissect out the smaller fragment(s) and reattach the appropriate structures to the patella, using drill holes and taking care not to drill through the articular cartilage. This repair may be patellar tendon to patella, quadriceps tendon to patella or medial or lateral retinaculum to the patella. Very firm fixation with mattress sutures through bone will permit early mobilization.

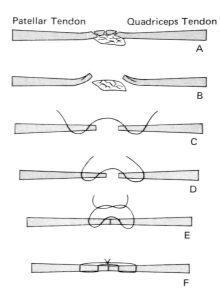

28

29 & 30

Capsulorrhaphy

The medial parapatellar incision is used, beginning at the top of the patella, extending along the edge of the patella and at the lower pole of the patella it swings across the tendon to the tuberosity and then swings medially to expose the anteromedial face of the upper tibia. In capsulorrhaphy the medial retinaculum is divided from the vastus medialis but including a portion of the vastus attachment down to the patellar tendon. To release the lateral side, the skin flap is reflected from the patella to expose the lateral side. Here the retinaculum is split along the edge of the patella, up into and including a portion of the attachment of the vastus lateralis to the patella to be sure that the patella is not tethered laterally. To complete the capsulorrhaphy on the medial side, decision must be made as to whether or not the vastus medialis is to be advanced, or is to be imbricated, or both. As a rule we use mattress sutures and imbricate the medial side about 1 cm. At the same time we possibly advance the vastus medialis attachment about 1 cm distally. The lateral release is not closed but the space is filled with the fat pad in order to prevent direct communication of the joint with the subcutaneous tissue.

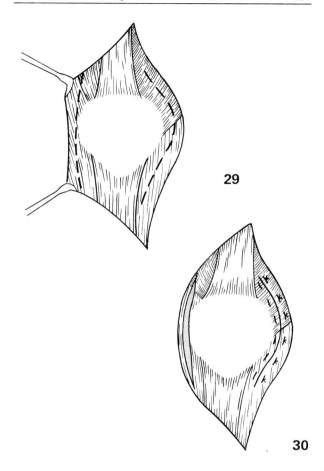

Transplantation of the patellar tendon

If it is necessary to carry out some procedure to re-align the patellar tendon, it is exposed at the distal end of the incision including the tuberosity and the medial face of the tibia. At this point exposure is adequate for any of one of the many methods of repositioning the patellar tendon's attachment to tibia to alter the alignment.

Exposure of the tibial tuberosity

If the exposure is of tuberosity alone, a transverse incision may be made directly across it and the skin retracted proximally and distally. The tendon can then be split to remove a loose fragment or to reduce the size of the tuberosity; an avulsed tubercle can also be replaced through this incision.

ANTERIOR (TRANSVERSE) INCISION

31

The transverse approach to the patella is suitable for removing both the broken and unbroken patella but it is ill suited for other conditions such as internal derangement, damaged ligaments, chondral fracture, etc. The tourniquet should be applied and then inflated with the knee at 90° flexion; the knee is then extended in the supine position. The skin is cut across the patella at the junction of the proximal and middle thirds.

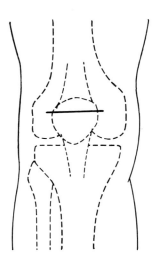

31

The prepatellar bursa is excised. If the patella is to be removed for chondromalacia, the incision is carried down to the underlying bone and the soft tissue is then carefully dissected toward the upper and lower poles of the patella. As this proceeds the quadriceps attachment is dissected from the proximal and the patellar tendon from the distal edge of the patella. The joint is explored as well as possible through this exposure. Then, mattress sutures are placed so as to approximate the quadriceps tendon to the patellar tendon. The flaps of tissue from the front of the patella can be utilized for re-inforcement but are usually quite inadequate. The suture is facilitated by placing a folded towel under the foot in order to hyperextend the knee.

Long leg stirrup splints are applied immediately after the operation and left on for 14 days. The leg is then measured for a long leg brace with adjustable flexion at the knee and at the ankle. If the wound is in satisfactory condition and the leg not too badly swollen, a long leg walking cast is applied for another 2 weeks. This makes a total of 4 weeks. During this period straight leg raising is not encouraged but isometric contraction of the quadriceps is. All other muscles are actively used by raising the limb sideways while lying on the uninvolved side and backwards while lying prone.

Weight-bearing in the cast is permitted but with crutches, in order to prevent a traumatic lurch. After the 4 weeks the cast is removed and active movement of the knee is encouraged. At this time the patient can usually flex the knee 30°—45° and is able to extend it fully. The brace is now applied; it is not for any lateral support of the knee but simply to prevent sudden forceful flexion beyond the attained range of motion. It does not prevent violent contraction of the quadriceps in the event of a stumble. Such a step may well disrupt the fresh repair, which is why it is wise to insist on the use of crutches. Physiotherapy is usually unnecessary but should be used if the patient is unable to obtain a satisfactory range. Manipulation under anaesthesia is rarely advisable.

The transverse incision is satisfactory for removing small prepatellar bursae, but not for large ones.

POSTEROMEDIAL APPROACH

32

This incision is suitable for removing the posterior horn of the medial meniscus when this cannot be done from the front; for removing foreign bodies from the posterior space and for removing exostoses from the back of the tibia, or, exceptionally, the femur. This approach is not suitable for repair of the posteromedial corner of the ligament nor of the posterior capsule, which will be discussed later. This incision is readily closed, the tissues falling together as they have been split.

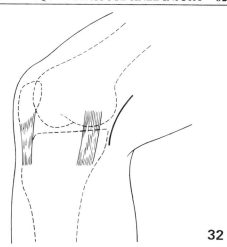

32

33, 34 & 35

The posteromedial incision is made with the knee flexed over the end of the table with means of flexing it even beyond this point. The place of incision is most easily chosen if a curved instrument is passed backwards through an anterior incision. Where the point is felt behind the medial ligament the incision is made about 8 cm long and parallel to the posterior edge of the tibia. The skin and subcutaneous flap should be reflected posteriorly, exposing the fascia of the thigh. This fascia should be split along the line of its fibres exposing the capsule of the knee. Just behind the heavy fibres of the medial capsular ligament is the 'soft spot', where the ligamentous structures are much thinner than those in front or behind. Careful splitting in the line of the fibres exposes the synovium, which can be divided along the line of the incision to enter the back of the joint. Using a flexible retractor, the posterior flap is retracted backward; it includes the capsule of the joint as far over as the neurovascular bundle, although it is usually unnecessary to go this far. The incision itself is not extended further but the retraction exposes the synovial fold behind the knee. Provided that the dissection remains intracapsular, the neurovascular bundle is not in danger. The meniscus blocks exposure into the knee joint. If it is abnormal and has been partially removed in front, it may be removed posteriorly by cutting along its attachment. This permits close examination of the posterior pouch and of the posterior part of the knee joint.

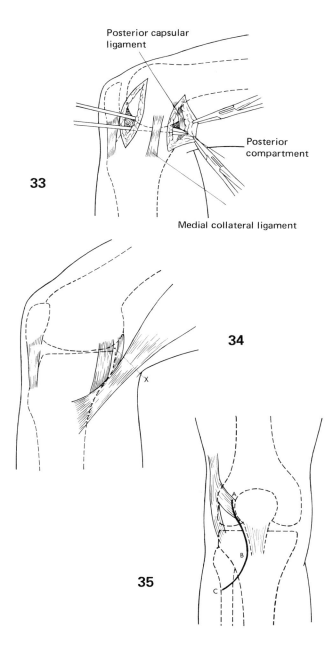

Posterior capsular
ligament

Posterior
compartment

Medial collateral ligament

33

34

35

ANTEROLATERAL APPROACH

36

The anterolateral incision is quite similar to the anteromedial incision, and is best used for lateral meniscectomy. It begins above the patella and crosses the knee joint in the interval between the tensor fasciae latae and the lateral retinaculum. The incision runs parallel to the iliotibial band to within a finger's breadth of the patella and then parallel to the patellar tendon. This permits the iliotibial band to be split and reflected backward giving good access to the lateral compartment. The cut must be extended downward and backward below the fibular head for repair of the lateral ligament, or for treatment of peroneal nerve injury. For access to the posterior compartment, a second incision (E to F) can be made just anterior to the biceps tendon and posterior to the fibular collateral ligament. There is often a very heavy decussating band of fibres extending from the iliotibial tract forward to the patella which needs to be divided. When this has been done the iliotibial tract falls backwards and allows excellent exposure of the lateral compartment of the knee when the synovium is cut in the line of the incision.

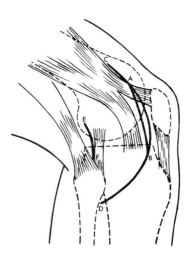

36

Access to the lateral compartment is hampered by the popliteus tendon, which passes between the lateral plateau of the tibia and the lateral ligament. If further treatment is indicated it may be necessary to extend this incision. To expose the lateral ligament the incision can be extended distally, passing downwards along the patellar tendon to the tuberosity, then angulating posteriorly to the level of the neck of the fibula. One must recall that the common peroneal nerve is behind the fibula and may be exposed by this approach. The flap can be reflected to re-attach the biceps to the fibula, the collateral ligament to the femur or to the fibula, or simply to repair it. The incision gives access to the posterior capsule either between the popliteus tendon and the lateral ligament or behind them.

37 & 38

Anterolateral approach for lateral meniscectomy

The anterolateral approach for lateral meniscectomy has been described. The synovium is divided along the line of the incision, it does involve some of the lateral portion of the fat pad, which is quite dense here. The first step should be to examine the joint for the *cruciate ligaments,* which are readily seen from this incision by retracting the fat pad forward and medially. The *patella* is examined by bringing the knee up to full extension and palpating the surface. The *femoral condyle* is examined for exostosis or for pannus, which frequently has grown over the condyle. The condyle and trochlear groove are examined for any chondral damage in the nature of osteochondral or chondral fractures. On exploring the *lateral meniscus,* it should be noted that the anterior end of the meniscus is fastened well back in the notch, lying adjacent to and alongside the anterior cruciate ligament. It has here a relatively long attachment that may be covered with synovium. There may be pannus growing over it, or it may be damaged. Fibrillation or any split or tear may be found along the arc of this curve. With a condylar retractor placed between the capsule and femoral condyle, a tenaculum is fastened to the lateral edge of the wound just above the meniscus and is pulled forward to permit inspection of the sulcus between the meniscus and the lateral capsule. Usually one can readily see back to the popliteal hiatus, where the popliteus tendon passes diagonally across, separating the capsule from the top of the tibia. This hiatus usually is 1—1·5 cm long and is a normal anatomical structure. If the cartilage feeler is slid along this sulcus it can be felt to drop into the popliteal hiatus and when pushed backwards for about 1—1·5 cm it comes against a definite stop. Care must be taken to keep this instrument horizontal because, if the handle is raised, the feeler may pass through the hiatus and go downwards along the popliteus tendon and lead the examiner to interpret this as a posterior tear.

Using a scalpel, the meniscus is separated from the capsule back as far as the hiatus. The posterior part is cut free with a Smillie knife, using it as a dissecting instrument, not as a guillotine, and the meniscus is gradually pulled over between the tibia and femur, the meniscus then acts as a retractor (or separator) so that the Smillie instrument can be pushed through

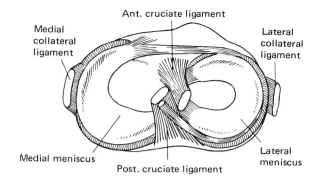

37

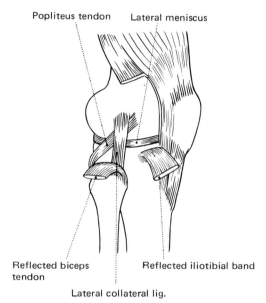

38

to divide the posterior attachment of the meniscus. At some point the meniscus will slip through into the notch, when careful dissection will free it from the bony attachment. Great care should be taken in this dissection not to damage the articular cartilage or the capsule or the cruciate ligaments. It is not necessary to damage any of these structures in a typical meniscectomy.

If there is no other abnormality the knee is carefully washed and closed in layers, using respectively 4/0 cotton, 2/0 cotton, 4/0 cotton and wire. Cotton cast fixation is applied and worn for 2 weeks. Immediate rehabilitative exercises are started the day after operation.

Further procedures through the limited anterolateral incision

If, after careful exploration of the meniscus, it is found that there is something else wrong with the knee, it can usually be managed through this incision. If there is an abnormality of the patella, the incision can be carried higher, the patella tilted and dealt with as required. If there is a small osteochondral fracture it is best treated by trephining and drilling, as described on page 620. Generalized softness of the articular cartilage can be treated by shaving. If there is damage to either facet, such as an avulsion fracture of a portion of the medial facet or fracture of the lateral facet is treated by removal of the loose fragment provided it does not include more than one-third of the width of the patella. Careful repair of the retinaculum to the patella permits rapid rehabilitation with no more immobilization than is used for the meniscus repair, namely, 2 weeks. If there is an osteochondral fracture on the femoral condyle and this is a large fragment, one may replace and hold it either with Smillie's nails, with small threaded Kirschner wires traversing the fragment and the lateral femoral condyle and pushed far enough to protrude under the skin of the lower part of the thigh, or with a screw. The objection to the screw is the metal in the joint, whereas the Kirschner wires can be cut off flush with the cartilage and taken out later through an incision on the medial side. If the fragment is small, shattered or does not contain bone, it can be removed and the loose fragments curetted down to fresh bone. Unless this bleeds the bone should be drilled with small Kirschner wires making multiple drill holes. All of this can be done through the lateral incision.

If the anterior cruciate has been pulled off the tibia it can be repaired, using drill holes in the top of the tibia. If it is torn off the femur, the lateral condyle is readily available through this incision and drill holes can be made through the femoral condyle into the notch. This procedure is described in more detail on page 616. If the posterior cruciate ligament is torn off the femur, a second incision on the medial epicondylar ridge will be required to make the parallel drill holes for the mattress sutures to pull the ligament up against the bony bed. This procedure is described on page 617. If this ligament has been torn off the tibia, it cannot be reached through this incision with intact collateral ligaments and a posterior incision will be necessary.

Lesions of the fat pad can be dealt with through either an anterolateral or an anteromedial incision. If exostoses are present along the lateral femoral condyle with chronic osteo-arthrosis they can be removed with a sharp osteotome, smoothed with a rasp and covered with bone wax; the vascular synovium should be coagulated. Such an operation requires no more immobilization than does meniscectomy. For

further details of the procedures other than meniscectomy, *see* page 618.

Anterolateral approach for the lateral epicondylar ridge

If the repair has been on the medial side and the lateral side has not been opened, a separate lateral incision will be required for re-attaching the anterior cruciate ligament to the femur. For this purpose, it is necessary to expose the lateral supracondylar ridge of the femur in order to place the two parallel drill holes to receive the mattress sutures that will hold the anterior cruciate ligament against the femoral condyle in the notch. If the knee opens up widely, the drills can be passed from inside the knee at the very back of the notch and out on the supracondylar ridge using a smooth, 3/32 inch (2 mm) pin. If this is not feasible, the opposite approach must be taken, drilling from the outside into the notch through the epicondyle.

39

An 8 cm incision should be made along the lateral supracondylar ridge. The skin is retracted and the iliotibial tract is split to expose the ridge. The vastus lateralis muscle should be retracted anteriorly to expose the bone; it is not necessary to cut into the muscle.

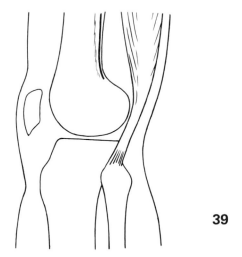

39

A smooth, 3/32 inch (2 mm) pin is drilled into the bone to emerge inside the knee on the medial side of the lateral condyle at the very posterior part of the intercondylar notch. The second drill hole is made 1 cm from the first and parallel to it. The drill holes in the notch should be at least 1 cm apart in order to avoid bunching the ligament with the mattress suture.

POSTEROLATERAL APPROACH

This approach gives access to the posterolateral compartment of the knee and, for example, to the posterior horn of the lateral meniscus, osteochondral foreign bodies and exostoses on the femur or tibia. It is not suitable for repair of the posterior capsule or the posterior cruciate ligament. It is most often used in conjunction with the limited anterolateral approach for exostoses, meniscectomy, synovectomy and in circumstances in which it does not seem necessary to make the much longer lateral approach extending down onto the leg.

40

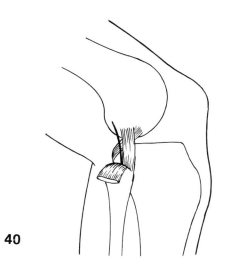

40

The patient lies on the operating table with the knee flexed 90° and the leg hanging vertically. The surgeon sits with the patient's foot between his knees. The incision lies slightly posterior to the fibular collateral ligament and enters the posterior compartment posterior to the popliteus tendon, which makes this incision more difficult to use than its counterpart on the posteromedial side of the knee. Careful palpation on the lateral side will identify the space between the biceps tendon posteriorly and the ilio-tibial band anteriorly. The curved skin incision runs parallel to the biceps tendon to below the fibula and extends from the fibula's head to a point about 7–8 cm above the joint line. Retraction of the skin flap exposes the deep fascia, which is incised along the line of its fibres. This exposes the synovial capsule, which in turn is divided along its fibres and retracted posteriorly. This retraction does not include the fibular collateral ligament. The popliteus tendon runs across this incision, closely hugging the tibial plateau as it passes behind the tibia. Usually the best access to the space is behind the popliteus tendon and the fibular collateral ligament. Although somewhat restricted here, the posterior space can be readily explored for the posterior horn of the meniscus, exostosis, ruptured popliteus, foreign bodies and osteochondral damage of the femoral condyle. The exposure is not adequate for repair of the fibular collateral ligament or lateral collateral ligament.

POSTERIOR APPROACH

41

Because of the important popliteal structures there has traditionally been a good deal of trepidation about approaching the knee from behind. Actually, the posterior approach is relatively atraumatic to the knee and it is entirely safe if one keeps in mind the anatomy of the area. The most satisfactory position is to place the patient prone with a folded sheet under the knee in order to extend the joint completely and outline the popliteal structures. The semitendinous tendon is located in the distal part of the thigh and followed up about 8 cm above the popliteal fold. From here the skin incision is made along the semitendinosus tendon until it reaches the popliteal fold. The incision at this point swings transversely across the popliteal fold until it reaches the biceps tendon, which it follows for about 8 cm. It is important to make the incision with the proximal end of it medial and the distal end of it lateral (for reasons which will be explained later).

42

The skin flaps are reflected to reveal the fascia of the popliteal area, which is quite thick and a definite structure.

The best landmark in this area is the posterior cutaneous nerve of the calf, which uniformly lies directly beneath the fascia coursing down between the two heads of the gastrocnemius muscle. The fascia should be split along this line for the full length of the incision. At the proximal end the posterior cutaneous nerve will be found to leave the sciatic very near the origin of the peroneal nerve as it passes down on the lateral side of the popliteal space.

Retraction of this fascia exposes the whole popliteal area. By careful dissection, the tibial nerve, which is located posterior and superficial to the artery and vein, can be followed down into the cleft between the two heads of the gastrocnemius. It is usually not necessary to dissect out the peroneal nerve since the retraction is going to go to that side, but it must be identified and protected. The medial head of the gastrocnemius is exposed at the proximal end of the incision and divided at its tendinous attachment to the back of the medial condyle, leaving enough tendon for resuture. The medial head of the gastrocnemius is then readily separated from the semimembranosus and the whole mass of the gastrocnemius can be retracted laterally. It must be emphasized that this cannot be done on the lateral side because the peroneal nerve is tethered so securely

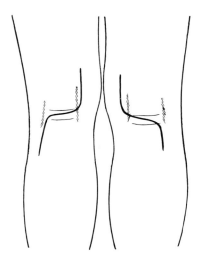

41

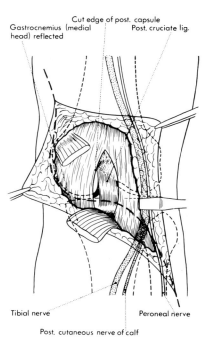

Cut edge of post. capsule
Gastrocnemius (medial   Post. cruciate lig.
head) reflected

Tibial nerve   Peroneal nerve

Post. cutaneous nerve of calf   **42**

behind the head of the fibula that it is not retractable. Having retracted the medial head of the gastrocnemius the neurovascular bundle can be readily retracted to the lateral side and the posterior capsule of the joint is exposed. The major vessels are protected by the retracted muscles. Although this incision is best done with a tourniquet, care must be taken to ligate any of the geniculate vessels which lie transversely across this space, but may not need to be sacrificed. It is not usually necessary to divide the superior geniculates because the division in the posterior capsule is not carried that far proximally.

43 & 44

This posterior approach is used for repair of the posterior cruciate ligament when it has been avulsed from the tibia and for repair of a torn *posterior ligament* of the joint which results from hypertension of the knee. The posterior ligament is a massive ligament which prevents hyperextension of the knee and may be avulsed from its attachment above the femoral condyles. It is very much more frequently torn from the tibia, less commonly directly across the joint line. If the ligament is found to have been torn directly across the joint line, it can be readily sutured; this is facilitated by removing the towel from under the knee and placing it under the foot to flex the knee and relax the posterior tissues. If the tear is across the joint line, retraction of its edges will reveal the *posterior cruciate ligament*, which has also been torn in most cases. If it is torn in the line of its fibres, the posterior capsule may have to be split further to give access for direct suture of the posterior cruciate ligament. If this ligament has been torn off the tibia the posterior capsule is retracted proximally to give access for repair, which can be done by drill holes (difficult), or by staples. Staples often work loose and have to be taken out again. For this reason the author prefers suture through drill holes in the tibia. Three or four holes are made about 1 cm apart just through the posterior cortex. The inset shows that by using a 1 cm curved needle, a suture can be passed through the ligament, through one drill hole and out of the next. Two or three mattress sutures hold the ligament securely in place. In certain instances there may be enough soft tissue to fasten to the tibia and so permit direct suture. If this is firm and secure, this is easier and just as satisfactory. If the posterior ligament and the posterior cruciate ligament have both been torn from the tibia, they can be repaired as a cuff.

If the posterior cruciate has been torn off the femur, the capsule must be split in the mid-line to the level of the gastrocnemius's attachment and then retracted laterally. This gives access to the medial side of the epicondylar ridge, where a vertical incision will expose the medial condyle, as described on page 617. Drill holes can be made through this condyle to the front of the notch. By use of the ligature carrier, mattress sutures are placed through the drill hole in the femur, through the posterior cruciate ligament, then back through a second drill hole. While difficult, this technique is not impossible; it requires patience as well as a curved needle holder and an adequate ligature carrier.

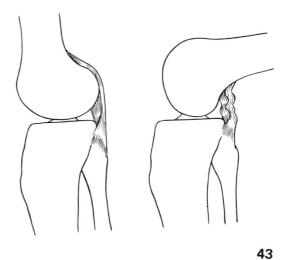

43

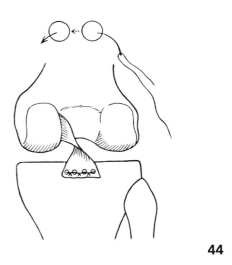

44

After all these ligatures have been placed and tied, the knee should be bent between 30° and 40°, the sutures tied, and immobilization secured in this position. Closure is very easy and the tendinous attachment of the gastrocnemius is readily sutured. When the popliteal fascia is closed, the whole area is pulled together.

It should be emphasized that this is not the proper approach to the posterior horn of the medial meniscus nor to remove foreign bodies from the back of the joint; these are more readily available from the postero-medial and posterolateral approaches.

POSTOPERATIVE CARE

If the repair includes the anterior cruciate ligament, the medial collateral ligament and posterior capsule, the limb should be supported by the thigh and by the foot to permit the tibia to drop backward and relax the tension on the anterior cruciate ligament. It is extremely important in positioning the foot that it be left in the weight-bearing position. It is very easy to apply the splint with the foot inverted, a position which is prone to cause contracture and complicate the rehabilitation. Attendants should carefully maintain the position until the stirrup splints are applied. A heavy plaster splint is applied from the gluteal fold, down the back of the leg and foot to beyond the toes. This is wrapped in place with a gauze bandage. Then a stirrup is placed beginning near the perineum, extending down the medial side of the leg, around under the heel, and back up the lateral side to the trochanter and is then wrapped in place with gauze bandage. In the case of the young athlete with strong muscles it seems better to protect a little more than this during the immediate post-operative stage, so a single layer of 6 inch plaster is wrapped around the area of the knee, over a layer of sheet wadding. This layer is taken off that evening or at least by the next morning and sooner if there is any complaint of pressure.

If the injury has involved the posterior cruciate ligament the support should be under the calf and under the foot, letting the thigh drop backward so as to relax the posterior cruciate. If both cruciates have been involved and repaired, the support should be equally distributed between the tibia and thigh. A careless flop of the foot toward extension may pull out the stitches in the cruciate ligaments. If the repair has been of the posterior capsule and posterior cruciate ligament, the posterior splint should be applied with the patient prone. Only when the plaster has set firmly should he be turned over and the stirrup applied.

The advantage of the stirrup splint is that it can be readily loosened if swelling occurs and readily be tightened if swelling subsides. If there is any doubt about the tightness of the dressing, it should be split. The split should be made for the entire length from the toes to the groin and down to the skin, otherwise swelling will occur in the lower part of the leg. If it is necessary to inspect the wound because of severe pain or suspicion of a haemarthrosis, the splint can be opened up, the stirrup removed and the leg left resting in the posterior splint for whatever procedure needs to be done to the knee itself.

Usually by 2 weeks the wound is well healed. Then a long leg plaster cast is applied with the knee flexed about $15°-20°$, depending on the type of repair. If the patient is responsible and if the thigh is relatively long and well-muscled, this may be a walking cast but he should be advised never to walk without crutches lest the lurching gait put stress on the knee. He wears this case or a replacement for a total of 8 weeks postoperatively.

[*The illustrations for this Chapter on Surgical Technique for Acute Knee Injury were drawn by Mr. F. Price.*]

Treatment of Tibial Condylar Fractures

Poul S. Rasmussen, M.D.
Orthopaedic Surgeon, County Hospital, Hellerup, Denmark

INTRODUCTION

An intra-articular fracture of the tibial condyles is a complex injury involving both skeletal and soft tissue structures, the integrity of which is essential to satisfactory joint function. A fracture of the tibial plateau may derange the congruency of the articulating surface, thereby often disturbing the stability and axial alignment of this heavily loaded joint. The immediate result of this derangement is impaired function, the late result frequently a pain-ful osteo-arthrosis. A third cause of functional impairment is post-traumatic stiffness, often resulting from too long immobilization. From this it appears that in the treatment of these fractures we have four main problems to solve:

(1) restoration of stability;
(2) restoration of axial alignment;
(3) restoration of motion;
(4) prevention of post-traumatic osteo-arthrosis.

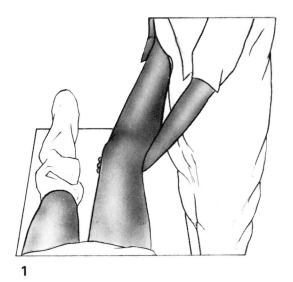

1

1

Instability

An important feature of about half of these fractures is that they produce instability of the joint. This is tested by trying to bend the fully extended joint sideways. Unstable fractures and none other should be treated operatively.

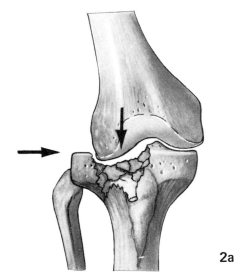

2a

2a-e

Pathogenesis and classification

Most of these fractures are produced by valgus and hyperextension forces to which is added a varying amount of vertical load. (*a*) The result of this is to crush and split one or other (usually the lateral) condyle and sometimes both. We may thus classify the fractures topographically into lateral (*b*), medial or bicondylar (*c* and *d*) and morphologically into split or wedge fractures as one type and compression fractures as another (*e*). A central compression is often associated with one or more marginal fragments.

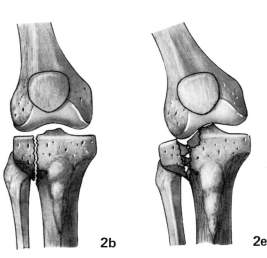

2b

2e

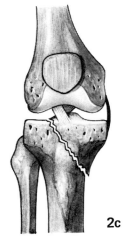

2c

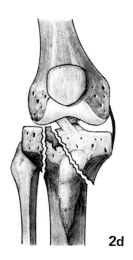

2d

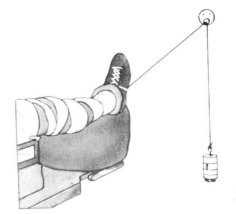

3

SURGICAL TECHNIQUE

Two different methods of open repair may be used:
   (1) closed reduction with internal fixation by means of a wire loop (Moberg);
   (2) open reduction with reconstruction of the joint surface by means of transplanted bone (Palmer).

3, 4 & 5

In the first method, which is recommended in very comminuted bicondylar cases the fracture is reduced manually and by strong traction on the extension table. Two Kirschner wires, the pointed ends of which are perforated, are passed from lateral to medial through the tibial plateaux parallel to the joint surface, taking care to avoid the peroneal nerve. The location of the guide pins should be verified by x-rays and the skin between them incised. A stainless steel wire of 1 mm thickness is drawn through the tibial head from medial to lateral by means of the guide pins. The steel wire should be placed under the periosteum so as not to constrict the soft tissues. The free ends of the steel wire are twisted tightly together and buried in a drill-hole through the cortex.

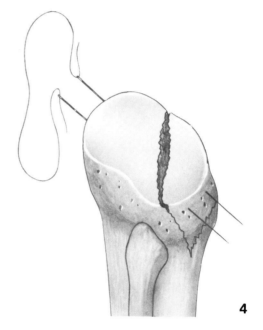

4

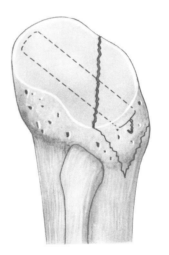

5

6,7 & 8

When instability is caused by a central compression closed reduction is impossible. In such cases the knee joint is exposed through a lateral lazy S incision. The lateral meniscus, which is usually torn, may be removed without ill-effects. This greatly facilitates the exposure.

The depressed part of the joint surface is elevated by inserting a chisel through a small cortical window or in cases combined with fracture of the cortical ring by passing it through the fracture.

The empty space below the reduced joint surface is filled with bone blocks from the iliac crest.

In cases of central compression with marginal split fragments the bone block reconstruction may be secured by applying a wire loop.

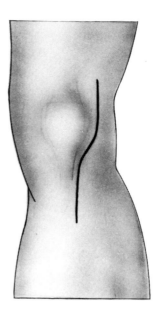

6

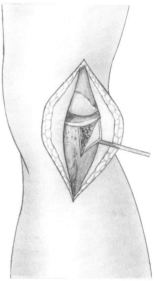

7

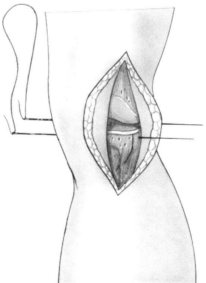

8

After treatment

The knee joint is immobilized in a circular plaster cast from the groin to the ankle for 6 weeks. Removal of the plaster is followed by 2–3 weeks' exercises without weight-bearing. Restricted weight-bearing is allowed for another 2 weeks after which full weight-bearing is permitted.

9a & b

Non-operative treatment

Though significant complications are rare after the operative procedures described here it should be pointed out that good functional results may be obtained even in unstable cases by the method of tibial traction and early movement described by Apley (1956). Such a method will, however, cause an unsightly valgus deformity in a considerable number of cases and the stay in hospital is much longer.

Fractures that cause no impairment of stability demand very little treatment. A plaster cast for 2 weeks followed by 2–4 weeks of restricted weight-bearing is a safe programme of treatment.

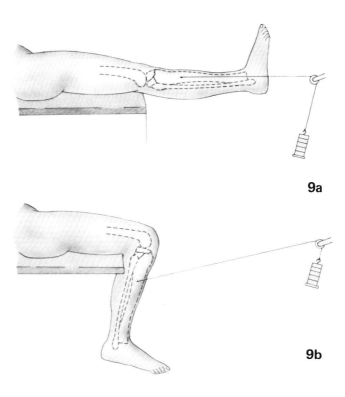

9a

9b

References

Apley, A. G. (1956). 'Fractures of the lateral tibial condyle, treated by skeletal traction and early mobilization. A review of sixty cases with special reference to the long-term results.' *J. Bone Jt Surg.* **38B**, 699
Moberg, E. (1961). *Dansk Kirurgisk Selskab, Nordisk Med.* **66**, 1595
Palmer, Ivar (1951). 'Fractures of the upper end of the tibia.' *J. Bone Jt Surg.* **33B**, 160
Rasmussen, Poul S. (1973). 'Tibial condylar fractures.' *J. Bone Jt Surg.* **55A**, 1331

[*The illustrations for this Chapter on Treatment of Tibial Condylar Fractures were drawn by Mr. F. Price.*]

Repair of the Tendo Achillis

P. S. London, M.B.E., F.R.C.S.
Surgeon, Birmingham Accident Hospital.

PRE-OPERATIVE

Indications for repair

If the tendon has been cut it should be repaired, but if it has sustained closed rupture opinions are divided between carrying out surgical repair and allowing the tendon to heal on its own. If guidance is required, it is suggested that for the young and vigorous, repair is likely to give a better result than spontaneous healing, particularly if there is a palpable gap in the tendon.

Position of patient

The patient should be prone with the foot resting on the table so that the ankle is comfortably flexed.

THE OPERATION

1

The incision

This should not lie directly over the tendon because the seam puckers when the ankle is flexed and it should not cross the prominent superolateral corner of the calcaneus. If there is a more or less transverse wound this should be extended so that the lower limb lies just medial to the tendon, which is the preferred side for access.

The cut is deepened to lay open the well marked sheath of the tendon and should be long enough to give comfortable access to the two ends — 4 inches (10 cm) is often enough.

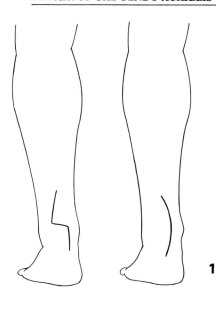

2

The cut tendon

If the distal end is an inch or so long the simple double right-angled stitch can be used.

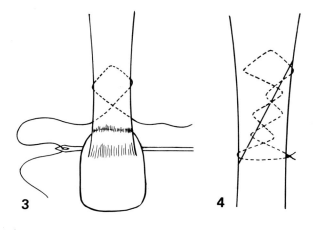

3 & 4

If the tendon has been cut very close to the bone the proximal end should be held by a simple criss-cross stitch, which is then passed through the calcaneus by means of an awl.

If the tendon has been cut obliquely a criss-cross stitch may be used but there may be advantage in making it lie not in one plane but on a spiral or staggered.

Closed rupture

5

In the elderly the tendon may be pulled off the bone and show little of the fraying that characterizes rupture of the younger tendon. This enables it to be repaired in much the same way as a cut tendon. When the two ends are frayed, however, any attempt at direct repair ends up as an untidy cobbling in which there is very little holding power. A more secure grip is obtained if the stitch can be passed criss-cross through the unfrayed parts and also through the sheath, especially where this lies opposite the frayed ends.

6 & 7

In order to avoid such cobbling some surgeons have used grafts taken from the tendon. A central strip of the intact part of the tendon can be slid down and laid across the frayed stretch or it can be left attached at its lower end and its upper end turned downwards. The best reason for using such a graft is to span a gap that may occur if repair is undertaken late or if part of the tendon has been lost for one reason or another.

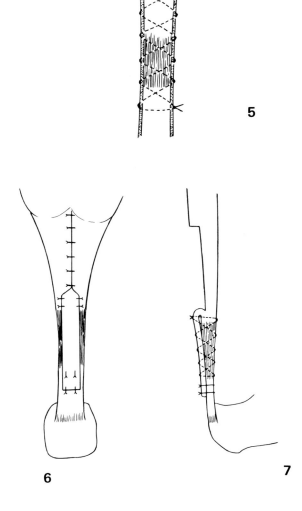

Closing the sheath

Whether or not the sheath is incorporated in the repair of the tendon, it should be carefully closed around the tendon, particularly if this has been frayed.

Closing the skin

Because the flexed position of the ankle creases the skin over the tendon, particular care is necessary when closing the skin; everting stitches are usually necessary.

After operation

The dressing is applied with the foot held up by the toes, which maintains the position for releasing the tendon and keeps the assistant out of the way. It is enough then to apply a simple slab to the front of the limb from the toes to the knee. It is not necessary to include the flexed knee in plaster unless there has been difficulty in closing a gap, as may occur when dealing with a chronic rupture.

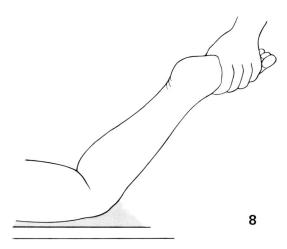

8

The stitches should be left for 2 weeks and after they have been removed a plaster slab is applied with the leg dangling and the foot pulled no more than comfortably up (extended) at the ankle. After another week the patient may be allowed to extend (pull the foot up) further and the limb in that position is encased in plaster from the knee down. The patient walks in plaster, with sticks or crutches if necessary, for another 3 weeks, after which the limb is set free and the patient regains his use of it with such physiotherapeutic supervision as his temperament makes necessary.

[The illustrations for this Chapter on Repair of the Tendo Achillis were drawn by Mr. F. Price.]

Emergency Operations on the Ankle

P. S. London, M.B.E., F.R.C.S.
Surgeon, Birmingham Accident Hospital

INTRODUCTION

Apart from wounds of the skin and tendons and occasionally of the nerves and blood vessels, emergency operations on the ankle are performed because of fracture or dislocation. Although the details of repair vary a good deal according to the details of the injury there are certain basic steps that can be combined in whichever way suits the injury. The well known patterns of fracture will not be considered as such, but some of them will be referred to as examples of the ways in which particular steps can be taken.

The basic steps fall into two groups — approaches and repair.

APPROACHES

1

Lateral incisions

These are used mainly for the exposure of the lower end of the fibula and ligaments attached to it.

Incision 1 is the lateral approach described by Kocher; it gives a good exposure of the fibula and the lateral side of the heel, but if one needs to get to the front of the joint the undermining required may kill the most sharply curved part of the flap.

Incision 2 is inclined forward so that it gives good access to the back of the fibula above and to the anterior, inferior tibiofibular ligament below. It is, therefore, particularly suitable for most of the fractures of the fibula and it can be extended onto the foot, but it may form a slight but noticeable web where it crosses the hollow in front of and below the lateral malleolus (shown dotted).

Incision 3 gives equally good access to the fibula without the liability to form a web, but it is more likely to damage the cutaneous branch of the musculo-cutaneous nerve.

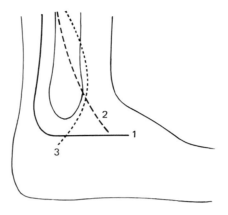

1

2, 3 & 4

Posterolateral incisions

Incision 1 gives good access to the posterolateral fractures of the tibia that occur in the so-called trimalleolar fractures, but it does not allow the fracture of the lateral malleolus to be dealt with unless it is extended as Kocher's incision.

Incision 2 is longer and gently curved and the skin in front of it can quite safely be undermined and lifted forwards far enough to expose the anterior, inferior tibiofibular region.

In either case, the fragment of the tibia is exposed by retracting the fleshy mass of flexor hallucis longus medially and the tendons of peronei longus and brevis laterally. Occasionally, the peroneal artery is quite large, so it should be looked for and protected in the angle behind the tibia and fibula.

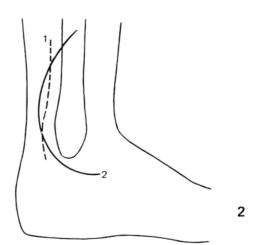

2

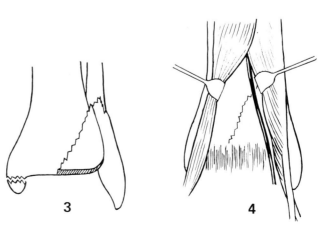

3   **4**

5

Medial incisions

It is usually sufficient to make a straight vertical cut (*incision 1*) that is centred on the tip of the medial malleolus and varies from 3 to 5 or 6 inches (7·5 – 12·5 cm or 15 cm) in length, according to the fatness of the patient. Its centring should be noted because if a screw is to be driven more or less upwards the operator needs room below the tip of the malleolus.

If it should be necessary to get at the back of the tibia the curved *incision 2* should be used.

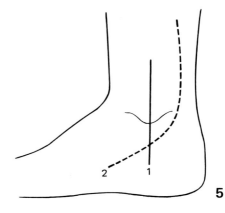

6 & 7

Anterior incisions

These are used in the case of repairable comminution of the lower end of the tibia in which some of the most important fragments are in front. They should be straight or gently sinuous about a vertical line and the bone should be approached between the extensor tendons. There is no special need to preserve the anterior tibial artery and nerve if doing so impedes access to the fragments.

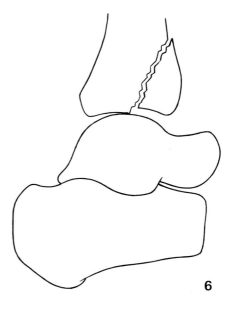

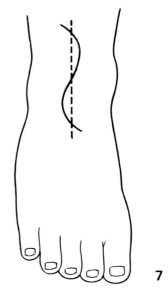

REPAIR OF LIGAMENTS

8

The lateral ligament of the ankle joint

This is the only ligament for which formal repair is likely to be required. In those cases in which repair is required there will have been rupture of the anterior and middle bands of the ligament, but it is open to doubt whether there is much advantage in the long run in going to the trouble of diagnosing and then repairing ruptures of this ligament. The author has yet to see a patient with an unstable ankle joint that was the result of unhealed rupture of the ligament, which is to be distinguished from recurrent inversion of the foot that occurs with an intact lateral ligament.

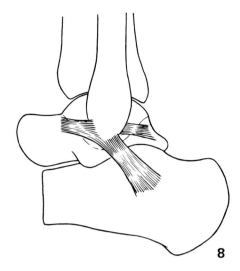

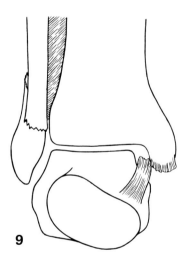

9

The medial ligament

This ligament is occasionally tucked between the talus and the medial malleolus, in which case there is likely to be difficulty in achieving accurate reconstruction of the lateral malleolus. In such a case, a medial incision should be made and the ligament held in its correct position by a stitch passed through a drill hole in the bone.

10-13

The anterior, inferior tibiofibular ligament

This is merely the most obvious and easily accessible of the three ligamentous bonds between the lower ends of the tibia and fibula and the surgeon's objective should be to restore this bond rather than to try to repair a thin and usually frayed sheet of tissue. The bond may be sundered in one of two ways — by simple diastasis, that is separation of the bones without fracture, or by fracture with more or less extensive tearing of ligament. In this case, the interosseous part of the ligament remains largely or wholly intact and the obvious tear is in the anterior part.

Occasionally, and usually in children in their early teens, the anterior, inferior tibiofibular ligament pulls out a block of bone from the anterolateral corner of the tibia (Tillaux's fracture).

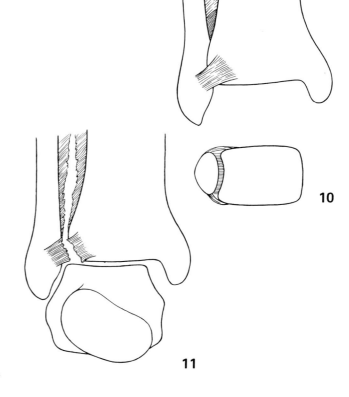

10

11

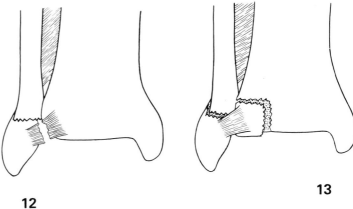

12

13

Restoration of the bond

14, 15 & 16

With screws

The essential step is to fix the fibula to the tibia. If there is diastasis (*see Illustration 11*) a fibulotibial screw is all that is required. It makes little difference whether it is oblique or horizontal, whether it has a full or a partial thread and whether or not it engages the medial cortex of the tibia. The necessary step is to ensure that the screw presses the fibula firmly against the tibia, which requires it to engage the tibia but not the fibula. Note that with fully threaded screws (*Illustration 14*) the tibia is drilled to the core diameter and the fibula to the full diameter of the screw whereas with partly threaded screws both bones are drilled only to the core diameter (*Illustration 15*). It is preferable in each case to tap the holes to take the thread.

If the screw is driven transversely it should be fairly close to the ankle joint so as to avoid the risk of bowing the fibula (*Illustration 16*).

Although it has been stated that passing a screw across the inferior tibiofibular joint causes bony ankylosis the author has not known this to happen. A suitably small screw can also be used to secure a block of bone pulled out by the anterior inferior tibiofibular ligament (*Illustration 15*).

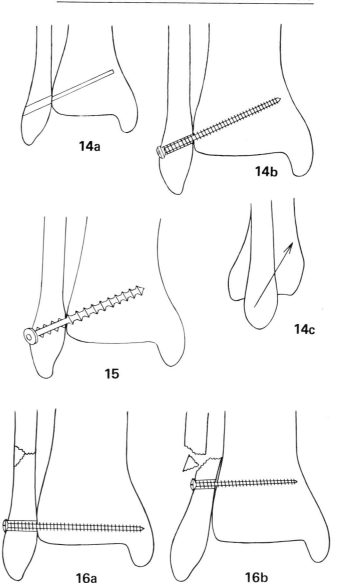

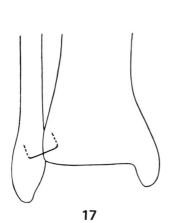

17

With staples

A 0·75 inch staple can be used to hold the fibula to the tibia.

The posterior, inferior tibiofibular ligament is much stronger and less easily accessible than the anterior and does not need to be repaired.

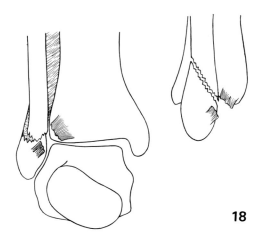

18

REPAIR OF BONES

THE FIBULA

18,19 & 20

Fractures of the fibula fall into three main patterns.

(*1*) The low spiral fracture that results from lateral rotation of the talus within the mortice of the ankle. The anterior inferior tibiofibular ligament is torn, but the main interosseous ligament is not. If the lateral malleolus is fixed securely to the rest of the fibula the mortice is fully restored.

(*2*) The interosseous ligament as well as the anterior inferior tibiofibular ligament is torn and for the security of the mortice to be restored the fracture of the fibula must be fixed and the fibula must be fixed to the tibia.

(*3*) A more nearly transverse fracture several inches up from the ankle; the tibiofibular ligaments may or may not be ruptured.

Fixation of the fibula to the tibia has already been considered; which remain to be considered are methods of fixing the pieces of fibula together.

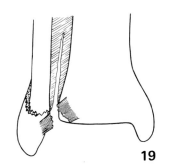

19

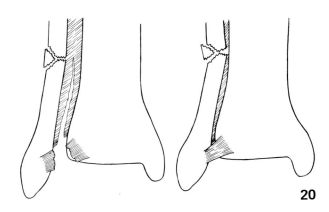

20

EMERGENCY OPERATIONS ON THE ANKLE 651

21

Binding with wire loops

If both steps have to be taken this one should precede
the fixing together of fibula and tibia because if there
is comminution of the fibula it can happen that the
malleolus is screwed back at the wrong level unless
the pieces of fibula have already been accurately re-
assembled.

Essential features of this procedure are:

(*1*) Perfect apposition of the fragments. The top-
most spike (arrowed) of the lower main piece must
be seen, preserved and set perfectly in place. This
may be helped by pulling on the lower piece with a
bone hook as shown and it is important so to support
the heel and ankle as to bring gravity to one's aid. The
fragments are held together with a suitable tool while
the wire is passed round the bone.

(*2*) Each piece of wire should be passed twice round
the bone and with long spiral fractures a pair of such
loops may be used, especially if there is splintering.

(*3*) The wire must be very tight. It is important to
recognize that wire loops cause trouble when they are
loose, not when they are tight. If wire has to be
applied where the bone is tapering sharply it can be
prevented from slipping if it lies in notches cut in
the bone.

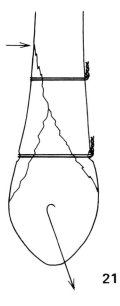

21

22

Screwing oblique fractures

Small cancellous, partly threaded screws designed by
A.O. serve this purpose very well.

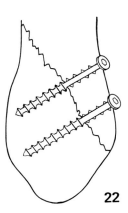

22

23, 24 & 25

Screwing the marrow cavity

This is satisfactory when the interosseous tibiofibular ligament is intact, but there are technical difficulties to bear in mind.

(*1*) The marrow cavity of the shaft of the fibula may be too narrow to admit a screw unless it is reamed out.

(*2*) The marrow cavity is too large or the fracture is too high to grip the screw firmly.

(*3*) The fibula is bowed, not straight.

(*4*) Apart from bowing, the screw may be driven in off the line of the fibula.

(*5*) There is too little clearance on the lateral side of the heel for the screw to be inserted.

(*6*) Unless the fracture is transverse it is usually unwise to use the screw to apply compression because this can distort the fracture and misplace the malleolus.

Intramedullary nails, being smooth, can slide out and are not recommended.

Plating the fibula

In some cases this is easier and more reliable than driving a screw up the fibula, but a bulky plate on the fibula can be very uncomfortable.

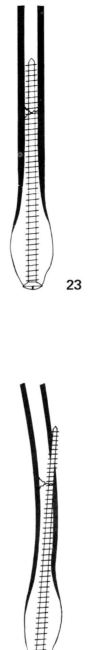

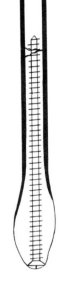

23

24

25

THE TIBIA

The medial malleolus

26 & 27

If there is a fracture of only the medial malleolus it does not need to be operated on unless it is badly displaced. Bony healing may be very slow but it usually comes about and even if it does not, an ununited medial malleolus does not matter if the lateral side of the mortice is secure. When both malleoli are broken the speed of recovery is much greater if both malleoli are fixed than if only the medial is screwed.

The incision should allow two things: (*1*) clear exposure of the ends of the fracture line and (*2*) easy insertion of the screw along a steeply inclined course.

Points *a* and *b* in *Illustration 26* are precisely identifiable as respectively the anterior articular margin and the attachment of the flexor retinaculum. The soft tissues should be stripped for a millimetre or two so as to leave no doubt about the accuracy of replacement of the fragment and all loose fragments of bone and articular cartilage or fringes of ligament and other soft tissues must be removed from between the fragments.

In the manipulation of what may be quite a small piece of bone pointed or edged tools such as bone hook, awl and periosteal elevator may be very useful.

Whatever sort of screw is used it should give compression at the fracture.

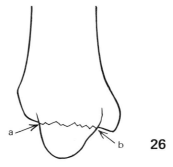

26

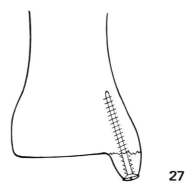

27

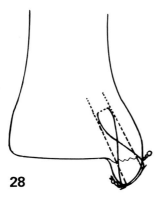

28

28

If the fragment(s) is (are) too small to be screwed the combination of Kirschner's wires and wire loops may be used.

The figure-of-8 passes through a drill hole in cortical bone and is pulled tightly round the protruding ends of two Kirschner's wires, which are then cut short, bent over and driven flush with the bone. The twisted ends of the wire should be placed where they will be least obtrusive.

29 & 30

'Posterior malleolus'

This fragment is usually integral with the fibula and stays in place if the fibula is fixed in place and it is very rarely necessary to operate on it. The necessity arises only when the fragment is very large or when it is not possible to keep it in place in any other way.

A posterolateral approach is used (*see Illustration 2*). The fracture is usually hidden by the intact periosteum that it has stripped from the posterior surface of the tibia. It is not necessary to cut through this in every case and if there is any doubt about the accuracy of replacement, x-rays can be used. The fixing screw or screws may be inserted from behind or from in front (but not in both directions in the one case) and should provide compression.

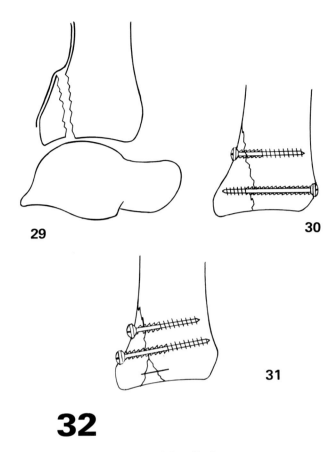

29

30

31

31

Anterior fragments

There are often more and smaller fragments than x-ray films have suggested and restoring the articular surface of the tibia can require much patience, skill and ingenuity. Small pieces of bone of particular importance can sometimes be held in place by fine wires while the main fragments are brought together around them.

32

Small fragments and fragile bones

There are occasions when screws are too coarse and one may then be obliged to resort to Kirschner's wires and wire sutures and accept a less secure reconstruction.

Apart from the difficulties of fixing small and delicate fragments of bone in place there may be considerable difficulty in setting them in place. Bone hooks can tear out, edged tools pressing a fragment into place may sink into it and bone-holding forceps and screws may do the same. Extreme care is necessary in such cases to avoid creating an even more comminuted and less manageable fracture than existed in the first place. Similar difficulties can arise if operation has been delayed for 2 or 3 weeks, after which time bone has softened and soft tissues have stiffened.

It may be necessary to supplement internal by external splintage and forego the undoubted advantage of early movement of the injured joint. Another useful method for occasional use is temporary transfixion of a joint that cannot otherwise be kept in place. Any stiffness resulting from transfixion is likely to be much less of a handicap than the effects of malunion.

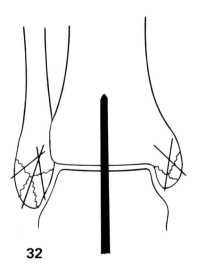

32

[*The illustrations for this Chapter on Emergency Operations on the Ankle were drawn by Mr. F. Price.*]

Fractures and Dislocations in the Foot

P. S. London, M.B.E., F.R.C.S.
Surgeon, Birmingham Accident Hospital

In practice one comes to recognize three main groups of injuries that require prompt operation: (*1*) crush injuries of the toes; (*2*) fractures and dislocations of the talus and calcaneus and; (*3*) disruptive injuries of the tarsometatarsal region.

CRUSH INJURIES OF THE TOES

1

Subungual bruise

The pain can be alleviated by perforating the nail with a red hot paper clip.

The operation is painless. A dressing should be worn until the haematoma is dry.

Open fractures

Careful toilet and closure will often be followed by healing by first intention but too often the toes are treated much more casually than the fingers and the results are consequently poor. An advantage with injured toes is that there need be less reluctance to sacrifice parts of them than parts of fingers in order to be sure of prompt healing.

2

For the sake of comfort in shoes, it may be desirable to fix fractures of toes and metatarsals so that they will heal in good position. Kirschner's wires are particularly useful for this purpose and can safely be driven across joints. Whenever possible, wires should first be driven distally from fractures because this is so much easier than trying to drive them proximally from the tip of a toe.

Wires that are going to have to stay in place for several weeks should, whenever possible, not be left sticking out through the skin to provide portals of bacterial entry.

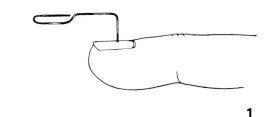

1

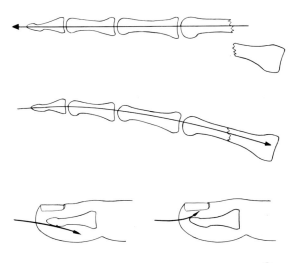

2

SOME PRINCIPLES FOR TREATMENT

In general, it may be proposed that, as far as it is possible to do so, the uninjured joints of an injured foot should be kept in motion from the beginning. If this is accepted, it follows that external splintage should be avoided whenever internal fixation can be carried out. A further proposition is that if a foot is to be stiffened by the effects of injury it should be as nearly as possible of normal shape. If, on the other hand, deformity is inevitable it is particularly important to preserve as much movement as possible.

3, 4 & 5

Surgical approaches in the foot

A useful general purpose incision follows a line from in front of the lateral malleolus to the cleft between the first two toes.

It can, if necessary, be extended upwards to give access to the ankle (*see* page 645, incision 1 in *Illustration 1*). It allows thorough decompression of the dorsum of the foot and, if there has been disruption in the metatarsus, it permits the plantar haematoma to be removed. It allows both the medial and lateral sides of the foot to be seen and although it may not provide enough room for Kirschner's wires to be inserted through the incision, there is no objection to driving these through the skin while they are directed by eye through the appropriate bones and joints. The extensors of the toes can be retracted *en masse* or separately in either direction and there is no objection to dividing one or both extensor retinacula in order to displace the long tendons more effectually.

In other cases, shorter incisions over one or two injured joints will suffice, but it may then be necessary to confirm with the aid of x-rays that the parts have been correctly restored. Such incisions should generally be longitudinal.

Other incisions for special purposes will be described in the relevant sections.

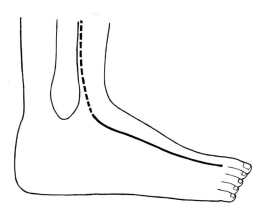

3

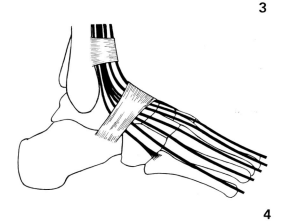

4

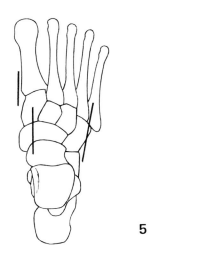

5

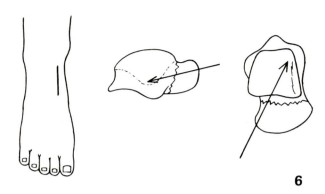

6

6, 7 & 8

Fracture of the neck of the talus

If there is more than a crack through the neck or the body of the bone, there is much to be said for fixing it with Kirschner's wire rather than putting the foot in plaster.

If fluoroscopy is not available it is easiest to do this by exposing the bone and seeing where to insert the wires. There is in many cases no need to remove the wires and so, for the sake of comfort and convenience, their ends should be within the skin. There are two simple ways of doing this. One is to measure the length of wire required and mark this with a notch made by rotating the wire within the lightly closed jaws of a wire cutter. The wire is inserted at the chosen place, driven in until the notch is level with the bone and then snapped off. Alternatively, an unnotched wire can be driven in nearly as far as is necessary, cut off flush with the skin and then driven home by means of a punch with a slightly cupped end that is fine enough to follow the wire through the skin.

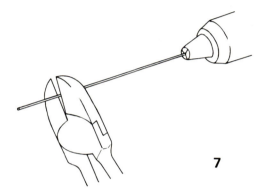

7

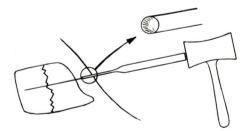

8

9 & 10

Fracture-dislocation of the talus

The experienced eye can usually identify the main features of a confusing jumble of shadows in the x-ray appearances of this injury, in which the body of the bone is expelled from its normal resting place along a curved and twisting course to the inner side of the heel, where it lies under tightly stretched skin that needs early relief from pressure. Although it may be possible to replace the displaced bone by pulling the heel downwards (by skeletal traction if necessary) so as to open the tibiocalcanean gap and then pushing the body upwards, forwards and inwards, it is undesirable to persist in such efforts and the further damage that they may inflict upon the skin that is already, and literally, hard-pressed. (Note that the wire through the heel is fairly far back.)

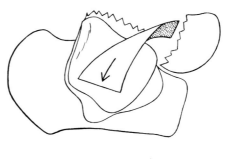

9

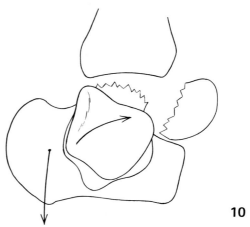

10

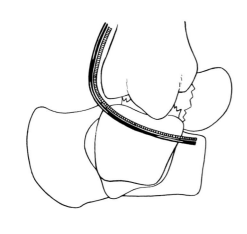

11

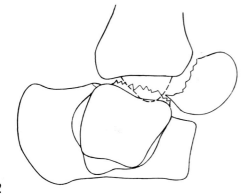

12

11 & 12

If closed manipulation fails the bone should be exposed by a gently curved cut across the prominence it causes but this must be done with great care because the posterior tibial nerve and vessels lie between the much thinned skin and the bone immediately beneath it. A bone hook, rather than a Kirschner wire through the bone, can be used to pull the calcaneus away from the tibia and it may then be quite easy to push the displaced body into place. This may, however, be prevented by tendons or capsule and sometimes by a spike of bone that sticks up from the neck. Although the medial malleolus may hide this cause of obstruction, if the soft tissues are carefully retracted it can be seen and the spike can then be tilted downwards and out of the way. It should be mentioned that it is rarely necessary to divide any soft tissues other than the skin; retraction is usually possible and effective in the absence of the bony obstruction just described. Once the body has been accurately replaced it should be fixed to the head by one or two Kirschner wires.

13 & 14

Total dislocation of the talus

This is the result of violent inversion of the foot that causes the talus to be thrust right out of its socket to lie on the outer side of the foot, with its upper surface tightly stretching the skin below the lateral malleolus. In some cases the skin splits so that the bone falls out and may be lost.

If the talus can be returned to its socket without having to cut the skin, it is probably wise to do so so as to avoid adding surgically to the damage that the skin has already suffered, but it must be understood that the bone has no blood supply and that there is in consequence a strong likelihood that it will have to be operated on later.

If, on the other hand, the skin has already given way, the bone should not be replaced and if conditions are favourable primary tibiocalcanean fusion can be carried out by cutting the bones to fit in a position of 10° or so of equinus and then clamping or screwing them together. Note that the navicular bone should stand clear of the tibia. With the heel of the shoe raised 0·5 inches or so this operation gives a useful foot and the generous trimming of crushed and torn skin allowed by the loss of bone favours uneventful healing of the wound.

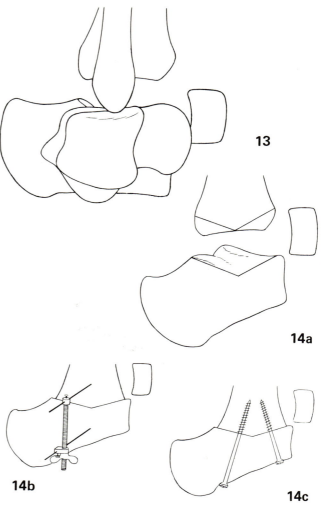

13

14a

14b

14c

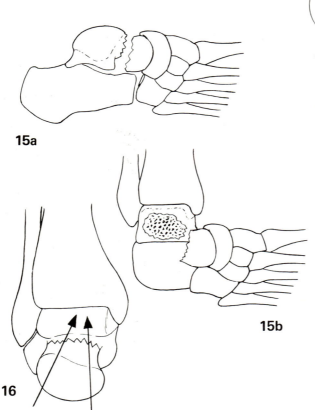

15a

15b

16

15 & 16

Inversion fracture of the talus

As well as the injuries that have already been described, fracture of the talus can occur as a result of supination or inversion, with the sharp, broken edge of the body of the talus blanching the skin in front of the ankle. The deformity is often easily corrected but best maintained by one or two Kirschner's wires.

17 & 18

Fracture of the lateral process of the talus

This injury is included not because it constitutes an emergency or because it occurs frequently but because it is often unrecognized and can give rise to disability that could have been prevented by timely operation. The patient is thought to have sprained the ankle and x-ray examination may support that diagnosis. Even if the films are examined with particular care the fracture may not be recognized in the ordinary anteroposterior and lateral views. The condition should be suspected when there is acute tenderness just below the tip of the lateral malleolus with an effusion into the ankle joint. The fracture is most easily seen in an anteroposterior view made with the foot at a right angle to the leg and rotated inwards by 10°–20°.

Large fragments should be fixed in place with Kirschner's wire and if the fracture is comminuted the fragments should be removed and the soft tissues repaired snugly.

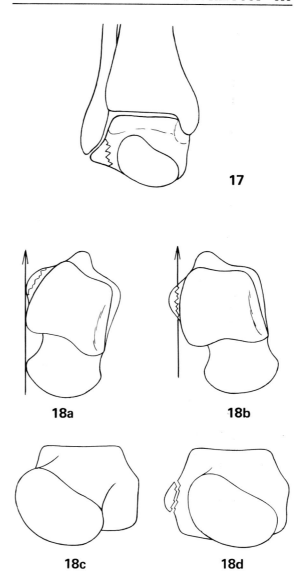

INJURIES OF THE CALCANEUS

Fractures for which early operation may be advantageous are the posterior avulsion ('beak') fractures and the crush fractures that affect particularly the posterior part of the talocalcanean joint.

19 & 20

Beak fractures

Although the smooth surface for a bursa extends quite a long way down the back of the calcaneus these are in fact avulsion fractures and the principal reason for operating on them promptly is that the sharp edge of the displaced fragment is liable to blanch the skin over it.

The incision should be vertical and on the medial side of the tendo Achillis so as to avoid the pressure that is applied to the lateral side of the heel. A coarsely threaded screw passed downwards has the advantage over a staple in that it is not liable to come out.

Crush fractures

There is still much argument about the best way to treat these fractures. It is a matter of common experience that a useful foot with no more than tolerable discomfort can co-exist with severe deformation of the heel. Success depends upon immediate, determined and continuing efforts to reduce swelling and to restore movement. On the other hand, there is marked deformation of the shoe and there may be

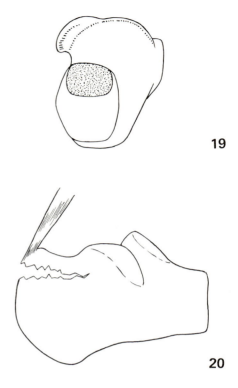

19

20

discomfort caused by pressure between the lateral malleolus and the outward bulge of the subjacent calcaneus. Each surgeon must decide for himself whether to operate on these fractures and, if so, by what method.

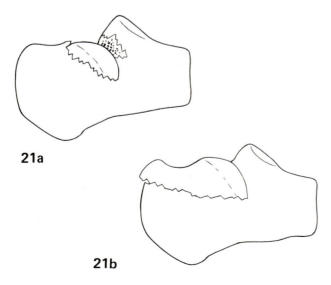

21a

21b

21a & b

The fractures fall into two groups, according to whether or not the fragment carrying the posterior articular facet for the talus has a backward extension to the tendo Achillis.

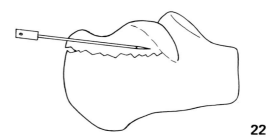

22

22-25

Correction of deformity by indirect methods

If there is a backward extension, this can be used as a handle for the articular surface by driving a spike into it from behind. With the patient prone, the flexed knee raised from the table by one hand under the spike and the other as close to the front of the ankle as possible. The weight of the limb causes the fragment to return to its correct position and by removing it from the body of the bone it makes it possible to correct the broadening of the heel that is an essential part of the injury. This can be done quite easily by squeezing the heel firmly between two hands; it is not necessary to use a powerful clamp. The corrected position is maintained by a plaster cast that includes the spike but leaves both the ankle and the talocalcanean joints free to be exercised.

This method can be very successful in restoring the shape of the foot and maintaining some movement at the talocalcanean joint in persons under 50 years of age but more or less displacement can recur and there is the risk of infection.

Direct methods of correcting deformity

These methods have to be used when the depressed articular facet has no backward extension and they can be used when it has.

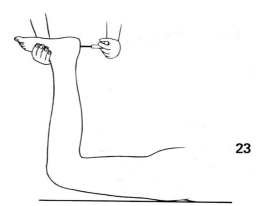

23

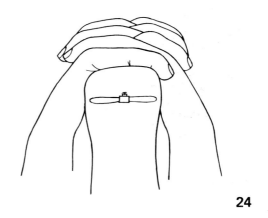

24

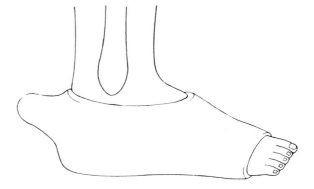

25

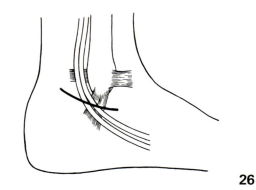

26

26, 27 & 28

Lateral approach

The skin is cut just below the lateral malleolus; it should expose the calcaneofibular ligament but it should not be necessary to divide it. The peroneal tendons may be pulled downwards if necessary.

The depressed facet is partly buried in the body of the bone and while it remains there it maintains the outward bulge. It is put back in place by levering up its anterolateral edge, which causes it to swing and twist up to fit accurately against the talus. The broadening of the heel can then be corrected easily by hand.

The depressed fragment can be propped up by a strong spike driven up from behind and below or by Kirschner's wires that fix it to the talus. Transfixing the talocalcanean joint adds negligibly to the damage that has already been done. Once the depressed fragment has been fixed in place the other fragments may not require any fixation, but there need be no hesitation about using other wires, screws or staples to prevent them from displacing. Although bone grafts have been recommended for the purpose of filling the gap caused by crushing of cancellous bone they are not essential.

If a strong spike is used a plaster slipper should be applied but it is convenient rather than necessary if Kirschner's wires have been used, with or without supplementary fixation. The wires transfixing the talocalcanean joint can be removed after 4–6 weeks.

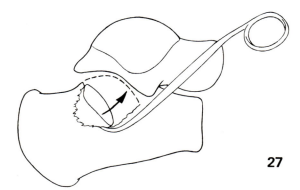

27

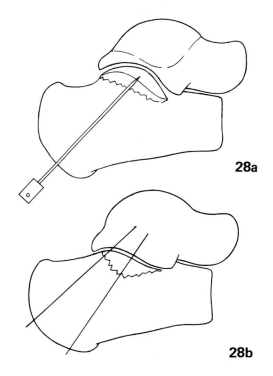

28a

28b

29 & 30

Removing the calcaneus

This is a successful way of dealing with a fracture that is too comminuted for internal fixation and particularly if the fracture is also open. The patient should be prone and the heel is opened by a straight, longitudinal ('cloven hoof') incision after which the bone should be removed piecemeal from the surrounding soft tissues. The tendo Achillis should be stitched to the plantar fascia, with the foot in 20° or 30° of equinus. It is advisable to use suction-drainage. The deformity is less than might be supposed and the patient walks with a normal heel-and-toe gait, though lacking spring. It is advisable to pad the heel of the shoe.

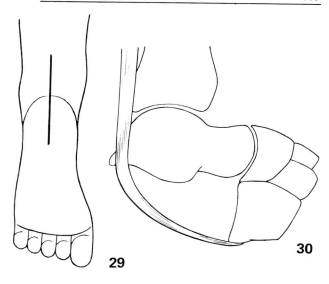

29 **30**

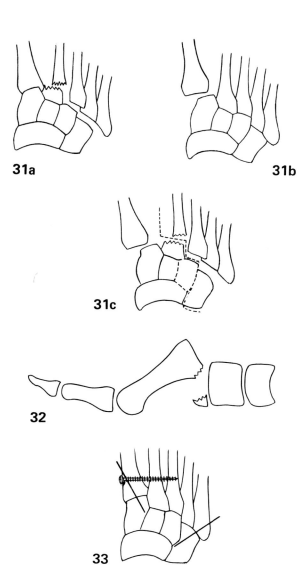

31a **31b**

31c

32

33

MAJOR DISRUPTIVE LESIONS OF THE FOOT

Although the x-ray appearances may be very confusing, these injuries fall into a few fairly well-defined patterns, albeit with variations in detail. The first requirement is to recognize that serious injury has occurred — failure of diagnosis is not all that rare. It is necessary to understand these patterns in order to treat the injuries successfully which in most cases is best done by internal fixation. If fluoroscopy is available it may not be necessary to open some of these injuries but there need be no hesitation to open the foot for reasons that have already been stated.

31, 32 & 33

Tarsometatarsal disruption

The four, or fewer of, the lateral metatarsals may be displaced laterally and the first may be displaced medially either as a separate injury or in combination with the foregoing. The lateral line of disruption often follows the line of tarsometatarsal joints but may follow an irregular course through the tarsus.

Occasionally, there is an isolated dorsal fracture-dislocation of the base of the first metatarsal bone, which is accompanied by hyperextension of the metatarsophalangeal joint.

Fixation can usually be achieved with the aid of Kirschner's wires and sometimes by screws, which it is not always necessary to remove.

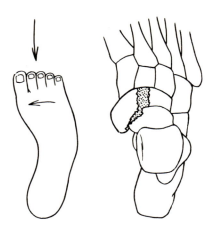

34

Disruption of the tarsus

34 & 35

Talonavicular fracture-subluxation

This injury occurs when the forepart of the foot is swung inwards with simultaneous longitudinal compression. It is usually sufficient to transfix the talonavicular joint with a wire or a screw but if there are also fractures of metatarsals it may be advisable to fix them as well.

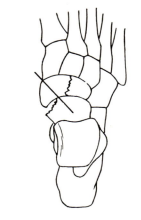

35

36

Talonavicular dislocation

Violent pronation may displace the navicular bone towards the sole. It is not usually necessary to operate on this injury but sometimes correction of the deformity is prevented by soft tissues — the figure shows how the tendon of tibialis anterior may act in this way.

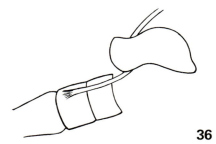

36

[*The illustrations for this Chapter on Fractures and Dislocations in the Foot were drawn by Mr. F. Price.*]

Index